# Dietary Patterns and Health: A Nutrition Science Approach

# Dietary Patterns and Health: A Nutrition Science Approach

Edited by Rebecca Matthews

MURPHY & MOORE
www.murphy-moorepublishing.com

Published by Murphy & Moore Publishing,
1 Rockefeller Plaza,
New York City, NY 10020, USA
www.murphy-moorepublishing.com

**Dietary Patterns and Health: A Nutrition Science Approach**
Edited by Rebecca Matthews



International Standard Book Number: 978-1-63987-161-2 (Hardback)



**Cataloging-in-Publication Data**

Dietary patterns and health : a nutrition science approach / edited by Rebecca Matthews.
p. cm.
Includes bibliographical references and index.
ISBN 978-1-63987-161-2
1. Diet. 2. Food habits. 3. Health. 4. Nutrition. I. Matthews, Rebecca.
TX357 .D54 2022
613.2--dc23

# TABLE OF CONTENTS

# PREFACE

The science of interpreting the relationship of nutrients of food with growth, reproduction, health, maintenance and disease of an organism is known as nutrition. The field also studies the processes of assimilation, excretion, biosynthesis, ingestion and catabolism. The total amount of nutrients that a person or an organism takes in is known as diet. It is taken to enhance and maintain optimal level of health. A healthy diet pattern requires intake of vitamins, minerals, fats, proteins and carbohydrates in the right amount. Nutrition science aims to improve the quality of life, longevity and health of an individual. It also focuses on reducing risks of chronic diseases like diabetes, cancer and multiple cardiovascular diseases. This book studies, analyses and upholds the pillars of nutrition science and its utmost significance in modern times. Also included herein is the detailed explanation of various concepts and applications related to this discipline. Those in search of information to further their knowledge will be greatly assisted by this book.

This book has been the outcome of endless efforts put in by authors and researchers on various issues and topics within the field. The book is a comprehensive collection of significant researches that are addressed in a variety of chapters. It will surely enhance the knowledge of the field among readers across the globe.

It gives us an immense pleasure to thank our researchers and authors for their efforts to submit their piece of writing before the deadlines. Finally in the end, I would like to thank my family and colleagues who have been a great source of inspiration and support.

**Editor**

# 1

# Associations of childhood, maternal and household dietary patterns with childhood stunting in Ethiopia: proposing an alternative and plausible dietary analysis method to dietary diversity scores

Yohannes Adama Melaku[1,2*], Tiffany K. Gill[2], Anne W. Taylor[2], Robert Adams[3], Zumin Shi[2] and Amare Worku[1]

## Abstract

**Background:** Identifying dietary patterns that consider the overall eating habits, rather than focusing on individual foods or simple counts of consumed foods, better helps to understand the combined effects of dietary components. Therefore, this study aimed to use dietary patterns, as an alternative method to dietary diversity scores (DDSs), and investigate their associations with childhood stunting in Ethiopia.

**Methods:** Mothers and their children aged under 5 years ($n = 3788$) were recruited using a two-stage random cluster sampling technique in two regions of Ethiopia. Socio-demographic, dietary and anthropometric data were collected. Dietary intake was assessed using standardized dietary diversity tools. Household, maternal and child DDSs were calculated and dietary patterns were identified by *tetrachoric* (factor) analysis. Multilevel linear and Poisson regression analyses were applied to assess the association of DDSs and dietary patterns with height-for-age z score (HAZ) and stunting, respectively.

**Results:** The overall prevalence of stunting among children under-five was 38.5% ($n = 1459$). We identified three dietary patterns each, for households ("fish, meat and miscellaneous", "egg, meat, poultry and legume" and "dairy, vegetable and fruit"), mothers ("plant-based", "egg, meat, poultry and legume" and "dairy, vegetable and fruit" and children ("grain based", "egg, meat, poultry and legume" and "dairy, vegetable and fruit"). Children in the third tertile of the household "dairy, vegetable and fruit" pattern had a 0.16 (β = 0.16; 95% CI: 0.02, 0.30) increase in HAZ compared to those in the first tertile. A 0.22 (β = 0.22; 95% CI: 0.06, 0.39) and 0.19 (β = 0.19; 0.04, 0.33) increase in HAZ was found for those in the third tertiles of "dairy, vegetable and fruit" patterns of children 24–59 months and 6–59 months, respectively. Those children in the second (β = −0.17; 95% CI: -0.31, −0.04) and third (β = −0.16; 95% CI: -0.30, −0.02) tertiles of maternal "egg, meat, poultry and legume" pattern had a significantly lower HAZ compared to those in the first tertile. No significant associations between the household and child "egg, meat, poultry and legume" dietary patterns with HAZ and stunting were found. Statistically non-significant associations were found between household, maternal and child DDSs, and HAZ and stunting.

(Continued on next page)

* Correspondence: adamayohannes@gmail.com
[1]Department of Public Health Sciences, Addis Continental Institute of Public Health, Addis Ababa, Ethiopia
[2]Adelaide Medical School, The University of Adelaide, Adelaide, Australia
Full list of author information is available at the end of the article

(Continued from previous page)

**Conclusion:** A higher adherence to a "dairy, vegetable and fruit" dietary pattern is associated with increased HAZ and reduced risk of stunting. Dietary pattern analysis methods, using routinely collected dietary data, can be an alternative approach to DDSs in low resource settings, to measure dietary quality and in determining associations of overall dietary intake with stunting.

**Keywords:** Dietary data analysis, Dietary diversity score, Dietary pattern, Stunting

## Background

Although the global burden of stunting decreased between 1990 and 2015 by more than 25%, it has continued to be a major nutrition-related risk factor causing 257 deaths per 100,000 globally [1]. In sub-Saharan Africa, 11.8 disability-adjusted life years (DALYs) and 136,455 childhood deaths in 2015 were attributable to stunting [2]. In Ethiopia, 38% of children under-five years of age were stunted [3] and it was a risk factor for 960,742 DALYs and 11,065 deaths in 2015 [2]. Stunting also halts the development of societies by negatively affecting mental and physical health [4]. Suboptimal nutrition is a major contributor to stunting in developing countries [5], although there are other causal and contextual factors [4].

Although there are well-established methods, collation and analysis of dietary data have remained challenging in low-income countries (LICs) for various reasons, including high costs, lack of centralized platforms for dietary data, little investment in research, low capacity and technical complexity [6]. As a result, dietary assessment is mainly dependent on approaches which require low cost and provide low quality. Dietary diversity assessment has remained the most commonly used method of data collection, analysis and interpretation approach in LICs. Dietary diversity scores (DDSs) of households, women and children [7–9] are important tools and the most commonly used indicators of assessing the adequacy of nutrient intake. In many studies, it has been also demonstrated that DDSs were useful indicators of micronutrient status [10–13] and a higher DDS is associated with a lower risk of stunting [14–16]. The indicators are relatively simple and suitable for use in large surveys [3]. However, data collected for the purpose of DDS analysis are qualitative, and in most cases, they are dichotomized (yes/no) [8] restricting further analyses. Thus, the analyses depend on a simple count of food groups and do not consider the correlations of the food groups and their impact on nutritional (disease) outcomes. In addition, because the main purpose of DDS analysis is on the number, rather than the type of foods consumed, this may ignore the antagonist, additive and synergistic effect of food groups.

Currently the focus of nutritional epidemiology is to investigate the patterns of multiple food and nutrient intakes without ignoring the interactions. Methodological development over the last two decades enables us to explore the association between diet and disease outcomes through a systematic consideration of the correlation between the components of the overall diet, that is dietary patterns [17, 18]. A study by *Humphries* et al. reported that total food expenditures (using food groups for child DDSs) did not significantly predict HAZ in Ethiopia. In this study, household food group expenditure index, determined by factor analysis of disaggregated food expenditure, was found to be a significant predictor for HAZ [19]. This leads to a premise that a mere aggregate availability and accessibility of the included food groups are not the determining factors for HAZ, rather the specific types of food groups available and their consumption pattern. Another study in the same cohort strengthens this conclusion [20]. Therefore, identifying dietary patterns that consider the overall eating habits, rather than focusing on individual foods (simple counting of consumed foods), better reflect the complexity of dietary intakes and help to understand the combined effect of diet components [21]. In this study, we aimed to identify household, maternal and child dietary patterns and investigate their associations with childhood stunting in Ethiopia using the same dietary data collected for determining DDS. In addition, the study compares the findings with the estimates of associations between DDSs and stunting. To the best of our knowledge, this is the first study investigating the aforementioned objectives.

## Methods

### Study area and participants

A cross-sectional study was conducted in the South Nations, Nationalities and People (SNNP) and Tigray (northern Ethiopia) regions between June and September 2014. The two regions are geographically located at opposite ends of Ethiopia, in the south and north, with differences in agroecology, subsistence farming being the most common occupation in both regions. The SNNP is a larger geographic area and has a greater population size compared to the Tigray region. This study was part of a larger project of the Alive and Thrive's (A&T) impact evaluation for community-based interventions. The major objectives of the evaluation included assessment of infant and young child feeding (IYCF) practices and stunting prevalence. The baseline and progress evaluation of the project were conducted between June and September 2010 and 2013, respectively.

### Sample size calculation and sampling technique

The sample size was calculated based on the 2010 baseline and 2013 progress evaluation surveys' estimates. It took into account an intracluster correlation of 0.03–0.04. A total of 75 clusters (enumeration areas [EAs]), a one-sided test, a power of 80%, and a significance level of $\alpha = 0.05$ were included in the calculations. Based on these considerations, a minimum sample size of 2950 was required (Table 1). However, in total, data were collected from 3788 children and their mothers.

A two-stage cluster sampling technique was used to select households with children under five. In the first stage (primary sampling unit), EAs were selected from 89 districts (the second smallest administrative units in Ethiopia). The EA is a geographical unit devised by the Central Statistical Authority (CSA) of Ethiopia, which consists of 150–200 households. This is the smallest cluster used in Demographic and Household Surveys and roughly coincides with the *kebele* (the smallest administrative units) boundaries (Fig. 1). A total of 75 EAs (26 from Tigray and 49 from SNNP), from 56 districts (19 from Tigray and 37 from SNNP) were selected using probability proportional to size (PPS) sampling in relation to the population of the EAs.

In the second stage, children between 0 to 59.9 months ($n = 3788$) were selected. A complete household listing with the number of children residing in each household, in each selected cluster, was developed in collaboration with the local health and administrative offices. This list included identification of all eligible candidates for the survey (mothers of those children under 60 months of age). From this list, three sampling frames were developed: children aged 0–5.9 months, 6–23.9 months, and 24–59.9 months. From each sampling frame, study subjects were selected using a systematic random sampling (SRS). Households selected to participate in one age category were not included in the other sampling frames, even if there were other eligible children in a household.

### Data collection

All data (interview and anthropometric) were collected by trained data collectors who had bachelor degrees or above. To maintain the data quality, demonstrations and pilot testing were conducted during the training period. Trained supervisors oversaw and monitored the data collectors during the field work. The supervisors also checked 5–10% of the anthropometric and interview data to ensure reliability.

### Anthropometry data collection

The length or height of children was measured to the nearest 0.1 cm using the United Nations International Children's Emergency Fund (UNICEF) recommended wooden board with an upright wooden base and movable headpieces. Children ≥24 months were measured while standing upright while those less than 24 months in the recumbent position. Weight was measured to the nearest 0.1 kg using UNICEF's scale [22]. Immunization cards or home records of the date of birth, if available, were used to determine the age of the children. In the case of absence of these documents, mother's recall was taken using the local calendar and then converted to the Gregorian calendar. Adult weighing and height scales were used to measure maternal weight and height, respectively. Mothers were asked to remove shoes and heavy cloths before weight and height were measured. Weight and height were recorded to the nearest 0.1 kg and 1.0 cm, respectively.

### Dietary data collection

Dietary data for children [7] and women [8] and household dietary and food insecurity data [9, 23] were assessed using standard tools. Dietary intake was assessed for the preceding day (24 h). For children aged 6–23 months, seven food groups (grains, roots and tubers; legumes and nuts; dairy products (milk, yogurt, cheese); flesh foods (meat, fish, poultry and liver/organ meats); eggs; vitamin-A rich fruits and vegetables; and other fruits and vegetables) were included [7]. For children 24–59 months, an additional two food groups (oils and fats and independent categories of other fruits and vegetables) were included.

**Table 1** Sample size calculation, 2014

| | Baseline (2010) rate (%) | Expected endline rate (%) | Percentage point (pp) or change in mean z-score | Power | Intra-class correlation at baseline (2010) | Intra-class correlation at 2013 progress evaluation survey | Minimum sample size required |
|---|---|---|---|---|---|---|---|
| Stunting (24-59 m) | 55.9 | 48.9 | 7 pp | 0.8 | 0.032 | NA | 1450 |
| Exclusive breast feeding (0–5.9 m) | 72.4 | 79.4 | 7 pp | 0.8 | 0.026 | 0.005 | 600 |
| Minimum dietary diversity (6–23.9 m) | 6.3 | 11.3 | 5 pp | 0.8 | 0.038 | 0.125 | 900 |
| Minimum total sample size required | | | | | | | 2950 |

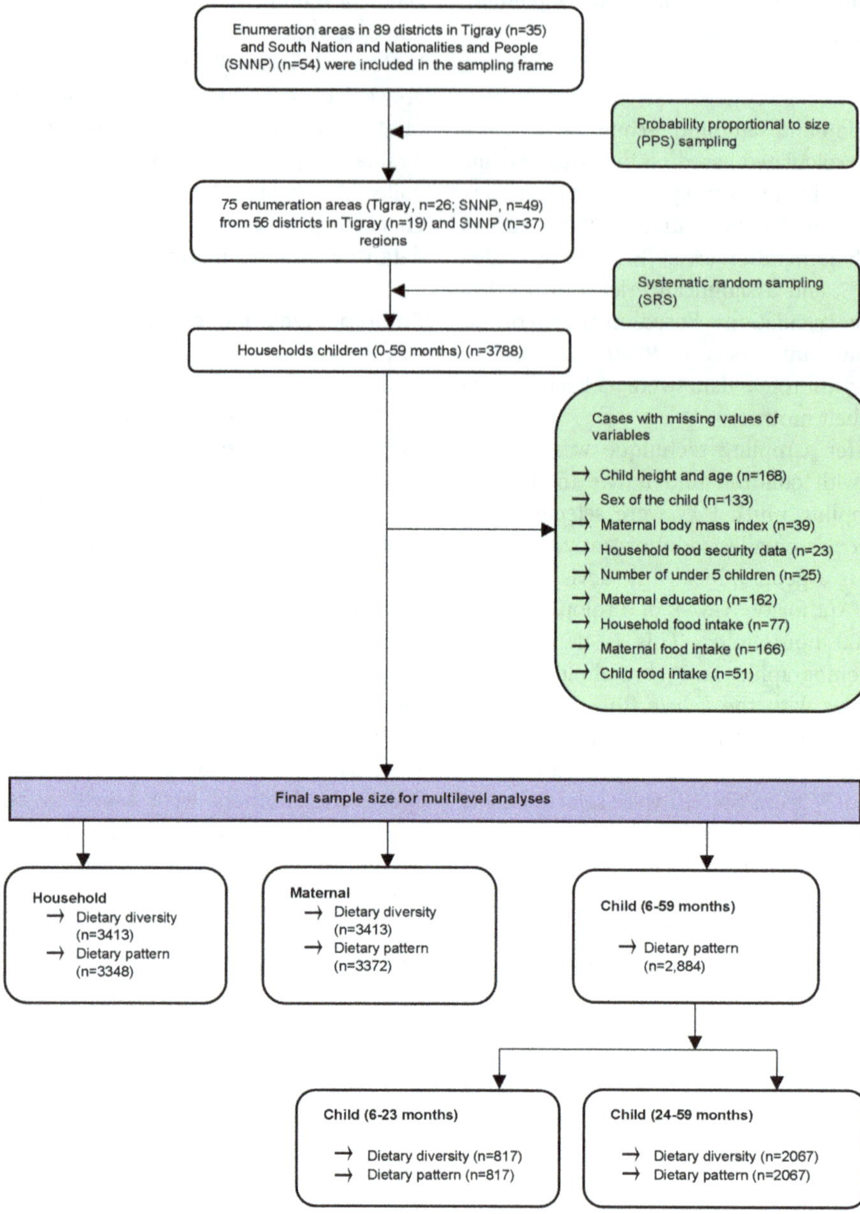


**Fig. 1** Sample description

The maximum dietary diversity for women of reproductive age (MDD-W) assessment includes 10 food groups (grains, white roots and tubers, and plantains; pulses (beans, peas and lentils); nuts and seeds; dairy; meat, poultry and fish; eggs; dark green leafy vegetables; other vitamin A-rich fruits and vegetables; other vegetables; other fruits). Consumption of food by any of the household member from any of 12 food groups in the last 24 h was also assessed and the household DDS was determined. The food groups were cereals; roots and tubers; vegetables; fruits; meat, poultry, offal; eggs; fish and seafood; pulses/legumes/nuts; milk and milk products; oils/fats; sugar/honey and miscellaneous [23].

### Other covariates

Data including socio-demographic (such as maternal age, maternal education, sex of the head of the household and paternal education), economic (household asset), environmental factors (such as water source and latrine type), health service utilization (such as place of delivery for index child), and household characteristics (such as the number of under-five children living in a household) were collected. Different socio-economic indicators were combined using principal component analysis to construct household wealth. The factor scores were divided into quantiles (poorest, poorer, middle, richer and richest) to indicate the relative socio-economic status of the

**Table 2** Characteristics of study participants by age of children in Ethiopia, 2014

| Characteristics | Overall | 0–5 months | 6–23 months | 24–59 months | *p*-value |
|---|---|---|---|---|---|
| N | 3788 | 601 | 896 | 2287 | |
| Sex of children | | | | | |
| Male | 1850 (48.8%) | 284 (47.3%) | 438 (48.9%) | 1126 (49.2%) | 0.680 |
| Female | 1805 (47.7%) | 294 (48.9%) | 433 (48.3%) | 1076 (47.0%) | |
| Missing | 133 (3.5%) | 23 (3.8%) | 25 (2.8%) | 85 (3.7%) | |
| Sex of household head | | | | | |
| Male | 3438 (90.8%) | 560 (93.2%) | 820 (91.5%) | 2055 (89.9%) | 0.098 |
| Female | 231 (6.1%) | 26 (4.3%) | 53 (5.9%) | 151 (6.6%) | |
| Missing | 119 (3.1%) | 15 (2.5%) | 23 (2.6%) | 81 (3.5%) | |
| Number of under 5 children in the household | | | | | |
| One Child | 2353 (62.1%) | 259 (43.1%) | 505 (56.4%) | 1585 (69.3%) | <0.001 |
| Two children | 1313 (34.7%) | 300 (49.9%) | 372 (41.5%) | 641 (28.0%) | |
| More than three children | 97 (2.6%) | 40 (6.7%) | 18 (2.0%) | 39 (1.7%) | |
| Missing | 25 (0.7%) | 2 (0.3%) | 1 (0.1%) | 22 (1.0%) | |
| Maternal age, median (IQR) | 29.0 (25.0, 35.0) | 27.0 (23.0, 32.0) | 28.0 (23.0, 33.0) | 30.0 (25.0, 35.0) | <0.001 |
| Maternal education | | | | | |
| No education | 2069 (54.6%) | 274 (45.6%) | 454 (50.7%) | 1339 (58.5%) | <0.001 |
| Primary | 1364 (36.0%) | 265 (44.1%) | 351 (39.2%) | 746 (32.6%) | |
| Secondary and above | 193 (5.1%) | 41 (6.8%) | 50 (5.6%) | 102 (4.5%) | |
| Missing | 162 (4.3%) | 21 (3.5%) | 41 (4.6%) | 100 (4.4%) | |
| Paternal education | | | | | |
| No education | 1283 (33.9%) | 177 (29.5%) | 282 (31.5%) | 823 (36.0%) | 0.004 |
| Primary | 1644 (43.4%) | 293 (48.8%) | 397 (44.3%) | 952 (41.6%) | |
| Secondary and above | 417 (11.0%) | 73 (12.1%) | 106 (11.8%) | 238 (10.4%) | |
| Missing | 444 (11.7%) | 58 (9.7%) | 111 (12.4%) | 274 (12.0%) | |
| Maternal body-mas index (kg/m$^2$), mean (SD) | 20.2 (2.4) | 20.9 (2.4) | 20.0 (2.3) | 20.1 (2.4) | <0.001 |
| Maternal Height (meter), mean (SD) | 1.6 (0.1) | 1.6 (0.1) | 1.6 (0.1) | 1.6 (0.1) | 0.550 |
| Place of delivery | | | | | |
| Home | 2371 (62.6%) | 263 (43.8%) | 483 (53.9%) | 1623 (71.0%) | <0.001 |
| Health facility | 1346 (35.5%) | 327 (54.4%) | 398 (44.4%) | 619 (27.1%) | |
| Other | 71 (1.9%) | 11 (1.8%) | 15 (1.7%) | 45 (2.0%) | |
| Water source | | | | | |
| Piped water | 1694 (44.7%) | 279 (46.4%) | 399 (44.5%) | 1014 (44.3%) | 0.740 |
| Other improved | 1104 (29.1%) | 168 (28.0%) | 253 (28.2%) | 683 (29.9%) | |
| Unimproved | 990 (26.1%) | 154 (25.6%) | 244 (27.2%) | 590 (25.8%) | |
| Latrine type | | | | | |
| Traditional pit latrine | 3087 (81.5%) | 493 (82.0%) | 735 (82.0%) | 1857 (81.2%) | 0.015 |
| Improved latrine | 25 (0.7%) | 10 (1.7%) | 3 (0.3%) | 12 (0.5%) | |
| No facility/bush/field | 676 (17.8%) | 98 (16.3%) | 158 (17.6%) | 418 (18.3%) | |
| Income quantile | | | | | |
| Poorest | 603 (15.9%) | 87 (14.5%) | 151 (16.9%) | 364 (15.9%) | 0.470 |
| Poorer | 602 (15.9%) | 96 (16.0%) | 134 (15.0%) | 372 (16.3%) | |
| Middle | 602 (15.9%) | 84 (14.0%) | 142 (15.8%) | 376 (16.4%) | |
| Richer | 602 (15.9%) | 109 (18.1%) | 136 (15.2%) | 356 (15.6%) | |

**Table 2** Characteristics of study participants by age of children in Ethiopia, 2014 *(Continued)*

| Characteristics | Overall | 0–5 months | 6–23 months | 24–59 months | *p*-value |
|---|---|---|---|---|---|
| Richest | 602 (15.9%) | 106 (17.6%) | 144 (16.1%) | 351 (15.3%) | |
| Missing | 777 (20.5%) | 119 (19.8%) | 189 (21.1%) | 468 (20.5%) | |
| Stunted | | | | | |
| No | 2161 (57.0%) | 510 (84.9%) | 539 (60.2%) | 1109 (48.5%) | <0.001 |
| Yes | 1459 (38.5%) | 45 (7.5%) | 330 (36.8%) | 1084 (47.4%) | |
| Missing | 168 (4.4%) | 46 (7.7%) | 27 (3.0%) | 94 (4.1%) | |
| Height-for-age z-score, mean (SD) | −1.6 (1.8) | 0.0 (1.6) | −1.5 (1.6) | −2.0 (1.6) | <0.001 |
| Underweight | | | | | |
| No | 2986 (78.8%) | 563 (93.7%) | 704 (78.6%) | 1715 (75.0%) | <0.001 |
| Yes | 802 (21.2%) | 38 (6.3%) | 192 (21.4%) | 572 (25.0%) | |
| Weight-for-age z-score, mean (SD) | −1.0 (2.3) | 0.2 (3.7) | −1.0 (2.3) | −1.3 (1.6) | <0.001 |

participants. The highest level of education achieved was categorized into no education, primary, and secondary and above. Water source was classified as piped, other improved and unimproved. The type of functional latrine used in the household was categorized into traditional pit latrine, improved latrine and no facility/bush/field.

### Anthropometry and dietary data analyses

Height-for-age z score (HAZ), an indicator of linear growth, was compared with reference data from the World Health Organization (WHO) Multicentre Growth Reference Study Group, 2006 [24] using the ENA (Emergency Nutrition Assessment) SMART (Standardized Monitoring and Assessment of Relief and Transitions) 2011 software. Children whose HAZ is <−2 SD from the median of the WHO reference population were considered stunted (short for their age). In our analysis, both HAZ (continuous) and stunting (categorical; stunted = 1/ not stunted = 0) were used as outcome variables. Maternal body mass index (BMI) was calculated based on the measured weight (kg) and height (meters) (weight [kg]/ $(\text{height[meters]})^2$).

For children aged 6 to 23, and 24 to 59 months, the minimum acceptable DDS was defined as consuming food from four or more of the standardized set of seven (6 to 23 months) or nine (24 to 59 months) food groups on the preceding day of the survey [7, 25]. For women (mothers/ caregivers of the index children), a threshold of at least 5 food groups of the 10 was considered acceptable [8]. The scores of household DDS were continuous, ranging from 0 to 12, based on whether any of the members of the household consumed any of the 12 food groups. Minimum household DDS was not determined because a dichotomous indicator has not been developed [8, 23]. However, we assumed that consumption of food groups above the median number as adequate. Nine Household Food Insecurity Access Scale (HFIAS) generic questions were used with a dichotomized response (0 = no/1 = yes) to assess food insecurity [9]. Each of the questions were asked with a recall period of four weeks (30 days). If a respondent answers "yes" to any of the above nine questions, frequency-of-occurrence questions were asked to determine whether the condition happened rarely (1 = once or twice), sometimes (2 = three to ten times) or often (3 = more than ten times). The insecurity status was categorized into four groups (secured, mild, moderate, and severe) using the Food and Nutrition Technical Assistance (FANTA) algorithm [9].

Dietary patterns were identified by *polychoric (tetrachoric)* analysis—a family of factor analysis which uses a *tetrachoric* correlation matrix to construct latent variables from dichotomized (binary) observed data [26]. For each of the dietary patterns, factor scores were assigned for all study participants. Factor scores show the relative position of the study participants in each of the identified patterns, thus reflecting adherence to the patterns. Pattern-specific factor scores are calculated as the sum of the products of the factor loading coefficients and standardized daily consumption of food and nutrient groups related to the pattern. The factor scores were orthogonally (varimax) rotated to create less correlation among the patterns and to facilitate their interpretability. Participants were then assigned into tertiles (first [lowest adherence]; second; and third [highest adherence] tertiles) based on their factor scores. Eigenvalues (>1), scree plots, and interpretability of the factors were used to determine the number of dietary and nutrient patterns. Factor loadings (the correlation between each pattern and the food and nutrient groups) were calculated. Percentages of variances (the variations that were explained by the identified dietary and nutrient patterns) were also computed.

### Statistical analyses

The chi-square (categorical variables), ANOVA (normally distributed continuous variables) and Kruskal-Wallis

| Household dietary pattern | Pattern 1 ("Fish, meat and miscellaneous") | Pattern 2 ("Egg, meat, poultry and legume") | Pattern 3 ("Dairy, vegetable and fruit") | Number of households(%), n=3788 |
|---|---|---|---|---|
| Fish and seafood | 1.40 | 0.02 | 0.01 | 10 (0.3%) |
| Fruits | -0.49 | 0.39 | 0.32 | 782 (20.7%) |
| Miscellaneous (Spices and commandments) | 0.48 | 0.26 | 0.32 | 3619 (95.8%) |
| Eggs | 0.05 | 0.68 | 0.09 | 576 (15.2%) |
| Meat, poultry, offal | 0.13 | 0.67 | 0.01 | 349 (9.2%) |
| Legumes | 0.02 | 0.61 | -0.14 | 2187 (58.0%) |
| Oils and Fats | 0.06 | 0.53 | 0.30 | 683 (18.1%) |
| Sugar/honey | 0.06 | 0.51 | 0.14 | 1190 (31.5%) |
| Cereals | -0.06 | 0.48 | -0.09 | 3411 (90.3%) |
| White tubers and roots | 0.01 | -0.31 | 0.51 | 1199 (31.7%) |
| Vegetables | 0.08 | 0.18 | 0.50 | 2826 (74.8%) |
| Milk and milk products | -0.02 | 0.13 | 0.43 | 1237 (32.7%) |

| Maternal dietary pattern | Pattern 1 ("Plant based") | Pattern 2 ("Egg, meat, poultry and legume") | Pattern 3 ("Dairy, vegetable and fruit") | Number of women (%), n=3788 |
|---|---|---|---|---|
| Eggs | -0.09 | 0.84 | 0.20 | 473 (12.5%) |
| Meat, poultry and fish | -0.06 | 0.82 | 0.02 | 347 (9.2%) |
| Other fruits | -0.07 | 0.23 | 0.63 | 604 (16.0%) |
| Other vitamin A-rich fruits and vegetables | 0.08 | 0.29 | 0.49 | 803 (21.3%) |
| Dairy | 0.21 | 0.17 | 0.45 | 1058 (28.0%) |
| Other vegetables | 0.01 | 0.04 | 0.34 | 2425 (64.1%) |
| Grains, white roots and tubers, and plantains | 0.64 | -0.09 | 0.19 | 1191 (31.5%) |
| Nuts and seeds | -0.50 | 0.23 | 0.34 | 3388 (89.6%) |
| Pulses (beans, peas and lentils) | -0.47 | 0.37 | 0.2 | 2179 (57.8%) |
| Dark green leafy vegetables | 0.33 | 0.12 | 0.31 | 951 (25.2%) |

| Child dietary pattern | Pattern 1 ("Grain based") | Pattern 2 ("Egg, meat, poultry and legume") | Pattern 3 ("Dairy, vegetable and fruit ") | Number of children (6-23 months, n=896) (%) | Number of children (24-59 months) months, n= 2287) (%) |
|---|---|---|---|---|---|
| Grains, roots and tubers | 2.99 | 0.02 | 0.02 | 802 (89.5%) | 2248 (98.3%) |
| Flesh foods (meat, fish, poultry and liver/organ meats) | 0.07 | 0.69 | -0.05 | 34 (3.8%) | 176 (7.7%) |
| Eggs | 0.11 | 0.68 | 0.01 | 170 (19.0%) | 337 (14.7%) |
| legumes and nuts | 0.18 | 0.58 | 0.04 | 318 (35.5%) | 1129 (49.4%) |
| Oils and fats | 0.18 | 0.51 | 0.29 | | 1512 (66.1%) |
| Other fruits | 0.12 | -0.02 | 0.87 | 231 (25.8%) | 921 (40.3%) |
| Other vegetables | 0.29 | 0.02 | 0.38 | 26 (2.9%) | 63 (2.8%) |
| Dairy products (milk, yogurt, cheese) | 0.03 | 0.16 | 0.31 | 268 (29.9%) | 688 (30.1%) |
| Vitamin-A rich fruits and vegetables | 0.08 | 0.29 | 0.31 | 71 (7.9%) | 251 (11.0%) |

**Fig. 2** Household, maternal and child dietary patterns and corresponding factor loadings and proportion of food groups. The colour gradation reflects how large and in which direction was the correlation between the food groups and the dietary patterns. Deep green colour refers a relatively higher correlation (a higher intake) of the food groups with the corresponding patterns. Deep red refers relatively a lower correlation (a lower intake) of the food groups with the corresponding dietary patterns

(continuous but not normally distributed) tests were used to compare differences of proportions, means and medians, respectively, between groups. Principal component analysis (PCA) was used to compute economic status (in quintiles) of households.

To assess the associations of household, maternal and child dietary diversity and patterns with HAZ and childhood stunting, β coefficients and the prevalence ratio (PR) with their corresponding 95% confidence intervals (CIs) were determined using multilevel linear and Poisson regression models, respectively [27]. Since the data were collected using a multi-stage cluster sampling technique, stunting could potentially be correlated in clusters (EAs). We, therefore, used a two-level model with individual factors as level 1 and geographical areas (EAs) at level 2 (random effects). A stepwise backward elimination of covariates in the models was conducted and potential factors were retained at *p-value* $< 0.20$. This method was used for both individual and community level factors. Dietary diversity and pattern scores were treated as categorical (model 1) and continuous (model 2) variables. Estimates of associations were adjusted for socio-demographic factors (child age, sex, maternal age and education, number of under-five children in a household), maternal anthropometry (height and BMI), infant and young child feeding practices (exclusive breastfeeding) and household food security at level 1. At level 2, water source was included. Model fit was assessed using Akaike's (AIC) and Bayesian (BIC) information criteria. We tested interactions between DDSs, dietary patterns, other covariates with HAZ and stunting using multiplicative terms. We conducted sensitivity analysis: 1) by labelling missing values of covariates as "missing" and including in the models; 2) by including and excluding covariates (such as household wealth, paternal education, place of delivery and latrine type). Further, the association between joint classifications of tertiles of dietary patterns and HAZ was explored. Statistical analyses were performed using Stata version 14.1 (Stata Corporation, College Station, TX, USA). A 2-sided *t-test* value of $P < 0.05$ was considered statistically significant.

## Results

### Participant characteristics

Almost half of the children (1805, 47.7%) were female. Only 3.1% of the households had a female head. In 2353 (90.8%) of households, there was only one child aged under five. The median maternal age was 29.0 years (IQR = 25.0, 35.0). More than half (2069; 54.6%) of the mothers were illiterate. The mean maternal BMI was 20.2 kg/m$^2$ (SD = 2.4). Almost two-thirds (2371; 62.6%) of mothers delivered the index child at home. The prevalence of stunting among children aged 0–59 months was 38.5% with a mean (SD) HAZ of 1.6 (1.8). A fifth (777; 20.5%) of the study participants had missing values of household income (Table 2).

### Dietary patterns

Figure 2 depicts household, maternal and child dietary patterns and corresponding factor loadings. For each, we identified three dietary patterns. Pattern 2 ("egg, meat, poultry and legume") and pattern 3 ("dairy, vegetable and fruit pattern") were similar for all groups. The "egg, meat, poultry and legume pattern" was characterized by a high intake of eggs, meats, legumes, cereals, oils, fats and sweets. The "dairy, vegetable and fruit based" pattern was characterized by a high intake of fruits tubers, roots, vegetables and milk and milk products. A "plant-based pattern" and a "dairy, vegetable and fruit pattern"

**Table 3** Household, maternal and child dietary diversity scores, food security and breastfeeding by stunting status in Ethiopia, 2014

| Characteristics | Total | Normal | Stunted | *p*-value |
|---|---|---|---|---|
| N | 3788 | 2161 | 1459 | |
| Household dietary diversity score (HDDS), median (IQR) | 5.0 (4.0, 7.0) | 5.0 (4.0, 7.0) | 5.0 (4.0, 6.0) | 0.004 |
| HDDS category | | | | |
| < =5 HDDS | 2031 (53.6%) | 1131 (52.3%) | 813 (55.7%) | 0.045 |
| > 5 HDDS | 1757 (46.4%) | 1030 (47.7%) | 646 (44.3%) | |
| Women (DDS-W), median (IQR) | 3.0 (2.0, 4.0) | 3.0 (2.0, 5.0) | 3.0 (2.0, 4.0) | <0.001 |
| DDS-W category | | | | |
| < 5 DDSW | 2859 (75.5%) | 1595 (73.8%) | 1137 (77.9%) | 0.005 |
| > =5 DDSW | 929 (24.5%) | 566 (26.2%) | 322 (22.1%) | |
| DDS 6–23 months, median (IQR) | 2.0 (1.0, 3.0) | 2.0 (0.0, 3.0) | 2.0 (2.0, 3.0) | <0.001 |
| DDS 6–23 months category | | | | |
| 0–3 food groups | 779 (86.9%) | 474 (87.9%) | 282 (85.5%) | 0.552 |
| 4–7 food groups | 117 (13.1%) | 65 (12.1%) | 48 (14.6%) | |
| Child DDS (24–59 months), median (IQR) | 3.0 (1.0, 4.0) | 2.0 (0.0, 4.0) | 3.0 (2.0, 4.0) | <0.001 |
| Child DDS (24–59 months) category | | | | |
| 0–3 food groups | 1411 (61.7%) | 661 (59.6%) | 684 (63.1%) | 0.054 |
| 4–9 food groups | 876 (38.3%) | 448 (40.4%) | 400 (36.9%) | |
| Household food security | | | | |
| Food Secure | 1744 (46.0%) | 1026 (47.5%) | 621 (42.6%) | 0.005 |
| Mildly Food Insecure Access | 344 (9.1%) | 201 (9.3%) | 133 (9.1%) | |
| Moderately Food Insecure Access | 1103 (29.1%) | 626 (29.0%) | 438 (30.0%) | |
| Severely Food Insecure Access | 574 (15.2%) | 298 (13.8%) | 256 (17.5%) | |
| Missing | 23 (0.6%) | 10 (0.5%) | 11 (0.8%) | |
| Exclusive breast feeding | 2719 (71.8%) | 1592 (73.7%) | 998 (68.4%) | 0.001 |

*HDDS* household dietary diversity score, *DDSW* women dietary diversity score

**Table 4** Stunting prevalence among children across tertiles of household, maternal and child nutrient pattern scores in Ethiopia, 2014

| | Tertiles of dietary patterns | | | |
|---|---|---|---|---|
| | T1 | T2 | T3 | |
| Household dietary patterns | | | | |
| | Pattern 1 ("fish, meat and miscellaneous") | | | |
| n | 1298 | 1259 | 1154 | |
| Normal | 715 (55.1%) | 734 (58.3%) | 668 (57.9%) | 0.097 |
| Stunted | 533 (41.1%) | 472 (37.5%) | 424 (36.7%) | |
| Missing | 50 (3.9%) | 53 (4.2%) | 62 (5.4%) | |
| | Pattern 2 ("egg, meat, poultry and legume") | | | |
| n | 1327 | 1291 | 1093 | |
| Normal | 760 (57.3%) | 762 (59.0%) | 595 (54.4%) | 0.044 |
| Stunted | 516 (38.9%) | 464 (35.9%) | 449 (41.1%) | |
| Missing | 51 (3.8%) | 65 (5.0%) | 49 (4.5%) | |
| | Pattern 3 ("dairy, vegetable and fruit") | | | |
| n | 1441 | 1052 | 1218 | |
| Normal | 776 (53.9%) | 584 (55.5%) | 757 (62.2%) | <0.001 |
| Stunted | 599 (41.6%) | 425 (40.4%) | 405 (33.3%) | |
| Missing | 66 (4.6%) | 43 (4.1%) | 56 (4.6%) | |
| Maternal dietary patterns | | | | |
| | Pattern 1 ("plant-based") | | | |
| n | 1270 | 1232 | 1235 | |
| Normal | 683 (53.8%) | 701 (56.9%) | 749 (60.6%) | 0.002 |
| Stunted | 529 (41.7%) | 481 (39.0%) | 431 (34.9%) | |
| Missing | 58 (4.6%) | 50 (4.1%) | 55 (4.5%) | |
| | Pattern 2 ("egg, meat, poultry and legume") | | | |
| n | 1264 | 1291 | 1182 | |
| Normal | 755 (59.7%) | 714 (55.3%) | 664 (56.2%) | 0.020 |
| Stunted | 447 (35.4%) | 528 (40.9%) | 466 (39.4%) | |
| Missing | 62 (4.9%) | 49 (3.8%) | 52 (4.4%) | |
| | Pattern 3 ("dairy, vegetable and fruit") | | | |
| n | 1262 | 1233 | 1242 | |
| Normal | 679 (53.8%) | 708 (57.4%) | 746 (60.1%) | 0.002 |
| Stunted | 530 (42.0%) | 476 (38.6%) | 435 (35.0%) | |
| Missing | 53 (4.2%) | 49 (4.0%) | 61 (4.9%) | |
| Child dietary patterns (6–59 months of age) | | | | |
| | Pattern 1 ("grain-based") | | | |
| | 1274 | 950 | 963 | |
| Normal | 649 (50.9%) | 509 (53.6%) | 493 (51.2%) | 0.430 |
| Stunted | 584 (45.8%) | 409 (43.1%) | 421 (43.7%) | |
| Missing | 41 (3.2%) | 32 (3.4%) | 49 (5.1%) | |
| | Pattern 2 ("egg, meat, poultry and legume") | | | |
| n | 1255 | 999 | 933 | |
| Normal | 640 (51.0%) | 538 (53.9%) | 473 (50.7%) | 0.249 |
| Stunted | 561 (44.7%) | 422 (42.2%) | 431 (46.2%) | |

**Table 4** Stunting prevalence among children across tertiles of household, maternal and child nutrient pattern scores in Ethiopia, 2014 *(Continued)*

| | Tertiles of dietary patterns | | | |
|---|---|---|---|---|
| | T1 | T2 | T3 | |
| Missing | 54 (4.3%) | 39 (3.9%) | 29 (3.1%) | |
| | Pattern 3 ("dairy, vegetable and fruit") | | | |
| n | 1136 | 1029 | 1022 | |
| Normal | 577 (50.8%) | 499 (48.5%) | 575 (56.3%) | 0.002 |
| Stunted | 505 (44.5%) | 494 (48.0%) | 415 (40.6%) | |
| Missing | 54 (4.8%) | 36 (3.5%) | 32 (3.1%) | |

were identified for mothers. While these two patterns appeared to be similar, the "plant-based" pattern was however characterized by a high intake of grains, tubers and leafy vegetables. Individual food items used for food groupings and the proportion of food groups consumed by households, mothers and children are depicted in Additional file 1: Tables S1, S2 and S3.

### DDSs, dietary patterns, household food security and stunting

Table 3 and Additional file 1: Table S4 show the DDSs of households, mothers and children by whether or not stunting was present. Three-quarters (2859; 75.5%) of the mothers had a DDS less than five. Only 13.1% of children aged 6–23 months had a DDS greater than or equal to four. The proportion of children aged 24–59 months who had a DDS less than or equal to three was 61.7% (1411). The proportion of food secure households was 46.0% (1744). A marginally significant statistical difference in the proportion of stunting was found between those children with a household DDS < =5 and >5 ($p = 0.045$). The prevalence of stunting was significantly different by maternal DDS ($p = 0.005$). No significant difference in the prevalence of stunting was found between the DDSs of children aged 6–23 and 24–59 months.

Except for the "fish, meat and miscellaneous" dietary pattern ($p = 0.097$), there were significant differences in the prevalence of stunting across the tertiles of the other household dietary patterns. The prevalence of stunting (41.6%) in the first tertile of household "dairy, vegetable and fruit" dietary pattern was higher compared to the third tertile (33.3%) ($p < 0.001$). Children in the third tertile of maternal and child "dairy, vegetable and fruit" dietary pattern were less likely to be stunted compared to the first and second tertiles ($p = 0.002$) (Table 4).

### Associations of DDSs and dietary patterns with HAZ and stunting

After adjusting for potential individual and community level factors, no significant associations between household, maternal and child DDSs with stunting (HAZ) was found. Children in the third tertile of the household "dairy, vegetable and fruit" pattern had a 0.16 ($\beta = 0.16$; 95% CI: 0.02, 0.30) increase in HAZ compared to those in the first tertile. Similarly, the prevalence of stunting among children in the third tertile of the pattern was lower (PR = 0.83; 95% CI: 0.72–0.95) compared to those in the first tertile. Those children in the second ($\beta = -0.17$; 95% CI: -0.31, −0.04) and third ($\beta = -0.16$; 95% CI: -0.30, −0.02) tertiles of maternal "egg, meat, poultry and legume" pattern had a significantly lower HAZ compared to those in the first tertile (Table 5 and Additional file 1: Table S5).

A 0.22 ($\beta = 0.22$; 95% CI: 0.06, 0.39) and 0.19 ($\beta = 0.19$; 95% CI: 0.04, 0.33) increase in HAZ was found for those in the third tertiles of the "dairy, vegetable and fruit" patterns for children 24–59 months and 6–59 months, respectively. The AIC and BIC were significantly lower for the household and maternal dietary patterns compared to the corresponding DDSs (Table 5). In the joint classification, children in the first tertile of maternal "egg, meat, poultry and legume" and the third tertile of child "dairy, vegetable and fruit" patterns had a 0.31 ($\beta = 0.31$; 95% CI: 0.05, 0.57) increase in HAZ compared to the respective third and first tertiles of the patterns. A 0.29 ($\beta = 0.29$; 95% CI: 0.07, 0.50) increase in HAZ was found for those children in the third tertiles of both the maternal and child "dairy, vegetable and fruit" dietary patterns, compared to the first tertiles of the patterns (Fig. 3).

The sensitivity analysis, which was undertaken by labelling missing values as "missing" and including them in the analysis, as well as incorporating additional covariates, did not change the findings materially. There were no significant interactions between the DDSs and dietary patterns, and the other covariates and HAZ (stunting). The interactions among dietary patterns for each of the levels (household, maternal and children) were also not significant (data not shown).

## Discussion

For households, mothers and children, we computed the DDSs and identified three dietary patterns for each. At all levels, a dietary pattern characterized by high intake

**Table 5** Adjusted β coefficients (95% confidence interval) for the associations of household, maternal and child dietary diversity scores and tertiles of dietary pattern scores with childhood height-for-age z score in Ethiopia, 2014

| | Adjusted β coefficient (95% confidence interval) for height-for-age z score | | | | |
|---|---|---|---|---|---|
| Household | | | | | |
| Dietary diversity score | <=4 | > = 5 | | *P* value | AIC (BIC) |
| | Reference | 0.03 (−0.80, 0.14) | | 0.624 | 12,722 (12850) |
| | Tertiles | | | | |
| Dietary patterns | T1 | T2 | T3 | P for trend | AIC (BIC) |
| Pattern 1 ("fish, meat and miscellaneous") | Reference | −0.01 (−0.15, 0.12) | −0.07 (−0.21, 0.07) | 0.312 | 12,466 (12600) |
| Pattern 2 ("egg, meat, poultry and legume") | Reference | −0.001 (−0.14, 0.13) | −0.03 (−0.19, 0.12) | 0.681 | 12,467 (12601) |
| Pattern 3 ("dairy, vegetable and fruit") | Reference | 0.07 (−0.07, 0.20) | 0.16 (0.02, 0.30)* | 0.026 | 12,462 (12597) |
| Maternal | | | | | |
| Dietary diversity score | <=4 | > = 5 | | P value | AIC (BIC) |
| | Reference | 0.03 (−0.10, 0.16) | | 0.672 | 12,722 (12851) |
| | Tertiles | | | | |
| Dietary patterns | T1 | T2 | T3 | P for trend | AIC (BIC) |
| Pattern 1 ("plant-based") | Reference | 0.07 (−0.07, 0.20) | 0.09 (−0.06, 0.23) | 0.229 | 12,564 (12699) |
| Pattern 2 ("egg, meat, poultry and legume") | Reference | −0.17 (−0.31, −0.04)* | −0.16 (−0.30, −0.02)* | 0.025 | 12,558 (12693) |
| Pattern 3 ("dairy, vegetable and fruit") | Reference | 0.06 (−0.07, 0.20) | 0.10 (−0.05, 0.25) | 0.229 | 12,564 (12698) |
| Children aged 6–23 months | | | | | |
| Dietary diversity score | <=3 | > = 4 | | P value | AIC (BIC) |
| | Reference | −0.26 (−0.61, 0.78) | | 0.130 | 3107 (3196) |
| | Tertiles | | | | |
| Dietary patterns | T1 | T2 | T3 | P for trend | AIC (BIC) |
| Pattern 1 ("grain-based") | Reference | 0.07 (−0.18, 0.32) | −0.20 (−0.50, 0.10) | 0.290 | 3124 (3219) |
| Pattern 2 ("egg, meat, poultry and legume") | Reference | 0.03 (−0.30 (0.32) | −0.02 (−0.27, 0.24) | 0.892 | 3127 (3222) |
| Pattern 3 ("dairy, vegetable and fruit") | Reference | −0.001 (−0.25, 0.25) | 0.02 (−0.27, 0.32) | 0.890 | 3128 (3222) |
| Children aged 24–59 months | | | | | |
| Dietary diversity score | <=3 | > = 4 | | P value | AIC (BIC) |
| | Reference | 0.12 (−0.02, 0.27) | | 0.095 | 7641 (7748) |
| | Tertiles | | | | |
| Dietary patterns | T1 | T2 | T3 | P for trend | AIC (BIC) |
| Pattern 1 ("grain-based") | Reference | 0.08 (−0.09, 0.25) | 0.04 (−0.14, 0.21) | 0.685 | 7663 (7776) |
| Pattern 2 ("egg, meat, poultry and legume") | Reference | 0.13 (−0.3, 0.30) | −0.05 (−0.23, 0.13) | 0.668 | 7659 (7772) |
| Pattern 3 ("dairy, vegetable and fruit") | Reference | −0.03 (−0.20, 0.14) | 0.22 (0.06, 0.39)** | 0.007 | 7654 (7766) |
| Children aged 6–59 months | | | | | |
| | Tetiles | | | | |
| Dietary patterns | T1 | T2 | T3 | P for trend | AIC (BIC) |
| Pattern 1 ("grain-based") | Reference | 0.10 (−0.04, 0.25) | −0.04 (−0.19, 0.11) | 0.643 | 10,746 (10871) |
| Pattern 2 ("egg, meat, poultry and legume") | Reference | −0.07 (−0.7, 0.21) | −0.02 (−0.17, 0.13) | 0.841 | 10,748 (10874) |
| Pattern 3 ("dairy, vegetable and fruit") | Reference | −0.02 (−0.16, 0.13) | 0.19 (0.04, 0.33)* | 0.014 | 10,741 (10867) |

The β coefficients were adjusted for both individual (maternal body mass index, age (if applicable), household food security, number of under-five children in a household, maternal education, maternal height, exclusive breast feeding) and community-level patterns (water source)

*P* for trend was determined by including the tertiles of dietary patterns as continuous variables

*AIC* Akaike's information criterion, *BIC* Bayesian information criterion

*$p < 0.05$; **$p < 0.01$

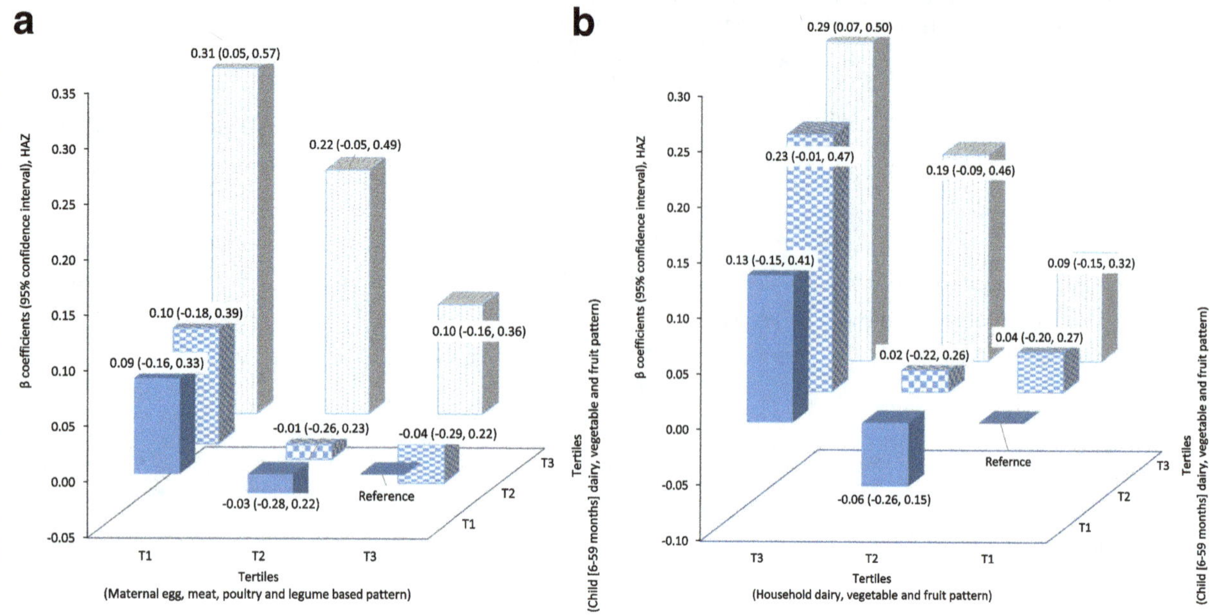


**Fig. 3** Multivariable adjusted β coefficient and 95% confidence interval of fractures in joint classified participants across nine strata formed with the tertiles of dietary patterns. The β coefficients were adjusted for both individual (maternal body mass index, age (if applicable), household food security, number of under-five children in a household, maternal education, maternal height, exclusive breast feeding) and community-level patterns (water source)

of dairy, vegetables and fruits was positively associated with HAZ and inversely related to stunting. In addition, a maternal "plant-based" pattern (characterized by high intake of grains, white tubers, roots, plantains and dark leafy vegetables) was inversely and significantly associated with childhood stunting. Statistically non-significant associations were found between household, maternal and child DDSs and stunting.

Dietary patterns show a better picture of eating habits compared to DDSs by reflecting mainly the behavioural aspect of food consumption that has a synergistic effect on health. Evidence shows that dietary patterns identified by factor analysis are associated with several non-communicable diseases [28, 29], highlighting the plausibility and validity of the approach. In low- and middle-income countries, a study also indicated that the application of factor analysis, using disaggregated food expenditure data to explore food consumption patterns, is an important approach to identify patterns and food groups that predict children's nutritional status [19]. The dietary patterns are defined based on the factor loadings of individual food items which contribute at different levels. Unlike DDSs, factor analysis is an a posteriori statistical analysis method that creates unrelated food patterns that could potentially be associated with an outcome [17]. In addition, using this approach, it is possible to assess the relative intake level of the individual food groups within a dietary pattern. Dietary patterns defined the overall characteristics of the dietary habits of the study groups. In this study, we found that the "dairy, vegetable and fruit" pattern was a common feature of household, maternal and childhood dietary habits.

The results indicate that a pattern characterised by a high intake of dairy, vegetables and fruits was positively associated with HAZ (inversely related to stunting). However, the proportion of households (32.7%), mothers (28.0%) and children (30.0%) consuming dairy products was low. In a recent study in Malawi, it was reported that frequent milk intake during pregnancy was positively associated with birth size [30]. In Ethiopia, a higher intake of cow's milk, in addition to cereals and/or legumes, was associated with a higher length-for-age z-scores among children aged 5–11 months [31]. In our study area, cow's milk is the most commonly consumed type of dairy product. It is believed that the milk contains important nutrients, including protein, calcium and vitamin A, which are important for development and bone growth [32]. A systematic review of dairy consumption and physical growth has shown that a daily intake of 245 ml of milk is associated with 0.4 cm increase in height per annum compared to non-consumers [33]. It was also reported that low consumption of vegetables and fruits was associated with stunting and poor linear growth in children aged 6–23 months [34]. This implies that, in addition to available interventions to increase dietary diversity, targeting to increase accessibility and consumption of dairy, vegetables and fruits specifically, could have an important contribution to the reduction of stunting prevalence.

Unlike other studies [14, 15, 35], we found a non-significant association of household, maternal and child DDSs with stunting. This difference could be explained by the differences in sample size, sampling and analysis methods. Particularly, with regard to the analysis methods, we used a multilevel Poisson regression model to determine the level of associations. This method allows for controlling for the geographical clustering effect of the samples, and accounting for potential correlations, under the premise that variations in childhood stunting could be due to both individual and community level factors [36]. Most studies that found a positive association between DDS and stunting did not consider this clustering effect [16, 37]. The association may also be confounded by income [38, 39]. However, in this study, even when we adjusted for income, the association still remained statistically non-significant.

A study by *Daniels* et al. suggested that the addition of portion size as part of data collection could improve the correlation of DDSs with nutrient adequacy [40]. Another study among Zambian infants suggested that although dietary diversity had a positive effect on linear growth, micronutrient adequacy among those who consumed fortified foods may be more accurately assessed using other food indicators [41]. In Eastern Kenya, a study reported that child DDS was not associated with childhood stunting [42]. In Ethiopia, while household food group expenditure index (identified using factor analysis) significantly predicted HAZ ($\beta = 0.067$; $p = 0.03$), dietary diversity was only marginally associated with HAZ ($\beta = 0.037$; $p = 0.05$) [19]. DDSs are important indicators of dietary quality in terms of micronutrient density and adequacy. However, DDSs only measure one dimension of dietary quality. Macronutrients (for instance, protein) also have an important role in growth and development in children [8]. Although DDS is an important approach to measure dietary quality, we recommend that the use of a posteriori dietary data analysis methods (such as factor analysis) as an alternative or complementary method, can give a further insight into the eating behaviours of a population group. These approaches are also important to understand the relative contribution of foods in a pattern that have a potential link with disease outcomes or nutritional status, eventually leading to identifying specific food items, which are most important in determining an outcome of interest (a disease or nutritional status).

Measures taken to ensure the quality of the data are a major strength of the study. Before, during and after the data collection, all possible quality control measures, including intensive training of data collectors, use of standard procedures and tools, intensive and supportive supervision and standardization of anthropometric measurements to minimize bias and associated errors were implemented. The use of qualitative dietary data without portion size and limited food items for the identification of dietary patterns in the factor analysis could be a limitation. Therefore, further validation studies are needed. In addition, due to the cross-sectional design, we cannot claim a cause-effect relationship between dietary patterns and stunting.

## Conclusions

Identification of dietary patterns using a posteriori dietary analysis methods can be an alternative and feasible method of diet quality assessment in LICs as an alternative approach to DDSs. We found that, while DDSs are not significantly associated with HAZ (stunting), a dietary pattern characterized by a high intake of dairy, vegetables and fruits by households, mothers and children is positively associated with HAZ and inversely associated with stunting. These findings could be of importance in developing food-based interventions targeting households, mothers and children. In addition, the study suggests an alternative approach of analysing dietary data to determine dietary quality using an a posteriori method with the same data collected for DDSs. More research is warranted to confirm the findings.

#### Abbreviations

AIC: Akaike's information criterion; BIC: Bayesian information criterion; BMI: Body mass index; *CI*: Confidence interval; DDS: Dietary diversity score; EA: Enumeration area; FANTA: Food and Nutrition Technical Assistance; HAZ: Height-for-age z score; LIC: Low income countries; PPS: Probability proportional to size; PR: Prevalence ratio; SNNP: South Nation and Nationalities and People; UNICEF: United Nations International Children's Emergency Fund; WHO: World Health Organization

#### Acknowledgments

We are thankful to Bill & Melinda Gates Foundation for funding (through Alive & Thrive, managed by FHI 360) this evaluation study. Additional financial support was obtained from the CGIAR Research Program on Agriculture for Nutrition and Health (A4NH), led by the International Food Policy Research Institute (IFPRI), for which are grateful. The authors express their gratitude to Addis Continental Institute of Public Health for collecting the data and thank all survey participants in the evaluation study. YAM is thankful for the support provided by the Australian Government Research Training Program Scholarship.

#### Authors' contribution

YAM and AW conceived the research idea. YAM analysed the data, interpreted the results and wrote the manuscript. AW gave critical comments at each stage of manuscript development. All authors critically reviewed the manuscript and approved for submission.

#### Funding

The Bill & Melinda Gates Foundation, through Alive & Thrive, managed by FHI 360 funded this evaluation study. Additional financial support was obtained from the CGIAR Research Program on Agriculture for Nutrition and Health (A4NH), led by the International Food Policy Research Institute (IFPRI). No financial support was received to write this specific paper.

**Authors' information**
YAM & AW: Department of Public Health Sciences, Addis Continental Institute of Public Health, Addis Ababa, Ethiopia; YAM, TKG, AWT and ZS: Adelaide Medical School, The University of Adelaide, Australia; RA: Health Observatory, Discipline of Medicine, The Queen Elizabeth Hospital Campus, The University of Adelaide, Adelaide, Australia.

**Competing interests**
The authors declare that they have no competing interests.

**Author details**
[1]Department of Public Health Sciences, Addis Continental Institute of Public Health, Addis Ababa, Ethiopia. [2]Adelaide Medical School, The University of Adelaide, Adelaide, Australia. [3]Health Observatory, Discipline of Medicine, The Queen Elizabeth Hospital Campus, The University of Adelaide, Adelaide, Australia.

**References**

1. Forouzanfar MH, Afshin A, Alexander LT, Anderson HR, Bhutta ZA, Biryukov S, Brauer M, Burnett R, Cercy K, Charlson FJ, et al. Global, regional, and national comparative risk assessment of 79 behavioural, environmental and occupational, and metabolic risks or clusters of risks, 1990–2015: a systematic analysis for the global burden of disease study. Lancet. 2015;388: 1659–724.
2. Institute for Health Metrics and Evaluation (IHME). GBD Compare. Seattle, WA: IHME, University of Washington, 2015. Available from http://vizhub.healthdata.org/gbd-compare. (Accessed [February 20,. 2016]).
3. Central Statistical Authority [Ethiopia] and ORC Macro. Ethiopia demographic and health survey 2016. Central statistical authority and ORC macro. Ethiopia and Calverton, Maryland, USA: Addis Ababa; 2016.
4. de Onis M, Branca F. Childhood stunting: a global perspective. Matern Child Nutr. 2016;12:12–26.
5. Shrimpton R, Yongyout MK. Analyzing the causes of child stunting in DPRK. UNICEF, New York: A report on the DPRK Nutrition Assessment; 2003.
6. Coates CJ, Colaiezzi AB, Bell W, Charrondiere RU, Leclercq C. Overcoming dietary assessment challenges in low-income countries: technological solutions proposed by the international dietary data expansion (INDDEX) project. Nutrients. 2017;9
7. World Health Organization. Indicators for assessing infant and young child feeding practices: part I. Geneva, Switzerland: WHO; 2008.
8. FAO and FHI 360, Minimum dietary diversity for women: A guide for measurement, 2016, FAO; Rome.
9. Coates J, Swindale A, Bilinsky P. Household food insecurity access scale (HFIAS) for measurement of food access: indicator guide. FANTA: New York, NY; 2007.
10. Kennedy GL, Pedro MR, Seghieri C, Nantel G, Brouwer I. Dietary diversity score is a useful indicator of micronutrient intake in non-breast-feeding Filipino children. J Nutr. 2007;137:472–7.
11. Moursi MM, Arimond M, Dewey KG, Trèche S, Ruel MT, Delpeuch F. Dietary diversity is a good predictor of the micronutrient density of the diet of 6-to 23-month-old children in Madagascar. J Nutr. 2008;138:2448–53.
12. Torheim L, Ouattara F, Diarra M, Thiam F, Barikmo I, Hatløy A, Oshaug A. Nutrient adequacy and dietary diversity in rural Mali: association and determinants. Eur J Clin Nutr. 2004;58:594–604.
13. Martin-Prével Y, Allemand P, Wiesmann D, Arimond M, Ballard T, Deitchler M, Dop MC, Kennedy G, Lee WT, Mousi M. Moving forward on choosing a standard operational indicator of women's dietary diversity. Rome: FAO; 2015.
14. Mahmudiono T, Sumarmi S, Rosenkranz RR. Household dietary diversity and child stunting in east java, Indonesia. Asia Pac J Clin Nutr. 2017;26:317–25.
15. Rah JH, Akhter N, Semba RD, Sd P, Bloem MW, Campbell AA, Moench-Pfanner R, Sun K, Badham J, Kraemer K. Low dietary diversity is a predictor of child stunting in rural Bangladesh. Eur J Clin Nutr. 2010;64:1393–8.
16. Moges T, Birks KA, Samuel A, Kebede A, Kebede A, Wuehler S, Zerfu D, Abera A, Mengistu G, Tesfaye B: Diet diversity is negatively associated with stunting among Ethiopian children 6–35 months of age. 2015.
17. Hoffmann K, Schulze MB, Schienkiewitz A, Nöthlings U, Boeing H. Application of a new statistical method to derive dietary patterns in nutritional epidemiology. Am J Epidemiol. 2004;159:935–44.
18. Thompson B. Exploratory and confirmatory factor analysis: understanding concepts and applications: American Psychological Association; 2004.
19. Humphries DL, Dearden KA, Crookston BT, Woldehanna T, Penny ME, Behrman JR. Household food group expenditure patterns are associated with child anthropometry at ages 5, 8 and 12 years in Ethiopia, India, Peru and Vietnam. Econ Hum Biol. 2017;26:30–41.
20. Humphries DL, Dearden KA, Crookston BT, Fernald LC, Stein AD, Woldehanna T, Penny ME, Behrman JR. Cross-sectional and longitudinal associations between household food security and child anthropometry at ages 5 and 8 years in Ethiopia, India, Peru, and Vietnam. J Nutr. 2015;145:1924–33.
21. Newby P, Tucker KL. Empirically derived eating patterns using factor or cluster analysis: a review. Nutr Rev. 2004;62:177–203.
22. World Health Organization. WHO Expert Committee on Physical Status. The Use and Interpretation of Anthropometry; Report of a WHO Expert Committee; World Health Organization: Geneva, Switzerland, 1995. Available online: http://apps.who.int/iris/bitstream/10665/37003/1/WHO_TRS_854.pdf (accessed on 14 March 2017).
23. Swindale A, Bilinsky P. Household Dietary Diversity Score (HDDS) for Measurement of Household Food Access: Indicator Guide VERSION 2. Washington, D.C.: Food and Nutrition Technical Assistance Project (FANTA); 2006. 2006/9 [cited 2017/2/2]; Available from: https://www.fantaproject.org/sites/default/files/resources/HDDS_v2_Sep06_0.pdf.
24. WHO/Multi Growth Resaerch Center Study Group (MGRSG. Complementary feeding in the WHO Multicentre Growth Reference Study. Acta Pediatrica. 2006;450:27–37.
25. Bandoh DA, Kenu E. Dietary diversity and nutritional adequacy of under-fives in a fishing community in the central region of Ghana. BMC Nutrition. 2017;3:2.
26. Uebersax JS. The tetrachoric and polychoric correlation coefficients. Statistical Methods for Rater Agreement. http://www.john-uebersax.com/stat/tetra.htm. Accessed 19 Apr 2017.
27. Barros AJ, Hirakata VN. Alternatives for logistic regression in cross-sectional studies: an empirical comparison of models that directly estimate the prevalence ratio. BMC Med Res Methodol. 2003;3:21.
28. Melaku YA, Gill TK, Adams R, Shi Z. Association between dietary patterns and low bone mineral density among adults aged 50 years and above: findings from the north West Adelaide health study (NWAHS). Br J Nutr. 2016;116:1437–46.
29. Drehmer M, Odegaard AO, Schmidt MI, Duncan BB, LdO C, SMA M, MdCB M, Barreto SM, Pereira MA. Brazilian dietary patterns and the dietary approaches to stop hypertension (DASH) diet-relationship with metabolic syndrome and newly diagnosed diabetes in the ELSA-Brasil study. Diabetol Metab Syndr. 2017;9:13.
30. Hjertholm KG, Iversen PO, Holmboe-Ottesen G, Mdala I, Munthali A, Maleta K, Shi Z, Ferguson E, Kamudoni P. Maternal dietary intake during pregnancy and its association to birth size in rural Malawi: a cross-sectional study. Matern Child Nutr. 2017;
31. Umeta M, West CE, Verhoef H, Haidar J, Hautvast JGAJ. Factors associated with stunting in infants aged 5–11 months in the Dodota-Sire District, rural Ethiopia. J Nutr. 2003;133:1064–9.
32. Yackobovitch-Gavan M, Phillip M, Gat-Yablonski G. How milk and its proteins affect growth, bone health, and weight. Horm Res Paediatr. 2017;
33. de Beer H. Dairy products and physical stature: a systematic review and meta-analysis of controlled trials. Econ Hum Biol. 2012;10:299–309.
34. Aguayo VM, Nair R, Badgaiyan N, Krishna V. Determinants of stunting and poor linear growth in children under 2 years of age in India: an in-depth analysis of Maharashtra's comprehensive nutrition survey. Matern Child Nutr. 2016;12(Suppl 1):121–40.
35. Darapheak C, Takano T, Kizuki M, Nakamura K, Seino K. Consumption of animal source foods and dietary diversity reduce stunting in children in Cambodia. Int Arch Med. 2013;6:29.
36. Haile D, Azage M, Mola T, Rainey R. Exploring spatial variations and factors associated with childhood stunting in Ethiopia: spatial and multilevel analysis. BMC Pediatr. 2016;16:49.
37. Motbainor A, Worku A, Kumie A, Stunting I. Associated with food diversity while wasting with food insecurity among Underfive children in east and west Gojjam zones of Amhara region, Ethiopia. PLoS One. 2015;10: e0133542.

38. Gebremedhin S, Baye K, Bekele T, Tharaney M, Asrat Y, Abebe Y, Reta N. Predictors of dietary diversity in children ages 6 to 23 mo in largely food-insecure area of south Wollo, Ethiopia. Nutrition. 2016;
39. Doan D. Does income growth improve diet diversity in China?Selected paper prepared for presentation at the 58 the AARES annual conference. New South Wales: Port Macquarie; 2014.
40. Daniels MC, Adair LS, Popkin BM, Truong YK. Dietary diversity scores can be improved through the use of portion requirements: an analysis in young Filipino children. Eur J Clin Nutr. 2007;63:199–208.
41. Mallard SR, Houghton LA, Filteau S, Chisenga M, Siame J, Kasonka L, Mullen A, Gibson RS. Micronutrient adequacy and dietary diversity exert positive and distinct effects on linear growth in urban Zambian infants. J Nutr. 2016; 146:2093–101.
42. Bukania ZN, Mwangi M, Karanja RM, Mutisya R, Kombe Y, Kaduka LU, Johns T. Food insecurity and not dietary diversity is a predictor of nutrition status in children within semiarid agro-ecological zones in eastern Kenya. J Nutr Metab. 2014;2014:907153.

2

# Dietary selenium intake based on the Chinese Food Pagoda: the influence of dietary patterns on selenium intake

Jing Wang[1,2], Linsheng Yang[1,2*], Hairong Li[1,2*], Yonghua Li[1] and Binggan Wei[1]

**Abstract**

**Background:** Selenium (Se) is essential for humans, with many critical roles in physiological and pathophysiological processes. Fish, eggs and meats are usually the rich food sources of Se. To improve the nutritional status of population, a new version of balanced dietary pattern in the form of the Chinese Food Pagoda (2016) was proclaimed. This study aimed to evaluate the contribution of this balanced dietary pattern to daily Se intake, and to assess Se intake status of Chinese residents under this Food Pagoda scenario.

**Methods:** Based on the food consumption recommended in the Food Pagoda, this study collected the data of Se contents in various food composites and estimated dietary Se intakes ($EI_{TDS}$) in 12 provinces from the 4th China Total Diet Study. The estimated Se intakes based on the Chinese Food Pagoda ($EI_{CHFP}$) in 12 provinces were calculated. $EI_{TDS}$ and $EI_{CHFP}$ in various food groups among different regions were compared.

**Results:** The average $EI_{CHFP}$ in all regions, within the range of 66.23–145.20 μg/day, was greater than the China recommended nutrient intake (RNI) (60 μg/day). None of the highest $EI_{CHFP}$ went beyond the tolerable upper intake level of Se (400 μg/day). Animal source foods should be the primary source of daily Se intake according to the $EI_{CHFP}$. The average $EI_{TDS}$ in China (88 μg/day) was in line with its range of $EI_{CHFP}$ (81.01–124.25 μg/day), but that in half of the regions failed to achieve their lowest $EI_{CHFP}$. Significant differences between $EI_{TDS}$ and $EI_{CHFP}$ were observed in cereal food, aquatic and dairy products ($P < 0.05$), among which Se intake from aquatic and dairy products presented seriously insufficient in almost all regions.

**Conclusions:** The ideal dietary pattern recommended in the Food Pagoda can meet the daily requirements of Chinese population for Se intake to maintain optimal health. From the perspective of the balanced diet and Se-rich sources, the consumption of aquatic products should be increased appropriately to improve the general Se intake level of Chinese population.

**Keywords:** Selenium, Dietary intake, Chinese Food Pagoda, China Total Diet Study

## Background

Selenium (Se) is an essential micronutrient for human health, with critical roles in redox homeostasis, antioxidant defense and immune system [1, 2]. Insufficient or excessive Se intakes are linked to many acute and chronic diseases [3–8]. In particular, problems related to Se deficiency are an emerging issue for human health worldwide [9]. It is estimated that 15% of the global population suffers Se deficiency of different degrees [10]. China as one of the 40 Se-deficient countries has over 105 million people facing adverse health impacts due to Se deficiency [11, 12]. Owing to large variations in food Se, the dietary Se intake varies considerably among regions, normally being consistent with Se distribution in the environment. In China, low Se intakes are primarily found in the low-Se geographic belt from northeast to southwest, with a mean of 27.6 μg/day; while high Se intakes are observed in Se-rich areas, with a mean of 85.5 μg/day; in some selenosis areas, the Se intake can even reach up to 1253.7 μg/day on average [12]. Considering its narrow range between the

* Correspondence: yangls@igsnrr.ac.cn; lihr@igsnrr.ac.cn
[1]Key Laboratory of Land Surface Pattern and Simulation, Institute of Geographical Sciences and Natural Resources Research, Chinese Academy of Sciences, 11 A Datun Road, Beijing 100101, People's Republic of China
Full list of author information is available at the end of the article

necessary and the toxic dose, an optimal daily Se intake is required to maintain public health.

A reasonable diet is the crucial determinant for daily Se intake [13]. It is well known that cereals, fish, eggs and meats are the major dietary sources of Se [12, 14, 15]. In response to stronger demands for healthy growth of people, the Chinese government proclaimed a new version of the Dietary Guidelines for Chinese Residents in the form of the Food Pagoda (Fig. 1), based on principles of nutritional science and the current national situation [16]. Five levels of the recommended consumption corresponding to five food groups are involved in the Food Pagoda, covering the essential foods we should consume in daily life [17]. This Pagoda recommends a relatively ideal dietary pattern to improve the general nutrition of Chinese residents. However, whether it can meet the daily requirements of Se intake for general population and achieve the optimal daily Se intake has yet to be ascertained.

In the past decades of China, Se deficiency diseases, for e.g. Kashin-Beck disease and Keshan disease, have been prevalent in low-Se areas, with particularly high morbidity in underdeveloped regions. Apart from low Se contents in local foods, unreasonable food consumption patterns were also considered as one of the main reasons for deficient Se intake [18]. A study on dietary Se intake in 1990s found that urban residents consumed more Se-rich foods such as meats, seafood, eggs and dairy products than rural residents, resulting in contrasting Se intakes between the two populations [18]. With the rapid growth of China's economy, food supply and diversity increased dramatically [19]. Since the balanced diet conforming to the Chinese Food Pagoda is deemed as an ideal dietary pattern to promote nutrition, it is necessary to assess the Se intake level under the scenario of this Food Pagoda, and to be clear about the gap between this level and the current Se intake status of Chinese population in different provinces. This is the first study to evaluate the Se intake of Chinese residents associated with the 2016 Chinese Food Pagoda and discuss the influence of dietary patterns on Se intake. It will be valuable for the future research on daily optimal Se intake and also for the government to put forward proper strategies on Se supplementation. Therefore, this study aimed to: 1) test whether compliance with the Food Pagoda could meet daily requirements of Se intake for Chinese residents; 2) make quantitative comparisons of the China Total Diet Study-based estimates of Se intake ($EI_{TDS}$) with the Food Pagoda-based estimates of Se intake ($EI_{CHFP}$) in different food groups.

## Methods

### Data source

The China TDS is a national survey to investigate the levels of various nutrients and chemical contaminants in foods and assess their dietary exposure for the Chinese population [20]. The data of food Se contents and the $EI_{TDS}$ in China and 12 provinces used in this study were directly obtained from results of the 4th China TDS in 2007 [21]. Hereinto, the analysis of food Se was conducted by the National Institute of Nutrition and Food Safety. $EI_{TDS}$ was calculated by multiplying determined food Se contents with the investigated food consumption data.

### Food consumption survey

The 4th China TDS was carried out in 2007, with a similar design and experimental methods to the 3rd China TDS in 1990 [22]. The Chinese Centre for Disease

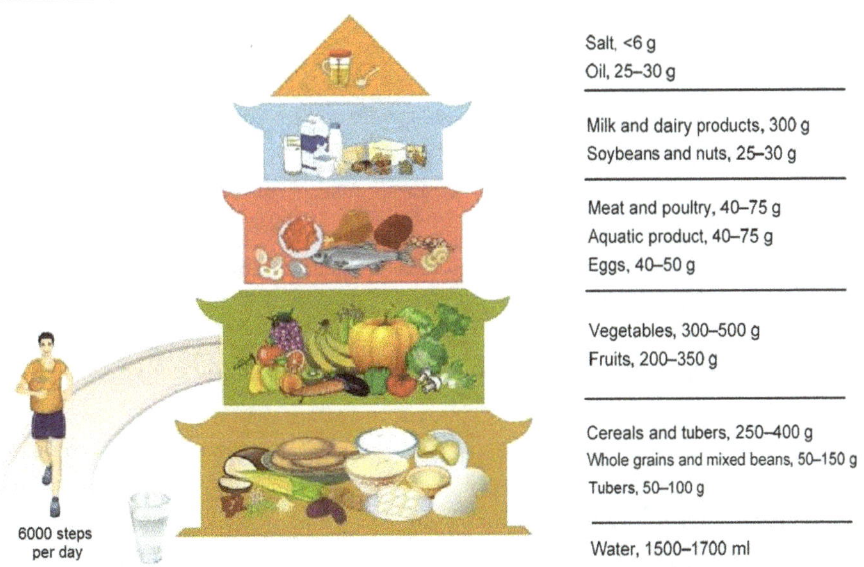
Salt, <6 g
Oil, 25–30 g
Milk and dairy products, 300 g
Soybeans and nuts, 25–30 g
Meat and poultry, 40–75 g
Aquatic product, 40–75 g
Eggs, 40–50 g
Vegetables, 300–500 g
Fruits, 200–350 g
Cereals and tubers, 250–400 g
Whole grains and mixed beans, 50–150 g
Tubers, 50–100 g
Water, 1500–1700 ml
6000 steps per day

**Fig. 1** Food Guide Pagoda for Chinese residents [16]

Control and Prevention organized the food consumption survey. Multistage random cluster sampling method and food composites approach were used in this survey. A total of 12 provinces were selected to represent the average dietary patterns of different areas of China, covering about 50% of the total Chinese population. These provinces consist of Heilongjiang (HLJ), Liaoning (LN), Hebei (HeB), Shaanxi (ShX), Ningxia (NX), Henan (HN), Shanghai (ShH), Fujian (FJ), Jiangxi (JX), Guangxi (GX), Hubei (HuB), and Sichuan (SC). Three survey sites (two rural counties and one urban city) were randomly selected in each province as food sampling sites, and 30 households were sampled randomly from each site. 1080 households in total were covered in the survey. The food consumption pattern in each province was determined by a 3-day household dietary survey (including weighing and recording) and 24-h recalls. The average daily consumption of each food category by a standard Chinese adult man (aged 18–45, 63 kg body weight, light physical activity) was used as the standard food consumption pattern, and was calculated from the total household food consumption [22].

### Samples collection and analysis

Food samples were collected from local food markets, grocery stores and rural households in each survey site. All food items were aggregated into 12 groups, including cereals, beans, tubers, meat and poultry, eggs, aquatic products, milk and dairy products, vegetables, fruits, sugars, water and beverages, and alcohol. These samples were cooked and prepared according to the local habits, and then blended to form composites with weights proportional to the average daily consumption for the province [21]. The prepared food composites were shipped to the National Institute of Nutrition and Food Safety for analysis [21]. Total Se content in food composites was determined by the inductively coupled plasma mass spectrometry (Agilent 7500a ICP-MS) after microwave digestion of 0.3–0.5 g (solid) or 4–5 mL (liquid) in a mixture of 6 mL of concentrated $HNO_3$ and 2 mL of 30% $H_2O_2$. Reagent blank, standard reference materials, and parallel samples were determined simultaneously to maintain the reliability of analysis. Limit of detection for Se was defined as three-times of the standard deviation of baseline value [21].

### Calculation of dietary se intake based on the Chinese food pagoda ($EI_{CHFP}$)

The ranges of $EI_{CHFP}$ in China and 12 provinces were calculated according to the following equation [20]:

$$EI_{CHFP} = C \times m,$$

where C (μg/g) is the concentration of Se in each food group determined in the 4th China TDS, including 12 food groups in 12 provinces (as listed in Table 1); m (g/d) is the consumption of corresponding food groups recommended in the Dietary Guidelines and Food Pagoda for Chinese Residents (2016) (as shown in Fig. 1). The lower and upper limits of recommended consumption were used for calculating the lowest and highest $EI_{CHFP}$, respectively. In terms of Se contents in food groups, the lowest values in staple food like cereals, beans and tubers were found in Hubei, Liaoning and Heilongjiang province, which was broadly consistent with the distribution of low-Se belt in China [23]. It can thus be confirmed that food Se contents determined in the TDS are reliable.

**Table 1** Concentrations of Se in various food groups in China and 12 provinces (μg/g)[a]

| Food Group | HLJ | LN | HeB | ShX | HN | NX | ShH | FJ | JX | HuB | SC | GX | AVG |
|---|---|---|---|---|---|---|---|---|---|---|---|---|---|
| Cereals | 0.004 | 0.003 | 0.028 | 0.062 | 0.010 | 0.036 | 0.013 | 0.008 | 0.031 | 0.003 | 0.020 | 0.016 | 0.020 |
| Beans | 0.027 | 0.022 | 0.022 | 0.048 | 0.023 | 0.017 | 0.012 | 0.020 | 0.011 | 0.028 | 0.043 | 0.053 | 0.027 |
| Tubers | 0.027 | 0.024 | 0.023 | 0.063 | 0.015 | 0.058 | 0.006 | 0.011 | 0.008 | 0.002 | 0.017 | 0.048 | 0.025 |
| Meat | 0.111 | 0.157 | 0.121 | 0.166 | 0.238 | 0.173 | 0.219 | 0.124 | 0.210 | 0.186 | 0.205 | 0.276 | 0.182 |
| Eggs | 0.172 | 0.146 | 0.338 | 0.549 | 0.266 | 0.120 | 0.291 | 0.276 | 0.164 | 0.285 | 0.375 | 0.249 | 0.269 |
| Aquatic product | 0.135 | 0.708 | 0.591 | 0.366 | 0.456 | 0.121 | 0.462 | 0.367 | 0.468 | 0.231 | 0.422 | 0.597 | 0.410 |
| Dairy product | 0.072 | 0.022 | 0.022 | 0.018 | 0.023 | 0.038 | 0.028 | 0.015 | 0.155 | 0.202 | 0.019 | 0.048 | 0.055 |
| Vegetables | 0.035 | 0.012 | 0.065 | 0.146 | 0.110 | 0.042 | 0.079 | 0.079 | 0.020 | 0.068 | 0.041 | 0.089 | 0.066 |
| Fruits | 0.002 | 0.002 | 0.002 | 0.002 | 0.022 | 0.008 | 0.002 | 0.002 | 0.002 | 0.002 | 0.002 | 0.025 | 0.006 |
| Sugars | 0.032 | 0.002 | 0.118 | 0.011 | 0.002 | 0.047 | 0.002 | 0.023 | 0.002 | 0.002 | 0.002 | 0.101 | 0.029 |
| Water | 0.002 | 0.005 | 0.002 | 0.002 | 0.002 | 0.004 | 0.002 | 0.002 | 0.002 | 0.002 | 0.002 | 0.002 | 0.002 |
| Alcohol | 0.006 | 0.005 | 0.002 | 0.002 | 0.002 | 0.002 | 0.009 | 0.008 | 0.002 | 0.004 | 0.002 | 0.008 | 0.004 |

Abbreviations: *HLJ* Heilongjiang, *LN* Liaoning, *HeB* Hebei, *ShX* Shaanxi, *NX* Ningxia, *HN* Henan, *ShH* Shanghai, *FJ* Fujian, *JX* Jiangxi, *GX* Guangxi, *HuB* Hubei, *SC* Sichuan, *AVG* average

[a]All the data of Se contents in different food groups were from the 4th China TDS [21]

### Statistical analysis

Data processing and chart production were mainly performed with the Microsoft Office Excel 2013 and SPSS 23.0. Coefficients of variation (CV) were calculated for the average $EI_{TDS}$ and $EI_{CHFP}$ in each food group. *T* test was used when comparing the difference between the average $EI_{TDS}$ and $EI_{CHFP}$ in various food categories.

## Results

### $EI_{CHFP}$ in China and different regions

Based on the concentrations of food Se in Table 1 and the food consumptions recommended in the Food Pagoda, results of the $EI_{CHFP}$ were shown in Table 2. It was observed that the average $EI_{CHFP}$ in 12 provinces were all greater than the China recommended nutrient intake (RNI) of Se (60 μg/day). The lowest $EI_{CHFP}$ was also higher than the RNI in almost all regions with the exception of Heilongjiang and Ningxia province which might be related to the relatively low Se levels in their local food (Table 1). None of the highest $EI_{CHFP}$ went beyond the tolerable upper intake level of Se (400 μg/day) set by the Chinese Nutrition Society [24]. Owing to the variation of Se levels in the local food, the average $EI_{CHFP}$ varied greatly among regions, ranging from 66.23 to 145.20 μg/day. The highest average $EI_{CHFP}$ was observed in Shaanxi province where Se levels in staple food and vegetables were the highest; while the lowest was found in Heilongjiang province where Se contents in all kinds of food groups were relatively low. It could be seen from Fig. 2 that differences of the average $EI_{CHFP}$ among regions mainly lay in dairy products (CV = 1.05), cereals, beans and tubers (CV = 0.70), as well as vegetables and fruits (CV = 0.56). Animal source foods including meat, eggs, aquatic and dairy products made the highest contribution to daily Se intake in all regions according to the Food Pagoda eating patterns, ranging from 41.8 to 81.9%.

**Table 2** The average $EI_{CHFP}$ and its ranges in China and different provinces (μg/day)

| Regions | The average $EI_{CHFP}$ [a] | The lowest $EI_{CHFP}$ | The highest $EI_{CHFP}$ |
|---|---|---|---|
| HLJ | 66.23 | 55.21 | 77.25 |
| LN | 79.75 | 60.90 | 98.60 |
| HeB | 105.32 | 79.39 | 131.25 |
| ShX | 145.20 | 112.65 | 177.75 |
| HN | 116.59 | 89.04 | 144.15 |
| NX | 74.41 | 58.92 | 89.90 |
| ShH | 100.32 | 77.59 | 123.05 |
| FJ | 84.81 | 65.05 | 104.58 |
| JX | 113.46 | 96.47 | 130.45 |
| HuB | 130.41 | 113.89 | 146.93 |
| SC | 86.75 | 67.42 | 106.08 |
| GX | 133.94 | 101.41 | 166.48 |
| AVG | 102.63 | 81.01 | 124.25 |

Abbreviations: *HLJ* Heilongjiang, *LN* Liaoning, *HeB* Hebei, *ShX* Shaanxi, *NX* Ningxia, *HN* Henan, *ShH* Shanghai, *FJ* Fujian, *JX* Jiangxi, *GX* Guangxi, *HuB* Hubei, *SC* Sichuan, *AVG* average, $EI_{CHFP}$ estimated Se intake based on the Chinese Food Pagoda

[a] The average $EI_{CHFP}$ = (the lowest $EI_{CHFP}$ + the highest $EI_{CHFP}$)/2

### $EI_{TDS}$ in China and different regions

According to the survey data from the 4th China TDS, the $EI_{TDS}$ of daily dietary Se in various food groups in 12 provinces were presented in Fig. 3. Generally, the level of average $EI_{TDS}$ for Chinese adults (88 μg/day) was slightly higher than the China RNI of Se (60 μg/day). Large geographical variation of dietary Se intake was observed among regions in China. As shown in Fig. 3, the highest $EI_{TDS}$ was found in Shaanxi province (135.31 μg/day) at 2.3 times of RNI, followed by Shanghai (134.58 μg/day); while the lowest $EI_{TDS}$ was observed in Heilongjiang province (43.86 μg/day), followed by Liaoning (53.35 μg/day), which were the only two provinces below the RNI. The $EI_{TDS}$ in most of the provinces, such as Hebei, Henan, Jiangxi, Hubei, Sichuan and Guangxi, was within the range of 71.5–95.72 μg/day. Great variations of $EI_{TDS}$ in food groups among regions were observed in aquatic products (CV = 1.17), dairy products (CV = 1.07), and cereals, beans and tubers (CV = 0.82), making differences in the major contributors to dietary Se intake in 12 provinces. Animal source food was found making the highest contribution to dietary Se intake in more than half of the regions, including Heilongjiang, Liaoning, Shanghai, Fujian, Hubei, Sichuan, and Guangxi province ranging from 38.1 to 69.4%. Particularly, aquatic products corresponded to the highest contributors in Fujian (45.4%) and Liaoning (30.9%) province. By contrast, cereals and tubers contributed the most to daily dietary Se intake in Shaanxi, Hebei, Ningxia, and Jiangxi province within the range of 41.6–61.9%. Vegetables made a predominant contribution to daily Se intake in Henan and Hubei province, accounting for 41.2 and 41.7% of the total intake respectively. Despite all this, it can be observed that animal foods and cereals are still the major sources of daily dietary Se intake in most regions of China, which is similar to previous studies in China [25].

### Comparison of $EI_{TDS}$ with $EI_{CHFP}$

Results of the comparison between total $EI_{TDS}$ and $EI_{CHFP}$ were depicted in Fig. 4. In terms of the whole country, the average $EI_{TDS}$ (88 μg/day) just fell into the range of its $EI_{CHFP}$ (81.01–124.25 μg/day). This indicated that the daily dietary Se intake of Chinese population was overall in line with the recommendation proposed by the Chinese Food Pagoda. However, similar situation was only found in Hebei, Shaanxi, Ningxia, and Sichuan province. The majority of regions including Heilongjiang, Liaoning, Henan, Jiangxi, Hubei, and Guangxi

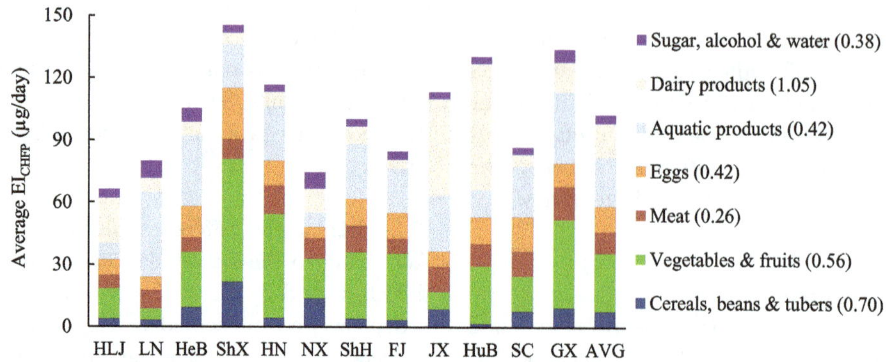


**Fig. 2** The average $EI_{CHFP}$ in different food groups in 12 provinces and China[a] Abbreviations: *HLJ* Heilongjiang, *LN* Liaoning, *HeB* Hebei, *ShX* Shaanxi, *NX* Ningxia, *HN* Henan, *ShH* Shanghai, *FJ* Fujian, *JX* Jiangxi, *GX* Guangxi, *HuB* Hubei, *SC* Sichuan, *AVG* average, *$EI_{CHFP}$* estimated Se intake based on the Chinese Food Pagoda.[a] Numbers in parentheses are coefficients of variation in each food group; the same as below

province had a lower $EI_{TDS}$ when compared with their corresponding lowest $EI_{CHFP}$. The gap between them ranged from 3.03 μg/day to 26.86 μg/day, with relatively bigger gaps in Hubei (26.86 μg/day) and Jiangxi (24.97 μg/day) province. By contrast, the $EI_{TDS}$ in Shanghai and Fujian province (134.58 and 111.31 μg/day) were even higher than their highest $EI_{CHFP}$ (123.05 and 104.58 μg/day). This comparison was just between the $EI_{TDS}$ and $EI_{CHFP}$ which were calculated under different food consumption patterns, regardless of the China RNI.

The $EI_{TDS}$ and their corresponding ranges of $EI_{CHFP}$ from each food category among different regions were calculated and integrated according to the five levels of food groups classified by the Food Pagoda. As listed in Table 3, $EI_{TDS}$ from the first level of the Food Pagoda (cereals, tubers and beans) in 12 provinces all exceeded their recommended ranges; while those from the fourth level (dairy products) were all far below their recommended amounts. This situation was more remarkable in Shaanxi, Hebei, Henan and Jiangxi province where the $EI_{TDS}$ from cereals, tubers and beans were more than 3 times of their highest $EI_{CHFP}$, while those from dairy products were substantially poor. Additionally, Se intake from the third level (meat, eggs and aquatic products) varied greatly among regions, where only Heilongjiang and Hubei province had appropriate Se intake from this level. Those in Shanghai and Fujian province were much higher than their upper limits of $EI_{CHFP}$, which might account for their higher $EI_{TDS}$ in Fig. 4. Almost all provinces had adequate Se intake from the second level of the Food Pagoda (vegetables and fruits) with the exception of Shaanxi, Henan and Guangxi province being slightly lower than their recommendations.

## Discussion

Compared with other countries in the world, the dietary Se intake of Chinese population (88 μg/day) was relatively moderate. It was higher than numerous countries throughout Europe (including the UK) and the Middle East where the reported daily Se intake were less than 55 μg/day [26], but lower than those from certain developed countries, such as the US where 133.5 μg/day of average Se intake for men was reported [27]. However, great geographical variations of Se intake still existed in China. There are many possible factors that can have an effect on Se intake and result in these variations. These

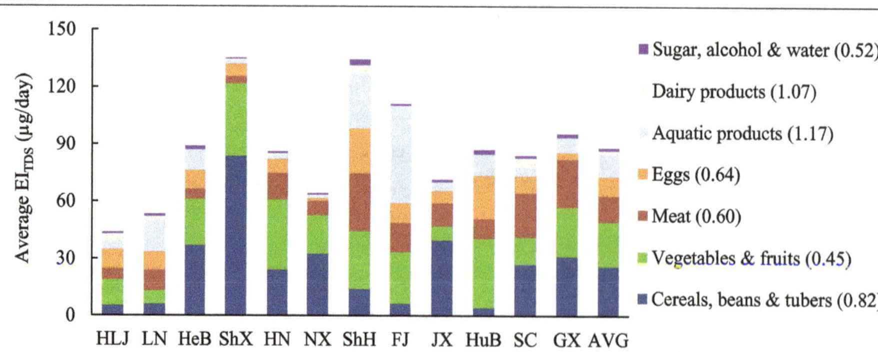


**Fig. 3** The average $EI_{TDS}$ in different food groups in 12 provinces and ChinaAbbreviations: *HLJ* Heilongjiang, *LN* Liaoning, *HeB* Hebei, *ShX* Shaanxi, *NX* Ningxia, *HN* Henan, *ShH* Shanghai, *FJ* Fujian, *JX* Jiangxi, *GX* Guangxi, *HuB* Hubei, *SC* Sichuan, *AVG* average, *$EI_{TDS}$* estimated Se intake based on the China Total Diet Study.

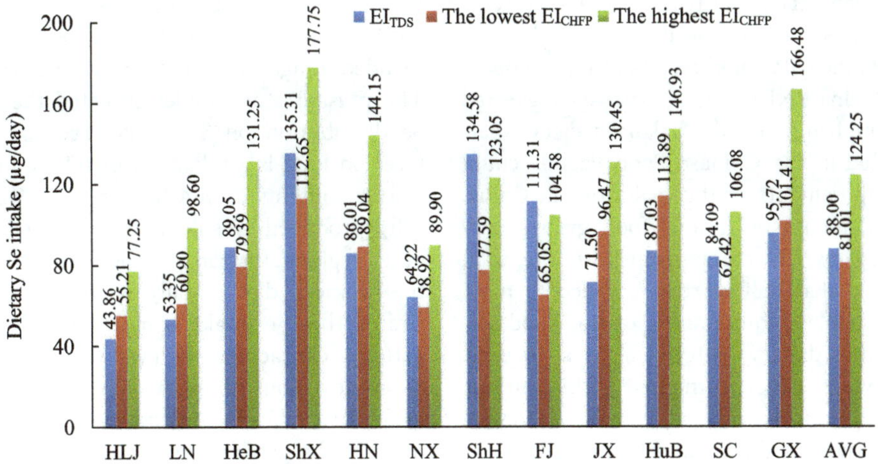


**Fig. 4** Comparison of daily dietary Se between $EI_{TDS}$ and $EI_{CHFP}$ in 12 provinces in ChinaAbbreviations: *HLJ* Heilongjiang, *LN* Liaoning, *HeB* Hebei, *ShX* Shaanxi, *NX* Ningxia, *HN* Henan, *ShH* Shanghai, *FJ* Fujian, *JX* Jiangxi, *GX* Guangxi, *HuB* Hubei, *SC* Sichuan, *AVG* average, $EI_{TDS}$ estimated Se intake based on the China Total Diet Study, $EI_{CHFP}$ estimated Se intake based on the Chinese Food Pagoda.

factors primarily include disparities in dietary patterns, consumption habits, food culture, economic levels, and also Se contents in food among different regions [18, 28, 29]. It is difficult to distinguish which factor plays a predominant role in dietary Se intake since the situation varies from regions to regions. For example, cereals and tubers made the highest contribution to daily dietary Se intake in Shaanxi, Hebei, Ningxia, and Jiangxi province, accounting for 41.6–61.9%; while 45.4 and 30.9% of daily Se intake were from aquatic products in Fujian and Liaoning province, making the highest contributors. The former is presumably ascribed to the relatively high Se levels in local crops (Table 1), as well as the food culture where tend to have large consumptions of flour or rice [21]; the latter, however, may be attributed to the consumption habits developed by their water-adjacent living environment. Correlations between Se contents and $EI_{TDS}$ in each food group also showed that highly significant correlations were only observed in foods with large consumptions, including cereals ($r = 0.936$, $P < 0.01$), tubers ($r = 0.787$, $P < 0.01$), vegetables ($r = 0.895$, $P < 0.01$) and fruits ($r = 0.769$, $P < 0.01$). Foods with relatively high Se contents but small consumptions, such as seafood, eggs, and meats, presented poor correlations with Se intake ($P > 0.05$). In this study, the influence of dietary patterns on Se intake was discussed separately by quantitative

**Table 3** $EI_{TDS}$ and $EI_{CHFP}$ in different food categories in 12 provinces of China (μg/day)[a]

| Food category | Cereals, tubers and beans | | Vegetables & Fruits | | Meat, eggs and aquatic products | | Dairy products | |
|---|---|---|---|---|---|---|---|---|
| | $EI_{TDS}$ | $EI_{CHFP}$ ranges | $EI_{TDS}$ | $EI_{CHFP}$ ranges | $EI_{TDS}$ | $EI_{CHFP}$ ranges | $EI_{TDS}$ | $EI_{CHFP}$ |
| HLJ | 5.55 | 2.83–5.25 | 13.50 | 10.90–18.20 | 19.96 | 16.72–27.05 | 4.09 | 21.60 |
| LN | 6.16 | 2.35–4.40 | 6.98 | 4.00–6.70 | 37.01 | 40.44–72.18 | 2.04 | 6.60 |
| HeB | 37.02 | 7.30–11.80 | 24.17 | 19.90–33.20 | 25.37 | 42.00–70.30 | 0.57 | 6.60 |
| ShX | 83.70 | 16.75–27.30 | 38.19 | 44.20–73.70 | 11.99 | 43.24–67.35 | 0.86 | 5.40 |
| HN | 24.41 | 3.33–5.65 | 36.72 | 37.40–62.70 | 23.30 | 38.40–65.35 | 0.73 | 6.90 |
| NX | 32.66 | 10.53–17.45 | 20.10 | 14.20–23.80 | 10.19 | 16.56–28.05 | 0.58 | 11.40 |
| ShH | 14.01 | 3.20–5.10 | 30.54 | 24.10–40.20 | 82.92 | 38.88–65.63 | 4.05 | 8.40 |
| FJ | 6.57 | 2.65–4.50 | 27.05 | 24.10–40.20 | 76.30 | 30.68–50.63 | 0.48 | 4.50 |
| JX | 39.61 | 6.88–10.65 | 7.48 | 6.40–10.70 | 23.16 | 33.68–59.05 | 0.05 | 46.50 |
| HuB | 4.31 | 1.40–2.50 | 36.43 | 20.80–34.70 | 43.99 | 28.08–45.53 | 0.22 | 60.60 |
| SC | 27.19 | 5.93–9.85 | 14.21 | 12.70–21.20 | 36.68 | 40.08–65.78 | 4.79 | 5.70 |
| GX | 31.35 | 6.93–12.25 | 25.77 | 31.70–53.25 | 36.48 | 44.88–77.93 | 0.22 | 14.40 |
| AVG | 26.05 | 5.93–9.85 | 23.43 | 21.00–35.10 | 35.61 | 34.44–57.85 | 1.56 | 16.50 |

Abbreviations: *HLJ* Heilongjiang, *LN* Liaoning, *HeB* Hebei, *ShX* Shaanxi, *NX* Ningxia, *HN* Henan, *ShH* Shanghai, *FJ* Fujian, *JX* Jiangxi, *GX* Guangxi, *HuB* Hubei, *SC* Sichuan, *AVG* average, $EI_{TDS}$ estimated Se intake based on the China Total Diet Study, $EI_{CHFP}$ estimated Se intake based on the Chinese Food Pagoda
[a]The data of $EI_{TDS}$ in different food categories were from the 4th China TDS [21]

comparison between $EI_{TDS}$ and $EI_{CHFP}$ which were calculated using the same food Se contents [21].

In the first place, the calculated results of $EI_{CHFP}$ being greater than the China RNI (Table 2) has well suggested that Se intake complying with the balanced dietary patterns recommended in the Chinese Food Pagoda could meet the daily requirements of the majorities in China, even though Se contents in various food groups vary greatly among regions. By comparison with the total $EI_{TDS}$, it was found that half of regions failed to meet the minimum Se intake requirements of the Food Pagoda, indicating that dietary patterns in these regions may exist irrationality. When compared within various food categories, it was noteworthy that significant differences between the average $EI_{CHFP}$ and $EI_{TDS}$ were found in cereals, tubers and beans ($t = -2.975$, $P = 0.007$), aquatic products ($t = 2.468$, $P = 0.021$) and dairy products ($t = 3.089$, $P = 0.005$). According to the average $EI_{CHFP}$ in the whole country, there should be 7.7% of Se intake contributed from staple food, 23.0 and 16.1% contributed from aquatic and dairy products. Clearly, the current Se intake from staple food has been sufficient, accounting for 29.6% of the average $EI_{TDS}$ in China; while that from aquatic and dairy products is largely deficient across the country, only accounting for 13.5 and 1.8% of the average $EI_{TDS}$ in China. In fact, Chinese population consumed very limited milk and dairy products every day, with an average of 28.4 g/day per capita according to the food consumption data in the 4th China TDS [21], far below 300 g/day per capita recommended in the Pagoda. The consumption of aquatic products (29.0 g/day per capita) was also less than the lower limit of the recommended amount (40 g/day per capita) [16, 21]. However, compared with other animal source foods, milk and dairy products are not very good sources for Se. The average Se content in dairy products was only 0.055 μg/g, far less than that in aquatic products (0.410 μg/g) [21]. Therefore, from the view of the balanced dietary pattern and Se sources, Se nutrition for the general population can be further improved by properly increasing the consumption of seafood and its by-products.

It is well known that human Se intake is closely associated with Se levels in foodstuffs and dietary pattern. The former is strongly dependent on the Se in soil which varies significantly across different regions of world [30]; the latter, however, can be changed with the increase of food supply and diversity as well as dietary habits. In the present study, for instance, in Heilongjiang and Liaoning province where $EI_{TDS}$ has not reached the China RNI, their Se intake can be further improved by slightly adjusting eating patterns on the basis of Food Pagoda, such as consuming more fish, milk and dairy products, and so on. Even in some regions where Se intake has achieved the RNI, it can still be supplemented by adjusting the consumption of Se-rich foods within the recommended ranges to obtain Se-associated health benefit. The present study underestimated the influence of soil Se distribution on Se intake, because even though Se levels in food is a reflection of soil Se in most instances, soil Se contents do not help in cases where the food locally produced is sold and consumed by residents in other regions. Instead, by calculating the contribution of the balanced diet to daily Se intake, this study demonstrated that Se intake complying with balanced dietary patterns can achieve or even exceed the China RNI in different regions no matter how greatly their Se contents in food vary. Thus, it is believed that the daily requirement of the general population for Se can be satisfied if the Chinese Dietary Guidelines and the Food Guide Pagoda are strictly obeyed.

## Conclusions

Attempts can be made to improve the general Se intake levels by adjusting eating patterns. The present study made it clear that the balanced dietary pattern based on the Chinese Dietary Guidelines and Food Pagoda could meet daily requirements of the majorities for Se in China under the current Se levels in food. However, the comparison between $EI_{TDS}$ and $EI_{CHFP}$ showed that Se intake in half of the regions could not achieve their lowest $EI_{CHFP}$. The differences between them among regions mainly lay in cereal food, aquatic and dairy products. Se intake from staple food for Chinese population may have been sufficient, and more Se nutrition can be taken from aquatic products in terms of a well-balanced diet.

#### Abbreviations

AVG: average; CV: coefficient of variation; $EI_{CHFP}$: Estimated Se intake based on the Chinese Food Pagoda; $EI_{TDS}$: Estimated Se intake based on the China Total Diet Study; FJ: Fujian; GX: Guangxi; HB: Hebei; HLJ: Heilongjiang; HN: Henan; HuB: Hubei; ICP-MS: inductively coupled plasma mass spectrometry; JX: Jiangxi; LN: Liaoning; NX: Ningxia; RNI: Recommended nutrient intake; SC: Sichuan; ShH: Shanghai; ShX: Shaanxi; TDS: Total diet study

#### Funding

This work was financially supported by the National Natural Science Foundation of China (41671500).

#### Authors' contributions

LSY designed the structure of this study; HRL helped to collect the data and contributed to revising the manuscript; JW analyzed the data and wrote the first draft. YHL and BGW had responsibility for final content. All authors read and approved the final manuscript.

### Competing interests

The authors declare that they have no competing interests regarding this study.


### Author details

[1]Key Laboratory of Land Surface Pattern and Simulation, Institute of Geographical Sciences and Natural Resources Research, Chinese Academy of Sciences, 11 A Datun Road, Beijing 100101, People's Republic of China. [2]College of Resources and Environment, University of Chinese Academy of Sciences, Beijing 100049, People's Republic of China.


### References


1. Rayman MP. Selenium and human health. Lancet. 2012;379:1256–68.
2. Kryukov GV, Castellano S, Novoselov SV, Lobanov AV, Zehtab O, Guigó R, et al. Characterization of mammalian selenoproteomes. Science. 2003;300: 1439–43.
3. Fairweather-Tait SJ, Bao YP, Broadley MR, Collings R, Ford D, Hesketh JE, et al. Selenium in human health and disease. Antioxid Redox Sign. 2011;14: 1337–83.
4. Méplan C, Hesketh J. Selenium and cancer: a story that should not be forgotten-insights from genomics. Cancer Treat Res. 2014;159:145–66.
5. Guo X, Ma WJ, Zhang F, Ren FL, Qu CJ, Lammi MJ. Recent advances in the research of an endemic osteochondropathy in China: Kashin-Beck disease. Osteoarthr Cartilage. 2014;22:1774–83.
6. Harthill M. Review: micronutrient selenium deficiency influences evolution of some viral infectious diseases. Biol Trace Elem Res. 2011;143:1325–36.
7. Wang XL, Yang TB, Wei J, Lei GH, Zeng C. Association between serum selenium level and type 2 diabetes mellitus: a non-linear dose-response meta-analysis of observational studies. Nutr J. 2016;15:48.
8. Manzanares W, Hardy G. Can dietary selenium intake increase the risk of toxicity in healthy children? Nutrition. 2016;32:149–50.
9. Reis ARD, El-Ramady H, Santos EF, Gratão PL, Schomburg L. Overview of selenium deficiency and toxicity worldwide: affected areas, selenium-related health issues, and case studies. In: Pilon-Smits E, Winkel L, Lin ZQ (eds) selenium in plants. Plant Ecophysiology 2017. 11:209–30.
10. Tan LC, Nancharaiah YV, van Hullebusch ED, Lens PNL. Selenium: environmental significance, pollution, and biological treatment technologies. Biotechnol Adv. 2016;34:886–907.
11. Xu ZC, Shao HF, Li S, Zheng C. Relationships between the selenium content in flue-cured tobacco leaves and the selenium content in soil in Enshi, China tobacco-growing area. Pak J Bot. 2012;44:1563–8.
12. Dinh QT, Cui ZW, Huang J, Tran TAT, Wang D, Yang WX, et al. Selenium distribution in the Chinese environment and its relationship with human health: a review. Environ Int. 2018;112:294–309.
13. Yu GH, Wen YM, He SY, Zhang L, Dong HY. Food selenium content and resident daily selenium intake in Guangzhou City. Chin J Appl Ecol. 2007;18: 2600–4.
14. Santos MD, Júnior FMRDS, Muccillo-Baisch AL. Selenium content of Brazilian foods: a review of the literature values. J Food Compos Anal. 2017;58:10–5.
15. Choi Y, Kim J, Lee HS, Kim C, Hwang IK, Park HK, et al. Selenium content in representative Korean foods. J Food Compos Anal. 2009;22:117–22.
16. The Chinese Nutrition Society. The Food Guide Pagoda for Chinese Residents. 2016. http://dg.cnsoc.org/upload/images/source/20160519163856103.jpg. Accessed 20 June 2016.
17. Wang SS, Lay S, Yu HN, Shen SR. Dietary guidelines for Chinese residents (2016): comments and comparisons. J Zhejiang Univ-Sci B (Biomed & Biotechnol). 2016;17:649–56.
18. Zhang ZW, Shimbo S, Qu JB, Watanabe I, Nakatsuka H, Matsuda-Inoguchi N, et al. Dietary selenium intake of Chinese adult women in the 1990s. Biol Trace Elem Res. 2001;80:125–38.
19. Ge KY. The transition of Chinese dietary guidelines and the food guide pagoda. Asia Pac J Clin Nutr. 2011;20:439–46.
20. Zhang L, Li JG, Liu X, Zhao YF, Li XW, Wen S. Dietary intake of PCDD/fs and dioxin-like PCBs from the Chinese total diet study in 2007. Chemosphere. 2013;90:1625–30.
21. Wu YN, Li XW. The fourth China Total diet study. 1st ed. Beijing: Chemical Industry Press; 2015.
22. Zhou PP, Zhao YF, Li JG, Wu GH, Zhang L, Liu Q, et al. Dietary exposure to persistent organochlorine pesticides in 2007 Chinese total diet study. Environ Int. 2012;42:152–9.
23. Tan JA, Zhu WY, Wang WY, Li RB, Hou SF, Wang DC, et al. Selenium in soil and endemic diseases in China. Sci Total Environ. 2002;284:227–35.
24. Cheng YY. A brief introduction to the 2013 revised "Chinese dietary reference intakes (DRIs)". Acta Nutrimenta Sinica. 2014;36:313–7.
25. Gao J, Liu Y, Huang Y, Lin ZQ, Bañuelos GS, Lam MHW, et al. Daily selenium intake in a moderate selenium deficiency area of Suzhou, China. Food Chem. 2011;126:1088–93.
26. Stoffaneller R, Morse NL. A review of dietary selenium intake and selenium status in Europe and the Middle East. Nutrients. 2015;7:1494–537.
27. Chun OK, Floegel A, Chung SJ, Chung CE, Song WO, Koo SI. Estimation of antioxidant intakes from diet and supplements in U.S. adults. J Nutr. 2010; 140:317–24.
28. Wang ZH, Zhai FY, He Y, Wang HJ, Yu WT, Yu DM. Influence of family income on dietary nutrients intake and dietary structure in China. Journal of Hygiene Research. 2008;37:62–4.
29. Li SM, Banuelos GS, Wu LH, Shi WM. The changing selenium nutritional status of Chinese residents. Nutrients. 2014;6:1103–14.
30. Chen LC, Yang FM, Xu J, Hu Y, Hu QH, Zhang YL, et al. Determination of selenium concentration of rice in China and effect of fertilization of selenite and selenate on selenium content of rice. J Agric Food Chem. 2002;50: 5128–30.

# 3

# Development of a dietary index based on the Brazilian Cardioprotective Nutritional Program (BALANCE)

Jacqueline Tereza da Silva[1,2*], Ângela Cristine Bersch-Ferreira[1,2], Camila Ragne Torreglosa[1,2], Bernardete Weber[2] and Renata Bertazzi Levy[1,3]

## Abstract

**Background:** The diet of the Brazilian Cardioprotective Nutritional Program (BALANCE) classifies food into four groups and sets the daily amount to be consumed. The dietary approach of BALANCE is different from other dietary recommendations; therefore, it is not possible to use existing dietary indexes (DI) to assess patient's adequacy to BALANCE diet. For this reason, it is important to develop a specific dietary index based on BALANCE diet. This study aims to describe the development of the BALANCE DI, evaluate its internal consistency, construct and content validity and population characteristics associated with the index.

**Methods:** We analyzed baseline data from the BALANCE randomized clinical trial (https://www.clinicaltrials.gov/; NCT01620398). The four food groups of the diet were adopted as index components. Points ranging from 0 to 10 were given to each index component. Internal consistency was evaluated by correlation coefficients between total score and component scores, as well as Cronbach's Alpha. Content and construct validity were assessed by checking how nutrients are associated with the index and if the index could distinguish between groups with known differences in diet, respectively. Crude and adjusted linear regression analyses were performed to evaluate population characteristics associated with the index.

**Results:** The analysis included 2044 subjects (58.6% men). The average of the total index was higher among women ($p < 0{,}05$). The components of the index showed low correlations with each other. The correlations between each individual component with the total index were > 0.40. Cronbach's alpha coefficient was 0.66. High scores in the index were inversely associated ($p < 0{,}05$) with energy, total fat, monounsaturated fat (MUFA) and cholesterol; they were positively associated ($p < 0{,}05$) with carbohydrates and fiber. Hypertensive men and diabetic women had higher scores, while male smokers had lower scores.

**Conclusions:** The BALANCE DI showed reliability and construct validity similar to other DI. It also detected characteristics of individuals that are associated with higher or lower index scores.

**Keywords:** Dietary assessment, Nutritional index, dietary patterns, Reliability and validity, Cardiovascular disease

* Correspondence: jacsnt@yahoo.com.br
[1]Department of Nutrition, School of Public Health, University of São Paulo, Avenida Doutor Arnaldo, 715, São Paulo, SP 01246904, Brazil
[2]Research Institute, Hospital do Coração (HCor), Rua Abílio Sorares, 250, 12° andar, São Paulo, SP 04005-000, Brazil
Full list of author information is available at the end of the article

## Background

Dietary habits are important modifiable risk factors for cardiovascular diseases (CVD), the first cause of death and burden of disease worldwide and in Brazil [1, 2]. The World Health Organization (WHO) emphasizes that a healthy diet, able to prevent CVD, is influenced by many complex interactions (income, food availability and affordability, individual preferences and beliefs, cultural traditions, geographical, environmental, social and economic factors) [3]. To take these complex interactions into account, the choice of foods that compose a healthy and cardioprotective diet should be regionalized.

Brazil has a variety of food rich in cardioprotective components such as fiber, vitamins and bioactive compounds that could be used to promote cardiovascular protection and minimize the burden of CVD. The Brazilian Cardioprotective Nutritional Program (BALANCE) is an educational intervention aimed at improving the consumption of foods available in the country with a potential cardioprotective role. The Brazilian Ministry of Health has been assessing the effectiveness of the BALANCE program in a multicentric and randomized clinical trial since 2013 [4].

The dietary component of the BALANCE program ranked foods in groups represented by the colours of the Brazilian flag. As green is the most abundant colour in the flag, the items included in the green group should be eaten more often. Yellow is the second most abundant flag colour, thus the advice is to eat foods in the yellow group in moderation. Blue represents foods that should be consumed in smaller quantities. Ultra-processed foods are not recommended in the BALANCE diet and are represented by red, which is not in the Brazilian flag. Details about the food classification criteria have been published elsewhere [4].

Several dietary indexes (DI) have been developed to study associations between dietary patterns and CVD in different populations [5–10]. A DI combines the many aspects of a nutritional recommendation or guideline and uses them as the items of the index. These aspects are generally the amount of nutrients, foods or food groups to be eaten in each period of time (day/week/month). Since the dietary aspects of the BALANCE program are different from other cardioprotective dietary patterns, it is not possible to use existing DI to assess the role of the BALANCE diet on cardiovascular protection. We therefore aim to describe the development of the BALANCE DI, to assess its internal consistency, construct and content validity, and to evaluate the population characteristics associated with the index.

## Methods

### Study population

To develop the DI we used data from the BALANCE study (https://www.clinicaltrials.gov/; NCT01620398), a multicentric randomized clinical trial. The trial aims to assess the effects of the Brazilian Cardioprotective Nutritional Program in the secondary prevention of cardiovascular diseases. Between March 2013 and January 2015, 2535 adults over 44-years-old and with a personal history of cardiovascular disease were enrolled in the trial and followed-up until December 2017 in one of the 35 sites in Brazil. Details of the trial procedures are given elsewhere [4]. The 2044 individuals who had full dietary data at baseline were included in the present analysis, which was approved by the School of Public Health/University of São Paulo Research Ethics Committee.

### Data collection and description of variables

Data were collected in the 35 sites by trained researchers following standardized procedures. Details of the data collection are given in the BALANCE research protocol, available on request from the authors [4].

Dietary intake was assessed from a single 24-h recall collected by trained interviewers who asked for a detailed description of all foods and drinks consumed the day before the interview, following an adaptation of the Multiple-Pass Method steps [11]. A photographic album of food portion sizes was available to help with the estimation of quantities of food consumed [12]. The food intake data was recorded in Nutriquanti Software using household measures and then converted to grams. The software calculated the energy and nutrient amount using information from different food composition tables, including the Brazilian Food Composition Table and the USDA Food Composition Table. All the 24-h recalls that ranged over less than 1000 kcal or more than 3000 kcal were double-checked. Discrepant home measures, such as "zero tablespoon" and "150 teacups" were also double-checked. Records with less than the 1st or greater than the 99th percentile of energy were excluded [13]. The relative participation of macronutrients in the diet was expressed as the percentage of total energy intake. Cholesterol, sodium and fiber were presented as milligrams or grams per each 1000 kcal ingested.

Height was measured twice with wall-mounted stadiometers (0.5 cm precision) with the subject barefoot in a standing position. Weight was collected twice with calibrated scales (100 g precision) with the subject barefoot and wearing light clothes. Waist circumference (WC) was measured twice with an anthropometric tape in the midpoint between the lowest rib and the iliac crest. The average of the measurements was used. If the measurements differed more than 0.5 kg for weight, 0.5 cm for height and 1 cm for WC, the entire procedure was repeated until the difference between the two new measures was lower than the established cut-off. Body mass index (BMI) was calculated as weight divided by the square of height (kg/m$^2$) and classified according to age.

If age ≤ 59 years-old, underweight = BMI < 18.5 kg/m$^2$, normal weight = BMI ≥ 18.5 kg/m$^2$ and < 25 kg/m$^2$, overweight = BMI ≥ 25 kg/m$^2$ [14]. If age ≥ 60 years-old, underweight = BMI < 23 kg/m$^2$, normal weight = BMI ≥ 23 kg/m$^2$ and < 28 kg/m$^2$, overweight = BMI ≥ 28 kg/m$^2$ [14, 15].

A questionnaire was applied to investigate the personal history of CVD and smoking status. Diagnoses of diabetes, hypertension and dyslipidemia were self-reported.

### The dietary component of the BALANCE program

The dietary component of the BALANCE program [4] is designed to meet the nutritional recommendations proposed by the Brazilian Cardiovascular Guidelines [16–20]. To implement these recommendations on nutritional advice, we compiled a list of cardioprotective foods, based on a set of qualitative criteria defined by nutrition experts considering the most relevant aspects of Brazilian nutritional guidelines: a) no added sugar; b) low-calorie content; c) lack of nutrients that increase cardiovascular risk (cholesterol, saturated fat, and sodium); and d) presence of cardioprotective nutrients (antioxidants and dietary fiber). The result of the compilation was a list consisting of low-fat yoghurt and milk, fruits and vegetables, and beans cooked with garlic, onion, soybean oil (up to 1%) and refined salt (up to 0.5%).

Energy, saturated fat, cholesterol and sodium densities [21] of foods in the list were evaluated to create cutoff values for food classification into the green, yellow and blue groups. The maximum density values of the list were 1.11 kcal per gram, 0.01 g of saturated fatty acid per gram, 0.04 mg of cholesterol per gram, and 2.01 mg of sodium per gram. These values were applied in the food categorization as follows: foods with all 4 density values equal to or less than the cutoffs were assigned to the green group (vegetables, fruits, beans, low-fat milk and yoghurt); foods with one or two densities above the cutoffs were assigned to the yellow group (rice, bread, pasta, oats, couscous, nuts, vegetable oil); foods with three or four nutrient densities above the cutoffs were categorized into the blue group (meat, fish, cheese, eggs).

Finally, the BALANCE diet contains a red group. The cutoffs were not adopted as criteria for assigning foods in this group. Instead, foods lacking beneficial components such as vitamins, antioxidants and dietary fiber and known as sources of trans fats, refined sugar, artificial sweeteners, and preservatives – mainly ultra-processed foods - compose the red group.

### The BALANCE dietary index

We created the BALANCE DI considering the aspects of the existing DI that are used to analyze associations between dietary patterns and cardiovascular disease [7, 22–25]. The BALANCE Program recommends a number of servings in each food group depending on the energy level, as shown in Table 1. Energy need was calculated multiplying current body weight by 20 kcal in overweight or 25 kcal in normal weight or 32 kcal in underweight participants [17, 26]. Individuals with calculated need below 1400 kcal were set to 1400 kcal, those above 2400 kcal were set to 2400 kcal. Intermediate values were assessed accordingly to mathematical approximation rules. For example, if the calculated need is 1758 kcal, the nutritionist must assign into the 1800 kcal, the closest value.

The index has four components corresponding to the BALANCE food groups. The scoring criteria are summarized in Table 2 and were made a priori, based on the BALANCE principles and recommendations and the population distribution of consumed servings. Each component was given a score ranging from 0 (worst) to 10 (best), therefore the total score ranges from 0 to 40.

A score of zero is given to the green group when there is no consumption and a score of 10 when the consumption is equal or higher than the recommendation. A score of 10 is assigned to the yellow group when the number of servings is exactly that recommended. The minimum score is assigned to the yellow group when the number of servings is 50% over or below the recommendation. The blue and red groups received a reverse score (higher intakes are given lower scores). In the blue group, the maximum score is assigned to the number of servings equal to or lower than the recommendation

**Table 1** BALANCE recommendation of servings per day in each food group according to the energy-level[a]

| BALANCE food groups | Number of servings per day | | | | | |
|---|---|---|---|---|---|---|
| | 1400 Kcal | 1600 Kcal | 1800 Kcal | 2000 Kcal | 2200 Kcal | 2400 Kcal |
| Green (vegetables, fruits, beans and legumes, low-fat milk) | 9 | 11 | 11 | 12 | 14 | 16 |
| Yellow (rice, bread, pasta, oats, couscous, nuts, vegetable oil) | 6 | 7 | 9 | 10 | 11 | 13 |
| Blue (meat, fish, cheese, eggs) | 2 | 2 | 3 | 3 | 4 | 4 |
| Red (ultra-processed foods) | 0 | 0 | 0 | 0 | 0 | 0 |

BALANCE = Brazilian Cardioprotective Nutritional Program
[a]This content was published in the BALANCE research protocol, is reproduced with permission and available on request from the authors [14]

**Table 2** Scoring criteria for the BALANCE dietary index, mean score (95% confidence interval) among men and women with a history of cardiovascular disease

| Index component (BALANCE food group) | Criteria for 0 point* | Criteria for 10 point* | Score for men | Score for women |
|---|---|---|---|---|
| Green (vegetables, fruits, beans and legumes, low-fat milk) | 0 | ≥ the recommendation | 4.49 (4.34; 4.65) | 4.55 (4.36; 4.73) |
| Yellow (rice, bread, pasta, oats, couscous, nuts, vegetable oil) | 50% > or < the recommendation | = the recommendation | 3.50 (3.30; 3.69) | 3.52 (3.29; 3.74) |
| Blue (meat, fish, cheese, eggs)** | ≥ 2 beyond the recommended | ≤ the recommendation | 5.20 (4.95; 5.46) | 6.09 (5.80;6.38) |
| Red (ultra-processed foods)** | ≥ 4 | ≤ 0 | 5.37 (5.14; 5.61) | 5.90 (5.64; 6.16) |
| Total score (range)** | 0 | 40 | 18.56 (18.11; 19.02) | 20.05 (19.54; 20.56) |

BALANCE = Brazilian Cardioprotective Nutritional Program
*Servings/d between the minimum and maximum criteria were given the scores proportionally
**Statistical differences between means $p < 0.05$ (Mann-Whitney test)

and the minimum when there are at least two servings above the recommendation. Finally, in the red group, a score of 10 is assigned when there is no consumption, and a score of 0 is given to 4 or more reported servings. Those participants consuming intermediate amounts were scored proportionally.

To calculate the score, we classified all food items reported in the 24-h recalls into the BALANCE food groups and defined the size of a serving. Then, we calculated the number of servings consumed and the corresponding score for each component. Finally, we summarized the component values to obtain the total score.

Because the BALANCE DI was developed to assess the consistency with the BALANCE Program dietary component, we decided to follow the rationale of the Program and use the BALANCE food groups as the items of the score. The foods in the green group have low energy, saturated fat, cholesterol and sodium density and higher levels of cardioprotective compounds [4]. Furthermore, the consumption of these foods is low in the Brazilian population [27] and we aim to improve the intake of such foods. For this reason, we did not assign a penalty for overconsumption and used a monotonic function to score this component (higher levels of intake received higher scores).

As the yellow group is the major provider of energy intake, we believe the consumption should be neither higher nor lower than the recommendation, to maintain the energy balance. Hence, the scoring system has two directions with intakes under or above the recommendation being penalized.

The blue group is mainly responsible for the saturated fat, cholesterol and sodium intake and received a reverse score (higher intakes get lower scores). The red group is not recommended in the BALANCE diet and therefore also gets a reverse score. For these items in the index there is no clear scientific evidence determining what amount of intake should receive the minimum score of zero. To improve discriminatory power and the ability to detect differences in the population, we determined, as the cutoff, an approximate value of the 75th percentile of the population intake distribution. A similar strategy has been adopted in previous studies [28].

### Statistical analysis

The scores of the overall index and its components were described in mean and 95% confidence interval (95% CI) for males and females and differences were assessed by Mann-Whitney tests. Subsequent analyses were performed separately by sex because the scores differed among men and women.

To evaluate the internal consistency of the index we analyzed the inter-item correlation matrix, and calculated the Spearman rank correlation coefficients between the components and total index. We also estimated the Cronbach's coefficient alpha. Values higher than 0.70 indicated reliability (internal consistency).

To assess construct validity, we checked if the index could distinguish between groups with known differences in diet (men and women). To assess the content validity, we verified if the index was associated with key nutrients in an expected direction, dividing it into quartiles and calculating the mean and 95% CI of energy and selected nutrient intakes in each quartile. The fourth quartile indicated the highest adequacy with the BALANCE, whereas the first quartile indicated the lowest adequacy with the diet. Tests for linear trends were performed to compare the population intakes across the quartiles.

The population characteristics associated with the index were assessed by linear regression, crude and adjusted for age, BMI, waist circumference, hypertension, dyslipidemia, diabetes and smoking status. All the analyses were conducted in STATA software, version 12, and statistical significance was defined as $p < 0.05$.

## Results

The analysis included 2044 subjects with a mean (standard deviation) age of 63 [9] years. Among males (58.6% of the population), 88.3% were hypertensive, 78.5% dyslipidemic, 41.9% diabetic, 63.3% former smoker and 7.4% current smoker and the mean (SD) of BMI and WC was, respectively, 28.5 (4.4) Kg/m$^2$ and 101.1 (11.3) cm. Among females, 93.2% were hypertensive, 79.0% dyslipidemic, 45. 7% diabetic, 41.6% former smoker and 8.0% current smoker and the mean (SD) of BMI and WC was, respectively, 29.8 (5.5) Kg/m$^2$ and 97.9 (12.9) cm.

Table 2 describes the criteria for minimum and maximum score in each component of the BALANCE DI and shows the mean (95% CI) for the components and total score among men and women. The results differed between sexes, with females having higher scores in the total index, and in the blue and red components (Table 2). The findings for the green and yellow groups were similar in both sexes.

The correlations among BALANCE DI components and total index are shown in Table 3. The components of the index had low correlations among themselves ($r < 0.10$). The blue and red groups showed similar correlations with the total index ($r = 0.61$ and $r = 0.62$, respectively) and were more correlated with the total index than the other components, indicating that their variance contributes more to the total score. Nevertheless, the green and yellow groups do add important information to the total score as they show correlations higher than 0.40. The Cronbach's coefficient alpha of the BALANCE dietary index was 0.66.

Table 4 presents the mean (95% CI) of energy and selected nutrient intakes across quartiles of the BALANCE index among men and women. Higher scores were inversely associated with intakes of energy, total fat, MUFA and cholesterol and positively associated with intakes of carbohydrate and fiber. Among males, there was no difference in the consumption of proteins across the quartiles of the score and among females, the intake of protein was higher in the 4th quartile. No difference was observed in the intake of polyunsaturated fat and sodium.

Table 5 presents population characteristics associated with the index. In general, males with hypertension and females with diabetes had higher scores in the index, while male smokers had lower scores. On average, the adjusted analyses showed hypertensive men having 1.77 higher scores than non-hypertensives, male current smokers had 2.13 lower scores compared with males who never smoked and diabetic women had 1.56 higher scores than non-diabetics.

## Discussion

BALANCE DI was developed to reflect the recommendations of the dietary component of the BALANCE Program. The index showed reasonable internal consistency, construct and content validity and detected population characteristics associated with higher or lower scores.

The ability to detect known differences in the population corroborates the construct validity of a DI [25]. It is well known that women in general eat more healthily than men and the BALANCE DI found variations across sex, with women having higher scores in the total index. This finding is consistent with previous studies assessing different diet indexes, which also observed women having a more favorable diet [25, 28–30]. The higher consumption of fruits and vegetables by women is usually the reason they obtain better scores in DI [28]. However, our study showed no differences in the consumption of fruits and vegetables (green food group) across sex, but found lower consumption of meat (blue food group) and ultra-processed foods (red food group) among women. The BALANCE DI also detected differences in the diet between smoker and non-smoker males. On average, smokers had lower scores than non-smokers.

The Cronbach's coefficient alpha measures the internal consistency and values higher than 0.70 indicate accepted reliability. Similar to other studies which found alphas between 0.6 and 0.7 [25, 31], the alpha coefficient for the BALANCE DI was 0.66. According to Guenther and colleagues [25], given the complex and multidimensional construct of DI and because individuals do not fully meet and do not fully fail to meet all the dietary standards used in the indexes, an alpha coefficient slightly lower than 0.70 is expected. The low inter-item correlation ($r < 0.10$) and correlations ≥0.40 between each item and total index strengthen the reliability of the index.

**Table 3** Correlation between BALANCE diet components and total index

| | Green group | Yellow group | Blue group | Red group | Total index |
|---|---|---|---|---|---|
| Green group | 1 | | | | |
| Yellow group | 0.0113 | 1 | | | |
| Blue group | 0.0096 | 0.0053 | 1 | | |
| Red group | 0.0883 | 0.0430 | 0.0892 | 1 | |
| Total index | 0.4033 | 0.4594 | 0.6131 | 0.6157 | 1 |

BALANCE = Brazilian Cardioprotective Nutritional Program. Green group = vegetables, fruits, beans and legumes, fat free milk and yogurt. Yellow = rice, bread, pasta, oats, couscous, nuts, vegetable oil. Blue = meat, fish, cheese, eggs. Red = ultra-processed foods

**Table 4** Energy and selected nutrient intake (mean and 95% confidence interval) across quartiles of the BALANCE dietary index among men and women with a history of cardiovascular disease

| Dietary component | MEN | | | | WOMEN | | | |
|---|---|---|---|---|---|---|---|---|
| | 1 | 2 | 3 | 4 | 1 | 2 | 3 | 4 |
| n | 300 | 299 | 299 | 299 | 211 | 212 | 212 | 212 |
| BALANCE index range | 0; 13.31 | 13.32; 18.33 | 18.34; 24.79 | 24.80; 38.62 | 0; 14.51 | 14.52; 20.54 | 20.55; 25.59 | 25.61; 39.59 |
| Energy, Kcal | 1851 (1777; 1926) | 1629 (1560; 1697) | 1453 (1396; 1509) | 1345 (1293; 1398) | 1498 (1416; 1579) | 1279 (1206; 1351) | 1213 (1140; 1287) | 1169 (1116; 1221) |
| Protein, % Kcal | 19.2 (18.4; 20.0) | 19.2 (18.3; 19.8) | 19.2 (18.5; 19.9) | 18.3 (17.7; 18.9)[1] | 17.5 (16.6; 18.5) | 18.7 (17.9; 19.7) | 17.8 (17.1; 18.6) | 18.8 (18.1; 19.6) |
| Carbohydrate, % Kcal | 48.0 (46.6; 49.3) | 50.8 (49.6; 52.0) | 54.6 (53.4; 55.8) | 58.7 (57.5; 59.9) | 51.3 (49.8; 52.7) | 54.1 (52.7; 55.6) | 57.2 (55.6; 58.8) | 59.3 (57.8; 60.7) |
| Total fat, % Kcal | 32.9 (31.9; 33.8) | 30.8 (29.9; 31.8) | 27.2 (26.3; 28.1) | 24.9 (24.0; 25.8) | 31.7 (30.5; 32.9) | 28.2 (27.0; 29.4) | 26.9 (25.7; 28.2) | 24.1 (23.0; 25.2) |
| Saturated, % Kcal | 10.9 (10.5; 11.3) | 8.4 (9.4; 10.1) | 8.4 (8.0; 8.8) | 7.1 (6.8; 7.5) | 11.0 (10.5; 11.5) | 9.2 (8.7; 9.7) | 8.4 (7.9; 8.7) | 7.2 (6.8; 7.7) |
| Monounsaturated, % Kcal | 9.1 (8.7; 9.5) | 9.8 (8.2;9.0) | 7.7 (7.3; 8.1) | 6.9 (6.6; 7.2) | 8.8 (8.3; 9.2) | 7.5 (7.0; 7.9) | 7.3 (6.8; 7.8) | 6.9 (6.3; 7.4) |
| Polyunsaturated, % Kcal | 7.5 (7.1; 7.9) | 7.9 (7.5; 8.4) | 7.4 (7.1; 7.8) | 7.3 (7.0; 7.7)[1] | 6.9 (6.4;7.3) | 7.3 (6.8; 7.8) | 7.1 (6.6;7.6) | 6.7 (6.3; 7.1)[1] |
| Cholesterol, mg/1000 Kcal | 162 (149; 174) | 141 (130; 152) | 133 (121; 145) | 111 (102; 120) | 147 (134; 160) | 130 (119; 141) | 113 (101; 125) | 103 (94; 112) |
| Sodium, mg/1000 Kcal | 1922 (1845; 2000) | 1818 (1752; 1885) | 1860 (1800; 1920) | 2090 (1762; 2417)[1] | 1760 (1678; 1852) | 1873 (1748; 1999) | 1798 (1711; 1884) | 1777 (1690; 1863)[1] |
| Fiber, g/1000 Kcal | 10.1 (9.6; 10.6) | 12.3 (11.8; 12.9) | 14.5 (13.8; 15.1) | 17.8 (17.0; 18.6) | 10.2 (9.5; 10.9) | 13.2 (12.4; 13.9) | 15.0 (14.0; 16.0) | 17.2 ( 16.2; 18.2) |

BALANCE = Brazilian Cardioprotective Nutritional Program. [1]The *P*-value for linear trend was not significant (≥ 0,05). All others were significant, $P < 0,05$

The BALANCE DI showed association with energy and key nutrients in an expected direction, because it was inversely associated with intakes of energy, total fat, MUFA and cholesterol and it was positively associated with intakes of fiber and carbohydrate. These findings are consistent with previous diet quality indexes for Swedish, Australian and American population without cardiovascular disease [9, 29, 32], except the 14-point Mediterranean diet adherence screener which was inversely associated with carbohydrate and positively associated with MUFA [33]. In concordance with our findings, Mendes and colleagues found that higher intakes of total fat were significantly associated with lower index scores in the Healthy Eating Index for the Brazilian population [30].

The lower levels of MUFA in the highest quartile of the index were expected because the sources of MUFA in western diets are usually the same as the sources of

**Table 5** Association between the BALANCE dietary index and characteristics of men and women with history of cardiovascular diseases

| Population characteristics | MEN | | | | WOMEN | | | |
|---|---|---|---|---|---|---|---|---|
| | Crude | | Adjusted[a] | | Crude | | Adjusted[a] | |
| | Coefficient | 95% CI | Coefficient | 95% CI | Coefficient | 95% CI | Coefficient | 95% CI |
| Age, years (continuous) | 0.06 | 0.01; 0.11 | 0.04 | −0.01;0.10 | 0.05 | −0.01; 0.11 | 0.04 | −0.022; 0.10 |
| BMI, kg/m2 (continuous) | − 0.09 | − 0.20; 0.01 | − 0.02 | − 0.24; 0.20 | − 0.08 | − 0.17; 0.01 | 0.02 | − 0.16; 0.20 |
| Waist circumference, cm (continuous) | − 0.04 | − 0.08; 0.00 | − 0.04 | − 0.12; 0.05 | − 0.04 | − 0.08; 0.00 | − 0.06 | − 0.13; 0.02 |
| Hypertension (no = 0, yes = 1) | 1.77 | 0.35; 3.18 | 1.86 | 0.41; 3.32 | −2.38; | −2.26; 1.78 | − 0.37 | −2.46; 1.73 |
| Dyslipidemia (no – 0, yes – 1) | − 0.20 | – 1.30; 0.91 | 0.53 | 1.67; 0.61 | − 0.18 | − 1.43; 1.07 | − 0.39 | − 1.68; 0.90 |
| Diabetes (no = 0, yes = 1) | 0.37 | −0.55; 1.29 | 0.40 | − 0.54; 1.34 | 1.18 | 0.16; 2.20 | 1.56 | 0.48; 2.63 |
| Smoking status (never smoked = 0) | | | | | | | | |
| Former smoker | 0.01 | − 1.00; 1.03 | 0.01 | − 1.01; 1.03 | 0.30 | − 1.67; 2.27 | −0.12 | − 1.21; 0.96 |
| Current smoker | −2.53 | −4.41; − 0.66 | −2.13 | −4.03; − 0.22 | 0.64 | − 1.30; 2.58 | −0.15 | − 2.14; 1.84 |

BALANCE = Brazilian Cardioprotective Nutritional Program
*BMI* Body mass index
[a]Adjusted for age, BMI, waist circumference, hypertension, dyslipidemia, diabetes and smoking status

saturated fat [34] and they should be consumed in small quantities in the BALANCE diet. Furthermore, the BALANCE diet encourages the intake of foods available and accessible in Brazil, which are not beneficial sources of MUFA, contrary to the reality of the Mediterranean region [4, 35].

Nevertheless, the relative participation of carbohydrate increases as the score in the index increases. This could be explained by the lower relative participation of total fat in the higher levels of the score. Because the amount of fiber was also positively associated with the index, another explanation for the higher quantities of carbohydrate in the top levels of the index is the high intake of fruits in the BALANCE diet (data not shown), which has, as a benefit, elevated amounts of vitamins and bioactive compounds with a cardioprotective role [36].

The higher percentage of protein among women in the 4th quartile of the index is an unexpected result. We have two possible explanations for that. First, the macronutrients are presented as a percentage of energy, which means that if the percentage of one macronutrient changes the others will consequently change. Thus, the higher amount of protein could be explained by the lower relative participation of total fat in the highest quartile of the index. Second, an increase in protein intake from green group foods (beans and legumes, fat-free milk and yoghurt) may also have led to this result.

We were not able to detect associations between the index and the intake of sodium. A possible explanation is the fact that the sodium intake was estimated from 24-h recalls, which is not a robust instrument for estimating sodium intake. The gold standard method to estimate sodium intake is the 24-h urinary excretion, but these data were not available. A previous study estimated sodium intake from semi-quantitative food frequency questionnaire and was also unable to detect an association between the DI and the intake of sodium [27].

In our study, we observed lower index scores among males smoking and higher scores among males with hypertension and females with diabetes. Previous studies did not find associations between hypertension and diabetes diagnosis and conformance with DI [32, 37], but found associations between DI and BMI, WC and smoking status [29, 32, 33]. It is important to highlight that these studies included patients without previous CVD, while BALANCE included patients in the secondary prevention. Thus, subjects from BALANCE trial may have already received nutritional advice from dieticians, doctors, and nurses before being enrolled in the trial, making them aware of the eating choices they should make. This is a possible explanation for having hypertensive and diabetics subjects with better index scores.

The present study has limitations. The diagnoses of diabetes, hypertension and dyslipidemia were self-reported. However, this is unlikely to have added bias to the study because participants are in the secondary prevention of cardiovascular disease, which requires them to take some medications daily. By the type of taken medication (antihypertensive, for example) patients and interviewers know their health condition.

Although the dietary data were collected by trained interviewers following standardized procedures and were submitted to quality control, the usual intake could not be estimated because we had only one 24-h recall. Usually intake is estimated with at least two 24-h recalls to soften the effects of within-person variance in the assessment of the diet-disease relationship. The present study described the development of a dietary index based on the BALANCE diet and did not assess diet-disease relationships. Furthermore, a single 24-h recall can characterize the average consumption of a group and can be used when the sample size is large (higher than 1000) [38].

The number of servings in the blue group is an upper limit, i.e. if the recommendation is two servings then two servings or less should be eaten, while foods in the red group are not supposed to be part of the diet. Blue and red groups are given a reverse score and there is no clear scientific evidence or logical value clarifying how high an intake should be to deserve the minimum score of zero. Thus, we decided to use data-driven cut-offs to avoid giving the maximum or minimum score to a large proportion of the population. The decision to use data-driven cut-offs could compromise the external validity of the index. It is also important to note that our findings are derived from a Brazilian population aged 45 years or older with a personal history of major cardiovascular events (stroke, coronary heart disease, peripheral vascular disease) and the BALANCE dietary index can characterise the diet of similar populations.

## Conclusion

In this manuscript, we described the development of BALANCE DI and assessed some aspects of its validity, as well as population characteristics associated with higher or lower scores.

Regarding the internal consistency, BALANCE DI showed performance similar with other DI. The construct validity was corroborated by the ability to discriminate groups with known differences in the diet (males/females). The positive association with the consumption of carbohydrate and fiber, probably reflecting the intake of fruits, and the inverse association with intakes of energy, total fat, MUFA and cholesterol reinforces the content validity. Concerning population characteristics, we observed that diabetic women and hypertensive men were more likely to have higher index scores while smoking males were more likely to have lower scores.

The BALANCE DI has several potential uses: evaluation of the BALANCE Program dietary intervention; monitoring trial participants' compliance with the diet during the follow-up period; assessment of the association between the BALANCE diet and major CVD events; prediction of CVD risk (future). Before applying the index for all these purposes, we suggest studies with longitudinal designs to assess the validity of the index against health outcomes and its performance in detecting the relationship between overall diet and health.

#### Abbreviations

BALANCE: Brazilian Cardioprotective Nutritional Program; BMI: Body mass index; CI: Confidence interval; CVD: Cardiovascular disease; DI: Dietary index; MUFA: Monounsaturated fatty acids; SD: Standard deviation; USDA: United States Department of Agriculture; WC: Waist circumference; WHO: World Health Organization


#### Acknowledgements

We thank all the researchers who work in the BALANCE trial. We thank Camila Zancheta Ricardo, Giovanna Calixto Andrade, Priscila Pereira Machado, Leandro Fornias Machado de Rezende and Lucas Damiani for their comments and contributions on the statistical analysis.

#### Funding

This manuscript reports a substudy of the BALANCE Program trial, which was funded by the Brazilian Ministry of Health in Partnership with the Research Institute of Hospital do Coração (HCor) — "Programa de Apoio ao Desenvolvimento Institucional do SUS (Brazilian Public Health System): PROADI-SUS". The funder had no influence on the study execution or manuscript writing.


#### Authors' contributions

JTS conceived and conducted the present study, analyzed data, drafted the manuscript and has primary responsibility for the final content. ACBF, CRT and BW provided the database from the BALANCE trial and contributed to the development of the dietary index. RBL designed the research, analysed data, performed statistical analysis, and critically revised the manuscript for important intellectual content. All authors have read and approved the final manuscript.

#### Competing interests

The authors declare that they have no competing interests.


#### Author details

[1]Department of Nutrition, School of Public Health, University of São Paulo, Avenida Doutor Arnaldo, 715, São Paulo, SP 01246904, Brazil. [2]Research Institute, Hospital do Coração (HCor), Rua Abílio Sorares, 250, 12° andar, São Paulo, SP 04005-000, Brazil. [3]Department of Preventive Medicine, School of Medicine, University of São Paulo, Avenida Doutor Arnaldo, 455, São Paulo, SP 01246903, Brazil.


#### References


1. World Health Statistics. Geneva: World Health Organization; 2015.
2. Mansur AP, Favarato D. Trends in mortality rate from cardiovascular disease in Brazil, 1980-2012. Arq Bras Cardiol. 2016;107:20–5.
3. Burlingame B, Dernini S. Sustainable diets and biodiversity: directions and solutions for policy, research and action. Rome, Italy: Nutrition and Consumer Protection Division FAO; 2012.
4. Weber B, Bersch-Ferreira Â, Torreglosa CR, Ross-Fernandes MB, da Silva JT, Galante AP, et al. The Brazilian Cardioprotective nutritional program to reduce events and risk factors in secondary prevention for cardiovascular disease: study protocol (the BALANCE program trial). Am Heart J. 2016;171:73–81. e2
5. Stefler D, Pikhart H, Jankovic N, Kubinova R, Pajak A, Malyutina S, et al. Healthy diet indicator and mortality in eastern European populations: prospective evidence from the HAPIEE cohort. Eur J Clin Nutr. 2014;68:1346–52.
6. Bach A, Serra-Majem L, Carrasco JL, Roman B, Ngo J, Bertomeu I, et al. The use of indexes evaluating the adherence to the Mediterranean diet in epidemiological studies: a review. Public Health Nutr. 2006;9:132–46.
7. Fung TT, Chiuve SE, McCullough ML, Rexrode KM, Logroscino G, Hu FB. Adherence to a DASH-style diet and risk of coronary heart disease and stroke in women. Arch Intern Med. 2008;168:713–20.
8. Roy R, Hebden L, Rangan A, Allman-Farinelli M. The development, application, and validation of a healthy eating index for Australian adults (HEIFA-2013). Nutrition. 2016;32:432–40.
9. Drake I, Gullberg B, Ericson U, Sonestedt E, Nilsson J, Wallström P, et al. Development of a diet quality index assessing adherence to the Swedish nutrition recommendations and dietary guidelines in the Malmö diet and Cancer cohort. Public Health Nutr. 2011;14:835–45.
10. McCullough ML, Feskanich D, Stampfer MJ, Giovannucci EL, Rimm EB, Hu FB, et al. Diet quality and major chronic disease risk in men and women: moving toward improved dietary guidance. Am J Clin Nutr. 2002;76:1261–71.
11. Moshfegh AJ, Rhodes DG, Baer DJ, Murayi T, Clemens JC, Rumpler WV, et al. The US Department of agriculture automated multiple-pass method reduces bias in the collection of energy intakes. Am J Clin Nutr. 2008;88:324–32.
12. Weber B, Berwanger O, Costa RP, Lara EMS, Fernandes MBR, Ferreira ÂCB, et al. Álbum fotográfico de medidas e porções de alimentos. São Paulo: Instituto de Ensino e Pesquisa do Hospital do Coração; 2012.
13. Nielsen SJ, Adair L. An alternative to dietary data exclusions. J Am Diet Assoc. 2007;107:792–9.
14. Physical status: the use and interpretation of anthropometry: report of a WHO Expert. Geneva: World Health Organization; 1995.
15. Anales da 36ª Reunión del Comité Asesor de Investigaciones en salud. Encuesta multicentrica: salud, bien estar y envejecimiento (SABE) en America Latina y el Caribe.mayo 2001; Washington (DC): Wold Health Organization.
16. Sociedade Brasileira de Cardiologia. IV Diretriz da Sociedade Brasileira de Cardiologia sobre Tratamento do Infarto Agudo do Miocárdio com Supradesnivel do Segmento ST. Arq Bras Cardiol. 2009;93(Suppl 2):179–264.
17. Sociedade Brasileira de Hipertensão, Sociedade Brasileira de Cardiologia, Sociedade Brasileira de Endocrinologia e Metabologia, et al. I Brazilian guidelines on diagnosis and treatment of metabolic syndrome. Arq Bras Cardiol. 2005;84(Suppl 1):1–28.
18. Sociedade Brasileira de Cardiologia. V Diretriz Brasileira Sobre Dislipidemias e Prevenção da Aterosclerose Departamento de Aterosclerose da Sociedade Brasileira de Cardiologia. Arq Bras Cardiol. 2013;101(Suppl1):1–22.
19. Sociedade Brasileira de Cardiologia, Sociedade Brasileira de Hipertensão, Sociedade Brasileira de Nefrologia. VI Brazilian guidelines on hypertension. Arq Bras Cardiol. 2010;95(Suppl 1):1–51.
20. Sociedade Brasileira de Diabetes. Diretrizes da Sociedade Brasileira de Diabetes (2015-2016). São Paulo: Sociedade Brasileira de Diabetes; 2016.
21. Drewnowski A, Fulgoni VL. Nutrient density: principles and evaluation tools. Am J Clin Nutr. 2014;99(Suppl):1223–8.
22. Miller PE, Cross AJ, Subar AF, Krebs-Smith SM, Park Y, Powell-Wiley T, et al. Comparison of 4 established DASH diet indexes: examining associations of index scores and colorectal cancer. Am J Clin Nutr. 2013;98:794–803.
23. Kennedy ET, Ohls J, Carlson S, Fleming K. The healthy eating index: design and applications. J Am Diet Assoc. 1995;95:1103–8.
24. Panagiotakos DB, Pitsavos C, Stefanadis C. Dietary patterns: a mediterranean diet score and its relation to clinical and biological markers of cardiovascular disease risk. Nutr Metab Cardiovasc Dis. 2006;16:559–68.
25. Guenther PM, Kirkpatrick SI, Reedy J, Krebs-Smith SM, Buckman DW, Dodd KW, et al. The healthy eating Index-2010 is a valid and reliable measure of diet quality according to the 2010 dietary guidelines for Americans. J Nutr. 2014;144:399–407.
26. Najas M. I Consenso Brasileiro de Nutrição e Disfagia em Idosos Hospitalizados. Barueri, SP: Sociedade Brasileira de Geriatria e Gerontologia; 2011.
27. Brasil, Ministério da Saúde. Vigitel Brazil 2014: protective and risk factors for chronic diseases by telephone survey. Brasília: Ministério da Saúde; 2015.
28. Guenther PM, Reedy J, Krebs-Smith SM. Development of the healthy eating Index-2005. J Am Diet Assoc. 2008;108:1896–901.

29. McNaughton SA, Ball K, Crawford D, Mishra GD. An index of diet and eating patterns is a valid measure of diet quality in an Australian population. J Nutr. 2008;138:86–93.
30. Mendes A, Gavioli L, Previdelli AN, Fisberg RM, Marchioni DML. The diet quality index evaluates the adequacy of energy provided by dietary macronutrients. Revista de Nurição. 2015;28:7.
31. de Andrade SC, Previdelli AN, Marchioni DML, Fisberg RM. Avaliação da confiabilidade e validade do Índice de Qualidade da Dieta Revisado. Rev Saude Publica. 2013;47:8.
32. Fogli-Cawley JJ, Dwyer JT, Saltzman E, McCullough ML, Troy LM, Jacques PF. The 2005 dietary guidelines for Americans adherence index: development and application. J Nutr. 2006;136:2908–15.
33. Schroder H, Fito M, Estruch R, Martinez-Gonzalez MA, Corella D, Salas-Salvado J, et al. A short screener is valid for assessing Mediterranean diet adherence among older Spanish men and women. J Nutr. 2011;141:1140–5.
34. Schwingshackl L, Hoffmann G. Monounsaturated fatty acids, olive oil and health status: a systematic review and meta-analysis of cohort studies. Lipids Health Dis. 2014;13:154.
35. Estruch R, Ros E, Salas-Salvadó J, Covas MI, Corella D, Arós F, et al. Primary prevention of cardiovascular disease with a Mediterranean diet. N Engl J Med. 2013;368:1279–90.
36. Alissa EM, Ferns GA. Functional foods and nutraceuticals in the primary prevention of cardiovascular diseases. J Nutr Metab. 2012; https://doi.org/10.1155/2012/569486.
37. Bhupathiraju SN, Lichtenstein AH, Dawson-Hughes B, Tucker KL. Adherence index based on the AHA 2006 diet and lifestyle recommendations is associated with select cardiovascular disease risk factors in older Puerto Ricans. J Nutr. 2011;141:460–9.
38. Willett W. Nutritional epidemiology. 3rd ed. New York: Oxford University Press; 2012.

# 4

# Association of serum vitamin D concentrations with dietary patterns in children and adolescents

Vijay Ganji[1*], Bernadette Martineau[2] and William Edmund Van Fleit[3]

## Abstract

**Background:** Because children have been advised on the dangers of sun exposure, diet is an important contributor of serum 25 hydroxyvitamin D [25(OH)D] concentrations. Aim of this study was to determine whether serum 25(OH)D concentrations were associated with any specific dietary patterns in US children.

**Methods:** Data from 2 cycles of National Health and Nutrition Examination Survey (NHANES) 2003–2004 and 2005–2006 for individuals aged 2 to ≤19 y, were used to study relation between dietary patterns and serum 25(OH)D. We derived 2 major dietary patterns based on the food frequency questionnaire data. These were labeled as High-Fat-Low-Vegetable Dietary (HFLVD) pattern and Prudent Dietary (PD) pattern.

**Results:** In multivariate adjusted analysis, there was no significant relationship between serum 25(OH)D concentrations and tertiles of HFLVD and PD dietary pattern scores in all subjects, boys, and girls. When dietary patterns scores were used as a continuous variable in adjusted analysis, children (all) with higher PD contribution scores to overall diet showed a significant positive relation with serum 25(OH)D ($\beta = 59.1$, $P = 0.017$). When data were stratified by sex, a significant positive relation was observed in girls between serum 25(OH)D concentration and PD pattern scores ($\beta = 82.1$, $P = 0.015$). A significant negative relation was observed in girls between serum 25(OH)D and HFLVD pattern scores ($\beta = -88.5$, $P = 0.016$).

**Conclusion:** Overall, serum 25(OH)D were associated with PD pattern but not with HFLVD pattern in US children. In public health perspective, it is important to encourage children, especially girls who are consuming HFLVD pattern to shift to healthier diet.

**Keywords:** Dietary patterns, NHANES, Serum 25 hydroxyvitamin D, US children, Vitamin D

## Background

A classical function of vitamin D is to regulate extracellular calcium and phosphorus. Current evidence suggests that vitamin D may play a role in various non-bone diseases such as autoimmune disease [1, 2], cardiovascular disease [3, 4], type-2 diabetes mellitus (T2DM) [5], depression [6], and cancer [7]. Dietary vitamin D sources include oily fish such as salmon, mackerel, bluefish, sardines and tuna, shiitake mushrooms (fresh or sun-dried), and egg yolks. Fortified dietary sources of vitamin D include milk, orange juice, infant formulas, yogurts, butter, margarine, cheeses, and breakfast cereals [8].

Serum 25-hydroxyvitamin D [25(OH)D] is a commonly used marker of vitamin D nutritional status. Hypovitaminosis D is a widespread problem in the US, specifically in children and adolescents [9–12]. Prevention of suboptimal vitamin D status in childhood may reduce future adverse health conditions. The contribution of dietary sources to vitamin D status is not clearly known in children. Some studies have shown that dietary intake of certain vitamin D rich foods had a significant positive influence on serum 25(OH)D concentrations [13, 14], whereas other studies have shown that vitamin D intake did not affect serum 25(OH)D concentrations [15]. While sunlight exposure is the major

* Correspondence: vganji@qu.edu.qa
[1]Human Nutrition Department, College of Health Sciences, Qatar University, Doha, Qatar
Full list of author information is available at the end of the article

source of circulating serum 25(OH)D [16], children and adolescents have been advised on the dangers of sun exposure [17] and are exposed to increased use of sunscreen lotions and time spent indoors which has likely contributed to the increasing prevalence of low vitamin D status [18]. Therefore, diet is an important contributor of circulating serum 25(OH)D in the absence of or in the presence of reduced sunlight exposure.

To our knowledge, no data are available on the relation between dietary patterns and serum 25(OH)D in US children and adolescents. Studies that have looked at diet and vitamin D status have addressed associations between individual food sources such as fortified milk or fatty fish. However, people consume a variety of foods in combination [9]. Dietary pattern analysis, an alternative approach to traditional single nutrient epidemiology, takes into account all nutrient interactions and allows for a more comprehensive approach to study the relation between disease and dietary intake [19]. Therefore, the objective of this study was to determine whether serum 25(OH)D concentrations were associated with any specific dietary patterns in US children and adolescents using assay-adjusted data from the National Health and Nutrition Examination Survey (NHANES) 2003–2006.

## Methods

### Brief NHANES survey methods

The National Center for Health Statistics (NCHS) conducts large, nationally representative, sample surveys known as NHANES on the noninstitutionalized US civilian population. A sample representative of individuals aged > 2 months was selected by using a stratified, multistage, probability sample survey design. Beginning in 1999, NHANESs were conducted as annual surveys and data are released in 2-y cycles for public use. Certain subgroups including low-income persons, adolescents, persons aged ≥60 y, non-Hispanic black (NHB), and Hispanic/Mexican American (H/MA) are oversampled to yield more reliable estimates for these specific groups. The detailed descriptions of the survey design and methodologies are described elsewhere [20].

NHANES 2003–2004 was conducted between January 2003 and December 2004 in 12,761 individuals [9643 were examined in the Mobile Examination Centers (MEC)] and NHANES 2005–2006 was conducted between January 2005 and December 2006 in 12,862 individuals (9950 were examined in the MECs). Participants were interviewed in their homes to gather information on demographic characteristics, diet, and health. Additional health data were collected during a medical examination conducted in MECs. At the MECs, a physical exam, blood and urine sample collection, and other diagnostic measurements were performed. All NHANES protocols were approved by the NCHS Ethics Review Board prior to data collection. Detailed description of these protocols is found elsewhere [21].

Households were randomly selected and all members within the household were screened for demographic characteristics. One or more individuals within the household were then selected for sample based on age, sex, and race-ethnicity. NHANES 2003–2006 sample included individuals ≥2 mo old. Race-ethnicity was categorized as non-Hispanic white (NHW), NHB, H/MA, and Other. Participants self-reported their race-ethnicity status. Poverty income ratio (PIR) was calculated as the ratio of income to the family's appropriate poverty threshold. To avoid damage to the MECs, examination data in the North were collected in spring/summer (May 1–October 31) and in South were collected in fall/winter (November 1–April 30). Data for body mass index (BMI) were obtained from the medical examination component of NHANES. Supplement users were defined based on participants who answered 'yes' to the question "Did you take supplements in the past 30 d?" Participants were asked about hours spent watching television, playing video games, and using the computer.

Blood samples were collected by venipuncture from participants in MECs according to standard protocols. Detailed specimen collection and processing methods have been previously reported [22, 23]. Serum 25(OH)D concentrations were analyzed and determined at the National Center for Environmental Health, Centers for Disease Control and Prevention using the Diasorin Radioimmunoassay (Stillwater, MN).

Periodically, NHANES data files are updated by the NCHS, replacing previous data files. In November 2010, an update occurred for serum 25(OH)D data because of changes and drifts in serum 25(OH)D assay over time. This was likely due to method variation that resulted from reagent and calibration lot-to-lot variation. The NCHS released a data advisory for vitamin D and recommended use of the assay-adjusted data by investigators rather than previously available unadjusted data. A detailed description of this data advisory for serum 25(OH)D is described elsewhere [24].

A 216-item food frequency questionnaire (FFQ) component was newly added to NHANES 2003–2004 and was used to gather information on the frequency of food consumption of participants over the past 12 months. The questionnaire was developed, tested, and validated by the National Institutes of Health, National Cancer Institute. Participants were asked the average number of times foods were consumed over the past 12 months and for certain types of foods, their seasonal intake were also gathered. Participants reported the number of times/d, wk., mo, or never that a food was consumed. All foods' frequency of consumption was standardized to a monthly intake by using a conversion factor of 30.4 d/mo as this is the number of days in an average month. Frequency of consumption was collected for dairy products, meat, fish and seafood, poultry, eggs, fruits and juices, vegetables, grains and legumes, snacks and sweets, beverages, and added fats. Those participants who did not answer the FFQ were excluded from this study.

### Study sample

Two cycles of NHANES 2003–2004 and 2005–2006 were used in this study. Although serum 25(OH)D concentrations are available publically in NHANES 2001–2002, this survey was not included in this current study because FFQ data were not collected. Data on children between ages 2 to ≤19 y from NHANES 2003–2004 and 2005–2006 were concatenated into one master analytic database, NHANES 2003–2006 ($n = 8747$). Subjects with serum 25(OH)D concentration data were then selected to include in this study ($n = 7172$). Of the remaining 7172 participants, children < 2 y old were excluded from the data analysis due to lack of completed FFQ ($n = 2572$). Of the remaining 4600 children, 71 were excluded because they reported that they were lactating or pregnant, 45 were excluded due to lack of BMI measurement, 4 were excluded due to lack of calorie intake data, 3 were excluded due to lack of supplement use data, and 73 were excluded due to lack of screen viewing response. Thus, the final analytic sample consisted of 4404 children and adolescents (Fig. 1).

### Study variables

In this study, the foods from the FFQ were categorized into 30 food groups. These 30 food groups were low-fat and high-fat dairy products, dairy alternatives, fish and other seafood, eggs, meat, processed meat, poultry, creamed soups, other soups, pizza, mixed foods, cereals, refined grains, whole grains, nuts, legumes, tomatoes, cruciferous, starchy, and other vegetables, fruit, fruit juices, snacks and sweets, butter and margarine, other

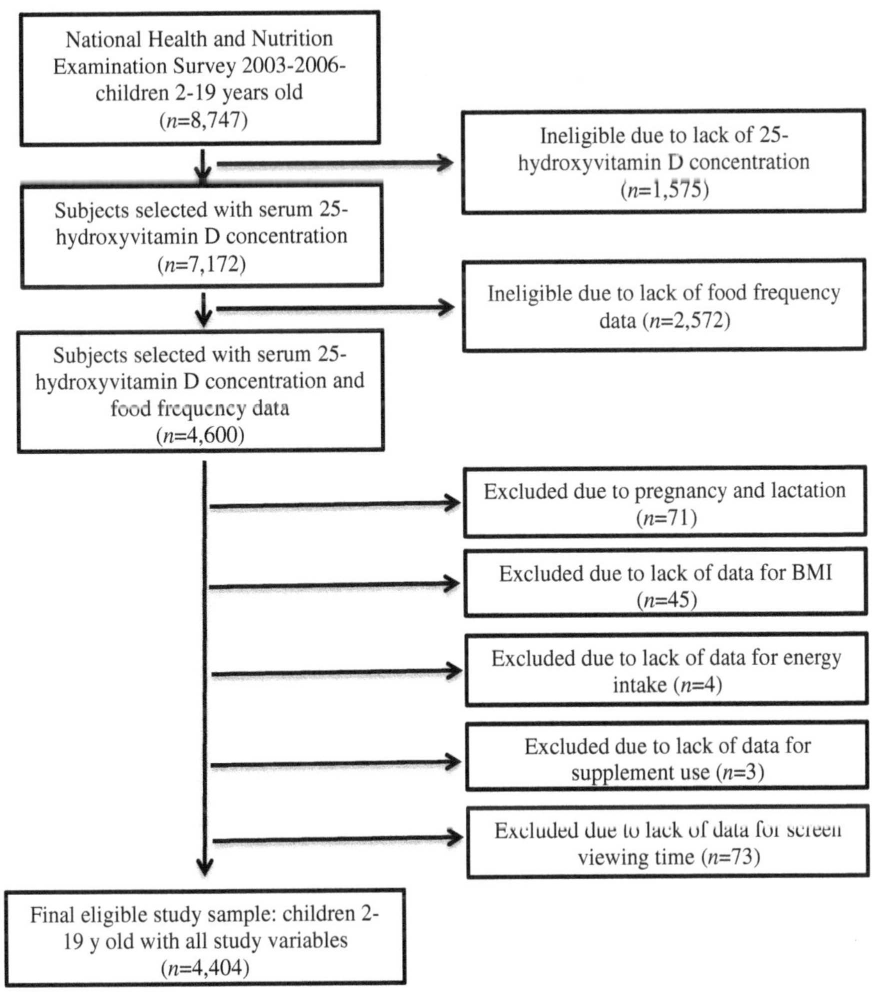


**Fig. 1** Study sample derivation after removing subjects for missing data for main variables and confounding variables sequentially (weighted $n = 60{,}274{,}698$)

fats, added sugars, coffee/tea, energy drinks (high or low), and alcohol (Table 1). Foods were categorized based on nutrient profiles or culinary use and were grouped similar to those used in other studies [25]. Frequency of dietary intake of these 30 food groups for each individual was used to identify major dietary patterns. Age, sex, race-ethnicity, BMI, PIR, time of examination, use of supplements, energy intake, and screen use hours were considered as potential confounding variables as these are known to affect serum 25(OH)D concentrations [18, 26]. Participants were categorized into 2–3 y, 4–8 y, 9–13 y, and 14–19 y old age groups. BMI was categorized as normal weight (<85th percentile) and overweight and obese (≥85th percentile) for age and sex. PIR was categorized as below poverty (< 1.0), middle income (1.0–2.5), higher income (> 2.5), and not reported. Combined television, computer, and video game use hours were categorized as ≤2 h, 3–4 h, or > 4 h/d. Smoking status and alcohol intake variables were also considered as potential confounding variables. However, smoking-related questions were only asked to children aged ≥12 y and alcohol-related questions were asked to adults aged ≥20 y; therefore, both were dropped from the analysis.

**Table 1** Food groups used in the dietary pattern analysis: NHANES 2003-2006[a]

| Food Groups[b] | Foods from Food-Frequency Questionnaire[c] |
|---|---|
| Low-fat dairy | 1, 2%, skim, nonfat, and evaporated milk; yogurt/frozen, low-fat cheese,and low-fat sour cream |
| High-fat dairy | Whole milk, cream, ice cream, pudding, cottage cheese, cheese, and sour cream |
| Dairy alternative | Soy, rice, and other milk; non-dairy creamer, and meal replacement beverage |
| Fish and other seafood | Oysters, clams, and shellfish; fish: fillets, sticks, tuna, salmon, and raw fish sushi |
| Eggs | Egg whites, whole egg, egg substitute, and egg salad |
| Meat | Beef, steak, roasts, hamburger, pork, ribs, and ham |
| Processed Meat | Bacon, Canadian bacon, sausage, hot dogs, luncheon meats, liver, and Liverwurst |
| Poultry | Chicken, all types; and turkey |
| Creamed soup | Creamed soups, all types; and chowders |
| Other soup | Broth-based soups and bean soups |
| Pizza | Pizza, all types |
| Mixed dishes | Casseroles, lasagna, macaroni and cheese, and chili |
| Cereal | Oatmeal, grits, and other cooked cereals; and cold cereal, all types |
| Refined grains | English muffin, bagel, roll, cracker, stuffing, cornbread, biscuit, pancake, waffle, pasta, and rice |
| Whole grains | Dark breads and rolls; brown rice, bulgur, cracked wheat and millet; and granola bars |
| Nuts | Peanuts, walnuts, and other nuts; seeds; and nut butters |
| Legumes | Pintos, kidney, blackeyed peas, lima, lentils, refried beans, baked beans, soybeans, and tofu |
| Starchy vegetables | White potatoes, french fries, and potato salad; squash, sweet potatoes, carrots, and yams |
| Tomatoes | Tomatoes, including fresh, tomato juice, and salsa |
| Cruciferous and green vegetables | Spinach, turnip, collard, chard, kale, broccoli, cabbage, cauliflower, Brussel sprouts, and lettuce |
| Other vegetables | Pickles, green beans, peas, peppers, onion, cucumber, corn, and mixed Vegetables |
| Fruit | Apples, pears, peaches, bananas,melons, strawberries, grapes, pineapple, and dried fruit |
| Fruit juices | Orange juice, grapefruit juice, apple juice, grape juice, and prune juice |
| Sweets and Snacks | Donuts, danish, cookie, brownie, cake, pie, cobbler, popcorn, pretzels, tortilla chips, and candy |
| Butter and Margarine | Butter and margarine, all types |
| Other fats | Olive oil, corn oil, canola oil, salad dressings, mayonnaise, and gravies |
| Condiments | Maple syrup, honey, jam, and jelly |
| Coffee/Tea | Coffee and tea, regular and decaffeinated |
| Energy drinks | Sodas and fruit drinks, including Hi-C, Kool-Aid, lemonade, and cranberry cocktail |
| Alcohol | Beer, wine, wine coolers, hard liquor, and mixed drinks |

[a]$n = 4404$; weighted $n = 60{,}274{,}698$. NHANES 2003–2004 and 2005–2006 were combined into one master database, NHANES 2003–2006
[b]Foods consumed by survey participants were categorized into 30 food groups based on nutrient profiles or culinary use
[c]Food consumption data were collected using a 216-item qualitative Food Frequency Questionnaire

**Data analysis**

Statistical analysis was performed using SAS statistical software (version 9.2, SAS Institute) as it is capable of handling the complex survey design of NHANES. The survey analysis procedures accounted for primary sampling unit, stratum, cluster, and observation weight in the calculation of variances used for interval estimation and hypothesis testing. The NOMCAR option was used in all analyses so that design variables with missing values are used in the domain analysis to estimate variances using Taylor series linearization method. Detailed guidelines on the sample weighting and the proper variance estimation procedures are outlined in the NHANES Analytic and Reporting Guidelines [20].

Factor analysis (principal component) was used to identify dietary patterns based on the frequency of dietary intake of the 30 predefined food groups. The PROC FACTOR procedure in SAS was used to conduct this analysis. The factors were rotated by orthogonal transformation to achieve a structure of independent factors with greater interpretability. The number of factors that were retained was determined based on an Eigenvalue (≥1.5), explained variance (≥5%), and Cattell scree plot. The remaining factors were considered the main dietary patterns and were labeled based on interpretation of the data. Factor loadings were derived for each of the 30 food groups across the extracted factors. For each dietary pattern, a factor score was calculated for each participant by combining the frequency of dietary intake of the food groups weighted by their factor loadings. Dietary pattern scores were then stratified into tertiles (low, medium, and high) based on the factor scores for each dietary pattern.

Chi-square tests were used to identify associations between demographic, lifestyle, and health characteristics among the dietary pattern tertiles. Multivariate-adjusted regression analysis was used to determine the associations between serum 25(OH)D concentrations and dietary patterns. Associations were analyzed according to the participants' factor scores for each dietary pattern divided into tertiles (low, medium, and high), and to the factor scores as a continuous variable. This analysis included sex, age, race-ethnicity, use of supplements, time of examination, BMI, PIR, and screen use hours as potential confounding variables. Variables found to be non-significant such as PIR and use of supplements were dropped from the model. Because previous studies found differences of serum 25(OH)D concentrations by sex [11, 26], the present analysis for the relation between serum 25(OH)D and dietary patterns was then stratified by sex. Univariate ANOVA was used to establish if serum 25(OH)D concentrations varied across dietary patterns for all subjects, boys, and girls in an unadjusted analysis. Analysis of covariance (ANCOVA) was utilized to establish if serum 25(OH)D concentrations varied across dietary patterns after adjusting for various confounding variables. Multiple comparisons among dietary patterns for serum 25(OH)D concentrations were made using independent unpaired t-tests with a Bonferroni correction. Serum 25(OH)D concentrations were presented as mean ± standard error (SE). Statistical significance was set at $\alpha = 0.05$.

## Results

**General demographic characteristics of study sample**

The sample consisted of 51.5% ($n = 2154$) boys and 48.5% ($n = 2250$) girls. Of the 4404 participants, 62.5% ($n = 1293$) were NHW, 15.3% ($n = 1428$) were NHB, and 13.3% ($n = 1323$) were H/MA. The participants were distributed across the age categories: 8.4% ($n = 399$) 2–3 y, 26.4% ($n = 924$) 4–8 y, 29.9% ($n = 1282$) 9–13 y, and 35.3% ($n = 1799$) 14–19 y olds. Of the study population, 34.1% ($n = 1133$) reported having taken a supplement 30 d prior to the completing the survey. The majority (61.1%, $n = 2215$) of the participants were examined in the summer. 84.8% ($n = 3626$) were classified as healthy weight and 15.2% ($n = 778$) as overweight and obese based on the BMI. The majority (49.9%, $n = 1984$) reported ≤2 h/d of television, computer, and video game usage, although 28.5% ($n = 1296$) reported between 3 and 4 h/d of usage and 21.6% ($n = 1124$) reported > 4 h/d of usage.

**Dietary patterns**

Two major dietary patterns were identified based on the factor analysis from the 30 predefined food groups (Table 1). Higher positive factor loading scores are interpreted to contribute most to the factor score, and conversely, higher negative factor loading scores contribute least to the factor score. The 1st factor had heavy factor loading scores for meats, snacks and sweets, condiments, mixed dishes, pizza, processed meats, refined grains, high fat dairy, coffee/tea, poultry, starchy vegetables, and fish and other seafood. Thus, the 1st factor was labeled as the High-Fat-Low-Vegetable Dietary (HFLVD) pattern. This was the most dominant dietary food pattern in the population and explained largest variance in food intake. The 2nd factor had heavy factor loading scores for all vegetable groups, fruit, other fats, mixed dishes, fish and other seafood, tomatoes, and meats. Thus, the 2nd factor was labeled as the Prudent dietary (PD) pattern. The detailed factor loading matrixes are listed in Table 2.

**Characteristics of study population by dietary pattern**

The sample distribution by characteristics of the study population across tertiles of each dietary pattern is presented in Table 3. Proportion of persons belonging to NHW and H/MA race-ethnicities tended to decrease, while proportion of persons belonging to NHB tended

**Table 2** Factor loading matrix for dietary patterns in National Health and Nutrition Examination Survey (NHANES) 2003-2006[a,b]

| Category[c] | Factor 1: HFLVD Pattern[d] | Factor 2: PD Pattern[d] |
|---|---|---|
| Cruciferous & green vegetables | 0.118 | 0.705 |
| Other vegetables | 0.144 | 0.734 |
| Tomatoes | 0.172 | 0.464 |
| Starchy vegetables | 0.514 | 0.518 |
| Fruit | 0.199 | 0.676 |
| Fruit juice | 0.364 | 0.243 |
| Nuts | 0.228 | 0.409 |
| Legumes | 0.085 | 0.406 |
| Fish & other seafood | 0.505 | 0.479 |
| Meat | 0.645 | 0.457 |
| Poultry | 0.519 | 0.392 |
| Processed Meat | 0.580 | 0.346 |
| Whole grains | −0.049 | 0.448 |
| Refined grains | 0.570 | 0.448 |
| Cereals | 0.084 | 0.347 |
| Eggs | 0.279 | 0.298 |
| Low fat dairy | −0.136 | 0.413 |
| High fat dairy | 0.543 | 0.133 |
| Dairy Alternative/Meal Replacement | 0.203 | 0.082 |
| Creamed soups | 0.163 | 0.196 |
| Other soups | 0.299 | 0.415 |
| Mixed dishes | 0.605 | 0.523 |
| Pizza | 0.604 | 0.089 |
| Snacks & sweets | 0.635 | 0.338 |
| Butter & Margarine | 0.423 | 0.288 |
| Other fats | 0.353 | 0.525 |
| Condiments | 0.632 | 0.173 |
| Energy drinks | 0.513 | −0.074 |
| Alcohol | 0.120 | −0.018 |
| Coffee/Tea | 0.523 | −0.078 |

[a]$n = 4404$; weighted, $n = 60{,}274{,}698$. Correlation coefficients
[b]Factor procedure, principal component analysis. Two factors with Eigenvalues ≥1.5 were rotated and extracted. Factors were labeled according to the foods found to have the highest correlation coefficients within each factor (dietary pattern). Positive factor scores indicate that those foods are more likely to be consumed in that dietary pattern. Lower negative scores indicate that those foods are least likely to be consumed in that dietary pattern
[c]Food categories were based on consumption data collected from a 216-item Food Frequency Questionnaire from NHANES 2003–2004 and 2005–2006. Individual foods were categorized into 30 food groups
[d]High-Fat-Low-Vegetable Dietary Pattern or Prudent Dietary Pattern

to increase across the tertiles of HFLVD pattern scores ($P < 0.001$). Proportion of children in the 14–19 y old age group tended to increase from tertile 1 (30.1%) to tertile 3 (40.6%) ($P = 0.003$), while their proportion tended to decrease from tertile 1 (48.8%) to tertile 3 (26.8%) ($P < 0.001$). In both the HFLVD and PD patterns, the proportion of children in the lowest PIR category tended to increase from the lowest tertile to the highest tertile pattern scores. In the HFLVD pattern, the proportion of children who viewed ≤2 h of combined television, computer, and video games tended to decrease from the lowest tertile (59.8%) to the highest tertile (41.6%) pattern scores ($P < 0.001$), while they tended to increase from the lowest (42.7%) to the highest tertile (55.4%) pattern scores ($P < 0.001$).

Subjects in the low-intake group of the HFLVD pattern ($P$ for trend = 0.003) and the high-intake group of the PD pattern ($P$ for trend< 0.001) were more likely to have consumed supplements. Subjects in the low-intake group of the PD pattern had a higher BMI ($P$ for trend < 0.001. Subjects in the high-intake group of the HFLVD pattern had higher combined usage of television, computer, and video games/d than those in the low-intake group (≤2 h/d) ($P$ for trend < 0.0001). Subjects in the high-intake group of the PD pattern had lower combined usage of television, computer, and video games/d ($P$ for trend < 0.0001).

**Relation between serum 25(OH)D and dietary patterns**

The relation of mean serum 25(OH)D concentrations and dietary pattern according to the tertiles of factor scores are presented in Table 4. In the unadjusted regression analysis, serum 25(OH)D concentrations differed significantly across the tertiles of the HFLVD pattern scores ($P = 0.003$) and PD pattern scores ($P = 0.012$). Subjects who had low-intake HFLVD pattern scores had greater serum 25(OH)D concentrations compared to those with medium and high-intake pattern scores (+ 1.2 ± 0.1 ng/mL and + 2.5 ± 0.01 ng/mL, respectively). When the model was adjusted to confounding variables, mean serum 25(OH)D concentrations of the boys and girls with low, medium, and high-intake HFLVD or PD patterns scores did not differ significantly. Girls with medium and high PD pattern scores had slightly higher mean serum 25(OH)D concentrations compared to those with low pattern score (21.5 ± 0.5 vs. 19.9 ± 0.6 ng/mL; $P = 0.064$).

The relation between serum 25(OH)D concentrations and dietary pattern scores as a continuous variable is presented in Table 5. In unadjusted analysis, subjects with higher HFLVD contributions scores to overall diet showed a significant negative relation to serum 25(OH) concentrations ($\beta = -135.56$; $P < 0.001$). In the same unadjusted analysis, subjects with higher PD contribution scores to overall diet did not show a significant association with serum vitamin D concentrations ($\beta = -57.1$; $P = 0.073$). However when subjects were stratified into

**Table 3** Sample distribution by demographic and health characteristics according to the tertiles of factor scores for dietary patterns: National Health and Nutrition Examination Survey (NHANES) 2003-2006[a, b]

| Characteristic | HFLVD Pattern Score[c] (n = 4404) | | | | PD Pattern Score[c] (n = 4404) | | | |
|---|---|---|---|---|---|---|---|---|
| | Low (<−0.003875) | Medium (−0.003875 to 0.000925) | High (> 0.000925) | P for Trend[d] | Low (< 0.004175) | Medium (− 0.004175 to 0.001912) | High (> 0.001912) | P for Trend[d] |
| N | 1338 | 1465 | 1601 | | 1523 | 1376 | 1505 | |
| Sex | | | | | | | | |
| Boys, % | 48.6 | 51.8 | 54.2 | 0.165 | 48.7 | 55.8 | 50.1 | 0.098 |
| Girls, % | 51.4 | 48.2 | 45.8 | | 51.3 | 44.2 | 49.9 | |
| Race-ethnicity | | | | | | | | |
| NHW, % | 70.0 | 62.2 | 55.2 | < 0.001 | 61.0 | 66.4 | 60.0 | 0.003 |
| NHB, % | 7.3 | 13.9 | 24.7 | | 18.0 | 13.2 | 14.7 | |
| H/MA, % | 14.3 | 14.1 | 11.5 | | 10.9 | 13.1 | 15.9 | |
| Other, % | 8.3 | 9.8 | 8.6 | | 10.9 | 7.3 | 9.4 | |
| Age | | | | | | | | |
| 2–3 y, % | 9.6 | 8.9 | 6.7 | 0.003 | 5.3 | 8.9 | 11.0 | < 0.001 |
| 4–8 y, % | 25.8 | 26.6 | 26.8 | | 18.6 | 30.0 | 30.4 | |
| 9–13 y, % | 34.6 | 29.4 | 25.8 | | 27.3 | 30.7 | 31.8 | |
| 14–19 y, % | 30.1 | 35.1 | 40.6 | | 48.8 | 30.4 | 26.8 | |
| Poverty income ratio[e] | | | | | | | | |
| < 1.0, % | 16.7 | 19.6 | 28.4 | < 0.001 | 20.4 | 20.0 | 24.3 | 0.001 |
| 1.0–2.5, % | 33.0 | 31.9 | 32.0 | | 32.5 | 29.8 | 34.7 | |
| ≥2.5, % | 48.1 | 44.7 | 37.2 | | 42.3 | 48.2 | 39.3 | |
| Not reported, % | 2.1 | 3.8 | 2.4 | | 4.8 | 2.0 | 1.6 | |
| Season of Examination[f] | | | | | | | | |
| Fall/Winter, % | 40.2 | 39.6 | 36.8 | 0.693 | 39.0 | 36.3 | 41.4 | 0.395 |
| Spring/Summer, % | 59.8 | 60.4 | 63.2 | | 61.0 | 63.7 | 58.6 | |
| Use of Supplements[g] | | | | | | | | |
| Yes, % | 38.4 | 35.3 | 28.5 | 0.003 | 27.0 | 36.4 | 38.9 | < 0.001 |
| No, % | 61.6 | 64.7 | 71.5 | | 73.0 | 63.6 | 61.1 | |
| Body mass index | | | | | | | | |
| <85th percentile, % | 86.0 | 84.0 | 84.5 | 0.610 | 81.8 | 86.2 | 86.4 | 0.028 |
| ≥85th percentile, % | 14.0 | 16.0 | 15.5 | | 18.2 | 13.8 | 13.6 | |
| Daily screen viewing[h] | | | | | | | | |
| ≤2 h, % | 59.8 | 48.4 | 41.6 | < 0.001 | 42.7 | 51.6 | 55.4 | < 0.001 |
| 3–4 h, % | 25.1 | 28.8 | 31.5 | | 30.2 | 27.8 | 27.4 | |
| > 4 h, % | 15.2 | 22.8 | 26.9 | | 27.0 | 20.6 | 17.3 | |

[a] $n = 4404$; weighted $n = 60{,}274{,}698$. NHANES 2003–2004 and 2005–2006 were combined into one master database, NHANES 2003–2006
[b] Dietary pattern scores were stratified into tertiles (low, medium, and high) based on factor scores for each dietary pattern
[c] High-Fat-Low-Vegetable Dietary pattern or Prudent Dietary pattern
[d] Significance determined by Rao-Scott chi-square test
[e] Ratio of income to the family's appropriate poverty threshold. A ratio of < 1.0 is characterized as below poverty
[f] Data collected during May 1–October 31 (spring/summer) and November 1–April 30 (fall/winter)
[g] Participants who took supplements 30 days before survey was conducted
[h] Data collected on the combined hours of television, computer, and video games usage per day

boys and girls, only girls showed significant relation with serum 25(OH)D concentrations for both dietary pattern scores. Girls with higher HFLVD contribution scores showed a significant negative relation ($\beta = -193$; $P < 0.001$) and girls with higher PD contribution scores showed a significant positive association to serum 25(OH)D concentrations ($\beta = 79.8$; $P = 0.035$).

In the adjusted multivariate regression analysis, all subjects with higher PD contribution scores to overall diet showed a significant positive relation with serum

**Table 4** Relation of serum 25(OH)D concentrations with dietary pattern scores: National Health and Nutrition Examination Survey (NHANES) 2003-2006[a,b]

| | HFLVD Pattern Score ($n = 4404$)[c, d] | | | | PD Pattern Score ($n = 4404$)[c, d] | | | |
|---|---|---|---|---|---|---|---|---|
| | Low (<− 0.003875) | Medium (− 0.003875 to 0.000925) | High (> 0.000925) | P- value[e] | Low (< 0.004175) | Medium (− 0.004175 to 0.001912) | High (> 0.001912) | P- value[e] |
| | ng/mL | ng/mL | ng/mL | | ng/mL | ng/mL | ng/mL | |
| Unadjusted analysis | | | | | | | | |
| All subjects ($n = 4404$) | 27.3 ± 0.5 | 26.1 ± 0.6 | 24.8 ± 0.7 | 0.003 | 24.7 ± 0.7 | 26.8 ± 0.5 | 26.7 ± 0.6 | 0.012 |
| Boys ($n = 2154$) | 27.4 ± 0.6 | 26.8 ± 0.7 | 25.8 ± 0.8 | 0.123 | 25.8 ± 0.7 | 26.9 ± 0.7 | 27.3 ± 0.7 | 0.151 |
| Girls ($n = 2250$) | 27.2 ± 0.7 | 25.2 ± 0.8 | 23.6 ± 0.8 | 0.003 | 23.6 ± 0.9 | 26.6 ± 0.6 | 26.1 ± 0.7 | 0.005 |
| Adjusted analysis | | | | | | | | |
| All subjects ($n = 4404$)[f] | 22.1 ± 0.4 | 22.1 ± 0.3 | 21.7 ± 0.5 | 0.594 | 21.4 ± 0.5 | 22.1 ± 0.3 | 22.5 ± 0.4 | 0.195 |
| Boys ($n = 2154$)[g] | 22.9 ± 0.5 | 23.3 ± 0.4 | 23.1 ± 0.6 | 0.810 | 23.0 ± 0.5 | 22.9 ± 0.4 | 23.5 ± 0.5 | 0.370 |
| Girls ($n = 2250$)[g] | 21.4 ± 0.5 | 20.9 ± 0.5 | 20.4 ± 0.7 | 0.529 | 19.9 ± 0.6 | 21.5 ± 0.5 | 21.5 ± 0.5 | 0.064 |

[a] $n = 4404$; weighted $n = 60{,}274{,}698$. NHANES 2003–2004 and 2005–2006 were combined into one master database, NHANES 2003–2006. Regression analysis of dietary patterns scores and serum 25(OH)D concentrations
[b] Dietary pattern scores were stratified into tertiles (low, medium, and high) based on factor scores for each dietary pattern
[c] Mean ± standard error
[d] High-Fat-Low-Vegetable Dietary Pattern or Prudent Dietary Pattern
[e] Significance determined by F-test in analysis of variance for unadjusted analysis and in analysis of covariance for adjusted analysis
[f] Analysis was adjusted for sex, race-ethnicity, age, season of examination, body mass index, and daily screen viewing. Poverty income ratio, supplement use, and energy intake were not found significant in this model and therefore those variables dropped
[g] Analysis was adjusted for race-ethnicity, age, time of examination, body mass index, and daily screen viewing. Poverty income ratio, supplement use, and energy intake were not found significant in this model and therefore these variables were dropped

25(OH)D ($\beta = 59.1$; $P = 0.017$). Similarly, when subjects were stratified into boys and girls in the adjusted analysis, only girls showed a significant relation with serum 25(OH)D concentrations for both pattern scores. Girls with higher HFLVD contribution scores showed a significant negative relation ($\beta = -88.5$; $P = 0.016$) and girls with higher PD contribution scores showed a significant positive association ($\beta = 82.1$; $P = 0.015$) to serum 25(OH)D concentrations.

## Discussion

To our knowledge, this is the most comprehensive study that investigated the relation between serum 25(OH)D concentrations and dietary patterns in children and adolescents in a nationally representative sample survey. Using factor analysis, we derived HFLVD and PD patterns. Serum 25(OH)D was significantly lower in HFLVD compared to PD pattern, and the highest serum 25(OH)D concentrations for all subjects were in those with low HFLVD or medium and high-intake PD patterns scores. In the multivariate adjusted analysis, a significant positive relation was found between PD pattern factor scores and serum 25(OH)D concentrations. When data were stratified by sex, a significant positive relation was observed in girls who consumed the PD dietary pattern and a significant negative relation was observed in girls who consumed the HFLVD dietary pattern.

Dietary patterns derived in this study were similar to the dietary patterns reported in the literature on US children [27]. Poti et al. [27] using the NHANES data derived Western and Prudent dietary patterns. Studies relating vitamin D intake with the vitamin D status have shown conflicting results [13, 15, 27]. We found that subjects with high PD pattern scores had significantly higher serum 25(OH) concentrations compared to those with HFLVD pattern scores. In contrast, Polish vegetarian children had 2-fold lower serum 25(OH)D concentrations than in their omnivorous counterparts [28]. While in this study those who consumed the PD pattern were not necessarily vegetarians, they did have higher factor scores for many similar type of foods found in a vegetarian diet and lesser factor scores for foods typical in an omnivorous diet. However Chan et al. [29] found no association between serum 25(OH)D and vegetarian status. Differences between studies may be due to differences in subject characteristics and confounding variables used in the statistical analysis.

The highest serum concentrations for all subjects were found in those with low-intake HFLVD scores or in those with medium- and high-intake PD pattern scores. In this analysis individuals were scored on each pattern, therefore a person's diet would be represented by a combination of both factors. A high factor score from one dietary pattern does not necessarily mean a low factor score from the other dietary pattern for an individual. However, these results seem to suggest that the greatest serum 25(OH)D concentrations occurred in individuals who consumed a healthier type diet that had a higher

**Table 5** Relation of serum 25(OH)D concentrations with dietary pattern scores: National Health and Nutrition Examination Survey (NHANES) 2003-2006[a,b]

| | β[c] | Standardized β | SE for β[d] | P-value[e] |
|---|---|---|---|---|
| Unadjusted analysis | | | | |
| HFLVD Pattern Score[f] | | | | |
| All subjects | −135.6 | −0.13 | 32.3 | < 0.001 |
| Boys | −81.4 | −0.08 | 47.8 | 0.099 |
| Girls | −193.0 | −0.19 | 36.7 | < 0.001 |
| PD Pattern Score[f] | | | | |
| All subjects | 57.12 | 0.06 | 30.8 | 0.073 |
| Boys | 36.13 | 0.04 | 31.8 | 0.265 |
| Girls | 79.75 | 0.08 | 36.1 | 0.035 |
| Adjusted analysis | | | | |
| HFLVD Pattern Score[f] | | | | |
| All subjects[g] | − 39.1 | −0.04 | 26.6 | 0.153 |
| Boys[h] | 17.7 | 0.02 | 36.3 | 0.631 |
| Girls[h] | − 88.5 | −0.09 | 34.6 | 0.016 |
| PD Pattern Score[f] | | | | |
| All subjects[g] | 59.1 | 0.06 | 23.5 | 0.017 |
| Boys[h] | 35.7 | 0.03 | 24.1 | 0.149 |
| Girls[h] | 82.1 | 0.08 | 31.8 | 0.015 |

[a]n = 4404; weighted n = 60,274,698. NHANES 2003–2004 and 2005–2006 were combined into one master database. NHANES 2001–2006
[b]Regression analysis using factor scores as continuous variable and dependent variable, serum 25(OH)D concentrations
[c]Multivariate regression coefficient
[d]Standard error for multivariate regression coefficient
[e]Significance between dietary patterns and serum 25(OH)D in the regression model
[f]High-Fat-Low-Vegetable Dietary pattern or Prudent Dietary pattern
[g]Analysis was adjusted for sex, race-ethnicity, age, season of examination, body mass index, and daily screen viewing. Poverty income ratio, supplement use, and energy intake were not found significant in this model, therefore those variables were dropped from the analysis
[h]Analysis was adjusted for race-ethnicity, age, season of examination, body mass index, and daily sun screen viewing. Poverty income ratio, supplement use, and energy intake were not found significant in this model, therefore those variables were dropped from the analysis

emphasis on vegetables, fruits, and some emphasis on mixed dishes, fish, and meats. The differences seen in serum 25(OH)D concentrations may be due to the factors other than diet; because when the analysis was adjusted for confounding variables, the association between serum 25(OH)D concentrations and dietary patterns was no longer present. This was seen in other studies such that other factors such as race, season, and sun exposure were more significant predictors of serum 25(OH)D concentrations than dietary intake [30, 31].

The higher serum 25(OH)D concentrations in those who adhere more closely to a PD pattern may be related to certain lifestyle and health-related factors. In this study, we found that children with high PD pattern scores had consumed more supplements compared to this with high HFLVD pattern scores. Consumption of dietary supplements has been associated with an increase of serum 25(OH)D concentration [32]. Children who consumed vitamin D supplements were less likely to be vitamin D deficient [9]. Additionally, it has been suggested that the bioavailability of vitamin D may be low in those who are overweight or obese because of excessive sequestering of vitamin D in adipose tissue [33]. Gordon et al. [12] found that a higher BMI and being African American was associated with decreased serum 25(OH)D. Similarly, we found that subjects with high HFLVD pattern scores were tend to be overweight or obese and NHB. This could be a possible explanation of the lower serum 25(OH)D concentrations in those who adhered more closely to the HFLVD pattern. Furthermore, greater indoor activity measured by hours spent watching television, using computers, or playing video games has also been found to be a factor associated with lower 25(OH)D concentrations [9]. In the present study, there was a greater proportion of children who had ≤2 h/d of screen viewing time had higher PD pattern scores compared to those with high HFLVD pattern score suggesting decreased overall screen viewing time is an important factor for the increased serum 25(OH)D concentrations in those who adhere to a PD.

Furthermore, the relation of serum 25(OH)D with both dietary patterns remained for girls only in the adjusted analysis. Nanri et al. [34] found higher serum 25(OH)D concentrations in women who had higher fish/shellfish consumption and lower BMI. They proposed the difference may be related to body composition of females compared to males. Because women generally have higher fat mass than men and vitamin D is fat-soluble, this could result in higher amounts being stored in the fat tissue of females and lower serum vitamin D concentrations. This could be a possible explanation for why in the present study we have observed girls who adhere most closely to the HFLVD pattern have significantly lower serum vitamin D concentrations.

The present study has several strengths that included a nationally representative survey with a large sample size of children and adolescents. Because of a wide range of data are available on demographic characteristics, dietary information, and other health-related factors, we were able to adjust serum 25(OH)D concentrations for several known confounding variables. Results in this study can be interpreted towards the general US children and adolescents population because NHANES is based on a probability sample survey design and is representative of the US population. Because of cross-sectional nature of this study, cause and effect measurement is not possible. In addition, dietary intakes of children estimated by a FFQ may be underreported due to subjects' inability to recall intakes accurately [35].

The errors in reporting food intakes may be minimal because the FFQ used in NHANES had been previously tested and validated by the National Cancer Institute.

## Conclusions

Overall, serum 25(OH)D concentration was associated with the PD pattern but not with the HFLVD pattern in US children and adolescents. When stratified by sex, the relation between dietary patterns and serum 25(OH)D was confined to only girls. Although vitamin D status has improved slightly recently, the hypovitaminosis D is still evident in US children and adolescents [36]. Because of hypovitaminosis D is linked to several chronic diseases [3–5], it is prudent to improve the vitamin D status of children to reduce the future risk for chronic diseases. In public health perspective, it is important to encourage children, especially girls who are consuming HFLVD pattern to shift to healthier diet.

#### Abbreviations

25(OH)D: 25-hydroxyvitamin D; ANCOVA: Analysis of Covariance; BMI: Body mass index; FFQ: Food frequency questionnaire; H/MA: Hispanic/Mexican American; HFLVD: High Fat-Low-Vegetable Dietary Pattern; MEC: Mobile Examination Centers; NCHS: National Center for Health Statistics; NHANES: National Health and Nutrition Examination Survey; NHB: non-Hispanic black; NHW: non-Hispanic white; PD: Prudent Dietary Pattern; PIR: Poverty Income Ratio; SE: Standard error; T2DM: type-2 diabetes mellitus

#### Authors' contributions

All authors substantially contributed to the conception, design, acquisition of data, analysis, and interpretation of results. VG and BM wrote the manuscript. WEVF was in charge of data management and data analysis. All authors reviewed, revised, and edited the manuscript. All authors read and approved the final manuscript.

#### Competing interests

The authors declare that they have no competing interests.

#### Author details

[1]Human Nutrition Department, College of Health Sciences, Qatar University, Doha, Qatar. [2]Children Healthcare of Atlanta, Emory University, Atlanta, GA, USA. [3]Georgia State University, Atlanta, GA, USA.

#### References

1. Pozzilli P, Manfrini S, Crinò A, Picardi A, Leomanni C, Cherubini V, et al. Low levels of 25-hydroxyvitamin D3 and 1,25-dihydroxyvitamin D3 in patients with newly diagnosed type 1 diabetes. Horm Metab Res. 2005;37:680–3.
2. Munger KL, Levin LI, Hollis BW, Howard NS, Ascherio A. Serum 25-hydroxyvitamin D levels and risk of multiple sclerosis. JAMA. 2006;296:2832–8.
3. Reis JP, von Mühlen D, Miller ER 3rd, Michos ED, Appel LJ. Vitamin D status and cardiometabolic risk factors in the United States adolescent population. Pediatrics. 2009;124:e371–9.
4. Ganji V, Zhang X, Shaikh N, Tangpricha V. Serum 25-hydroxyvitamin D concentrations are associated with prevalence of metabolic syndrome and various cardiometabolic risk factors in US children and adolescents based on assay-adjusted serum 25-hydroxyvitamin D data from NHANES 2001-2006. Am J Clin Nutr. 2011;94:225–33.
5. Nunlee-Bland G, Gambhir K, Abrams C, Abdul M, Vahedi M, Odonkor W. Vitamin D deficiency and insulin resistance in obese African-American adolescents. J Pediatr Endocrinol Metab. 2011;24:29–33.
6. Ganji V, Milone C, Cody MM, McCarty F, Wang YT. Serum vitamin D concentrations are related to depression in young adult US population: the third National Health and nutrition examination survey. Int Arch Med. 2010;3:29.
7. Sinha A, Avery P, Turner S, Bailey S, Cheetham T. Vitamin D status in paediatric patients with cancer. Pediatr Blood Cancer. 2011;57:594–8.
8. Holick MF. Vitamin D deficiency. N Engl J Med. 2007;357:266–81.
9. Kumar J, Muntner P, Kaskel FJ, Hailpern SM, Melamed ML. Prevalence and associations of 25-hydroxyvitamin D deficiency in US children: NHANES 2001-2004. Pediatrics. 2009;124:e362–70.
10. Mansbach JM, Ginde AA, Camargo CA Jr. Serum 25-hydroxyvitamin D levels among US children aged 1 to 11 years: do children need more vitamin D? Pediatrics. 2009;124:1404–10.
11. Saintonge S, Bang H, Gerber LM. Implications of a new definition of vitamin D deficiency in a multiracial us adolescent population: the National Health and nutrition examination survey III. Pediatrics. 2009;123:797–803.
12. Gordon CM, DePeter KC, Feldman HA, Grace E, Emans SJ. Prevalence of vitamin D deficiency among healthy adolescents. Arch Pediatr Adolesc Med. 2004;158:531–7.
13. Houghton LA, Gray AR, Szymlek-Gay EA, Heath A-LM. Ferguson EL vitamin D-fortified milk achieves the targeted serum 25-hydroxyvitamin D concentration without affecting that of parathyroid hormone in New Zealand toddlers. J Nutr. 2011;141:1840–6.
14. Xu C, Perera RA, Chan YH, Fang VJ, Ng S, Ip DK, et al. Determinants of serum 25-hydroxyvitamin D in Hong Kong. Br J Nutr. 2015;114:144–51.
15. Cole CR, Grant FK, Tangpricha V, Swaby-Ellis ED, Smith JL, Jacques A, et al. 25-hydroxyvitamin D status of healthy, low-income, minority children in Atlanta. Georgia Pediatrics. 2010;125:633–9.
16. Lehmann B, Meurer M. Vitamin D metabolism. Dermatol Ther. 2010;23:2–12.
17. American Academy of Pediatrics. Ultraviolet light: a hazard to children. American Academy of Pediatrics. Committee on Environmental Health. Pediatrics. 1999;104:328–33.
18. Misra M, Pacaud D, Petryk A, Collett-Solberg PF, Kappy M. Drug and therapeutics Committee of the Lawson Wilkins Pediatric Endocrine Society. Vitamin D deficiency in children and its management: review of current knowledge and recommendations. Pediatrics. 2008;122:398–417.
19. Kerver JM, Yang EJ, Bianchi L, Song WO. Dietary patterns associated with risk factors for cardiovascular disease in healthy US adults. Am J Clin Nutr. 2003;78:1103–10.
20. National Center for Health Statistics. National Health and Nutrition Examination Survey Analytic and Reporting Guidelines (2018) http://www.cdc.gov/nchs/data/nhanes/nhanes_03_04/nhanes_analytic_guidelines_dec_2005 pdf (accessed April 2018).
21. National Center for Health Statistics. National Health and Nutrition Examination Survey- Survey Brochures and Consent Documents (2018) https://wwwn.cdc.gov/nchs/nhanes/continuousnhanes/documents.aspx?BeginYear=2003 (accessed April 2018).
22. National Center for Health Statistics. National Health and Nutrition Examination Survey Laboratory Protocol 2003–2004 (2018) https://wwwn.cdc.gov/nchs/nhanes/continuousnhanes/labmethods.aspx?BeginYear=2003 (accessed February 2018).
23. National Center for Health Statistics. National Health and Nutrition Examination Survey Laboratory Protocol 2004–2006 (2018) https://wwwn.cdc.gov/nchs/nhanes/continuousnhanes/labmethods.aspx?BeginYear=2005 (accessed February 2018).
24. National Center for Health Statistics. Analytical Note for 25-Hydroxyvitamin D Data Analysis using NHANES III (1988-1994), NHANES 2001–2006, and NHANES 2007–2010 (2018) https://wwwn.cdc.gov/nchs/nhanes/vitamind/analyticalnote.aspx?h=/Nchs/Nhanes/2005-2006/VID_D.htm&t=VID_D%20Doc (accessed April 2018).
25. Hu FB, Rimm E, Smith-Warner SA, Feskanich D, Stampfer MJ, Ascherio A, et al. Reproducibility and validity of dietary patterns assessed with a food-frequency questionnaire. Am J Clin Nutr. 1999;69:243–9.

26. Ganji V, Zhang X, Tangpricha V. Serum 25-hydroxyvitamin D concentrations and prevalence estimates of hypovitaminosis D in the U.S. population based on assay-adjusted data. J Nutr. 2012;142:498–507.
27. Poti JM, Duffey KJ, Popkin BM. The association of fast food consumption with poor dietary outcomes and obesity among children: is it the fast food or the remainder of the diet? Am J Clin Nutr. 2014;99:162–71.
28. Ambroszkiewicz J, Klemarczyk W, Gajewska J, Chełchowska M, Laskowska-Klita T. Serum concentration of biochemical bone turnover markers in vegetarian children. Adv Med Sci. 2007;52:279–82.
29. Chan J, Jaceldo-Siegl K, Fraser GE. Serum 25-hydroxyvitamin D status of vegetarians, partial vegetarians, and nonvegetarians: the Adventist health Study-2. Am J Clin Nutr. 2009;89:1686S–92S.
30. Rajakumar K, Holick MF, Jeong K, Moore CG, Chen TC, Olabopo F, et al. Impact of season and diet on vitamin D status of African American and Caucasian children. Clin Pediatr (Phila). 2011;50:493–502.
31. Hall LM, Kimlin MG, Aronov PA, Hammock BD, Slusser JR, Woodhouse LR, et al. Vitamin D intake needed to maintain target serum 25-hydroxyvitamin D concentrations in participants with low sun exposure and dark skin pigmentation is substantially higher than current recommendations. J Nutr. 2010;140:542–50.
32. Burgaz A, Akesson A, Oster A, Michaëlsson K, Wolk A. Associations of diet, supplement use, and ultraviolet B radiation exposure with vitamin D status in Swedish women during winter. Am J Clin Nutr. 2007;86:1399–404.
33. Smotkin-Tangorra M, Purushothaman R, Gupta A, Nejati G, Anhalt H, Ten S. Prevalence of vitamin D insufficiency in obese children and adolescents. J Pediatr Endocrinol Metab. 2007;20:817–23.
34. Nanri A, Foo LH, Nakamura K, Hori A, Poudel-Tandukar K, Matsushita Y, et al. Serum 25-hydroxyvitamin D concentrations and season-specific correlates in Japanese adults. J Epidemiol. 2011;21:346–53.
35. Schaefer EJ, Augustin JL, Schaefer MM, Rasmussen H, Ordovas JM, Dallal GE, et al. Lack of efficacy of a food-frequency questionnaire in assessing dietary macronutrient intakes in subjects consuming diets of known composition. Am J Clin Nutr. 2000;71:746–51.
36. Schleicher RL, Sternberg MR, Lacher DA, Sempos CT, Looker AC, Durazo-Arvizu RA, et al. The vitamin D status of the US population from 1988 to 2010 using standardized serum concentrations of 25-hydroxyvitamin D shows recent modest increases. Am J Clin Nutr. 2016;104:454–61.

# 5

# Adaptation and validation of a food frequency questionnaire (FFQ) to assess dietary intake in Moroccan adults

Khaoula El Kinany[1,2], Vanessa Garcia-Larsen[3,4*], Mohamed Khalis[1], Meimouna Mint Sidi Deoula[1], Abdelilah Benslimane[1], Amran Ibrahim[1], Mohamed Chakib Benjelloun[5] and Karima El Rhazi[1]

**Abstract**

**Background:** To date, no culture-specific food frequency questionnaires (FFQ) are available in North Africa. The aim of this study was to adapt and examine the reproducibility and validity of an FFQ or use in the Moroccan population.

**Methods:** The European Global Asthma and Allergy Network (GA$^2$LEN) FFQ was used to assess its applicability in Morocco. The GA$^2$LEN FFQ is comprised of 32 food sections and 200 food items. Using scientific published literature, as well as local resources, we identified and added foods that were representative of the Moroccan diet. Translation of the FFQ into Moroccan Arabic was carried out following the World Health Organization (WHO) standard operational procedure. To test the validity and the reproducibility of the FFQ, 105 healthy adults working at Hassan II University Hospital Center of Fez were invited to answer the adapted FFQ in two occasions, 1 month apart, and to complete three 24-h dietary recall questionnaires during this period. Pearson correlation, and Bland-Altman plots were used to assess validity of nutrient intakes. The reproducibility between nutrient intakes as reported from the first and second FFQ were calculated using intra-class correlation coefficient (ICC). All nutrients were log-transformed to improve normality and were adjusted using the residual method.

**Results:** The adapted FFQ was comprised of 255 items that included traditional Moroccan foods. Eighty-seven adults (mean age 27.3 ± 5.7 years) completed all the questionnaires. For energy and nutrients, the intakes reported in the FFQ1 were higher than the mean intakes reported by the 24-h recall questionnaires. The Pearson correlation coefficients between the first FFQ and the mean of three 24-h recall questionnaires were statistically significant. For validity, de-attenuated correlations were all positive, statistically significant and ranging from 0.24 (fiber) to 0.93 (total MUFA). For reproducibility, the ICCs were statistically significant and ranged between 0.69 for fat and 0.84 for Vitamin A.

**Conclusion:** This adapted FFQ is an acceptable tool to assess usual dietary intake in Moroccan adults. Given its representativeness of local food intake, it can be used as an instrument to investigate the role of diet on health and disease outcomes.

**Keywords:** Food frequency questionnaire, Morocco, North Africa, Validity, Reproducibility, Diet, GA$^2$LEN

* Correspondence: vgla@jhu.edu
[3]Department of International Health, The Johns Hopkins Bloomberg School of Public Health, Baltimore, USA
[4]Population Health and Occupational Disease, NHLI, Imperial College London, London, UK
Full list of author information is available at the end of the article

## Background

The burden of chronic non-communicable diseases (NCD) in African countries continues to rise [1]. The epidemiological profile of North Africa increasingly mirrors that of more developed societies, where cancer, cardiovascular, and respiratory diseases represent a major societal and health burden. Prevalence of these, and other NCDs related to diet, has continuously increased in the last two decades [2–4], but there is scant scientific evidence on the role of dietary habits on disease risk and prevalence in the Moroccan population [5, 6].

Food frequency questionnaires (FFQs) are a helpful instrument to ascertain usual dietary intake and its relationship with health and disease outcomes [7, 8]. Although FFQs are widely used in Europe and America [9, 10], nutritional epidemiology in Morocco remains hindered by the lack of locally representative dietary questionnaires, particularly FFQs. We are only aware of one FFQ recently developed to ascertain usual fruit and vegetable intake in Moroccan adults [11]. To date, the vast majority of what we know about dietary habits and chronic disease in this country relates to their association with Ramadan and obesity [2, 12].

The rapid socio-economic transition in North Africa has been accompanied by changes in the way the population eat, which are not easily captured with dietary questionnaires from, for example, high income countries. Morocco is a fast-growing developing country with a diet characterised by intake of vegetable-based dish, spices, and meat [11–13], and a rich combination of very traditional dishes with a more modern cuisine. Having FFQs that reflect such transitions and cultural features are urgently needed to identify regionally and locally relevant dietary risk factors for health and disease outcomes. To implement these FFQs, the validity and reproducibility of the instrument needs to be assessed [14, 15].

Our study was aimed at adapting the international GA$^2$LEN FFQ to include staple foods consumed in Morocco, and at validating it in a sample of health Moroccan adults.

## Methods

### Participants

One hundred five adults working at Hassan II University Hospital Center of Fez were invited to answer the three 24-Hour Recall and the FFQ in two occasions. Eligibility to take part in the study was defined as having a regular diet over the previous 12 months and not have used any medications known to affect food intake or appetite during this period. The subjects had a stable weight. Data collection was conducted over a period of 4 months (July to October) in 2009.

### FFQ adaptation

The Global Asthma and Allergy Network (GA$^2$LEN) FFQ was adapted to reflect the Moroccan diet. The GA$^2$LEN FFQ was designed to be used as a single, common instrument to assess dietary intake across Europe [9]. It was initially piloted and validated in five European countries, and it has been subsequently used in several multi-national studies including high and low income countries [16].

To adapt the GA$^2$LEN FFQ to the Moroccan diet we compiled information published in the scientific literature on usual foods commonly consumed in Morocco and these were added to each section. In order to retain its international comparability, several food items from the original GA$^2$LEN FFQ were kept in each of the sections even though they were not necessarily relevant to the Moroccan diet (e.g. pork or alcohol intake).

The Standard Operational Procedure (SOP) of the World Health Organization [17] was followed for the forward and back translations from English to Moroccan Arabic. A first translation from English into Moroccan Arabic (*version 1*) was carried out by a bilingual person. This version was then tested amongst five people from the respiratory unit of the University Hospital of Fez. Doubts and difficulties in answering the questions were investigated and after this initial assessment, a second Arabic version was produced (*version 2*). To improve the identification of foods relevant to the Moroccan population, the research team in Fez also visited several local markets and supermarkets to identify common brand names and foods that could be relevant and were added accordingly, adding up to a total of 255 food items in the FFQ (Table 1). Subsequent back-translation into English was performed by another translator with a good knowledge of English but who had not seen the FFQ before. A final draft of the FFQ (*version 3*) was agreed in Moroccan Arabic and English (Table 1).

Each food item in the FFQ was assigned a portion size using standard local household units such as plate, bowl, spoons of different size (tablespoon, teaspoon), tea-pot, tea-glass, and glass of water, as well as using photographs from a booklet ('Food and typical preparations of the Moroccan population' [14].

Frequency of dietary intake reported in the FFQ was estimated by selecting one of eight categories: never, once to three times per month, once a week, twice to four per week, five to six times per week, once per day, twice to three times, more than four times.

### Validation of the FFQ

The FFQ was validated against the average of three 24-h recall questionnaires over a period of 1 month (Fig. 1). Participants were first asked to answer a 24-h recall questionnaire, where they reported all the foods and beverages consumed the day before, providing

**Table 1** Foods included in FFQ for Morocco

| Name |
|---|
| 1-Bread |
| Any type of bread |
| Bread, whole meal, average (Durum Wheat) |
| Bread, white, French stick |
| Bread of zouane (Rye) |
| Mllaoui/rghaif/mssemen/batbout/matlouaa |
| Bread of smida/harcha (Semolina) |
| Homemade bread |
| Other type of bread (barley) |
| 2-Breakfast with grains |
| Any type of grains |
| Assida/Smida |
| Dchicha/belboula |
| Porridge (herbel), mflak |
| All-Bran |
| Corn Flakes |
| 3-Couscous |
| Barley Couscous, cooked with meat, vegetables and dried grape |
| Barley Couscous, cooked with sugar and cinnamon |
| Wheat Couscous, cooked with meat, vegetables and dried grape |
| Wheat Couscous, cooked with sugar and cinnamon |
| Corn Couscous, cooked with meat, vegetables and dried grape |
| Corn Couscous, cooked with sugar and cinnamon |
| 4-Pasta |
| Any type of Pasta |
| Pasta white boiled (Spaghetti, Macaroni) |
| Pasta, whole meal, boiled |
| Pasta with meat vegetables and cheese |
| Chaaria Mhammsa |
| 5-Cake |
| Any type of cake, cherry |
| Madeleine cake |
| Cake with date |
| Croissants |
| Moroccan swetees |
| Basboussa Maqrout |
| Aassida |
| Doughnuts, ring |
| Rice pudding, canned |
| Pancake roll |
| Cake, coconut |
| Sellou Zammita |
| Chabbakia Mkharrka |
| 6-Rice |

**Table 1** Foods included in FFQ for Morocco *(Continued)*

| Name |
|---|
| Any type of rice, brown, boiled |
| Rice, white, easy cook, boiled |
| Rice, brown, boiled |
| Noodles, rice, dried |
| 7-Sugar |
| Sugar, white |
| Jam, fruit spread |
| Honey |
| Syrup, golden |
| 8-Sweets without chocolate |
| Chew sweets |
| Fudge |
| Toffees |
| Cereal chewy bar |
| Polo skimo glace |
| 9-Chocolate |
| Any type of chocolate |
| Chocolate covered bar with fruit/nut/bix |
| Natural white and black chocolate |
| 10-Vegetable oil |
| Oil, vegetable, blended, average |
| Oil, safflower |
| Oil, olive |
| Oil, Argan |
| Oil, corn |
| 11-Margarine and vegetable fat |
| Any margarine and vegetable fat, (except soya fat) |
| Light margarine or less fat (30% fat) |
| Margarine (from 40 to 60% fat) |
| Normal margarine (more than 70% fat) |
| Mixed fat (except soya) |
| Original fat of soya (any type) |
| 12-Butter and animals fat |
| Any animal fat (butter) |
| Butter with less fat (40% less fat) |
| Butter with less fat (from 40 to 60% fat) |
| Smen (traditional butter) |
| 13-Nuts |
| Any type of dried Fruit |
| Peanuts, plain |
| Cashew nuts, roasted & salted |
| Almonds toasted |
| Walnuts |
| Pistachio nuts, roasted & salted |

**Table 1** Foods included in FFQ for Morocco *(Continued)*

| Name |
|---|
| Chestnuts |
| Oak nut |
| 14-Legumes |
| Any legumes |
| white beans, boiled |
| Lentils, red, split, boiled |
| Chick peas, whole, dried, boiled unsal |
| Green beans/French beans, raw |
| Broad beans, frozen, boiled in unsalted |
| Soya beans, dried, boiled |
| Peas, raw |
| 15-Vegetables (mean dish) |
| Any vegetables except potatoes |
| Lettuce, average, raw |
| Spinach, raw |
| Fenugreek seeds |
| Rejla; Bakkoula |
| Mloukhia (jews Mallow) |
| Tomatoes, raw |
| Aubergine, raw (Eggplant) |
| Courgette, raw (squash) |
| Peppers, red, raw, yellow |
| Cucumber, raw |
| Carrots, raw |
| Parsnip, raw |
| Swede, raw |
| Artichoke globe, raw |
| Radish, white, mooli, raw |
| Beetroot, raw |
| Chilli peppers, green, raw |
| Sweet corn Kernels, raw |
| Asparagus, raw |
| Aromatic herbs (Mint basilica, parsley basil coriander) |
| Leeks, raw |
| Mushrooms, black, white |
| Onions, raw |
| Garlic, raw |
| Cauliflower, raw |
| Pumpkin red |
| Brussels sprouts, raw |
| Broccoli, green, raw |
| Cabbage white, red, green |
| Tomatoes stuffed with vegetables |
| Pickle, mixed veg |
| Ginger, root |
| 16-Potatoes (mean dish) |
| Any type of potatoes |
| Potatoes, old mashed with hard marg |
| Potatoes, old, baked, flesh & skin |
| Chips, homemade, fried in blended oil |
| Salad, potato with French dressing |
| Potato cakes fried in veg oil |
| Tortillas |
| Sweet potato |
| 17-Fruits (one unit) |
| Any type of fruits |
| Apples |
| Pears |
| Bananas |
| Peaches |
| Avocado |
| Cherries |
| Lemon pickles |
| Mulberries, raw, Blackcurrants, Raspberries |
| Watermelon |
| Grapes |
| Mangoes |
| Apricots |
| Nectarines |
| Plums |
| Dried mixed fruit |
| Pineapple |
| Kiwi Fruit |
| Juice, lemon |
| Oranges |
| Mandarine |
| Grapefruit |
| Fruit cocktail, conserved in syrup |
| Figs, raw, dried |
| Black or green olives |
| Raisins |
| Dates, dried with stones |
| 18-Juice |
| Orange juice (concentrate) |
| Pomegranate juice (pomegranate, raw) |
| Any other type of juice |
| 19-Non-alcoholic beverages |
| Lemonade |

**Table 1** Foods included in FFQ for Morocco *(Continued)*

| Name |
|---|
| Beet juice |
| Mineral water |
| 20-Coffee/Tea |
| Tea, infusion |
| Coffee, instant, made up |
| Zizwa (coffee, liquid) |
| Tea, Chinese, leaves, infusion |
| Mint, fresh |
| Other herbal infusions |
| 21-Beer |
| Any type of beer |
| 22-Wine |
| Any type of wine |
| Wine, red |
| Wine, white, dry |
| Wine, rose |
| 23- Other-alcoholic beverages |
| Port, sherry, liqueur, |
| Spirits 37.5% |
| 24-Red meat |
| Any type of red meat (beef, cow, lamb, goat) |
| Beef, fillet steak, forerib, lean & fat, roast, steamed, grilled |
| Beef in tagine |
| Minced meat of beef |
| Lamb, grilled, steamed, roasted |
| Lamb cooked in tagine, Mrouzia |
| Minced meat of lamb |
| Goat meat |
| Veal, fillet, roast |
| Camel meat |
| Rabbit, Duck, partridge |
| Sausage of beef, lamb, cow, chilled, fried |
| kocha or bread filled with meat |
| Kabab, chawarma |
| Pork |
| Khliaa/Dried meat |
| Khliaa (dried meat with salt and cooked with fat), cow |
| Khliaa (dried meat with salt and cooked with fat), sheep |
| Qaddid (dried meat with salt), cow, sheep |
| Dried pork meat |
| 25-Poultry |
| Any type of chicken |
| Chicken steamed |
| Chicken cooked in tagine |
| Chicken grilled and roasted |
| Turkey steamed |
| Turkey cooked in tagine |
| Turkey grilled and roasted |
| Sausage and skewer of turkey |
| Poultry smoked, conserved |
| Any poultry smoked, conserved (e.g. mortadella, casheer) |
| 26-Offal (sekat) |
| Liver of beef, lamb |
| Tongue, heart, kidney, head, brain, of cow or beef or sheep, lamb |
| 27-Fish |
| Any fish fresh, smoked, white, fat |
| Fresh fat fish (e.g. salamon, tuna, truite, sardine, bouri) |
| White fresh fish (e.g. sole, merlan) |
| Fresh fish / other sea foods (eggs of fish) |
| Seafood shrimp, squid, mussels |
| Frozen seafood |
| Frozen fat fish (e.g. salamon, tuna, truite, sardine, bouri) |
| Frozen white fish (e.g. sole, merlan) |
| Conserved fat fish (e.g. salamon, tuna, truite, sardine, bouri) |
| Fat fish dried or smoked (e.g. salamon, tuna, truite, sardine, bouri) |
| White fish dried or smoked (e.g. sole, merlan) |
| Conserved seafood shrimp, squid, mussels |
| 28-Eggs |
| Farmer eggs |
| Farmer egg boiled or sandwich |
| Farmer eggs's meals: Omlet, eggs with tomatos, eggs with pepper and tomatos |
| Dessert with Farmer eggs (Cake, egg tart) |
| Industrial eggs |
| Industrial egg boiled or sandwich |
| Industrial egg's meals: Omlet, eggs with tomatos, eggs with pepper and tomatos |
| Dessert with Industrial eggs (Cake, egg tart) |
| 29-Milk of cow/Milk of soya |
| Whole milk (milk,cow,whole,3,5%fat) |
| Lben (alone or with fruit) |
| Skimmed milk (Milk, cow, skimmed, 0,5% fat) |
| Semi skimmed milk (Milk, cow, partly skimmed, 1.5% fat) |
| Milk free fat |
| Raib |
| Soya milk |
| Saykook |
| Yaourt |
| Yaourt Activia |

**Table 1** Foods included in FFQ for Morocco *(Continued)*

| Name |
|---|
| Soya yaourt |
| 30-Cheese |
| Any type of cheese |
| Hard cheese (e.g. Cheddar, Parmesan) |
| Soft cheese (Camembert, Brie, Philadelphia) |
| Semi hard Cheese (Gouda, Emmental/Edam) |
| Jben (Natural or aromatic) |
| Fresh cheese (e.g. Vita, Mozarelle) |
| Others: La vache qui rit, Kiri, Coeur du lait, Junior |
| 31-Other dairy products |
| Ice cream |
| Cream |
| Fresh cream |
| Double cream |
| 32- Miscellaneous foods |
| Soup with vegetables and meat |
| Soup with vegetables and grains (e.g. Dchicha, Smida) |
| Soup with meat or offal |
| Soup with fish |
| Tagine with meat or poultry |
| Salt brik |
| Pizza |
| Sorghum |
| Chilli sauce |
| Ketchup |
| Salad sauce |
| Mayonnaise |
| Mustard |

qualitative (e.g. type of food) and quantitative (e.g. portions) details. Each of the three 24-h recall questionnaires was administered 10 days apart, on two working days and 1 week-end day. The recalled food items were assigned to the food groups of the adapted FFQ.

The FFQ was completed in two occasions, a month apart, a day after participants completed the first and last 24-h recall questionnaires.

### Nutritional composition data for Moroccan foods

Available Food Composition Tables from Morocco were used to derive nutrient composition for several traditional dishes and for some modern products [14, 15]. Additional information needed for non-traditional ('modern') foods was obtained from other regional sources of data, namely the Tunisian food composition table [18], the food composition table for African countries (FAO) [19], the French food composition table (CIQUAL) [20] and the United States department of agriculture nutrient database (USDA) [21].

To calculate total energy intake (TEI), macro-, and micro-nutrient intakes, we created a syntax using the SPSS.20 software. First, the amount of servings consumed was estimated using the standard food portion sizes and these were converted into grams per day [14]. For seasonal foods, participants were asked to answer the question based on intake when these foods were available. The daily intake was calculated according to the number of months per year that each seasonal food was available. TEI and nutrient intakes were calculated by multiplying the frequency of consumption of each food item by the content (per 100 g) and by the specified portion, and then adding the contribution from all food items.

### Socio-demographic characteristics

The FFQ had an additional section enquiring about general characteristics namely age, sex, educational level, and occupation. To estimate body mass index (BMI), height and weight were measured using a calibrated equipment (stadiometer and weighing scale, respectively) and BMI was derived using the formula weight (kg) divided by height$^2$ ($m^2$).

### Statistical analyses

Descriptive results were expressed as means standard deviations, or as percentages and frequencies for continuous and qualitative variables, respectively.

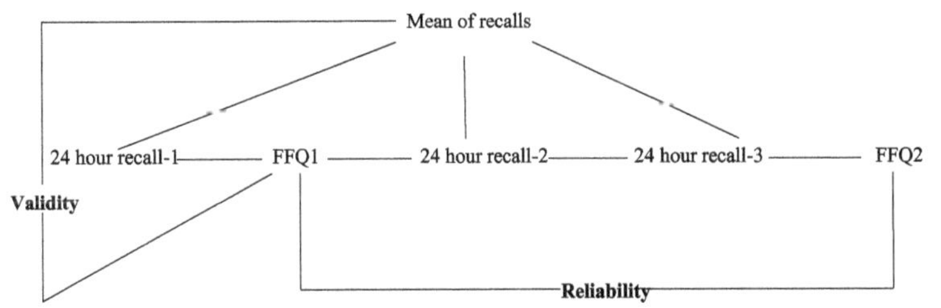


**Fig. 1** Schematic representation of the study aiming to test the relative validity and reliability of the Moroccan Food Frequency Questionnaire against 24-hour recalls

The mean daily intake of the three 24-h recall questionnaires was used as a representative average of the consumption reported in these questionnaires. Descriptive means and standard deviations of nutrient intakes estimated by the FFQ the first and second time (FFQ1 and, FFQ2), and the average of the three 24-h recall questionnaires are presented as untransformed values. As nutrient variables were not normally distributed these were log-transformed (log10) to reduce skewness and optimize the normality of the distribution.

Validity of the FFQ1 was compared with the average of three 24-h recall questionnaires using Pearson correlation coefficients. Adjustment correlation coefficients for TEI were calculated using the residual method [22] (with TEI as the independent variable and the nutrient as the dependent variable). Energy adjusted intakes were calculated by adding the mean nutrient intake to the residual derived from the regression analysis. The de-attenuated correlations [23] were calculated to remove the within-person variability found in the 24-h recall questionnaires using the following formula:

$$r_t = r_0\sqrt{1 + r/n}$$

$\mathbf{r_t}$ is the corrected correlation between the energy adjusted nutrient derived from the FFQ and 24-h recall questionnaires, $\mathbf{r_0}$ is the observed correlation, **r** is the ratio of estimated within-person and between- person variation in nutrient intake derived from the three 24-h recall questionnaires, and **n** is the number of replicated recalls ($n = 3$).

Bland–Altman plots [24, 25] were used to assess agreement between the two methods. For this analysis, the average values of FFQ1 and three 24 Hour Recalls ((FFQ1 + Mean 24 HRs)/2) were plotted against the difference in intake between the two methods, and the limits of agreements (mean difference ± 1.96 SD (differences)) were used to show how large the disagreements between the two methods.

For the reproducibility of the FFQ, the agreement between FFQ1 and FFQ2 was assessed by Pearson product-moment correlation coefficients and intra-class correlation coefficients (ICC) of transformed nutrients and energy-adjusted nutrient intakes. Statistical analyses were performed using SPSS 20.0.

### Participant's consent and ethics

All participants were informed about their role in the study and gave formal consent before being interviewed. The study was approved by the Ethics Committee at University of Fez.

## Results

The final version of the adapted FFQ contained 255 foods, which were classified into 32 groups as follows: (1) bread, (2) breakfast with grains, (3) couscous, (4) pasta, (5) cake, (6) rice, (7) sugar, (8) sweets without chocolate, (9) chocolate, (10) vegetable oil, (11) margarine and vegetable fat, (12) butter and animals fat, (13) dried fruit, (14) legumes, (15) vegetables, (16) potatoes, (17) fruits, (18) juice, (19) non-alcoholic beverages, (20) coffee/tea, (21) beer, (22) wine, (23) other-alcoholic beverages, (24) red meat, (25) poultry, (26) sekat (offal), (27) fish, (28) eggs, (29) milk of cow/milk of soya, (30) cheese, (31) other dairy products, and (32) miscellaneous foods (Table 1).

A total of 87 participants completed all the dietary questionnaires (two FFQs and three24-h recall questionnaires). Most of the participants were females (70.1%) and young adults (mean age 27.3 ± 5.7 years). Over two thirds of participants (70.6%) had a normal BMI (Table 2). Eighteen subjects did not complete the second FFQ, with the main reason being declining to participate again ($n = 12$), or not being available after several attempts were made to contact them ($n = 6$).

The mean intake of TEI, macro-nutrients and micro-nutrients measured by FFQ1, FFQ2, and the 24-h recall questionnaires are presented in Tables 3. For TEI and nutrients intakes, the means reported in the FFQ1 were higher than the means reported using the average of the three 24-h recall questionnaires. The Bland-Altman plots for energy, and macronutrients (carbohydrates, proteins, and fat) are shown in Fig. 2. The Bland Altman plots confirmed an over-estimation of nutrient intakes consumptions by the FFQ.

Correlations between nutrient intakes derived from the FFQ1 and the mean of the 24-hour recall questionnaires are presented in Table 4. Crude correlation coefficients between the two methods varied from 0.23 (fiber) to

**Table 2** Socio-demographic characteristics and anthropometric measurements of study participants ($N = 87$)

| Characteristics | Results |
|---|---|
| Age (mean ± SD) | 27.3 ± 5.6 |
| Gender (%) | |
| Female | 70.1 |
| Male | 29.9 |
| Education (%) | |
| Primary | 2.3 |
| Secondary | 10.3 |
| University | 87.4 |
| Body masse index category (%) | |
| Underweight (< 18.5) | 3.5 |
| Normal (18.5–24.9) | 70.6 |
| Overweight (25–29.9) | 22.4 |
| Obese (BMI ≥30) | 3.5 |

**Table 3** Daily consumption of nutrients estimated by the first and second Food Frequency Questionnaire and mean of three 24 Hour Recalls

| Nutrients | FFQ1 Mean ± SD | FFQ2 Mean ± SD | 24 Hour Recalls Mean ± SD |
|---|---|---|---|
| Energy (kcal) | 2546.5 ± 719.5 | 2392.5 ± 738.9 | 1926.2 ± 589.6 |
| Carbohydrates(g) | 452.1 ± 149.7 | 430.4 ± 148.6 | 321.9 ± 103.3 |
| Proteins (g) | 135.3 ± 61.6 | 128.9 ± 57.4 | 87.1 ± 38.2 |
| Fat (g) | 108.2 ± 39.9 | 103.9 ± 44.3 | 71.8 ± 39.0 |
| Total MUFA(g) | 110.2 ± 64.0 | 104.6 ± 57.8 | 45.8 ± 32.9 |
| Total PUFA(g) | 78.3 ± 53.8 | 72.5 ± 47.1 | 31.1 ± 29.9 |
| Total SFA(g) | 80.9 ± 55.6 | 75.6 ± 54.3 | 41.4 ± 33.1 |
| Vitamin A (μg) | 445.1 ± 220.9 | 439.9 ± 259.2 | 533.1 ± 680.8 |
| Vitamin C (mg) | 221.6 ± 141.6 | 196.3 ± 114.0 | 129.3 ± 93.4 |
| Vitamin E (mg) | 73.4 ± 53.1 | 70.1 ± 48.7 | 28.0 ± 30.2 |
| Selenium (μg) | 138.4 ± 74.0 | 144.7 ± 67.2 | 91.1 ± 63.7 |
| Magnesium (mg) | 567.3 ± 237.0 | 556.7 ± 230.3 | 324.7 ± 143.7 |
| Calcium (mg) | 1241.6 ± 600.6 | 1188.7 ± 576.2 | 755.0 ± 408.2 |
| Iron (mg) | 28.5 ± 22.4 | 26.7 ± 20.6 | 16.9 ± 11.4 |
| Fiber (g) | 49.4 ± 58.5 | 44.9 ± 52.1 | 26.3 ± 37.4 |

0.89 (total monounsaturated fatty acids [MUFA]), and were statistically significant. Adjusting for TEI was statistically significant for all nutrients but it decreased the value of correlation coefficients. However, de-attenuation (adjustment for residual measurement error) increased all correlation coefficients, ranging from 0.24 (fiber) to 0.93 (total MUFA).

The intra-class correlation coefficients (ICC) and Pearson's correlation coefficients for both the unadjusted and the energy adjusted nutrient intakes estimated from FFQ1 and FFQ2 were presented in Table 5. The Pearson correlations (unadjusted) between nutrient intakes assessed by two FFQ varied from 0.62 (carbohydrates) to 0.76 (Vitamin A). Adjusting for total energy intake decreased all correlation coefficients, ranging from 0.53 (fat) to 0.73 (Vitamin A). The ICCs unadjusted ranged from 0.76 (carbohydrates) to 0.86 (Vitamin A and Vitamin C). The ICCs energy adjusted ranged from 0.69 (fat) to 0.84 (Vitamin A). All correlations were statistically significant.

## Discussion

Our study described the process of adaptation of the international GA$^2$LEN FFQ for use in Moroccan adults, and its relative validity and reproducibility to estimate usual food intake. The adapted FFQ contained 255 items, including staple foods consumed by the Moroccan population. The FFQ was classified into 32 food groups or sections, to mirror the structure of the GA$^2$LEN FFQ, which facilitates international comparability. To our knowledge, this is the first FFQ in Morocco to include a

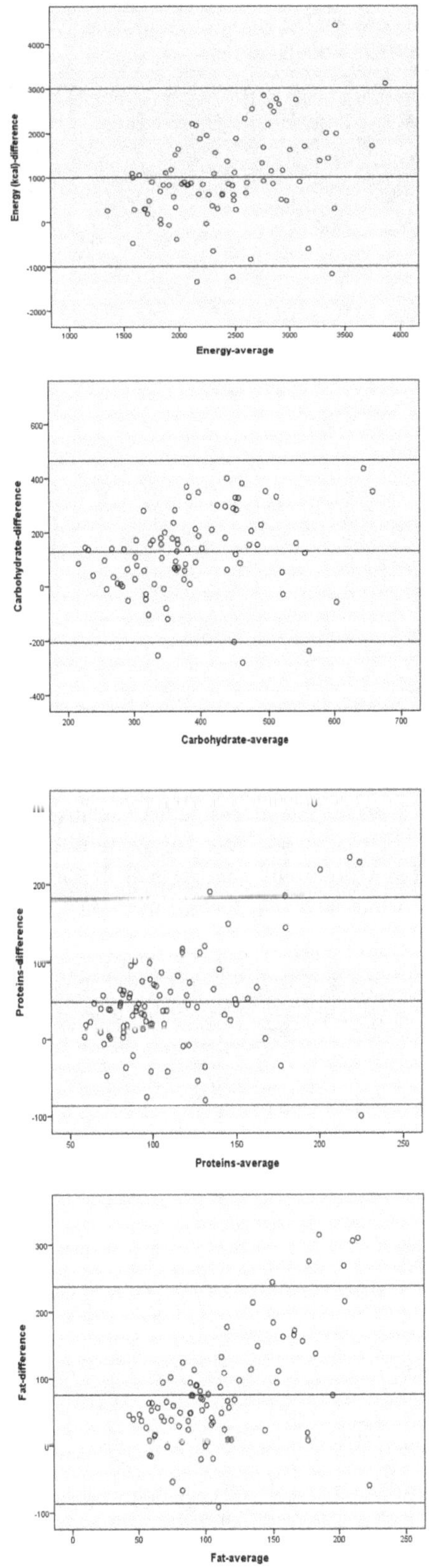


**Fig. 2** Bland altman plots of difference between energy and macronutrients (carbohydrate, proteins, and fat) as predicted by the first FFQ and the mean of three 24-hour recalls

**Table 4** Validity of Food Frequency Questionnaire: Pearson correlations between first food frequency questionnaire and mean of three 24 Hour Recalls

| Nutrients | 24 Hour Recalls Vs Food Frequency Questionnaire1 | | |
|---|---|---|---|
| | Unadjusted | Energy adjusted | De-attenuated |
| Energy (kcal) | 0.67* | – | 0.69* |
| Carbohydrates(g) | 0.63* | 0.60* | 0.66* |
| Proteins (g) | 0.34* | 0.29* | 0.35* |
| Fat (g) | 0.26* | 0.19* | 0.28* |
| Total MUFA(g) | 0.89* | 0.86* | 0.93* |
| Total PUFA(g) | 0.87* | 0.84* | 0.91* |
| Total SFA(g) | 0.79* | 0.82* | 0.90* |
| Vitamin A (μg) | 0.55* | 0.52* | 0.72* |
| Vitamin C (mg) | 0.62* | 0.40* | 0.63* |
| Vitamin E (mg) | 0.71* | 0.70* | 0.74* |
| Selenium (μg) | 0.36* | 0.33* | 0.38* |
| Magnesium (mg) | 0.56* | 0.43* | 0.66* |
| Calcium (mg) | 0.46* | 0.42* | 0.55* |
| Iron (mg) | 0.69* | 0.58* | 0.74* |
| Fiber (g) | 0.23* | 0.21* | 0.24* |

*Energy and nutrients were transformed (log10) to improve normality *$p \leq 0.01$

comprehensive list of both traditional and 'modern' foods, providing a reasonable assessment of relative dietary intake over a 1-year period. We are aware of another FFQ developed in Morocco by Landais et al., but it is limited to intake of fruits and vegetables only [11]. The energy adjusted Pearson correlation between the FFQ and the mean 24-HRs showed that the relative validity findings were moderately consistent across the majority of nutrients, they ranged between 0.19 for fat to 0.86 for total MUFA, and these observed values were comparable to other FFQs validation studies [26–28].

The nutrient intakes reported with the use of the FFQ were higher than those reported using the 24-h recall questionnaires. This over-reporting is not uncommon when validating an FFQ with a relatively large number of food items [26, 29–33]. We used the average of three 24-h recall questionnaires, which is considered an acceptable number of days to capture usual intake [34]. A systematic review found that 75% of validation studies use the 24-h recall questionnaires as reference method against FFQs [35], preferred for the accuracy to capture daily consumption of a varied diet, and for their relatively easier administration and analysis compared to other dietary questionnaires. The FFQ and the 24-h recall questionnaire have some differences in their error sources, which make them sufficiently independent [36]. Both instruments are prone to memory bias (long-term vs short term in the FFQ vs the 24-h recall questionnaire, respectively) and have differences in the perception of portion sizes (usually pre-defined in the FFQ) [35, 37, 38]. The 24-h recall questionnaire method is based on open-ended questions; while the FFQ is usually designed to have close-ended questions.

The acceptable correlations between the the FFQs and 24-HRs and the overestimation of energy and nutrient

**Table 5** FFQ reproducibility: Pearson correlation coefficients and intra-class correlation coefficients (ICC) for nutrient intake as reported in $FFQ_{t1}$ and $FFQ_{t2}$ in Moroccan adults

| Nutrients | Pearson correlation coefficient | | Intra-class correlation coefficient | |
|---|---|---|---|---|
| | Unadjusted | Energy-adjusted | Unadjusted | Energy-adjusted |
| Energy (kcal) | 0.73** | – | 0.84** | – |
| Carbohydrates(g) | 0.62** | 0.56** | 0.76** | 0.72** |
| Proteins (g) | 0.68** | 0.60** | 0.81** | 0.75** |
| Fat (g) | 0.69** | 0.53** | 0.81** | 0.69** |
| Total MUFA(g) | 0.71** | 0.61** | 0.82** | 0.76** |
| Total PUFA(g) | 0.70** | 0.61** | 0.83* | 0.76** |
| Total SFA(g) | 0.73* | 0.64** | 0.84** | 0.78** |
| Vitamin A (μg) | 0.76** | 0.73** | 0.86** | 0.84** |
| Vitamin C (mg) | 0.75** | 0.67** | 0.86** | 0.80** |
| Vitamin E (mg) | 0.71** | 0.60** | 0.83** | 0.75** |
| Selenium (μg) | 0.66** | 0.60** | 0.80** | 0.75** |
| Magnesium (mg) | 0.64** | 0.59** | 0.78** | 0.74** |
| Calcium (mg) | 0.69** | 0.64** | 0.81** | 0.78** |
| Iron (mg) | 0.71** | 0.66** | 0.83** | 0.80** |
| Fiber (g) | 0.72** | 0.65** | 0.84** | 0.79** |

*Energy and nutrients were transformed (log10) to improve normality; **$p \leq 0.001$

intakes between the two methods were confirmed by the Bland-Altman plots. These figures indicated a positive mean difference for TEI and macronutrients. These results are in agreement with those reported by other studies [39–41].

Since no dietary method can assess nutrient intake without error [35], we used energy adjusted nutrient estimates in our analyses as a way to reduce correlated errors between the two dietary methods [22, 38]. Energy-adjustment decreased correlation coefficients for all nutrients, which often happens when variability is more related to systematic errors of under/overestimation than to energy intake [42–44]. Similarly, other studies have not reported that energy-adjusted estimates improved crude correlations [45–47]. The de-attenuated correlations were increased because of the correction for the day to day variation in intakes.

The reproducibility of the FFQ was examined by the administration of the questionnaire in two occasions, 1 month apart. As reported in other studies [48, 49], we found that the estimates observed in FFQ1 were slightly higher than in the second FFQ. This could be partly explained by the level of engagement of the participants and the attention required to complete the FFQ in full. The ICCs showed a good level of agreement for the reporting of macro- and micronutrients, ranging from 0.69 (fat) to 0.75 (proteins for macro nutrients, and over 0.7 for most micro-nutrients, suggesting that the FFQ has a good repeatability and reproducibility [50].

Our study has several strengths. The structure of the FFQ was adapted from the international GA$^2$LEN FFQ, whose applicability has been demonstrated in multinational studies in high [9] and low income countries [51]. In order to make the FFQ representative of the Moroccan population, we endeavored to identify traditional foods that are part of the staple diet of the country, while also maintaining the international structure of the food classification to facilitate international comparisons. We followed a strict protocol to ensure the FFQ was correctly translated into Moroccan Arabic, which is different from the written and spoken Arabic in other North African countries. The FFQ also takes into account seasonal variations in food consumption, an important feature in North Africa where seasonality strongly influences dietary choices.

We acknowledge this validation study has some limitations. The FFQ captures usual intake of foods over a longer period of time than a 24-h recall questionnaire, which could lead to errors in the results. We compared the FFQ to the average intake reported in three 24-h recall questionnaires. Although this is an acceptable number of interviews, several studies recommend seven recall days (replicates) to capture a better estimate of the habitual intake. However, three recording days per subject are considered feasible and sufficient to estimate within-person variability (day-to-day variability). Due to the length of the validation study (1 month), some seasonal variations might not have been captured accurately with the 24-h recall questionnaire. This may negatively impact the correlation results, reflecting differences between the two instruments, rather than limitations of the FFQ. The length of the FFQ (255 food items) might have discouraged the participants to respond it fully. We designed the FFQ bearing in mind the current gap in nutritional epidemiology in North Africa, creating a tool that captures the usual diet of Morocco, and that it estimates intake of other foods that are associated with the nutritional transition of the region. Finally, the majority of the study sample was comprised of women with a high level of education. This does not represent the general population of Morocco, where illiteracy and poverty are common. The use of the FFQ in the general population would probably require a close interaction between an interviewer and the participant to overcome communication and educational limitations.

## Conclusions

This adaptation and validation study showed that the FFQ has a good relative validity and a good reproducibility for most nutrients. It is the first complete and validated tool to assess usual dietary intake in the Moroccan population that includes a wide range of traditional, as well as more 'modern' food items. Given its representativeness of local foods and habits, it can be used as an instrument to assess the relation of dietary habits and diseases in which diet might play a role.

### Abbreviations

BMI: Body mass index; EPIC: European Prospective Investigation into Cancer and Nutrition; FAO: Food and Agriculture Organization; FCT: Food composition table; FFQ: Food frequency questionnaire; GA$^2$LEN: The European Global Asthma and Allergy Network; ICC: Intra-class correlation coefficient; MUFA: Monounsaturated fatty acids; NCD: Non-communicable diseases; PUFA: Polyunsaturated fatty acids; SFA: Saturated fatty acids; SOP: The standard operational procedure; WHO: World Health Organization

### Acknowledgments

We are grateful to all subjects who participated in the study. We are also grateful to the GA$^2$LEN Scientific Steering Committee for facilitating the GA$^2$LEN FFQ and its methods as reference for our study. We also thank Dr. Inge Huybrechts, from Nutritional Epidemiology Group (NEP), International Agency for Research on Cancer, World Health Organization Lyon, France, for her pertinent remarks and comments to improve the manuscript during the drafting.

### Funding

The validation study did not receive funding. All participants voluntarily agreed to take part.

**Authors' contributions**
KE and VGL conceived the study idea, its design, and led the analyses and interpretation of the data. KR supervised the data collection. VGL wrote the final version of the manuscript. MK contributed to the conception and the design of the study. MMSD contributed to the conception of the study, and the acquisition of data. AB, AI, MMSD and MCB contributed to the study design and to the data collection. All authors have read and approved the manuscript.

**Competing interests**
The authors declare that they have no competing interests.

**Author details**
[1]Department of Epidemiology and Public Health, Faculty of Medicine and pharmacy of Fez, Sidi Mohamed Ben Abdellah University, Fez, Morocco. [2]Laboratory of Microbiology and Molecular Biology, Faculty of Science DharMehraz, Fez, Morocco. [3]Department of International Health, The Johns Hopkins Bloomberg School of Public Health, Baltimore, USA. [4]Population Health and Occupational Disease, NHLI, Imperial College London, London, UK. [5]Respiratory Department, Hassan II University Hospital Center of Fez, Fez, Morocco.

**References**

1. Reshma N, Toshiko K. Non-communicable diseases in Africa: youth are key to curbing the epidemic and achieving sustainable development. Policy Brief. 2015;
2. Belahsen R. Nutrition transition and food sustainability. Proc Nutr Soc. 2014; 73(3):385–8.
3. Boutayeb A, Boutayeb S. The burden of non communicable diseases in developing countries. Int J Equity Health. 2005;4(1):2.
4. El Rhazi K, Nejjari C, Zidouh A, Bakkali R, Berraho M, Barberger Gateau P. Prevalence of obesity and associated sociodemographic and lifestyle factors in Morocco. Public Health Nutr. 2011;14(1):160–7.
5. Afshin A, Micha R, Khatibzadeh S, Fahimi S, Shi P, Powles J, Singh G, Yakoob MY, Abdollahi M, Al-Hooti S, et al. The impact of dietary habits and metabolic risk factors on cardiovascular and diabetes mortality in countries of the Middle East and North Africa in 2010: a comparative risk assessment analysis. BMJ Open. 2015;5(5):e006385.
6. Mokhtar N, Elati J, Chabir R, Bour A, Elkari K, Schlossman NP, Caballero B, Aguenaou H. Diet culture and obesity in northern Africa. J Nutr. 2001;131(3): 887S–92S.
7. Cade JE, Burley VJ, Warm DL, Thompson RL, Margetts BM. Food frequency questionnaires: a review of their design, validation and utilisation. Nutr Res Rev. 2004;17(1):5–22.
8. Jee-Seon S, Kyungwon O, Hyeon Chang K. Dietary assessment methods in epidemiologic studies. Epidemiol Health. 2014;36:e2014009.
9. Garcia-Larsen V, Luczynska M, Kowalski ML, Voutilainen H, Ahlström M, Haahtela T, Toskala E, Bockelbrink A, Lee HH, Vassilopoulou E, et al. Use of a common food frequency questionnaire (FFQ) to assess dietary patterns and their relation to allergy and asthma in Europe: pilot study of the GA2LEN FFQ. Eur J Clin Nutr. 2011;65(6):750–6.
10. Subar AF, Thompson FE, Kipnis V, Midthune D, Hurwitz P, McNutt S, McIntosh A, Rosenfeld S. Comparative validation of the block, Willett, and National Cancer Institute food frequency questionnaires. The eating at America's table study. Am J Epidemiol. 2001;154(12):1089–99.
11. Landais E, Gartner A, Bour A, McCullough F, Delpeuch F, Holdsworth M. Reproducibility and relative validity of a brief quantitative food frequency questionnaire for assessing fruit and vegetable intakes in north-African women. J Hum Nutr Diet. 2014;27:152–9.
12. Benjelloun S. Nutrition transition in Morocco. Public Health Nutr. 2002; 5(1A):135–40.
13. Andersen LF, Solvoll K, Johansson LR, Salminen I, Aro A, Drevon CA. Evaluation of a food frequency questionnaire with weighed records, fatty acids, and alpha-tocopherol in adipose tissue and serum. Am J Epidemiol. 1999;150(1):75–87.
14. Neve J: Aliments et préparations typiques de la population marocaine: Outil pour estimer la consommation alimentaire.; 2008.
15. El Khayate R: Contribution à l'élaboration d'une table de composition des aliments au Maroc; 1948.
16. Palmer SC, Ruospo M, Campbell KL, Garcia Larsen V, Saglimbene V, Natale P, Gargano L, Craig JC, Johnson DW, Tonelli M, et al. Nutrition and dietary intake and their association with mortality and hospitalisation in adults with chronic kidney disease treated with haemodialysis: protocol for DIET-HD, a prospective multinational cohort study. BMJ Open. 2015;5(3):e006897.
17. World Health Organisation Regional Office of Africa: Standard Operating Procedures For AFRO Strategic Health Operations Centre (AFRO SHOC). 2014.
18. El Ati J., Béji C., Farhat A., Haddad S., Cherif S., Trabelsi T., Danguir J., Gaigi S., Le Bihan G., Landais E. et al: Table de composition des aliments tunisiens; 2007.
19. Food and Agriculture Organization of the United Nations: Food composition Table for Use in Africa. WT Wu Leung, FAO, Rome, Italy; US Dept Health, Education, and Welfare, Bethesda 1968.
20. The French Agency for Food, Environmental and Occup Health Saf (ANSES): Ciqual French Food Composition Table version. 2016.
21. USDA. Foods list. In: National Nutrient Database for standard reference, 24; 2012.
22. Willett WC, Howe GR, Kushi LH. Adjustment for total energy intake in epidemiologic studies. Am J Clin Nutr. 1997;65(4):1220S–8S. discussion 1229S–1231S
23. Rosner B, Willett WC. Interval estimates for correlation coefficients corrected for within-person variation: implications for study design and hypothesis testing. Am J Epidemiol. 1988;127(2):377–86.
24. Bartlett JW, Frost C. Reliability, repeatability and reproducibility: analysis of measurement errors in continuous variables. Ultrasound Obstet Gynecol. 2008;31(4):466–75.
25. Bland JM, Altman DG. Measuring agreement in method comparison studies. Stat Methods Med Res. 1999;8(2):135–60.
26. Shu XO, Yang G, Jin F, Liu D, Kushi L, Wen W, Gao YT, Zheng W. Validity and reproducibility of the food frequency questionnaire used in the shanghai Women's health study. Eur J Clin Nutr. 2004;58(1):17–23.
27. Liu L, Wang PP, Roebothan B, Ryan A, Tucker CS, Colbourne J, Baker N, Cotterchio M, Yi Y, Sun G. Assessing the validity of a self-administered food-frequency questionnaire (FFQ) in the adult population of Newfoundland and Labrador, Canada. Nutr J. 2013;12:49.
28. Jain MG, Rohan TE, Soskolne CL, Kreiger N. Calibration of the dietary questionnaire for the Canadian study of diet, Lifestyle and Health cohort. Public Health Nutr. 2003;6(1):79–86.
29. Fumagalli F, Pontes Monteiro J, Sartorelli DS, Vieira MN, de Lourdes Pires Bianchi M. validation of a food frequency questionnaire for assessing dietary nutrients in Brazilian children 5 to 10 years of age. Nutrition. 2008;24(5):427–32.
30. Osowski JM, Beare T, Specker B. Validation of a food frequency questionnaire for assessment of calcium and bone-related nutrient intake in rural populations. J Am Diet Assoc. 2007;107(8):1349–55.
31. Sevak L, Mangtani P, McCormack V, Bhakta D, Kassam-Khamis T, dos Santos Silva I. Validation of a food frequency questionnaire to assess macro- and micro-nutrient intake among south Asians in the United Kingdom. Eur J Nutr. 2004;43(3):160–8.
32. Jackson M, Walker S, Cade J, Forrester T, Cruickshank JK, Wilks R. Reproducibility and validity of a quantitative food-frequency questionnaire among Jamaicans of African origin. Public Health Nutr. 2001;4(5):971–80.
33. Jaceldo-Siegl K, Knutsen SF, Sabaté J, Beeson WL, Chan J, Herring RP, Butler TL, Haddad E, Bennett H, Montgomery S, et al. Validation of nutrient intake using an FFQ and repeated 24 h recalls in black and white subjects of the Adventist health Study-2 (AHS-2). Public Health Nutr. 2010;13(6):812–9.
34. Eck LH, Klesges RC, Hanson CL, Slawson D, Portis L, Lavasque ME. Measuring short-term dietary intake: development and testing of a 1-week food frequency questionnaire. J Am Diet Assoc. 1991;91(8):940–5.
35. Cade J, Thompson R, Burley V, Warm D. Development, validation and utilisation of food-frequency questionnaires – a review. Public Health Nutr. 2002;5(4):567–87.
36. Haftenberger M, Heuer T, Heidemann C, Kube F, Krems C, Mensink GB. Relative validation of a food frequency questionnaire for national health and nutrition monitoring. Nutr J. 2010;9:36.
37. Willett W. Nutritional epidemiology. New York: Oxford University Press; 1998.
38. Thompson FE, Byers T. Dietary assessment resource manual. J Nutr. 1994; 124(11 Suppl):2245S–317S.

39. Komatsul TR, Okul SK, Gimenoll SG, Asakuralll L, Coelhol L, Demézio d, Silvalv CV, AkutsuV R, Sachs A. Validation of a quantitative food frequency questionnaire developed to under graduate students. Revista Brasileira de Epidemiologia. 2013;16(4):898–906.
40. Streppel MT, de Vries JH, Meijboom S, Beekman M, de Craen AJ, Slagboom PE, Feskens EJ. Relative validity of the food frequency questionnaire used to assess dietary intake in the Leiden longevity study. Nutr J. 2013;12:75.
41. van Dongen MC, Lentjes MA, Wijckmans NE, Dirckx C, Lemaître D, Achten W, Celis M, Sieri S, Arnout J, Buntinx F, et al. Validation of a food-frequency questionnaire for Flemish and Italian-native subjects in Belgium: the IMMIDIET study. Nutrition. 2011;27(3):302–9.
42. Malekshah AF, Kimiagar M, Saadatian-Elahi M, Pourshams A, Nouraie M, Goglani G, Hoshiarrad A, Sadatsafavi M, Golestan B, Yoonesi A, et al. Validity and reliability of a new food frequency questionnaire compared to 24 h recalls and biochemical measurements: pilot phase of Golestan cohort study of esophageal cancer. Eur J Clin Nutr. 2006;60(8):971–7.
43. Rimm EB, Giovannucci EL, Stampfer MJ, Colditz GA, Litin LB, Willett WC. Reproducibility and validity of an expanded self-administered semiquantitative food frequency questionnaire among male health professionals. Am J Epidemiol. 1992;135(10):1114–26.
44. Beaton GH, Milner J, McGuire V, Feather TE, Little JA. Source of variance in 24-hour dietary recall data: implications for nutrition study design and interpretation. Carbohydrate sources, vitamins, and minerals. Am J Clin Nutr. 1983;37(6):986–95.
45. Dehghan M, del Cerro S, Zhang X, Cuneo JM, Linetzky B, Diaz R, Merchant AT. Validation of a semi-quantitative food frequency questionnaire for Argentinean adults. PLoS One. 2012;7(5):e37958.
46. Wang X, Sa R, Yan H. Validity and reproducibility of a food frequency questionnaire designed for residents in North China. Asia Pac J Clin Nutr. 2008;17(4):629–34.
47. Cardoso MA, Tomita LY, Laguna EC. Assessing the validity of a food frequency questionnaire among low-income women in São Paulo, southeastern Brazil. Cad Saude Publica. 2010;26(11):2059–67.
48. Marchionil DML, Voci SM, Leite de Lima FE, Fisberg RM, Slater B. Reproducibility of a food frequency questionnaire for adolescents. Cad Saúde Pública. 2007;23(9):2187–96.
49. Sue McPherson R, Hoelscher DM, Alexander M, Scanlon KS, Serdula MK. dietary assessment methods among school-aged children: validity and reliability. Prev Med. 2000;31(2):11–33.
50. Imaeda N, Goto C, Tokudome Y, Hirose K, Tajima K, Tokudome S. Reproducibility of a short food frequency questionnaire for Japanese general population. J Epidemiol. 2007;17(3):100–7.
51. Saglimbene VM, Wong G, Ruospo M, Palmer SC, Campbell K, Larsen VG, Natale P, Teixeira-Pinto A, Carrero JJ, Stenvinkel P, et al. Dietary n-3 polyunsaturated fatty acid intake and all-cause and cardiovascular mortality in adults on hemodialysis: the DIET-HD multinational cohort study. Clin Nutr. 2017;

# 6

# Maternal dietary patterns during pregnancy and preterm delivery: a large prospective cohort study in China

Min-Shan Lu[1,2,3†], Jian-Rong He[1,2†], Qiaozhu Chen[3†], Jinhua Lu[1,2], Xueling Wei[1,2], Qianling Zhou[1], Fanfan Chan[1,2], Lifang Zhang[1,2], Niannian Chen[1,2], Lan Qiu[1,2], Mingyang Yuan[1,2], Kar Keung Cheng[4], Huimin Xia[1,5*], and Xiu Qiu[1,2,3*], on behalf of the Born in Guangzhou Cohort Study Group

**Abstract**

**Background:** Evidence about the associations between maternal dietary patterns and preterm delivery is scarce in Eastern countries. The purpose of this study was to examine the associations between maternal dietary patterns during pregnancy and preterm delivery in a Chinese population.

**Methods:** A total of 7352 mothers were included in the Born in Guangzhou Cohort Study, a prospective study in China. A validated self-administered food frequency questionnaire (FFQ) was used to assess maternal diet at 24–27 weeks of gestation. Dietary patterns were identified by cluster analysis. Gestational age was obtained from routine medical records. Preterm delivery was defined as delivery before 37 completed weeks of gestation, and was further classified into spontaneous and iatrogenic preterm delivery, and also early/moderate and late preterm delivery. Associations between dietary patterns and preterm delivery outcomes were assessed using logistic regression analyses.

**Results:** Six dietary patterns were identified, including 'Milk', 'Cereals, eggs, and Cantonese soups', 'Meats', 'Fruits, nuts, and Cantonese desserts', 'Vegetables', and 'Varied'. There were 351 (4.8%) preterm deliveries in this study population. Among those of preterm delivery, 16.2 and 83.8% were early/moderate and late preterm delivery, respectively. Compared with women of 'Vegetables' pattern, those of 'Milk' pattern had greater odds of overall preterm delivery (adjusted odds ratio [OR] 1.59, 95% confidence interval [CI] 1.11, 2.29, $p < 0.05$), spontaneous preterm delivery (adjusted OR 1.73, 95% CI 1.14, 2.62, $p < 0.05$) and late preterm delivery (adjusted OR 1.73, 95% CI 1.08, 2.62, $p < 0.05$); those of 'Cereals, eggs, and Cantonese soups' and 'Fruits, nuts, and Cantonese desserts' patterns had greater odds of late preterm delivery (adjusted OR 1.54, 95% CI 1.01, 2.35 for 'Cereals, eggs, and Cantonese soups', adjusted OR 1.61, 95% CI 1.04, 2.50 for 'Fruits, nuts, and Cantonese desserts', respectively).

**Conclusion:** Maternal diet with frequent consumption of milk and less frequent consumption of vegetables during pregnancy might be associated with increased odds of preterm delivery. Future interventions should investigate whether increasing vegetable intake reduces preterm deliveries.

**Keywords:** Pregnant women, Dietary pattern, Preterm delivery, Cluster analysis, Birth cohort, Chinese women

* Correspondence: huimin.xia@bigcs.org; huimin.xia876001@gmail.com; xiu.qiu@bigcs.org; qxiu0161@163.com

†Min-Shan Lu, Jian-Rong He and Qiaozhu Chen contributed equally to this work.

[1]Division of Birth Cohort Study, Guangzhou Women and Children's Medical Center, Guangzhou Medical University, 9 Junsui Road, Zhujiang Newtown, Tianhe District, Guangzhou 510623, China

Full list of author information is available at the end of the article

## Background

Preterm delivery, defined as birth before 37 completed weeks of gestation, is associated with short-term and long-term neonatal morbidity, and is one of the leading causes of neonatal mortality [1, 2]. Women who deliver preterm have a higher risk of developing cardiovascular disease than those who deliver at full-term [3]. Maternal nutrition can directly affect the growing fetus [3, 4] and considerable amount of evidence has strongly supported the role of diet in preterm delivery [5, 6].

The incidence of preterm delivery is about 11.1% globally [2]. There are geographical variations of the prevalence of preterm delivery; and a maximum 10% of preterm births survive in low-resource settings compared with over 90% in high resource countries. China is one of the ten countries with the highest numbers of preterm deliveries [2]. The rate of preterm delivery in China was 7.1% in 2011 [7], and was estimated to increase in future years [8]. Country specific actions might be considered to tackle factors influencing preterm delivery.

As an important modifiable factor, maternal diet has received considerable amount of attention in previous studies of preterm delivery. However, these studies have mainly focused on assessing the associations between single foods or nutrients and preterm delivery, and yielded mixed results [9–11]. It is not yet known whether the associations between maternal nutrition and preterm delivery are due to overall nutrition or deficiency of a particular nutrient [11]. It is challenging to distinguish the specific effects of single foods or nutrients because of their highly interconnected nature [12]. It might therefore be more useful to assess the whole foods or dietary pattern [12], in order to obtain information valuable for nutrition interventions during pregnancy.

Dietary patterns can represent the combined effects of all foods consumed in a person's diet. To date, few studies investigated the associations between maternal dietary patterns and preterm delivery, and had varied findings [13–17]. Most of the evidence focused in western countries, including Denmark [13], Norway [14], America [15], and Australia [16]; while only one study was conducted among the Asian population [17]. Chia et al. in the Growing Up in Singapore Towards healthy Outcomes study (GUSTO) reported that vegetables, fruits, and white rice consumption is associated with a lower incidence of preterm delivery among a multiethnic sample in Singapore [17]. Dietary habits are population specific. Distinctive differences exist between the Chinese and the Western diets [18]. Chinese pregnant women have complex and diverse eating behaviors, and follow a set of dietary customs which are not extensively explored in the literature [19, 20]. The aim of this study is therefore to examine the associations between dietary patterns during pregnancy among the Chinese pregnant women and the incidence of preterm delivery.

## Methods

### Study design and population

The present study used data from the Born in Guangzhou Cohort Study (BIGCS), an ongoing prospective cohort study conducted in the Guangzhou Women and Children's Medical Center (GWCMC). The BIGCS aims to elicit the role of social, biological and environmental influences on pregnancy and child health and development. Methods of the BIGCS are detailed elsewhere [21]. Briefly, women were recruited during their first routine antenatal examinations (normally around 16 weeks, Q1) at two campuses of the GWCMC, and followed up at the second trimester (about 24 to 27 weeks, Q2) and at delivery. The inclusion criteria were women of less than 20 weeks gestation, of Chinese nationality, living in Guangzhou, intended to stay in Guangzhou with their child for at least three years after delivery. The protocols of the BIGCS were reviewed and approved in accordance with the standards of the Institutional Ethics Committee of the GWCMC. All participants gave written consent at the time of recruitment.

A flowchart of the selection process of the study population is shown in Fig. 1. During February 2012 and April 2015, 15,772 eligible pregnant women were invited and 11,859 (75.2%) of them agreed to participate in the BIGCS. After excluding participants who had missing Q1 data ($n = 545$), pre-pregnancy hypertension ($n = 10$), pre-pregnancy diabetes ($n = 23$), occurrence of twin pregnancy ($n = 228$) or dropped out ($n = 705$), missing Q2 data ($n = 2800$), implausible dietary data (a weekly intake frequency of < 32, $n = 45$), terminations of pregnancy ($n = 101$), and missing delivery data ($n = 50$), there were 7352 mothers included in this study. Compared to the remaining 7352 women in the present analysis, women who missed Q2 data were younger, and more likely to have lower levels of education, income and pre-pregnancy body mass index (BMI) (Additional file 1: Table S1).

### Dietary assessment

Information about dietary intake was obtained from a self-administered, non-quantitative food frequency questionnaire (FFQ) at the Q2 interview. This FFQ is a structured questionnaire on 64 specified food items (Additional file 1: Table S2), as well as additional questions regarding cooking oil, beverages, Chinese soup (normally cooked with meat and/or vegetables, of salty flavor and water-like texture [22]), processed meats (such as Lap-mei, Siu mei) and Cantonese desserts. For each food item, participants were asked to indicate their frequency of consumption 'in the past week'. The FFQ has previously been validated using the BIGCS cohort data [23]. Briefly, a subsample of cohort participants ($n = 210$) completed (1) the first FFQ (FFQ1) at 24–27 weeks of gestation, (2) three inconsecutive 24 h dietary recalls during 29–31 weeks of gestation, and (3) the second FFQ (FFQ2) at 33–35 weeks of gestation. The crude

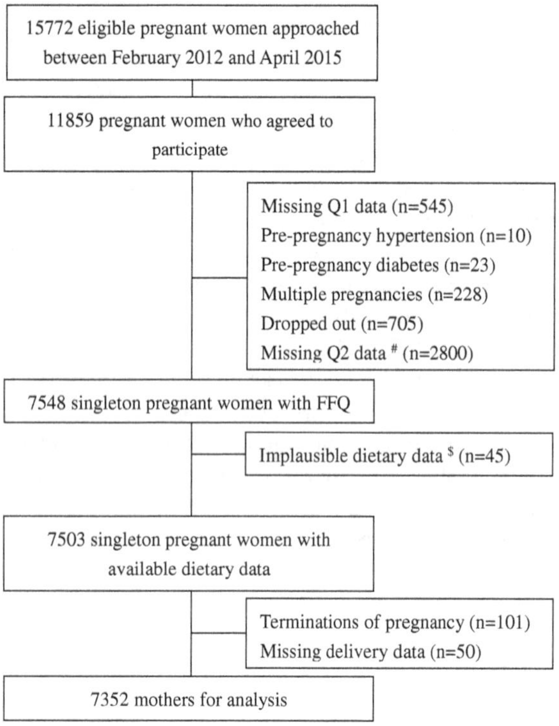


**Fig. 1** Selection process of study population in the BIGCS. # There are 2800 participants who did not attend our study clinic in their 24–27 gestational weeks and did not finish the Q2 questionnaire. However, these participants remained in the BIGCS cohort. We excluded them in the current analyses, as dietary information collected in Q2 was the key variable. $ A weekly intake frequency of less than 32 was considered as the 'implausible dietary intake' data

Spearman correlation coefficients for consumption frequencies of food groups between FFQ1 and FFQ2 (0.33–0.71) and between FFQ2 and the average of three 24 h dietary recalls (0.23–0.62) are considered acceptable for dietary assessment during pregnancy [23].

Individual food items were combined into 30 food groups according to a similar nutrient profile or culinary uses (Additional file 1: Table S3). The frequencies of intake of food groups were calculated by summing the weekly consumption frequencies of each food item in the group. The percentages (%) of weekly intake of the food groups were calculated as frequency of the food group intake divided by total frequencies of food intake for each participant. The variables of 'frequency' and 'percentage' reflect dietary intake from different perspectives. The variable 'frequency' reflects the exact frequency of individual food intake; while the variable 'percentage' considers the balance of frequencies from different food intakes. Both 'percentage' and 'frequency' variables were used to construct dietary pattern, respectively, with the application of cluster analysis. Since our purpose was to provide dietary advice for the general pregnant women, we believed the balancing of diet may be more informative than the specific frequency as the ideal amount of food intake should depend on individual energy expenditure status. Therefore, in this paper, results obtained from the 'percentage' variables were presented as the main results; while results obtained from the 'frequency' variables were presented as supplementary.

Cluster analysis was performed using the k-means procedure, as described elsewhere [24]. The K-means method was applied to classify participants into a predetermined number of mutually exclusive groups, by comparing Euclidean distances between each participant and each cluster center in an interactive process until no further changes occur. Several runs were conducted by varying the number of clusters from two to six, in order to identify the optimal one. The ratios of between-cluster variance to within-cluster variance for each food group [25] were compared across the number of clusters when the variables 'percentage' were used as input variables in cluster analysis (Additional file 1: Table S4). We believed that clusters identified from six-cluster solution could better reflect the diversity of participants' dietary characteristics and are more nutritional meaningful than that from three-cluster solutions. Based on the aforementioned determinations, we selected the six-cluster solution as the most appropriate solution when used 'percentage' variables as input variables. We also selected the six-cluster solution when used 'frequency' variables as input variables based on the nutritional meaningfulness of clusters. Cluster names were based on the food groups with highest content. These clusters are explained in the result section.

### Assessment of preterm delivery

The primary outcome of this study was preterm delivery, defined as delivery at $36^{+6}$ weeks or below. Gestational age was confirmed by ultrasound examination in the first- or early second-trimester, and was documented in the routine medical record. Secondary outcomes of this study included spontaneous, iatrogenic, early/moderate, and late preterm delivery. Preterm delivery was classified into spontaneous (spontaneous onset of preterm delivery) and iatrogenic (induced or caesarean delivery on maternal or fetal indications) preterm delivery. Preterm delivery was also categorized into early/moderate ($\leq 33^{+6}$ weeks) and late ($34^{+0}$ to $36^{+6}$ weeks) preterm delivery, according to the gestational age.

### Covariates

Information regarding potential confounders was assessed by self-reported comprehensive baseline questionnaire at Q1, including maternal age, education level (high school or below, vocational/technical college, undergraduate, postgraduate), monthly income (≤1500, 1501–4500, 4501–9000, or ≥ 9001 yuan), parity (primiparous, multiparous), passive smoking during pregnancy (no, yes), supplementation with folic acid (no, started during pregnancy, or started pre- conception), pre-pregnancy weight (kg) and height (m), previous preterm delivery (no, yes). Pre-pregnancy BMI (kg/m$^2$) was calculated by dividing weight in kilograms by height in meters squared. Study participants were divided into three groups as follows: BMI < 18.5 kg/m$^2$ (underweight), BMI 18.5–23.9 kg/m$^2$ (normal), BMI ≥ 24 kg/m$^2$ (overweight or obese), according to the Guidelines for Prevention and Control of Overweight and Obesity in Chinese Adults [26].

### Statistical analyses

Descriptive statistics (i.e., mean, standard deviation, frequencies, and percent frequencies) were reported for all socio-demographic factors (age, education level, and monthly income), health characteristics (parity, passive smoking during pregnancy, pre-pregnancy BMI, previous preterm delivery, and supplementation with folic acid). These variables were cross- tabulated by dietary patterns, and significant differences were assessed by ANOVA for continuous variables or chi-square tests for categorical variables. Logistic regression was conducted to assess the independent effect of dietary patterns on preterm delivery related outcomes, including overall preterm delivery, spontaneous preterm delivery, iatrogenic preterm delivery, early/moderate preterm delivery as well as late preterm delivery. All covariates described above were entered into each regression model as potential confounders. The firth's correction was applied to improve the accuracy of the logit coefficients in the adjusted models referring to iatrogenic preterm delivery and early/moderate preterm delivery.

$P < 0.05$ was considered statistically significant. Cluster analysis was performed by R version 3.2.3 [27], and the remaining analyses were performed using SPSS software version 20.0 (SPSS, Inc., Chicago, USA).

## Results

Six clusters of dietary pattern were identified (Table 1), namely the 'Milk' (n 1090, 14.8%), 'Cereals, eggs, and Cantonese soups' (n 1078, 14.7%), 'Meats' (n 1125, 15.3%), 'Fruits, nuts, and Cantonese desserts' (n 875, 11.9%), 'Vegetables' (n 1442, 19.6%), and 'Varied' (n 1742, 23.7%) patterns. 'Milk' had the most frequently consumed of milk products (including fresh milk, pasteurized milk, milk powder, and formula for pregnant women) and less frequently consumed of whole vegetables. 'Cereals, eggs, and Cantonese soups' had the most frequently consumed of staples such as rice, pasta, porridge, eggs, and Cantonese soups. 'Meats' had the most frequently consumed of red meat and processed meat. 'Fruits, nuts, and Cantonese desserts' had the most frequently consumed of fruits, nuts, and Cantonese desserts. 'Vegetables' had the most frequently consumed of leafy and cruciferous vegetables. 'Varied' was characterized by relatively frequent consumption of mixed foods, including noodles, bread, root vegetables, melon vegetables, mushrooms, sea vegetables, bean vegetables, processed vegetables, poultry, animal organ meat, fish, other seafood, bean products, yoghurt, sweet beverages, puffed food, confectioneries, and snacks.

Subject characteristics across the six dietary patterns are shown in Table 2. There were significant differences in maternal age, education level, monthly income, parity, and passive smoking during pregnancy among subjects in these six groups. No significant difference regarding supplementation with folic acid, pre-pregnancy BMI and previous preterm delivery was found among subjects in these six groups.

The gestational length range was $27^{+6}$ to $42^{+1}$ weeks in our study. There were 351 women delivered preterm, taking up 4.8% of the total participants. Among these 351 women, 262 (74.6%) were spontaneous preterm delivery, 62 (17.7%) were iatrogenic preterm delivery, and the rest 27 (7.7%) cases were either spontaneous or iatrogenic preterm delivery. We are unable to classify these 27 cases because they did not deliver their babies at the GWCMC. Among 351 women who delivered preterm, 294 (83.8%) were late preterm and 57 (16.2%) were moderately or early preterm. The incidence of preterm delivery was highest (66 cases, 6.1%) in the 'Milk' group. Table 3 shows associations between dietary patterns and preterm delivery. Because the beneficial value of vegetables, we selected 'Vegetables' pattern as reference pattern. Compared with women in the 'Vegetables' group (reference), those in the 'Milk' group had significantly higher odds of preterm delivery after adjustment for potential confounders (OR 1.59, 95% CI 1.11, 2.29, $p < 0.05$). No significant difference in the odds of preterm delivery was observed among subjects in other patterns neither in the crude nor adjusted models.

When we analyzed secondary outcomes individually, we found significantly greater odds of spontaneous preterm delivery for women in the 'Milk' groups in comparison to those in the 'Vegetables' groups (adjusted OR 1.73, 95% CI 1.14, 2.62, $p < 0.05$). No significant association was found between iatrogenic preterm delivery and maternal dietary pattern. We also found significantly greater odds of late preterm delivery for women in the 'Milk' (adjusted OR 1.73, 95% CI 1.08, 2.62, $p < 0.05$), 'Cereals, eggs, and Cantonese soups' (adjusted OR 1.54, 95% CI 1.01, 2.35, $p < 0.05$) and 'Fruits, nuts, and Cantonese desserts' (adjusted OR 1.61, 95% CI 1.04, 2.50, $p < 0.05$) groups in comparison to those in the 'Vegetables' groups. No significant association was found between moderately or early preterm delivery and maternal dietary pattern (Table 3).

By using 'frequencies' of 30 food groups as input variables in the cluster analysis, we also identified six dietary patterns and labeled them as 'Rich' (n 381, 5.2%), 'Milk-S'

**Table 1** Percentages (%) of weekly intake of 30 food groups assessed with a self-administered food frequency questionnaire across the six dietary patterns identified among 7352 pregnant Chinese women from the Born in Guangzhou Cohort Study

| | Dietary patterns | | | | | | | | | | | |
|---|---|---|---|---|---|---|---|---|---|---|---|---|
| | Varied (*n* = 1742) | | Milk (*n* = 1090) | | Pattern [a] (*n* = 1078) | | Meats (*n* = 1125) | | Pattern [b] (*n* = 875) | | Vegetables (*n* = 1442) | |
| Food groups [c] | Mean | SD | Mean | SD | Mean | SD | Mean | SD | Mean | SD | Mean | SD |
| Cereals | | | | | | | | | | | | |
| Rice | 8.1 | 2.8 | 10.9 | 3.4 | 16.4 | 3.8 | 12.5 | 3.2 | 10.4 | 3.4 | 12.0 | 3.5 |
| Pasta | 4.4 | 2.8 | 4.1 | 2.8 | 5.1 | 3.6 | 4.2 | 2.8 | 4.3 | 2.9 | 4.0 | 2.5 |
| Noodles | 2.8 | 3.0 | 1.6 | 2.0 | 2.3 | 2.6 | 2.0 | 2.1 | 2.4 | 2.6 | 2.0 | 2.1 |
| Porridge | 1.6 | 1.5 | 1.3 | 1.5 | 1.8 | 1.8 | 1.6 | 1.7 | 1.3 | 1.5 | 1.4 | 1.5 |
| Bread | 2.1 | 1.8 | 1.8 | 2.1 | 2.0 | 2.0 | 1.6 | 1.8 | 1.3 | 1.7 | 1.9 | 1.9 |
| Vegetables | | | | | | | | | | | | |
| Leafy and cruciferous vegetables | 10.1 | 3.0 | 10.7 | 3.4 | 7.8 | 2.9 | 10.5 | 3.7 | 9.3 | 3.4 | 17.9 | 3.8 |
| Root vegetables | 3.7 | 1.9 | 2.5 | 1.8 | 2.8 | 1.8 | 2.7 | 1.8 | 3.0 | 1.9 | 3.1 | 2.0 |
| Melon vegetables | 4.2 | 2.2 | 3.3 | 2.1 | 3.7 | 2.3 | 3.5 | 2.2 | 4.0 | 2.4 | 3.5 | 2.2 |
| Mushrooms | 1.5 | 1.2 | 1.0 | 1.1 | 1.1 | 1.1 | 1.0 | 1.0 | 1.2 | 1.1 | 1.1 | 1.1 |
| Sea vegetables | 1.0 | 1.0 | 0.6 | 0.8 | 0.7 | 0.9 | 0.6 | 0.9 | 0.7 | 0.9 | 0.6 | 0.9 |
| Bean vegetables | 1.6 | 1.2 | 1.2 | 1.2 | 1.3 | 1.3 | 1.3 | 1.2 | 1.3 | 1.1 | 1.3 | 1.1 |
| Processed vegetables | 0.6 | 1.0 | 0.3 | 0.7 | 0.5 | 0.9 | 0.4 | 0.8 | 0.4 | 0.9 | 0.4 | 0.8 |
| Fruits | 7.7 | 2.4 | 8.1 | 2.9 | 8.1 | 2.8 | 7.5 | 2.9 | 15.3 | 3.9 | 7.6 | 2.9 |
| Meats | | | | | | | | | | | | |
| Red meat | 7.1 | 2.5 | 7.7 | 3.0 | 6.8 | 2.7 | 14.4 | 3.4 | 7.1 | 3.1 | 7.6 | 3.0 |
| Poultry | 2.6 | 1.8 | 2.4 | 1.7 | 2.5 | 1.8 | 2.5 | 2.0 | 2.0 | 1.6 | 2.4 | 1.8 |
| Animal organ meat | 1.2 | 1.5 | 1.0 | 1.4 | 1.0 | 1.3 | 1.0 | 1.4 | 0.8 | 1.1 | 0.9 | 1.2 |
| Processed meat | 0.3 | 0.7 | 0.3 | 0.9 | 0.3 | 0.8 | 0.4 | 0.9 | 0.3 | 0.7 | 0.2 | 0.7 |
| Eggs | 5.3 | 2.2 | 5.8 | 2.5 | 5.8 | 2.9 | 5.5 | 2.8 | 5.3 | 2.5 | 5.0 | 2.3 |
| Fish | 3.1 | 1.9 | 3.0 | 2.1 | 3.0 | 2.0 | 2.9 | 2.0 | 2.7 | 1.8 | 2.9 | 1.8 |
| Other seafood | 1.2 | 1.3 | 0.9 | 1.1 | 1.0 | 1.2 | 0.9 | 1.1 | 1.0 | 1.2 | 0.9 | 1.2 |
| Bean products | 6.9 | 3.6 | 3.4 | 2.4 | 4.2 | 2.8 | 3.7 | 2.5 | 4.4 | 2.8 | 3.8 | 2.5 |
| Nuts | 4.3 | 2.4 | 4.1 | 2.6 | 3.8 | 2.7 | 3.3 | 2.5 | 4.6 | 3.1 | 3.5 | 2.5 |
| Milk | 5.1 | 2.7 | 13.0 | 4.1 | 5.9 | 3.0 | 5.4 | 2.9 | 5.9 | 3.2 | 5.1 | 2.9 |
| Yoghurt | 2.5 | 2.2 | 1.5 | 1.9 | 2.0 | 2.3 | 1.7 | 2.0 | 2.2 | 2.3 | 1.8 | 2.1 |
| Sweet beverages | 1.9 | 3.1 | 1.2 | 2.1 | 1.6 | 2.6 | 1.2 | 1.9 | 1.4 | 2.2 | 1.2 | 2.0 |
| Cantonese desserts | 0.3 | 0.9 | 0.3 | 1.0 | 0.2 | 0.7 | 0.2 | 0.8 | 0.4 | 1.1 | 0.2 | 0.7 |
| Cantonese soups | 3.1 | 2.1 | 3.6 | 2.3 | 4.0 | 2.5 | 3.7 | 2.3 | 3.1 | 2.3 | 3.2 | 2.1 |
| Puffed food | 0.3 | 0.7 | 0.2 | 0.5 | 0.2 | 0.6 | 0.2 | 0.5 | 0.2 | 0.5 | 0.2 | 0.5 |
| Confectioneries | 2.2 | 2.5 | 1.3 | 2.0 | 1.6 | 2.2 | 1.3 | 1.8 | 1.7 | 2.2 | 1.4 | 2.0 |
| Snack | 3.2 | 2.4 | 2.9 | 2.7 | 2.9 | 2.7 | 2.4 | 2.3 | 2.2 | 2.3 | 2.7 | 2.3 |

[a] "Cereals, eggs and Cantonese soups"
[b] "Fruits, nuts and Cantonese desserts"
[c] Percentage values (%), calculated as frequency of the food group intake divided by total frequencies of food intake. The highest mean values are underlined

(n 864, 11.8%), 'Fruits' (n 930, 12.6%), 'Meats-S' (n 975, 13.3%), 'Moderate' (n 1735, 23.6%), and 'Prudent' (n 2467, 33.6%) patterns (Additional file 1: Table S5). The letter "S" was added after the pattern name (e.g. "Milk-S" and "Meats-S") to separate supplementary (from 'frequency' variables) and main (from 'percentage' variables) results. Additional file 1: Table S6 presents subject characteristics across the six dietary patterns. No significant association was found between these dietary patterns and overall preterm delivery. Compared with women in other dietary patterns, women in the 'Milk-S' group had significantly higher odds of spontaneous preterm delivery (adjusted OR

**Table 2** Characteristics of the participants across the six dietary patterns identified by cluster analysis

| | | Dietary patterns | | | | | | $P_{value}$* |
|---|---|---|---|---|---|---|---|---|
| | Total | Varied | Milk | Cereals, eggs and Cantonese soups | Meats | Fruits, nuts and Cantonese desserts | Vegetables | |
| Characteristics | (*n* = 7352) | (*n* = 1742) | (*n* = 1090) | (*n* = 1078) | (*n* = 1125) | (*n* = 875) | (*n* = 1442) | |
| Age, years, mean ± SD | 29.1 ± 3.3 | 29.3 ± 3.3 | 29.0 ± 3.5 | 28.8 ± 3.3 | 29.0 ± 3.3 | 29.0 ± 3.2 | 29.3 ± 3.4 | 0.002 |
| Education level, n (%) | | | | | | | | < 0.001 |
| High school or below | 624 (8.5) | 117 (6.7) | 105 (9.6) | 110 (10.2) | 83 (7.4) | 79 (9.0) | 130 (9.0) | |
| Vocational/technical college | 1807 (24.6) | 338 (19.4) | 285 (26.1) | 309 (28.7) | 282 (25.1) | 213 (24.3) | 380 (26.4) | |
| Undergraduate | 4031 (54.8) | 986 (56.6) | 591 (54.2) | 569 (52.8) | 642 (57.1) | 461 (52.7) | 782 (54.2) | |
| Postgraduate | 890 (12.1) | 301 (17.3) | 109 (10.0) | 90 (8.3) | 118 (10.5) | 122 (13.9) | 150 (10.4) | |
| Monthly income, Yuan, n (%) | | | | | | | | < 0.001 |
| ≤ 1500 | 692 (9.4) | 161 (9.2) | 107 (9.8) | 93 (8.6) | 101 (9.0) | 92 (10.5) | 138 (9.6) | |
| 1501–4500 | 2274 (30.9) | 430 (24.7) | 402 (36.9) | 387 (35.9) | 383 (34.0) | 216 (24.7) | 456 (31.6) | |
| 4501–9000 | 3062 (41.6) | 754 (43.3) | 410 (37.6) | 441 (40.9) | 453 (40.3) | 396 (45.3) | 608 (42.2) | |
| ≥ 9001 | 1158 (15.8) | 353 (20.3) | 143 (13.1) | 140 (13.0) | 164 (14.6) | 150 (17.1) | 208 (14.4) | |
| Refused to answer | 166 (2.3) | 44 (2.5) | 28 (2.6) | 17 (1.6) | 24 (2.1) | 21 (2.4) | 32 (2.2) | |
| Parity, n (%) | | | | | | | | < 0.001 |
| Primiparous | 6430 (87.5) | 1501 (86.2) | 1002 (91.9) | 967 (89.7) | 956 (85.0) | 799 (91.3) | 1205 (83.6) | |
| Multiparous | 922 (12.5) | 241 (13.8) | 88 (8.1) | 111 (10.3) | 169 (15.0) | 76 (8.7) | 237 (16.4) | |
| Passive smoking during pregnancy, n (%) | 2222 (30.2) | 472 (27.2) | 322 (29.5) | 364 (33.8) | 384 (34.1) | 252 (28.8) | 428 (29.7) | < 0.001 |
| Supplementation with folic acid, n (%) | | | | | | | | 0.110 |
| No | 603 (8.2) | 128 (7.3) | 91 (8.3) | 96 (8.9) | 103 (9.2) | 66 (7.5) | 119 (8.3) | |
| Started during pregnancy | 3501 (47.6) | 811 (46.6) | 511 (46.9) | 535 (49.6) | 535 (47.6) | 392 (44.8) | 717 (49.7) | |
| Started pre conception | 3248 (44.2) | 803 (46.1) | 488 (44.8) | 447 (41.5) | 487 (43.3) | 417 (47.7) | 606 (42.0) | |
| Pre-pregnancy BMI, kg/m$^2$, n (%) | | | | | | | | 0.325 |
| < 18.5 | 1803 (24.5) | 414 (23.8) | 293 (26.9) | 274 (25.4) | 257 (22.8) | 212 (24.2) | 353 (24.5) | |
| 18.5–23.9 | 4608 (62.7) | 1114 (63.9) | 645 (59.2) | 682 (63.3) | 705 (62.7) | 563 (64.3) | 899 (62.3) | |
| ≥ 24 | 847 (11.5) | 189 (10.8) | 137 (12.6) | 110 (10.2) | 145 (12.9) | 93 (10.6) | 173 (12.0) | |
| Missing | 94 (1.3) | 25 (1.4) | 15 (1.4) | 12 (1.1) | 18 (1.6) | 7 (0.8) | 17 (1.2) | |
| Previous preterm delivery, n (%) | 53 (0.7) | 14 (0.8) | 9 (0.8) | 5 (0.5) | 8 (0.7) | 3 (0.3) | 14 (1.0) | 0.502 |

*ANOVA and Chi square tests were used to test differences between the patterns

1.44, 95% CI 1.02, 2.02, $p < 0.05$), while women in the 'Rich' group had significantly lower odds of spontaneous preterm delivery (adjusted OR 0.41, 95% CI 0.18, 0.93, $p < 0.05$) (Additional file 1: Table S7).

## Discussion

This is the first prospective study to examine the relationships between maternal dietary patterns and preterm delivery in a Chinese population with a relatively large sample size. Six dietary patterns of the Chinese were generated, represented by foods generally consumed by the Chinese frequently and the cultural Cantonese cuisine. Women in the 'Milk' group had greater odds of overall preterm delivery, spontaneous preterm delivery and late preterm delivery than those in the 'Vegetables' group. We also found that, compared with women in

**Table 3** Associations between dietary patterns and preterm delivery

| Preterm delivery | Dietary patterns | | | | | |
|---|---|---|---|---|---|---|
| | Varied | Milk | Cereals, eggs and Cantonese soups | Meats | Fruits, nuts and Cantonese desserts | Vegetables |
| Overall preterm delivery (n, %) | 85 (4.9) | 66 (6.1) | 54 (5.0) | 44 (3.9) | 43 (4.9) | 59 (4.1) |
| Crude OR (95% CI) | 1.20 (0.86–1.69) | 1.51 (1.05–2.17) * | 1.24 (0.85–1.80) | 0.95 (0.64–1.42) | 1.21 (0.81–1.81) | 1.00 (Reference) |
| Adjusted OR (95% CI) [a] | 1.27 (0.90–1.80) | 1.59 (1.11–2.29) * | 1.31 (0.89–1.92) | 1.01 (0.67–1.51) | 1.30 (0.87–1.96) | 1.00 (Reference) |
| Spontaneous preterm delivery (n, %) | 63 (3.7) | 52 (4.8) | 39 (3.7) | 32 (2.9) | 34 (3.9) | 42 (2.9) |
| Crude OR (95% CI) | 1.25 (0.84–1.86) | 1.67 (1.10–2.53) * | 1.25 (0.81–1.95) | 0.97 (0.61–1.55) | 1.35 (0.85–2.13) | 1.00 (Reference) |
| Adjusted OR (95% CI) [a] | 1.29 (0.86–1.92) | 1.73 (1.14–2.62) * | 1.30 (0.83–2.03) | 1.00 (0.63–1.60) | 1.41 (0.89–2.24) | 1.00 (Reference) |
| Iatrogenic preterm delivery (n, %) | 14 (0.8) | 9 (0.9) | 10 (1.0) | 5 (0.5) | 8 (1.0) | 16 (1.1) |
| Crude OR (95% CI) | 0.73 (0.36–1.50) | 0.76 (0.33–1.73) | 0.84 (0.38–1.87) | 0.40 (0.15–1.09) | 0.83 (0.35–1.95) | 1.00 (Reference) |
| Adjusted OR (95% CI) [a, b] | 0.79 (0.38–1.61) | 0.79 (0.34–1.74) | 0.90 (0.40–1.94) | 0.46 (0.16–1.14) | 0.87 (0.36–1.97) | 1.00 (Reference) |
| Late preterm delivery (n, %) | 73 (4.2) | 53 (4.9) | 47 (4.4) | 37 (3.3) | 40 (4.6) | 44 (3.1) |
| Crude OR (95% CI) | 1.38 (0.95–2.03) | 1.63 (1.08–2.45) * | 1.44 (0.95–2.19) | 1.08 (0.69–1.68) | 1.51 (0.98–2.34) | 1.00 (Reference) |
| Adjusted OR (95% CI) [a] | 1.46 (0.99–2.15) | 1.73 (1.08–2.62) * | 1.54 (1.01–2.35) * | 1.11 (0.73–1.79) | 1.61 (1.04–2.50) * | 1.00 (Reference) |
| Moderately or early preterm delivery (n, %) | 12 (0.7) | 13 (1.3) | 7 (0.7) | 7 (0.6) | 3 (0.4) | 15 (1.1) |
| Crude OR (95% CI) | 0.67 (0.31–1.43) | 1.17 (0.55–2.47) | 0.63 (0.26–1.55) | 0.60 (0.24–1.47) | 0.33 (0.10–1.15) | 1.00 (Reference) |
| Adjusted OR (95% CI) [a, b] | 0.73 (0.34–1.55) | 1.19 (0.56–2.50) | 0.68 (0.27–1.58) | 0.63 (0.25–1.48) | 0.42 (0.11–1.21) | 1.00 (Reference) |

[a] Adjusted for maternal age, education level, monthly income, parity, passive smoking during pregnancy, supplementation with folic acid, pre-pregnancy BMI, and previous preterm delivery

[b] The firth's correction was applied to improve the accuracy of the logit coefficients

* $P_{value} < 0.05$

the 'Vegetables' group, those in the 'Cereals, eggs, and Cantonese soups' and 'Fruits, nuts, and Cantonese desserts' groups had increased odds of late preterm delivery.

Our findings implied that maternal diet with frequent consumption of vegetables might contribute to lower odds of preterm delivery. Similarly, several studies suggested that vegetables are important components of protective dietary patterns to which women adhere may have lower odds of preterm delivery. In a large prospective cohort study in Norway, diets rich in vegetables and fruits, known as the prudent diet, are associated with a lower incidence of preterm delivery [14]. Another study in Singapore has shown that a dietary pattern high in vegetables, fruits, and white rice is associated with a lower incidence of preterm delivery [17]. Low vegetables intake might induce to inadequacy of antioxidants, which can reduce both systemic and local inflammation [28] and hence the risk of preterm premature rupture of membranes [29]. Insufficient intake of vegetables inhibits peristalsis and might lead to constipation during pregnancy [30, 31], which might further impair fetal growth [32].

Frequent consumption of milk and less frequent consumption of vegetables in our study was found to have higher odds of preterm delivery. Similarly, increased odds of preterm delivery were also found for a diet high in whole milk in the American population [15]. Our findings could be explained from the following aspects. Firstly, dairy is not consumed on a regular or daily basis for most of the Chinese [19]. The variety of dairy products in China is not as much as that in the Western countries. Milk (mainly cow's milk), including fresh milk and milk powder, is the main source of dairy products in China [18]. Yoghurt consumption is increasing in China; however, there is still a gap to catch up with the Western world. Dairy products (e.g. milk, cheese and yoghurt), high in dietary protein and calcium, are essential for fetal growth and skeletal development [33, 34]. Dairy is thus recommended in pregnancy dietary guidelines in different countries including China [35, 36]. Women in the 'Milk' group tended to consume whole milk more frequently, milk powder while they had yoghurt less frequently in their diet (Table 1). Yoghurt products enriched with probiotics have been reported to be associated with a reduced risk of preterm delivery [9, 37]. Another possible explanation is that women having a frequent consumption of milk in our study might thus consider their diet healthy enough, without paying attention to the context of a balanced diet and the whole vegetables consumption.

In the subgroup analyses, we only found a significant association between dietary pattern and spontaneous preterm delivery for women in the 'Milk' groups in comparison to those in the 'Vegetables' groups. Our supplementary results obtained from 'frequency' variable support such finding. After stratification of preterm delivery according to gestational age, we only found significantly greater odds of late preterm delivery for women in the 'Milk,' 'Cereals, eggs, and Cantonese soups' and 'Fruits, nuts, and Cantonese desserts' groups in comparison to those in the 'Vegetables' groups. In agreement with our study, several studies also showed that the significant association was primarily driven by the higher incidence of spontaneous preterm delivery [14, 15, 17] and late preterm delivery [14]. It is speculated that dietary factors might only marginally reduce the progression to preterm delivery and the effect is therefore most easily detectable in late preterm delivery [14]. It appears that there is no significant association between maternal diet and iatrogenic preterm delivery or early/moderately preterm delivery in our study. Notably, only a single measure of dietary intake obtained from an FFQ was used in this study, limiting the validity of the finding.

This is the first prospective study to examine the relationship between maternal dietary patterns and preterm delivery in a Chinese population with a relatively large sample size. The high participation rate in the cohort study and the availability of ultrasound data to confirm gestational age are additional major strengths. Previous studies exploring maternal dietary patterns and preterm delivery have mostly been conducted by using factor analysis to identify dietary patterns. Instead, we used cluster analysis, which can provide a clear description of exactly what is frequently consumed [38]. Our findings might thus be more valuable for a nutrition intervention design to target pregnant women in need. In addition, patterns obtained from cluster analysis in our study appear to better reflect the Asian dietary pattern than that from factor analysis conducted by He et al. in the same cohort [39].

The present study had some limitations. Firstly, we did not collect data on food servings or portion sizes of food items, and were unable to calculate the amount of food consumption and adjust the total energy intake. However, it was suggested that individuals are generally incapable to describe food portions accurately [40], and there are sustainable within subject variations in the indication of food quantities [41]. In contrast, a simple FFQ is sufficient to indicate actual intakes [42]. As previous studies [39, 43], frequencies of food intake were used as a proxy for a quantitative indicator. Secondly, we assessed food intake 'in the past week' at 24–28 week of gestation. The information during this short period might not be representative of dietary habits throughout pregnancy. However, previous studies have suggested that overall dietary patterns differed minimally during pregnancy [44, 45]. Thirdly, we could not precisely distinguish women who were on special diets, which might affect the findings. However, such case is estimated to be rare in our study, as we have excluded women with pre-pregnancy hypertension or diabetes. Only four participants were reported as 'vegan'. Fourthly, more than 20% of the participants missed Q2 data. Finally, owing to the nature of the observational study design, we are unable to identify the causality between preterm delivery and diet. Residual confounders are likely to exist even after we have adjusted for several factors in the statistical analysis.

## Conclusions

In conclusion, a maternal pregnancy diet with frequent consumption of milk and less frequent consumption of vegetables is found to be associated with increased odds of preterm delivery among Chinese women in the current large-scale birth cohort. Frequent consumption of vegetables should be recommended during pregnancy to prevent preterm delivery.

## Additional file

**Additional file 1: Table S1.** Comparison of characteristics among women remained in the present study and those who missed Q2 data. **Table S2.** Food List in the food frequency questionnaire (FFQ) of BIGCS. **Table S3.** List of food items included in the 30 main food groups. **Table S4** The ratios of between-cluster variance to within-cluster variances for each food group across clusters from two to six. **Table S5.** Frequencies of weekly intake of 30 food groups assessed with a self-administered food frequency questionnaire across the six dietary patterns identified among 7352 pregnant Chinese women from the Born in Guangzhou Cohort Study. **Table S6.** Characteristics of the participants across the six dietary patterns identified by cluster analysis. **Table S7.** Associations between dietary patterns and preterm delivery.

#### Abbreviations

ANOVA: One-way analysis of variance; BIGCS: Born in Guangzhou cohort study; BMI: Body mass index; CI: Confidence interval; FFQ: Food frequency questionnaire; GWCMC: Guangzhou women and children's medical center; OR: Odds ratios; SD: Standard deviation

#### Acknowledgements

The authors are grateful to the pregnant women who participated in the BIGCS and all obstetric care providers who assisted in the implementation of the study. We also thank the Born in Guangzhou Cohort Study Group, including Yashu Kuang, Bing Huang, Shenghui Li, Xiaoyan Xia, Yanyan Wu, Songying Shen, Wanqing Xiao, Huiyun Xiao, Huihui Liu, Fengjuan Zhou, Si Tu, Dongmei Wei, Zhaohuan Gui, Yanfei Xing, Lisha Zhu, Xian Liu, Yan Hu, Ying Ma, Weidong Li, Yan Li, Xingwen Zou, Lin Jiang, Jing Zhao, and Yi Hu.

**Funding**
The present study was supported by the grants from the National Natural Science Foundation of China (81673181, 81703244), Guangzhou Science Technology and Innovation Commission (201508030037), and Guangdong Provincial Department of Science and Technology (2014A020213022).

**Authors' contributions**
KKC, HX and XQ conceived and designed the study; ML, JH and QC conceived and designed the study, analyzed and interpreted the data, and drafted the manuscript; JL and XW analyzed and interpreted the data; QZ helped draft the manuscript; FC, LZ, NC, LQ and MY collected and assembled the data. All authors performed critical revision for important intellectual content and approved the final version of the manuscript.

**Competing interests**
The authors declare that they have no competing interests.

**Author details**
[1]Division of Birth Cohort Study, Guangzhou Women and Children's Medical Center, Guangzhou Medical University, 9 Junsui Road, Zhujiang Newtown, Tianhe District, Guangzhou 510623, China. [2]Department of Woman and Child Health Care, Guangzhou Women and Children's Medical Center, Guangzhou Medical University, Guangzhou, China. [3]Department of Obstetrics and Gynecology, Guangzhou Women and Children's Medical Center, Guangzhou Medical University, Guangzhou, China. [4]Institute of Applied Health Research, University of Birmingham, Birmingham, UK. [5]Department of Neonatal Surgery, Division of Birth Cohort Study, Guangzhou Women and Children's Medical Center, Guangzhou Medical University, 9 Junsui Road, Zhujiang Newtown, Tianhe District, Guangzhou 510623, China.

**References**
1. Petrini JR, Dias T, McCormick MC, Massolo ML, Green NS, Escobar GJ. Increased risk of adverse neurological development for late preterm infants. J Pediatr. 2009;154:169–76.
2. Blencowe H, Cousens S, Oestergaard MZ, Chou D, Moller AB, Narwal R, Adler A, Vera Garcia C, Rohde S, Say L, Lawn JE. National, regional, and worldwide estimates of preterm birth rates in the year 2010 with time trends since 1990 for selected countries: a systematic analysis and implications. Lancet. 2012;379:2162–72.
3. Tanz LJ, Stuart JJ, Williams PL, Rimm EB, Missmer SA, Rexrode KM, Mukamal KJ, Rich-Edwards JW. Preterm delivery and maternal cardiovascular disease in young and middle-aged adult women. Circulation. 2017;135:578–89.
4. Nnam NM. Improving maternal nutrition for better pregnancy outcomes. Proc Nutr Soc. 2015;74:454–9.
5. Dean SV, Mason E, Howson CP, Lassi ZS, Imam AM, Bhutta ZA. Born too soon: care before and between pregnancy to prevent preterm births: from evidence to action. Reprod Health. 2013;10(Suppl 1):S3.
6. Requejo J, Merialdi M, Althabe F, Keller M, Katz J, Menon R. Born too soon: care during pregnancy and childbirth to reduce preterm deliveries and improve health outcomes of the preterm baby. Reprod Health. 2013; 10(Suppl 1):S4.
7. Zou L, Wang X, Ruan Y, Li G, Chen Y, Zhang W. Preterm birth and neonatal mortality in China in 2011. Int J Gynaecol Obstet. 2014;127:243–7.
8. Blencowe H, Cousens S, Chou D, Oestergaard M, Say L, Moller AB, Kinney M, Lawn J. Born too soon: the global epidemiology of 15 million preterm births. Reprod Health. 2013;10(Suppl 1):S2.
9. Myhre R, Brantsaeter AL, Myking S, Gjessing HK, Sengpiel V, Meltzer HM, Haugen M, Jacobsson B. Intake of probiotic food and risk of spontaneous preterm delivery. Am J Clin Nutr. 2011;93:151–7.
10. Baron R, Te Velde SJ, Heymans MW, Klomp T, Hutton EK, Brug J. The relationships of health behaviour and psychological characteristics with spontaneous preterm birth in nulliparous women. Matern Child Health J. 2016;21:873–82.
11. Bloomfield FH. How is maternal nutrition related to preterm birth? Annu Rev Nutr. 2011;31:235–61.
12. Hu FB. Dietary pattern analysis: a new direction in nutritional epidemiology. Curr Opin Lipidol. 2002;13:3–9.
13. Rasmussen MA, Maslova E, Halldorsson TI, Olsen SF. Characterization of dietary patterns in the Danish national birth cohort in relation to preterm birth. PLoS One. 2014;9:e93644.
14. Englund-Ogge L, Brantsaeter AL, Sengpiel V, Haugen M, Birgisdottir BE, Myhre R, Meltzer HM, Jacobsson B. Maternal dietary patterns and preterm delivery: results from large prospective cohort study. BMJ. 2014;348:g1446.
15. Martin CL, Sotres-Alvarez D, Siega-Riz AM. Maternal dietary patterns during the second trimester are associated with preterm birth. J Nutr. 2015;145:1857–64.
16. Grieger JA, Grzeskowiak LE, Clifton VL. Preconception dietary patterns in human pregnancies are associated with preterm delivery. J Nutr. 2014; 144:1075–80.
17. Chia AR, de Seymour JV, Colega M, Chen LW, Chan YH, Aris IM, et al. A vegetable, fruit, and white rice dietary pattern during pregnancy is associated with a lower risk of preterm birth and larger birth size in a multiethnic Asian cohort: the growing up in Singapore towards healthy outcomes (GUSTO) study. Am J Clin Nutr. 2016;104:1416–23.
18. Yang SS, Zhang YX. The reseach of the differences between Chinese and western diet cultures. Cross-cultural communication. 2010;6:75–83.
19. Gao H, Stiller CK, Scherbaum V, Biesalski HK, Wang Q, Hormann E, Bellows AC. Dietary intake and food habits of pregnant women residing in urban and rural areas of Deyang City, Sichuan Province, China. Nutrients. 2013;5:2933–54.
20. Tian HG, Nan Y, Hu G, Dong QN, Yang XL. A dietary survey of the Chinese population in urban and rural areas of Tianjin. Asia Pac J Clin Nutr. 1996;5:229–32.
21. Qiu X, Lu JH, He JR, Lam KH, Shen SY, Guo Y, et al. The born in Guangzhou cohort study (BIGCS). Eur J Epidemiol. 2017;32:337–46.
22. Chen TM. A tradition of soup: flavors from China's Pearl River Delta. Berkeley: North Atlantic books; 2009.
23. Yuan MY, He JR, Chen NN, Lu JH, Shen SY, Xiao WQ, et al. Validity and reproducibility of a dietary questionnaire for consumption frequencies of foods during pregnancy in the born in Guangzhou cohort study (BIGCS). Nutrients. 2016;8
24. Lu MS, Chen QZ, He JR, Wei XL, Lu JH, Li SH, et al. Maternal dietary patterns and fetal growth: a large prospective cohort study in China. Nutrients. 2016;8
25. Lo Siou G, Yasui Y, Csizmadi I, McGregor SE, Robson PJ. Exploring statistical approaches to diminish subjectivity of cluster analysis to derive dietary patterns: the tomorrow project. Am J Epidemiol. 2011;173:956–67.
26. Chen C, Lu FC. The guidelines for prevention and control of overweight and obesity in Chinese adults. Biomed Environ Sci. 2004;17(Suppl):1–36.
27. The R project. http://www.r-project.org.
28. Jeffery IB, O'Toole PW. Diet-microbiota interactions and their implications for healthy living. Nutrients. 2013;5:234–52.
29. Romero R, Chaiworapongsa T, Espinoza J. Micronutrients and intrauterine infection, preterm birth and the fetal inflammatory response syndrome. J Nutr. 2003;133:1668S–73S.
30. Anderson AS, Whichelow MJ. Constipation during pregnancy: dietary fibre intake and the effect of fibre supplementation. Hum Nutr Appl Nutr. 1985;39:202–7.
31. Derbyshire E, Davies J, Costarelli V, Dettmar P. Diet, physical inactivity and the prevalence of constipation throughout and after pregnancy. Matern Child Nutr. 2006;2:127–34.
32. Blackburn S. Maternal, Fetal, & neonatal physiology - E-book: a clinical perspective. 5th ed. St. Louis: Elsevier Health Sciences; 2017.
33. Brantsaeter AL, Olafsdottir AS, Forsum E, Olsen SF, Thorsdottir I. Does milk and dairy consumption during pregnancy influence fetal growth and infant birthweight? A systematic literature review. Food Nutr Res. 2012;56
34. Chang SC, O'Brien KO, Nathanson MS, Caulfield LE, Mancini J, Witter FR. Fetal femur length is influenced by maternal dairy intake in pregnant African American adolescents. Am J Clin Nutr. 2003;77:1248–54.
35. Ortega RM. Dietary guidelines for pregnant women. Public Health Nutr. 2001;4:1343–6.
36. Society TCN. The Chinese dietary guideline. Available from http://dg.cnsoc.org/. 2016.
37. Stojanovic N, Plecas D, Plesinac S. Normal vaginal flora, disorders and application of probiotics in pregnancy. Arch Gynecol Obstet. 2012;286:325–32.
38. Tucker KL. Dietary patterns, approaches, and multicultural perspective. Appl Physiol Nutr Metab. 2010;35:211–8.
39. He JR, Yuan MY, Chen NN, Lu JH, Hu CY, Mai WB, et al. Maternal dietary patterns and gestational diabetes mellitus: a large prospective cohort study in China. Br J Nutr. 2015;113:1292–300.

40. Guthrie HA. Selection and quantification of typical food portions by young adults. J Am Diet Assoc. 1984;84:1440–4.
41. Hunter DJ, Sampson L, Stampfer MJ, Colditz GA, Rosner B, Willett WC. Variability in portion sizes of commonly consumed foods among a population of women in the United States. Am J Epidemiol. 1988;127:1240–9.
42. Tjonneland A, Haraldsdottir J, Overvad K, Stripp C, Ewertz M, Jensen OM. Influence of individually estimated portion size data on the validity of a semiquantitative food frequency questionnaire. Int J Epidemiol. 1992;21:770–7.
43. Yu C, Shi Z, Lv J, Du H, Qi L, Guo Y, et al. Major dietary patterns in relation to general and central obesity among Chinese adults. Nutrients. 2015;7:5834–49.
44. Cuco G, Fernandez-Ballart J, Sala J, Viladrich C, Iranzo R, Vila J, Arija V. Dietary patterns and associated lifestyles in preconception, pregnancy and postpartum. Eur J Clin Nutr. 2006;60:364–71.
45. Crozier SR, Robinson SM, Godfrey KM, Cooper C, Inskip HM. Women's dietary patterns change little from before to during pregnancy. J Nutr. 2009;139:1956–63.

# 7

# Environmental footprints of food consumption and dietary patterns among Lebanese adults

Farah Naja[1], Lamis Jomaa[1], Leila Itani[2], Jeremy Zidek[4], Sibelle El Labban[1], Abla Mehio Sibai[3] and Nahla Hwalla[1*]

**Abstract**

**Background:** Following the release of the Sustainable Development Goals, dietary patterns and guidelines are being revised for their effect on the environment in addition to their health implications. The objective of this study was to evaluate and compare the Environmental Footprints (EFPs) of food consumption patterns among Lebanese adults.

**Methods:** For this study, data for adults aged > 18 years ($n = 337$) were drawn from a previous national survey conducted in Lebanon (2008–2009), where dietary intake was assessed using a 61-item Food Frequency Questionnaire. Dietary patterns previously derived in the study sample included: Western, Lebanese-Mediterranean and High-Protein. In this study, food consumption and dietary patterns were examined for their EFPs including water use, energy use, and greenhouse gas (GHG) emissions, using review of life cycle analyses.

**Results:** In the study population, the EFPs of food consumption were: water use: 2571.62 ± 1259.45 L/day; energy use: 37.34 ± 19.98 MJ/day and GHGs: 4.06 ± 1.93 kg CO2 eq / day. Among the three dietary patterns prevalent in the study population, the Lebanese-Mediterranean diet had the lowest water use and GHG per 1000 Kcal (Water (L/Kg): 443.61 ± 197.15, 243.35 ± 112.0, 264.72 ± 161.67; GHG (KG CO2 eq/day) 0.58 ± 0.32, 0.38 ± 0.24, 0.57 ± 0.37, for the Western, Lebanese-Mediterranean and High- Protein, respectively). The scores of the High-Protein dietary pattern were associated with higher odds of the three EFPs, whereas the Lebanese-Mediterranean dietary pattern was associated with lower odds of energy use. Furthermore, scores of the Western pattern were associated with higher water use.

**Conclusions:** The findings of this study showed that, among Lebanese adults, the Western and High-Protein dietary patterns had high EFPs, whereas the Lebanese-Mediterranean dietary pattern had lower water use and GHG emissions. Coupled to our earlier findings of the Lebanese-Mediterranean pattern's beneficial effects on health, the findings of this study lend evidence for the notion that what is healthy for people may also be healthy for ecosystems and highlight the need for nutrition recommendations to take into consideration the nexus of water, food, energy, in addition to health.

**Keywords:** Dietary patterns, Environmental footprint, Mediterranean, Sustainability, Lebanon

## Background

The Middle East and North Africa (MENA) region suffers from a high prevalence of non-communicable diseases (NCDs) constituting 47% of the region's burden of diseases, and this rate is expected to rise up to 60% by 2020 [1]. Such a high burden of NCDs is possibly brought about by a shift in dietary habits and a remarkable nutrition transition [2].

* Correspondence: nahla@aub.edu.lb
[1]Nutrition and Food Sciences Department, Faculty of Agriculture and Food Sciences, American University of Beirut, PO Box 11-0236, Riad El Solh, Beirut 11072020, Lebanon
Full list of author information is available at the end of the article

This nutrition transition is characterized by a rapid shift in dietary intake from traditional, diverse and balanced diets towards more 'westernized' diets [1], specifically a high consumption of 'harmful' foods and low consumption of 'protective' foods [3]. This situation has triggered national and regional efforts to develop dietary guidelines and recommendations that promote the consumption of balanced diets known for their protective effects against NCDs [4, 5]. However, these efforts did not consider the environmental impact of such guidelines in a region that suffers of depleted resources, in terms of water scarcity, land degradation and high energy use [2]. These issues have been raised by the released Sustainable Development Goals (SDGs) which called for sustainable consumption and production and brought "sustainable diets" to the forefront of the sustainability agenda [6, 7]. 'Sustainable diets,' according to the Food and Agriculture Organization (FAO) (2012), are *those diets with low environmental impacts that contribute to food and nutrition security and to healthy life for present and future generations. Sustainable diets are protective and respectful of biodiversity and ecosystems, culturally acceptable, accessible, economically fair and affordable; nutritionally adequate, safe and healthy; while optimizing natural and human resources* [8]. Accordingly, United Nations Environment Program (UNEP) (2016), called to reexamine food-based dietary guidelines, not only for their health outcomes but also with respect to their environmental sustainability, given the considerable impact of dietary choices and food consumption on the environment [9]. Efforts to quantify environmental impacts of food consumption led to the development of environmental footprint indicators, spanning multiple dimensions and including greenhouse gas emissions (carbon footprint), nitrogen release (nitrogen footprint), water use (blue and green water footprint) and land use (land footprint) [10].

Accordingly, a growing body of research explored the previously recommended diets and dietary patterns in terms of their impact on environmental footprints and depletion of natural resources [11, 12]. Results from these studies suggested that plant-based dietary patterns, which are primarily based on fruits, vegetables, legumes, whole grains, nuts and seeds, have a more positive impact on health and a lower environmental impact than animal-based dietary patterns. Nevertheless, these findings need to be considered through a context-specific lens to account for regional and local variations in agricultural practices, environmental resources, local food systems and cultural preferences of diverse populations [13].

Lebanon is a middle income country in the MENA region, which, similar to other neighboring countries, is witnessing an increase in the prevalence of diet-related diseases, a rapid nutrition transition coupled with scarcity and poor management of natural resources [1, 14]. Previous research in the country has studied dietary intake and food consumption patterns in terms of their effect on health and wellbeing. The results of these investigations consistently identified two main dietary patterns: 'Western' and 'Lebanese- Mediterranean,' where, the Western pattern has been associated with adverse health outcomes, including obesity, hypertension, and metabolic syndrome. On the other hand, the Lebanese-Mediterranean pattern showed protective effects against metabolic abnormalities and type 2 diabetes [14–18]. These findings provided evidence for recommendations to limit consumption of the Western dietary pattern and encourage adherence to the Lebanese-Mediterranean diet in order to combat the rising epidemic of NCDs in the country. However, such dietary recommendations and guidelines were not examined in terms of their environmental sustainability, as called upon by the international community and the SDGs, in a country and a region where environmental issues are paramount. The aim of the present study was to evaluate the environmental footprints (EFPs) of overall food consumption and to examine the association of these EFPs with dietary patterns previously identified in Lebanon. Contributions of foods and food groups to the EFPs of each pattern were also examined.

## Methods

### Study design, participants and data collection

Data for this study were drawn from the cross-sectional National Nutrition and Non-Communicable Disease Risk Factor Survey (2008–2009). Details describing the sampling frame and techniques are described elsewhere [19]. In brief, the households which were considered as primary sampling units were selected, using a stratified cluster random sampling frame. The numbers of households from each cluster were proportional to the cluster's size. Within each household, one adult with no history of chronic diseases (> 18 years of age) was randomly chosen and was invited to participate in the survey. At the participants' homes, data collection was conducted following the WHO STEPwise approach to Surveillance (STEPS) [20] and included socio-demographic and lifestyle questionnaires, anthropometric measurements, biochemical assessment, as well as a food frequency questionnaire (FFQ) for the evaluation of dietary intake ($n = 337$) [21]. The study protocol was reviewed and approved by the Institutional Review Board of the American University of Beirut, and informed consent was obtained from all participants in the study.

For the purpose of this study, survey data pertaining to the participants' socio-demographic and lifestyle characteristics as well as dietary intake were used. Socio-demographic characteristics included age, sex, crowding index, marital status, and education level. Crowding index (CI), defined as the average number of people per room, excluding the kitchen and bathroom, was used as a proxy for socioeconomic status, whereby a lower CI was associated with a higher socio economic status [22]. Earlier investigations showed that CI was associated with adherence to certain dietary patterns in Lebanon [19, 23, 15].The lifestyle factors considered in this study were related to smoking and physical activity. Physical activity was assessed using the short Arabic version of the International Physical Activity Questionnaire [24]. Using metabolic equivalents mins per week, three levels of physical activity were determined (low, moderate, high). Dietary intake of study participants was assessed using a 61-item FFQ. These foods are listed in Additional file 1. This FFQ measured dietary intake over the 1 year preceding the interview. For each food item listed in the FFQ, a standard portion size was specified and five frequency choices were given (never, daily, weekly, monthly or yearly). This FFQ was designed by a panel of nutritionists and included culture specific dishes and recipes. It was tested on a convenient sample of Lebanese adults to check for clarity and cultural sensitivity. Further details about this FFQ are found elsewhere [15].

#### Dietary patterns in the study population

Previous work by our research group derived dietary patterns prevalent among the survey participants ($n = 337$) [19, 21], whereby the 61 food items listed in the FFQ were grouped into 25 food groups based on similarities in ingredients, nutrient profile, and/or culinary usage [25] and were entered in the factor analysis. Food items having a unique composition (e.g. eggs, olives, and mayonnaise) were classified individually. Furthermore, certain food items such as falafel sandwiches, though made of legumes, were entered separately from this food group given that falafel is a fried form of legumes and the sandwiches are usually eaten out of home, unlike other legume-based dishes that are mainly consumed in stew form and prepared at home. The total intake for each group (expressed as daily gram intake) was calcualted by summing the daily gram intake of each food within the group. For example, the daily gram intake from the food group 'Dried fruits' was calculated by adding the daily gram intake of dried raisins, dried apricots and dried prunes. Further details about the derivation of these patterns are presented elsewhere [21]. In brief, three dietary patterns were identified using factor analysis: Western, Lebanese-Mediterranean, and High-Protein. The Lebanese-Mediterranean deitary pattern was previously proposed as a variant of the Mediterranean diet [26]. The factor scores for each of the identified pattern were calculated by multiple regression approach whereby independent variables in the regression equation are the standardized observed values of the food items in the estimated patterns. These predictor variables are weighted by regression coefficients, which are obtained by multiplying the inverse of the observed variable correlation matrix by the matrix of factor loadings. The factor scores are the dependent variables in the regression equation [27]. Each individual received a factor score for each dietary pattern. The obtained scores were normally distributed with a mean of zero and standard deviation equal 1. These scores indicated the degree to which each participant's diet corresponds to the identified pattern. In this study, these scores were used to examine the association of dietary patterns with the EFP. The foods/ food groups that consituted these patterns and their factor loadings are described in Table 1.

#### Derivation of environmental foot prints (EFPs)

For the purpose of this study, metrics for three EFPs were calculated including water use, energy use and GHGs (Additional file 1). The mapping of dietary patterns to their associated EFPs required the estimation of metrics for the EFPs of each of the 61 items listed in the FFQ which made up the food groups of these patterns. These metrics were estimated based on a review of previously published Life Cycle Assessment (LCAs) analyses. LCA is an internationally recognized method employed to estimate the impact of resource use at all stages of a product's existence from creation to end of life [25]. The LCAs reviewed in this study followed the ISO 14040 and 14,044 [28]. LCAs conducted in Mediterranean or neighboring countries with similar climates to Lebanon were prioritized over LCAs conducted in countries of other regions in the world. For each EFP metric, the origins of LCA data (local, regional or international) used in its estimation are described in Additional file 2. In this appendix, the references used in estimating the EFPs for each food item are also listed. For each food item, LCAs that covered processes from cradle to market (or distribution point) were selected. LCAs that included use phase impacts (such as cooking, heating or refrigeration) were not considered in this study. In this study, the functional unit considered was 1.0 kg of food consumed. The functional unit is defined as a representative, reference measure of the studied system to which all inputs and outputs can be related [29]. For wine/beer, some LCAs report results in liters instead of Kg. Results in these studies were recalculated to a per kg basis assuming a density of 1.0 kg/l. For milk and milk products, though most LCAs report their results in Kg of milk, the percentage fat and protein in the milk could vary. Therefore the outcomes of the LCAs used for milk were adjusted to reflect the standard fat and protein corrected milk values of 3.5% fat and 3.2% and was used as fat-protein corrected milk (FPCM), a common practice in dairy LCAs, using the following formula: FPCM(kg) = 0.149 * milk kg + 5.89 * fat kg. + 3.48 * protein kg [30].

#### *Water use*

The water use environmental metric consisted of the total water use in liters (blue and green water combined) per kilogram of food consumed. Two important elements were considered in the calculation of the water use metric:

1) Consideration of the domestically produced vs imported proportion of each foods: The Food and Agriculture Organization (FAO) data [31] and the United Nations Comtrade database [32] were used to identify foods that are produced locally versus those that are imported. In addition, for imported foods, we have considered the top two countries by amount from where a certain food is imported.
2) Use of a water stress-based impact assessment method: Following step (1), water use was adjusted for each country using the water stress index (WSI)

**Table 1** Food items/groups constituting the dietary patterns prevalent in the study population[ab]

| Western | Lebanese-Mediterranean | High-Protein |
|---|---|---|
| Pizza, pies and refined grains (0.63) | Fruits (0.64) | Poultry (0.69) |
| Fast food sandwiches(0.57) | Legumes (0.56) | Meat (0.63) |
| Sweets (0.53) | Whole dairy products (0.53) | Fish (0.59) |
| Regular soda (0.51) | Olives (0.47) | Low fat dairy products (0.55) |
| Mayonnaise (0.45) | Vegetables (0.45) | Hot drinks (0.35) |
| Nuts and Seeds (0.43) | Burghol (whole wheat parboiled and crushed) (0.34) | Breakfast cereals (0.22) |
| Eggs(0.4) | Dried fruits (0.29) | Light soda (0.22) |
| Fats and oils(0.37) | Traditional suits (0.25) | |
| Ice cream(0.31) | | |
| Bottled fruit juices(0.23) | | |
| Alcoholic beverages (0.21) | | |

[a]Factor loading of the various food groups/items are presented in ()
[b]The dietary patterns and the food items-and their factor loading- making up these patterns were taken from data of Matta et al. (2016) [21]

developed by Pfister et al., 2009 [33].WSI is considered an impact assessment component that allows accounting for crop production in water stressed areas.

In light of these two aforementioned considerations, the water use metric estimation in this study was adjusted using the below formula:

$$\text{Water use (adjusted)} = (\text{Water use}^{*}\%\text{produced}^{*}\ \text{WSILebanon}) + (\text{Water Use}^{*}\%\text{importedTotal}^{*}\%\text{importedCountry1}^{*}\ \text{WSICountry1}) + (\text{Water Use}^{*}\%\text{importedTotal}^{*}\%\text{importedCountry2}^{*}\ \text{WSICountry2})$$

### *GHGs*

The GHG metric was calculated in kg CO2 eq/kg food consumed. Most LCAs used in this study reported GHG emissions in terms of CO2 eq. However, a few LCAs reported $CH_4$ and $N_2O$ separately, in addition to $CO_2$. For these LCAs, emissions from $N_2O$ and $CH_4$ were converted to kg CO2 eq using the following two equations [34]:

$$CO_{2eqN2O} = X_{N2O} * GWP_{N2O}$$

$$CO_{2eq\ CH4} = X_{CH4} * GWP_{CH4}$$

where $X_{N2O}$ is the amount of $N_2O$ released in kg, $X_{CH4}$ is the amount of $CH_4$ released in kg, $GWP_{N2O}$ is the 100-year global warming potential of $N_2O$, and $GWP_{CH4}$ is the 100-year global warming potential of $CH_4$, $GWP_{N2O} = 265$, and $GWP_{CH4} = 28$ [34].

The total CO2 eq was calculated by adding $CO_{2eq\ N2O}$ and $CO_{2eq\ CH4}$ to the $CO_2$ emissions. It is important to note that CH4 emissions from decomposing organic waste in landfills was not directly considered in this analysis due to a lack of specific data for each food item. Fluorinated gases are also not considered as their contributions to the accumulated GHGs of food products may be considered negligible [35].

### *Energy use*

In this paper, 'energy use' referred to industrial energy consumption while 'energy intake' referred to human energy consumption. Energy use was estimated in MJ/kg food consumed. For all foods considered in this study, energy values and GHG emissions were sourced separately.

### Statistical analysis

Socio-demographic characteristics of the study population were described using proportions. For each food item listed in the FFQ, the EFPs metrics corresponding to each participant's dietary intake was estimated using the below formula:

$$\sum_{i=1}^{n} consumed_i * impact_i$$

where $n$ is the food item number, $consumed_i$ is the amount of food consumed in kg- as obtained from the FFQ, and $impact_i$ is the EFPs per unit kg consumed for each food. The EFPs per unit Kg of food item are presented in Additional file 1. For example, the 'rice and rice products' food item is estimated to have a GHG impact of 2.05 kg $CO_{2eq}$ / $kg_{consumed}$. Therefore, if a survey participant consumed an average of one serving of rice (75 g) per day, then rice would contribute 0.15 kg $CO_{2eq}$ to the overall GHG footprint of the diet of this participant. Accordingly, for each of the 61 food items, study participants had estimated metrics for the 3 EFPs that corresponded to their dietary intake (Additional file 1). The Means ± SD of EFP metrics for water use, energy use and GHGS were calculated for the overall dietary intake in the study population. In addition the EFPs of each of the three patterns were calculated by adding the EFPs of the food groups making up these patterns. To adjust for dietary energy intake, the EFPs for the various dietary patterns were also reported per 1000 Kcal and were compared using repeated measure ANOVA. The effects of adherence to any of the dietary patterns on the odds of having a high EFPs were estimated using multiple logistic regression models. For each dietary pattern, three separate regression models were built, each model corresponding to one of the three EFP metrics considered in this study. In each of these models, the independent variable was the score of one of the dietary patterns and the dependent variable was high EFPs. The latter was defined as belonging to the top 20% of the respective EFPs. These models were adjusted for age, sex and energy intake.

## Results

Table 2 describes the characterstics of the study popualtion, in terms of sociodemographic, lifestyle and dietary intake. Over 60% of the study population had a crowding index greater than 1 and were married. As for education, 34% of the study sample had a university level. Mean dietary energy intake was 2638.87 ± 1231.08 Kcal, with carbohydrates, proteins and fats contributing 49.06%, 15.71% and 36.48% respectively. (Table 2).

Table 3 presents the EFP of dietary intake in the study sample, as a total and by dietary pattern. Overall dietary intake of survey participants has the following EFPs (mean ± SD): Water use: 2571.62 ± 1259.45 L/day; Energy use: 37.34 ± 19.98 MJ/day GHG: 4.06 ± 1.93 kg $CO_{2eq}$/day.

After adjustment for energy (/1000 Kcal), for both water use and GHGs, the Lebanese-Mediterranean pattern had the lowest EFP ($p < 0.05$), while no significant difference was noted between the Western and the High-Protein patterns. For energy use, the highest EFP was that of the Western diet, followed by the Lebanese-Mediterranean diet and the High-Protein, with significant differences between these patterns at $p < 0.05$. (Table 3).

Table 4 shows the results of the multiple logistic regression of the effect of adherence to each of the dietary patterns on the odds of high EFPs, controlling for age, sex and dietary energy intake. For water use, adherence to both the Western pattern and High-Protein dietary patterns was associated with higher odds of having a high water use footprint, while no association was noted with the Lebanese-Mediterranean dietary pattern. The magnitude of the association between a high EFP of water use with the Western dietary pattern was higher than that with the High-Protein dietary pattern (OR: 2.56 and OR 1.93 respectively). As for energy use, while the High-Protein dietary pattern was associated with higher odds of having high EFP for this metric (OR: 1.90, 95% CI: 1.00–4.00), a Lebanese-Mediterranean dietary pattern was associated with significantly lower odds (OR: 0.95, 95%CI: 0.92–0.98). For GHG, the High-Protein dietary pattern was significantly associated with having a high EFP for this metric (OR: 3.22, 95%CI: 1.96–5.28). (Table 4).

Table 5 presents the percent contributions of various food or food groups to the 3 EFPs of each of the dietary patterns. The total EFPs of each pattern was based on

**Table 2** Characteristics of the study population ($n = 337$)[a]

| | Study population ($n = 337$) |
|---|---|
| Demographic characteristics | |
| Age (years) | |
| 18–30 | 111(32.9) |
| 31–40 | 103(30.6) |
| ≥ 41 | 123(36.5) |
| Sex | |
| Males | 168 (49.8) |
| Females | 169 (50.2) |
| Social and lifestyle characteristics | |
| Crowding index | |
| < 1 | 122(36.4) |
| ≥ 1 | 213(63.6) |
| *p*-value | |
| Marital status | |
| Single | 129(38.3) |
| Married | 208(61.7) |
| Education | |
| Up to High school | 231(68.5) |
| University level | 106(31.5) |
| Smoking | |
| No | 231(68.5) |
| Yes | 106(31.5) |
| Physical activity level | |
| Low | 122(36.2) |
| moderate | 68(20.2) |
| High | 147(43.6) |
| Dietary intake characteristics | |
| Energy intake (Kcal) | 2638.87 ± 1231.08 |
| Carbohydrates (% of total energy) | 49.06 ± 7.03 |
| Proteins (% of total energy) | 15.71 ± 2.90 |
| Fats (% of total energy) | 36.48 ± 6.90 |

[a]Values in this table represent n(%) and mean ± SD for categorical and continuous variables respectively

**Table 3** Environmental Footprints of dietary intake in the study sample: Total and by dietary pattern §

| | Total | Western | Lebanese-Mediterranean | High-Protein |
|---|---|---|---|---|
| Water use (L / day) | 2571.62 ± 1259.45 | 1231.02 ± 937.23[a] | 602.06 ± 330.70[b] | 653.87 ± 452.92[b] |
| Water use (L/day) per 1000 Kcal | 951.68 ± 216.26 | 443.61 ± 197.15[a] | 243.35 ± 112.0[b] | 264.72 ± 161.67[a] |
| Energy use (MJ / day) | 37.34 ± 19.98 | 20.53 ± 17.50[a] | 10.82 ± 6.27[b] | 5.00 ± 4.41[c] |
| Energy use (MJ / day)/1000 Kcal | 14.25 ± 5.76 | 7.55 ± 4.85[a] | 4.60 ± 2.87[b] | 2.09 ± 1.84[c] |
| GHG (KG CO2 eq/day) | 4.06 ± 1.93 | 1.58 ± 1.23[a] | 0.90 ± 0.56[b] | 1.40 ± 0.99[c] |
| GHG (KG CO2 eq/day)/1000 Kcal | 1.53 ± 0.51 | 0.58 ± 0.32[a] | 0.38 ± 0.24[b] | 0.57 ± 0.37[a] |

§Values with different superscripts are significantly different at $p < 0.05$
Values with different superscripts (a, b) are significantly different

the sum of EFPs of food groups making up this pattern. Within the Western pattern, the highest contributor to all EFPs was 'All grains' (water use: 22.67%; energy use: 32.80% and GHGs: 29.22%). For the Lebanese-Mediterranean dietary pattern, compared to other food/food groups making up this pattern, whole dairy products had the highest percentage contribution to water use (43.01%). 'Vegetables' contributed most to energy use (60.12%) and GHG (50.75%) of this pattern. Within the High-Protein pattern, the highest contributor to all three EFPs was 'Meat' (water use: 69.30%, energy use: 50.87% and GHG: 73.08%). (Table 5).

## Discussion

The results revealed comparable levels of water use, energy use, and GHG emission for food consumption of Lebanese adults to estimates of other countries. Furthermore, comparing dietary patterns, the Lebanese- Mediterranean diet had the lowest EFPs for water use and GHGs. In terms of associations between adherence (higher scores) to various dietary patterns and having a high EFP (belonging to the top 20% of the population), the results of this study suggested that adherence to either the Western or the High-Protein led to an increase in the odds for water use, the High-Protein pattern was also associated with higher odds for energy use and GHGs, while the Lebanese-Mediterranean was associated with lower odds for energy use.

For comparison purposes of the EFP of the Lebanese food consumption to other countries, the EFPs were calculated based on an intake of 2500 kcal/person. For water use, in this study, the average per-person water use (2451 L/day) was slightly lower than the global average (2799 L/day [36] and similar to estimates obtained for Finland (2377 L/day) [37]. Water use of food consumption in the United States and Italy had higher estimates (3998 L/day and 3469 L/day, respectively) [37]. Though within range, the water use estimated for average food consumption in Lebanon ought to be taken into consideration especially in view of the scarcity of natural resources. Lebanon together with other countries of the MENA region are among the most water stressed areas of the world, whereby the water availability per person is more than six times below the global average (1383 $m^3$ to 8462 $m^3$) [38]. The within-range estimate for water use associated with food consumption in this study coupled with water scarcity in the country is alarming in view of the high water cost of agricultural production, especially that the forecasted climate change is expected to further reduce rainfall by 6–8%, snow cover by 40%, and prolong drought periods for every 1 °C of temperature rise [39]. Regarding energy, the estimate obtained in this study (35 MJ/day) is higher than that of the United States (28 MJ/day) [40], this finding is alarming especially that Lebanon relies almost solely on imported energy, whether in the form of gas or oil, while its average citizen consumes greater kWh as compared to global estimate (3563 kWh in Lebanon vs 3030 kWh per person globally) [41]. As for GHGs associated with food consumption in Lebanon, the results of the study revealed an estimate (3.9 Kg CO2 eq/day) that is similar to other Mediterranean countries such as Greece (3.6 Kg CO2 eq/day) [42] and to the United States (3.56 Kg CO2 eq/day) [43] and lower than estimates reported in France (4.8 Kg CO2 eq/day) [44]. Such differences could be explained by variations in processes of agricultural practices/food production [45, 46] or composition of food consumption. Regarding the latter, Mediterranean countries tend to consume lower meat and

**Table 4** Multiple logistic regression for the association between dietary patterns and the odds of high EFPs scores in the study population ($n = 377$) [ab]

| Dietary patterns | Water use (L / day) | Energy use (MJ / day) | GHG (kg CO2 eq / day) |
|---|---|---|---|
| Western | 2.56 (1.13–5.18) | 0.96 (0.93–1.00) | 1.32 (0.62–2.81) |
| Lebanese-Mediterranean | 1.01 (0.97–1.04) | 0.95 (0.92–0.98) | 1.26 (0.86–1.85) |
| High-Protein | 1.93 (1.26–2.96) | 1.90 (1.00–4.00) | 3.22 (1.96–5.28) |

[a]High environmental foot print is defined as belonging to the top 20% of each footprint
[b]The logistic regression models were adjusted for age, sex, and energy intake

**Table 5** Percentage contribution (mean ± SD) of food/food groups to EFP metric of the dietary patterns

| Dietary patterns | Water use (L / day) | Energy use (MJ / day) | GHG (kg CO2eq / day) |
|---|---|---|---|
| Western | | | |
| Pizza, pies and refined grains | 25.88 ± 14.39 | 5.88 ± 5.39 | 4.11 ± 3.87 |
| Fast food sandwiches | 11.59 ± 10.98 | 5.06 ± 6.25 | 21.62 ± 18.02 |
| Sweets | 14.67 ± 14.64 | 6.89 ± 7.36 | 5.75 ± 5.97 |
| Regular Soda | 8.26 ± 11.26 | 10.68 ± 14.03 | 4.81 ± 7.24 |
| Mayonnaise | 0.39 ± 0.82 | 0.34 ± 0.75 | 0.37 ± 0.85 |
| Nuts and seeds | 10.83 ± 13.36 | 0.93 ± 2.18 | 0.96 ± 2.02 |
| Eggs | 4.84 ± 7.66 | 1.47 ± 4.71 | 5.42 ± 7.91 |
| Fats and oils | 9.62 ± 8.01 | 12.24 ± 9.18 | 6.97 ± 6.35 |
| Ice cream | 0.32 ± 0.44 | 1.32 ± 1.79 | 1.98 ± 2.67 |
| Bottled fruit juices | 13.18 ± 17.30 | 21.31 ± 24.43 | 16.37 ± 20.40 |
| Alcohol beverages | 0.43 ± 2.23 | 1.08 ± 3.58 | 2.43 ± 6.90 |
| Lebanese-Mediterranean | | | |
| Fruits | 20.69 ± 14.09 | 10.62 ± 9.19 | 10.23 ± 8.73 |
| Legumes | 13.11 ± 9.59 | 0.81 ± 0.93 | 6.90 ± 6.39 |
| Whole dairy products | 43.01 ± 19.05 | 21.04 ± 18.73 | 22.02 ± 20.32 |
| Olives | 8.39 ± 11.33 | 3.27 ± 5.79 | 6.55 ± 10.04 |
| Vegetables | 10.29 ± 7.68 | 60.12 ± 20.49 | 50.75 ± 21.08 |
| Burghol (whole wheat parboiled and crushed) | 2.13 ± 4.42 | 3.18 ± 5.01 | 2.16 ± 3.81 |
| Dried fruits | 0.29 ± 1.06 | 0.36 ± 1.27 | 0.33 ± 1.19 |
| Traditional sweets | 2.09 ± 2.89 | 0.60 ± 0.92 | 1.07 ± 1.55 |
| High-Protein | | | |
| Poultry | 19.21 ± 14.27 | 18.21 ± 12.48 | 14.98 ± 12.44 |
| Meat | 69.30 ± 21.29 | 50.87 ± 22.73 | 73.08 ± 20.79 |
| Fish | 3.22 ± 7.76 | 19.50 ± 17.89 | 6.86 ± 11.06 |
| Low fat dairy products | 4.88 ± 12.31 | 6.02 ± 16.59 | 3.56 ± 11.58 |
| Hot drinks | 0.55 ± 2.17 | 0.03 ± 0.10 | 0.01 ± 0.03 |
| Breakfast cereals | 0.38 ± 5.45 | 0.56 ± 5.52 | 0.35 ± 5.45 |
| Light Soda | 2.47 ± 8.86 | 4.80 ± 14.15 | 1.16 ± 6.23 |

meat products (main contributors to GHGs) as compared to Europe and the Unites States [47]. Despite the lower GHGs associated with food consumption in some Mediterranean countries (including Lebanon) as compared to Western countries, the recent review of the link between global diets, environmental sustainability and health suggested that adherence to a typical Mediterranean diet results in even lower estimate for GHGs (2.6 Kg CO2 eq/day), lending evidence for future research for dietary intake recommendations to lower the GHG associated in Mediterranean countries. Such research ought to consider the evaluation and implementation of dietary recommendation within the tightly linked diet–environment–health trilemma [48].

In this study, the results indicated that the Lebanese-Mediterranean dietary pattern had the lowest levels of water use and GHG emissions, as compared to the Western and the High-Protein patterns. The lower EFPs of the Lebanese-Mediterranean diet were also observed for other traditional diets in Japan [49], South Asia [50] and among indigenous people in Italy [51]. This finding is also in line with those of a previous investigation of the EFPs of dietary patterns in Spain which showed that adherence to a Western dietary pattern led to a significant increase in GHG, agricultural land use, energy as well as water consumption, while adherence to the Mediterranean diet reduced the impact on all EFPs metrics considered in that study [52]. Furthermore, a recent systematic review of studies examining dietary patterns and their environmental sustainability concluded that adherence to Mediterranean style diets has a less negative impact on the environment than current average dietary intakes in the United States [12]. In fact, within the definition of sustainable diets, the FAO and *Biodiversity*

*International* in collaboration with other organizations acknowledged the Mediterranean diet as an example of sustainable diets with four main themes which related not only to health and wellbeing, but also to environment and sustainability, economy as well as well as culture [53, 54]. It is important to note that the Lebanese-Mediterranean shares many characteristics of the Mediterranean diet including high consumption of fruits, vegetables, and olive oil and olives. Hence the Lebanese- Mediterranean was previously proposed as a variant of the Mediterranean diet from the eastern side of the Mediterranean basin [26]. Similar to the other Mediterranean and traditional diets, the lower EFPs of the Lebanese-Mediterranean diet observed in this study could be due to the fact that limited intake of animal food and higher consumption of plant foods (vegetables, cereals and legumes), which are characteristics of this diet, have lower GHG emissions [55, 56]. The present study's findings that the Lebanese-Mediterranean diet had lowest water and GHGs footprints, while the Western dietary pattern had high EFPs are of particular concern as the country is undergoing nutrition transition towards a more westernized dietary consumption. The ongoing nutrition transition would lead to intensification in EFPs and potentially impacting the available natural resources in a region facing significant water scarcity, climate, and landscape and ecosystems threats [53].

When the associations between the various patterns and EFPs were investigated, the results showed a direct association between a higher adherence with the High-Protein pattern and all three EFPs considered in this study. This finding echoes previous reports documenting that the consumption of animal-based food groups has the highest impact on the environment, including water use, energy use and GHGs [48].

In this study, the EFPs of dietary patterns were further characterized whereby the main contributors, in terms of foods and food groups, to the EFPs within these patterns were identified. Within the Western pattern, grains, fast food sandwiches and bottled juices contributed most to EFPs. The Fast food sandwiches of the Western pattern were composed of processed meat-based fillings, such as 'Chawarma' and hamburger. In many countries, red meat was identified as the greatest contributor to diet-related as well as overall agricultural GHG emissions [57–62]. In accordance with the results of this study, Hendrie et al. (2014) showed that red meat and non-core foods (which included processed meats, hot drinks and other energy-dense food items) in the Average Australian Diet accounted for the greatest contribution to GHG emissions [63]. The high contribution of bottled fruit juices to water use in the Western pattern, is in agreement with the reportedly high water footprint of apple and orange juice (200–230 L of water/200 ml glass or 1020–1140 L of water/L of juice) [64]. Interestingly in the Western pattern grains contributed most to the EFPs of this pattern. Although in general, grains are reported to be low on environmental impact [65], however, their high consumption by Lebanese adults led to their large contribution to the EFPs of this pattern. Within the Lebanese-Mediterranean pattern, dairy products alone contributed over 40% of the total water use of this pattern, 21% of energy use and 22% of its GHGs. Though not a common element of the Mediterranean diets, dairy products were part of the Lebanese-Mediterranean pattern. Lebanon, as well as other countries of the Levant including Syria and Jordan, traditionally consumes large quantities of dairy products, which are typically consumed as fermented milk products such as yogurt, strained yogurt (labneh) and white cheese in brine [66]. This finding is in line with other studies which showed that dairy products, principal sources of animal protein in some Mediterranean diets, presented high environmental footprints possibly due to the low consumption of meat and meat products in general in these diets [52, 67]. It is noteworthy that the vegetables group contributed to 60% of energy use and 51% of GHG in this pattern. These results could be explained by 1) the relatively high consumption of vegetables within the Lebanese diet and 2) the fact that production of vegetables requires more energy and GHGs than grains and fruits [48, 68]. In light of these findings, it appears sensible to recommend limiting dairy and increasing fruit consumption within the Lebanese-Mediterranean pattern. However future studies are needed to examine such recommendations taking into consideration the nexus of water, food, energy, as well as health. Policies focusing on one dimension of this nexus ignore the potential tradeoffs among the different impacts and may inadvertently strain resources [10]. For the High-Protein pattern, meat and poultry has the highest contribution to the EFPs of this pattern. As indicated earlier in this section, most research investigating the EFP of food consumption concluded that animal-based food groups, including meat and poultry pose the highest burden on the environment, including high water use, energy use and GHGs [48].

The strength of this study lies in it being the first in the MENA to examine EFPs of food consumption and dietary patterns and as such it could constitute a model for other countries in the region to emulate. The findings of this study ought to be considered in light of a few limitations. First, in the context of this study, metrics derived through the use of LCAs are to be interpreted with caution. LCAs allow for measuring the ecological footprint of each food or food category throughout its life cycle, which typically includes agricultural production and processing [12]. However most of the LCAs are conducted in high income countries with very few based in middle or low income countries. In this study, effort was exerted to use local and regional LCAs. If not available, LCAs from high income countries with similar climate and environmental conditions were used. Second, although this study addressed three EFPs, other elements of environmental sustainability such as soil erosion, biodiversity, pollution, farm management and ecosystem services were not considered in this study. It is important to note that the lack of a detailed inventory of agricultural and production practices in Lebanon and other countries of the region limit the feasibility of a comprehensive assessment of environmental footprints of food consumption.

## Conclusion

The findings of this study showed that, among Lebanese adults, food consumption in general and the Lebanes e-Mediterranean dietary pattern had the lowest estimates for water and GHGs footprints, while the Western and High- Protein patterns had higher EFPs. Coupled to our earlier findings of the Lebanese-Mediterranean pattern's beneficial effects on health and the Western pattern's deleterious effects on health, the findings of this study lend evidence for the notion that what is healthy for people may also be healthy for ecosystems. These EFPs estimates associated with food consumption patterns in the country could be used to inform policies vis-a-vis agricultural production, type of production, food imports, subsidies and recommendations for sustainable food consumption. This study is a first step towards the formulation of sustainable diets for the Lebanese population. Further studies are needed to examine the nutrition value, quantity and quality of the food items comprising the identified patterns in order to achieve this goal and help countries address the SDGs.

### Abbreviations

CH4: Methane; CI: Crowding index; CO2eq: Carbon dioxide equivalent; EFP: Environmental Footprints; FFQ: Food Frequency Questionnaire; GHG: Greenhouse Gas; GWPCH4: Global warming potential of methane; GWPN2O: Global warming potential of nitrous oxide; ha: Hectar; LCA: LIfe cycle analysis; MENA: Middle East and North Africa Region; MJ: Mega Joules; N2O: Nitrous oxide; NCD: Non-Communicable Diseases; NRI: Natural Resources Inventory; SDG: Sustainable Development Goals; t: Metric Ton; UNEP: United Nations Environment Program; WHO: World Health Organization

### Funding

This research did not receive any specific grant from external funding agencies in the public, commercial or not-for-profit sectors. Internal funding from the American University of Beirut supported the data analysis included in this research.

### Authors' contributions

FN led the write-up of the manuscript and supervised data analysis and interpretation; LJ, contributed to the interpretation of the results and the write up of the manuscript; LI was responsible for the statistical analysis of dietary data. JZ was responsible for the derivation of the EFPs metrics. AS contributed to the analysis of dietary data; NH was responsible for the conceptualization of the study objectives, provided valuable input for data interpretation and has critically reviewed the manuscript. All authors have approved the final article.

### Competing interests

The authors declare that they have no competing interests.

### Author details

[1]Nutrition and Food Sciences Department, Faculty of Agriculture and Food Sciences, American University of Beirut, PO Box 11-0236, Riad El Solh, Beirut 11072020, Lebanon. [2]Department of Nutrition & Dietetics, Faculty of Health Sciences, Beirut Arab University, PO Box 11-5020, Riad El Solh, Beirut 11072809, Lebanon. [3]Department of Epidemiology and Population Health, Faculty of Health Sciences, American University of Beirut, PO Box 11-0236, Riad El Solh, Beirut 11072020, Lebanon. [4]Futura Food LLC, 113 Creekside Drive, State College, PA 16801, USA.

### References

1. Mehio Sibai A, Nasreddine L, Mokdad AH, Adra N, Tabet M, Hwalla N. Nutrition transition and cardiovascular disease risk factors in Middle East and North Africa countries: reviewing the evidence. Ann Nutr Metab. 2010; 57:193–203.
2. Hwalla N, Bahn R and El Labban S, "Sustainable food consumption in Arab countries" 2015, https://pdfs.semanticscholar.org/99a7/57dc14fadc9d9e23955e04ef610e9cd5b5c6.pdf. Accessed May 4 2017.
3. Afshin A, Micha R, Khatibzadeh S, Fahimi S, Shi P, Powles J, et al. The impact of dietary habits and metabolic risk factors on cardiovascular and diabetes mortality in countries of the Middle East and North Africa in 2010: a comparative risk assessment analysis. BMJ Open. 2015;5(5):e006385.
4. Bach-Faig A, Berry EM, Lairon D, Reguant J, Trichopoulou A, Dernini S, et al. Mediterranean diet pyramid today. Science and cultural updates. Public Health Nutr. 2011;14(12A):2274–84.
5. Fischer CG and Garnett T, "Plates, pyramids, planet: developments in national healthy and sustainable dietary guidelines: a state of play assessment" 2016, http://www.fao.org/3/a-i5640e.pdf. Accessed 23 Apr 2017.
6. United Nations Development Programme (UNDP), "Sustainable Development Goals," 2016, http://www.undp.org/content/undp/en/home/sustainable-development-goals/. Accessed 21 Apr 2017.
7. Meybeck A, Gitz V. Sustainable diets within sustainable food systems. Proc Nutr Soc. 2017;76(1):1–11. https://doi.org/10.1017/S0029665116000653. PubMed PMID:28195528.
8. Food and Agriculture Organization of the United Nations(FAO), "Sustainable diets and biodiversity: directions and solutions for policy, research and action.," 2012, http://www.fao.org/docrep/016/i3004e/i3004e.pdf. Accessed 21 Apr 2017.
9. United Nations Environment Programme (UNEP), "Sustainable Development Goals (SDGs)," 2016, http://www.un.org/sustainabledevelopment/. Accessed 18 Apr 2017.
10. Gephart JA, Davis KF, Emery KA, Leach AM, Galloway JN, Pace ML. The environmental cost of subsistence: optimizing diets to minimize footprints. Sci Total Environ. 2016;553:120–7.
11. Johnston JL, Fanzo JC, Cogill B. Understanding sustainable diets: a descriptive analysis of the determinants and processes that influence diets and their impact on health, food security, and environmental sustainability. Adv Nutr. 2014;5(4):418–29.
12. Nelson ME, Hamm MW, Hu FB, Abrams SA, Griffin TS. Alignment of healthy dietary patterns and environmental sustainability: a systematic review. Adv Nutr. 2016;7(6):1005–25.
13. Jones AD, Hoey L, Blesh J, Miller L, Green A, Shapiro LF. A systematic review of the measurement of sustainable diets. Adv Nutr. 2016;7(4):641–64.
14. Nasreddine L, Naja F, Sibai A-M, Helou K, Adra N, Hwalla N. Trends in nutritional intakes and nutrition-related cardiovascular disease risk factors in Lebanon : the need for immediate action. J Med Liban. 2014;62(2):83–91.

15. Naja F, Hwalla N, Itani L, Karam S, Sibai AM, Nasreddine L. A Western dietary pattern is associated with overweight and obesity in a national sample of Lebanese adolescents (13–19 years): a cross-sectional study. Br J Nutr. 2015;114(11):1909–19.
16. Nasreddine L, Naja F, Sibai A-M, Hwalla N, Itani L, Dimassi H. Dietary patterns in cardiovascular diseases prevention and management: review of the evidence and recommendations for primary care physicians in Lebanon. J Med Liban. 2014;62(2):92–9.
17. Naja F, Hwalla N, Itani L, Salem M, Azar ST, Zeidan MN, et al. Dietary patterns and odds of type 2 diabetes in Beirut, Lebanon: a case–control study. Nutr Metab. 2012;9(1):111.
18. Naja F, Nasreddine L, Itani L, Chamieh MC, Adra N, Sibai AM, et al. Dietary patterns and their association with obesity and sociodemographic factors in a national sample of Lebanese adults. Public Health Nutr. 2011;14(9):1570.
19. Naja F, Nasreddine L, Itani L, Adra N, Sibai A, Hwalla N. Association between dietary patterns and the risk of metabolic syndrome among Lebanese adults. Eur J Clin Nutr. 2013;52(1):97–105.
20. Bonita R, De Courten M, Dwyer T, Jamrozik K and Winkelmann R, "Surveillance of risk factors for noncommunicable diseases: the WHO STEPwise approach: summary," 2001, http://www.who.int/ncd_surveillance/media/en/269.pdf. Accessed April 17 2017.
21. Matta J, Nasreddine L, Jomaa L, Hwalla N, Mehio Sibai A, Czernichow S, et al. Metabolically healthy overweight and obesity is associated with higher adherence to a traditional dietary pattern: a cross-sectional study among adults in Lebanon. Nutrients. 2016;8(7):432.
22. Rahmouni K, Correia ML, Haynes WG, Mark AL. Obesity-associated hypertension. Hypertension. 2005;45(1):9–14.
23. Jomaa L, Hwalla N, Itani L, Chamieh MC, Mehio-Sibai A, Naja F. A Lebanese dietary pattern promotes better diet quality among older adults: findings from a national cross-sectional study. BMC Geriatr. 2016;16(1):85.
24. "INTERNATIONAL PHYSICAL ACTIVITY QUESTIONNAIRES (IPAQ)," http://www.sdp.univ.fvg.it/sites/default/files/IPAQ_English_self-admin_short.pdf. Accessed 30 July, 2018.
25. Scientific Applications International Corporation (SAIC), Curran MA. Life-cycle assessment: principles and practice. Cincinnati; National Risk Management Research Laboratory, Office of Research and Development, US Environmental Protection Agency. 2006. pp. 1–80.
26. Naja F, Hwalla N, Itani L, Baalbaki S, Sibai A, Nasreddine L. A novel Mediterranean diet index from Lebanon: comparison with Europe. Eur J Clin Nutr. 2015;54(8):1229–43.
27. DiStefano C, Zhu M, Mindrila D. Understanding and using factor scores: considerations for the applied researcher. Pract Assess Res Eval. 2009;14(20):1–11.
28. Finkbeiner M, Inaba A, Tan R, Christiansen K, Klüppel H-J. The new international standards for life cycle assessment: ISO 14040 and ISO 14044. Int J Life Cycle Assess. 2006;11(2):80–5.
29. Weidema B, Wenzel H, Petersen C, Hansen K. The product, functional unit and reference flows in LCA. Environmental News. 2004;70:1–46.
30. Tyrrell H, Reid J. Prediction of the energy value of Cow's Milk1, 2. J Dairy Sci. 1965;48(9):1215–23.
31. Food and Agriculture Organization of the United Nations (FAO), "FAOSTAT," 2017, http://www.fao.org/faostat/en/#data. Accessed Apr 27 2017.
32. United Nations, "UN Comtrade database," 2014-2017, https://comtrade.un.org/. Accessed 26 Apr 2017.
33. Pfister S, Koehler A, Hellweg S. Assessing the environmental impacts of freshwater consumption in LCA. Environmental science & technology. 2009;43(11):4098–104.
34. Forster P, Ramaswamy V, Artaxo P, Berntsen T, Betts R, Fahey DW, et al., Changes in atmospheric constituents and in radiative forcing. Chapter 2, in Climate change 2007. The physical science basis. 2007.
35. U.S. Energy Information Administration, "Carbon Dioxide Emission Estimates," 2016, https://www.eia.gov/environment/emissions/co2_vol_mass.cfm. Accessed March 15.
36. Jalava M, Kummu M, Porkka M, Siebert S, Varis O. Diet change—a solution to reduce water use? Environ Res Lett. 2014;9(7):074016.
37. Capone R, Iannetta M, El Bilali H, Colonna N, Debs P, Dernini S, et al. A preliminary assessment of the environmental sustainability of the current Italian dietary pattern: water footprint related to food consumption. J Food Nutr Res. 2013;1(4):59–67.
38. Jemmali H, Sullivan CA. Multidimensional analysis of water poverty in MENA region: an empirical comparison with physical indicators. Soc Indic Res. 2014;115(1):253–77.
39. MoE/UNDP, "Impacts of Climate Change on Water," 2014, http://climatechange.moe.gov.lb/water. Accessed April 25.
40. Alexandrou A, Tenbergen K, Adhikari D. Energy balance of a typical US diet. Foods. 2013;2(2):132–42.
41. International Energy Agency, "Lebanon: Indicators for 2014," 2017, http://www.iea.org/statistics/?country=LEBANON&year=2014&category=Key%20indicators&indicator=TPESbySource&mode=chart&categoryBrowse=true&dataTable=BALANCES&showDataTable=false. Accessed 25 Apr 2017.
42. Abeliotis K, Costarelli V, Anagnostopoulos K. The effect of different types of diet on greenhouse gas emissions in Greece. International Journal on Food System Dynamics. 2016;7(1):36–49.
43. Heller MC, Keoleian GA. Greenhouse gas emission estimates of US dietary choices and food loss. J Ind Ecol. 2015;19(3):391–401.
44. Vieux F, Darmon N, Touazi D, Soler LG. Greenhouse gas emissions of self-selected individual diets in France: changing the diet structure or consuming less? Ecol Econ. 2012;75:91–101.
45. Hoekstra AY and Chapagain AK, Water footprints of nations: water use by people as a function of their consumption pattern, in Integrated assessment of water resources and global change. 2006, Springer. p. 35–48.
46. Smith P, Martino D, Cai Z, Gwary D, Janzen H, Kumar P, et al. Contribution of working group III to the fourth assessment report of the intergovernmental panel on climate change. Cambridge: Cambridge University Press; 2007.
47. Donini LM, Dernini S, Lairon D, Serra-Majem L, Amiot M-J, del Balzo V, et al. A consensus proposal for nutritional indicators to assess the sustainability of a healthy diet: the mediterranean diet as a case study. Front Nutr. 2016;3.
48. Tilman D, Clark M. Global diets link environmental sustainability and human health. Nature. 2014;515(7528):518–22.
49. Gabriel AS, Ninomiya K, Uneyama H. The role of the Japanese traditional diet in healthy and sustainable dietary patterns around the world. Nutrients. 2018;10(2):173.
50. Rasul G. Managing the food, water, and energy nexus for achieving the sustainable development goals in South Asia. Environmental Development. 2016;18:14–25.
51. Kuhnlein HV. Food system sustainability for health and well-being of indigenous peoples. Public Health Nutr. 2015;18(13):2415–24.
52. Sáez-Almendros S, Obrador B, Bach-Faig A, Serra-Majem L. Environmental footprints of Mediterranean versus Western dietary patterns: beyond the health benefits of the Mediterranean diet. Environ Health. 2013;12(1):118.
53. FAO/CIHEAM. Towards the Development of Guidelines for Improving the Sustainability of Diets and Food Consumption Patterns in the Mediterranean Area.Available: http://www.fao.org/docrep/016/ap101e/ap101e.pdf. Accessed 25 April 2017.
54. Dernini S, Meybeck A, Burlingame B, Gitz V, Lacirignola C, Debs P, et al. Developing a methodological approach for assessing the sustainability of diets: the Mediterranean diet as a case study. New Medit. 2013;12(3):28–36.
55. Carlsson-Kanyama A, González AD. Potential contributions of food consumption patterns to climate change. Am J Clin Nutr. 2009;89(5):1704S–9S.
56. Fara G. Nutrition between sustainability and quality. Ann Ig. 2015;27(5):693–704.
57. Tukker A, Goldbohm RA, De Koning A, Verheijden M, Kleijn R, Wolf O, et al. Environmental impacts of changes to healthier diets in Europe. Ecol Econ. 2011;70(10):1776–88.
58. Weber CL, Matthews HS. Food-miles and the relative climate impacts of food choices in the United States. Environ Sci Technol. 2008;42:3508–13.
59. Berners-Lee M, Hoolohan C, Cammack H, Hewitt C. The relative greenhouse gas impacts of realistic dietary choices. Energy Policy. 2012;43:184–90.
60. Wolf O, Pérez-Domínguez I, Rueda-Cantuche JM, Tukker A, Kleijn R, de Koning A, et al. Do healthy diets in Europe matter to the environment? A quantitative analysis. J Policy Model. 2011;33(1):8–28.
61. Kim B, Neff R. Measurement and communication of greenhouse gas emissions from US food consumption via carbon calculators. Ecol Econ. 2009;69(1):186–96.
62. Scarborough P, Allender S, Clarke D, Wickramasinghe K, Rayner M. Modelling the health impact of environmentally sustainable dietary scenarios in the UK. Eur J Clin Nutr. 2012;66(6):710–5.
63. Hendrie GA, Ridoutt BG, Wiedmann TO, Noakes M. Greenhouse gas emissions and the Australian diet—comparing dietary recommendations with average intakes. Nutrients. 2014;6(1):289–303.
64. Water Footprint Network, "Product Gallery," n.d, http://waterfootprint.org/en/resources/interactive-tools/product-gallery/. Accessed April 26 2017.
65. Barilla Center for Food and Nutrition(BCFN). Double Pyramid 2016 – A more sustainable future depends on us.Available: https://www.barillacfn.com/m/

publications/doublepyramid2016-more-sustainable-future-depends-on-us.pdf. Accessed April 26 2017.
66. Alqaisi O, Ndambi OA, Uddin MM, Hemme T. Current situation and the development of the dairy industry in Jordan, Saudi Arabia, and Syria. Trop Anim Health Prod. 2010;42(6):1063–71.
67. Serra-Majem L. The Mediterranean diet as an example of environmental sustainability. Omega International. 2016;2(5):1–8.
68. Scarborough P, Appleby PN, Mizdrak A, Briggs AD, Travis RC, Bradbury KE, et al. Dietary greenhouse gas emissions of meat-eaters, fish-eaters, vegetarians and vegans in the UK. Clim Chang. 2014;125(2):179–92.

# 8

# Population-based studies of relationships between dietary acidity load, insulin resistance and incident diabetes in Danes

Joachim Gæde[1†], Trine Nielsen[1†], Mia L. Madsen[1], Ulla Toft[2], Torben Jørgensen[2,3,4], Kim Overvad[5], Anne Tjønneland[5], Torben Hansen[1], Kristine H. Allin[1,6] and Oluf Pedersen[1*]

## Abstract

**Background:** It has been suggested that the acidity of the diet may be related to increased risk of type 2 diabetes. To investigate this hypothesis, we tested if the acidity of the diet, measured as the Potential Renal Acid Load (PRAL) score, was associated with incident diabetes and diabetes-related intermediary traits.

**Methods:** A total of 54,651 individuals from the Danish Diet, Cancer and Health (DCH) cohort were included in the prospective cox regression analyses of incident diabetes over a 15 years follow-up period. Moreover, 5724 Danish individuals with baseline data from the Inter99 cohort were included in the cross sectional, multivariate and logistic regression analyses of measures of insulin sensitivity, insulin release and glucose tolerance status derived from an oral glucose tolerance test (OGTT).

**Results:** In the DCH cohort a trend analysis showed that quintiles of PRAL score were, after multifactorial adjustment, associated with a higher incidence of diabetes ($p_{trend} = 6 \times 10^{-7}$). HR for incident diabetes was 1.24 (1.14; 1.35) ($p = 7 \times 10^{-7}$) between first and fifth PRAL score quintile.
In Inter99 higher PRAL score associated with insulin resistance as estimated by lower BIGTT-Si (an OGTT-derived index of insulin sensitivity) ($p = 4 \times 10^{-7}$) and Matsuda index of insulin sensitivity ($p = 2 \times 10^{-5}$) as well as higher HOMA-IR ($p = 0.001$). No association was observed for measures of insulin release, but higher PRAL score was associated with lower OGTT-based disposition index.

**Conclusions:** A high dietary acidity load is associated with a higher risk of diabetes among middle-aged Danes. Although adjustment for BMI attenuated the effect sizes the association remained significant. The increased risk of diabetes may be related to our finding that a high dietary acidity load associates with impaired insulin sensitivity.

**Keywords:** Dietary acid load, PRAL, Glucose, Insulin resistance, Disposition index, Type 2 diabetes

## Background

Accumulating evidence suggests that a high dietary acidity load results in chronic tissue metabolic acidosis which, in turn, may contribute to the development of insulin resistance and type 2 diabetes (T2D) [1–5].

Observational studies report that a high dietary acidity load associates with the risk of developing T2D: an epidemiological study of ~66,000 middle-aged French women, including 1372 incident T2D cases, reported a higher incidence of T2D during 14 years of follow-up in those study participants with a high dietary acidity load [6]. Also, in an analysis combining data from three observational studies of American health professionals with a total of 15,305 cases of T2D in 4,025,131 person years of follow-up, the authors reported an increased risk of T2D with a higher PRAL score [7]. Yet, this finding could not be reproduced in a Swedish study of 911 elderly men with 115 cases through 18 years of follow-up [8]. Gender discrepancies have been suggested since a study of 1191 incident cases of T2D among ~65,000 Japanese showed an association with T2D in men only

* Correspondence: Oluf@sund.ku.dk
†Joachim Gæde and Trine Nielsen contributed equally to this work.
[1]The Novo Nordisk Foundation Center for Basic Metabolic Research, Section of Metabolic Genetics, Faculty of Health and Medical Sciences, University of Copenhagen, Blegdamsvej 3B, DK-2200 Copenhagen, Denmark
Full list of author information is available at the end of the article

during 5 years of follow-up [9]. Finally, higher dietary acidity load was reported to associate with increased insulin resistance in a study of 1732 Japanese (> 90% men) [10].

A widely used approach to estimate dietary acidity load is the Potential Renal Acid Load (PRAL) score which is a validated proxy for renal net acid excretion [11]. Another estimation for the acidity of the diet is the NEAP score (Net Endogenous Acid Production). Both estimates seem to reflect a similar risk of incident diabetes [6, 7, 9, 10].

The PRAL score is based on dietary intake of protein and various micronutrients, phosphorus, potassium, calcium and magnesium, and takes into account the absorption rate of the nutrients in the gut, unlike the NEAP score, which only operates with potassium and protein intake [6]. A negative PRAL score reflects an alkalizing potential of the diet whereas a positive PRAL score reflects an acidifying potential of the diet.

The aim of the present study was to substantiate and elaborate previous findings and test if PRAL score associates with impaired glucose tolerance and incident diabetes in our study sample of middle-aged people from the general Danish population. Furthermore, in a cross sectional study of middle-aged individuals from the Danish general population, we aimed to test the hypothesis that a higher PRAL score associates with diabetes-related intermediary traits, including impaired beta-cell function and insulin resistance, derived from Oral Glucose Tolerance Tests (OGTT).

## Methods

The present study is based on two Danish population-based cohorts: the Diet, Cancer and Health cohort (DCH) and the Inter99 cohort (ClinicalTrials.gov ID no. NCT00289237).

### Diet, Cancer and health cohort

During 1993 to 1997, 160,725 Danish men and women were invited to participate in the DCH cohort; the inclusion criteria being age 50–64 years, living in the greater Copenhagen and Aarhus areas, born in Denmark and not registered with a previous cancer diagnosis in the Danish Cancer Registry. In total, 27,178 men and 29,875 women participated. However, 574 individuals were excluded due to cancer diagnosis before baseline, leaving 56,479 participants available for analysis.

The present study is based on data from 25,808 men and 28,843 women after exclusion of patients with known diabetes at baseline ($n$ = 1371), participants with incomplete dietary registration ($n$ = 53), participants with extreme values of self-reported energy intake (< 1000 KJ/day ($n$ = 0) or > 20,000 KJ/day ($n$ = 197)) and participants with missing values for BMI and lifestyle characteristics (diet, smoking and physical activity) ($n$ = 207). Information on incident diabetes during the 15 years of follow-up was obtained from The National Diabetes Register [12] and dates of death were obtained from the Danish Civil Registration System. All other information was collected at baseline. A flowchart is given in Additional file 1: FigureS1.

In the DCH cohort, diet was monitored at recruitment by a 192-item FFQ that each participant received by mail before their visit to the study centre. The FFQ was designed specifically for this study population, aiming to capture the average intake of different food and beverage items over the past 12 months before study inclusion. Daily intakes of foods and nutrients were calculated for each participant by the software programme FoodCalc (www.ibt.ku.dk/jesper/foodcalc/). A description of the development and validation of this FFQ, and a detailed description of the estimation of the dietary intake of the population have been published [13–16]. Information on smoking habits and physical activity was obtained from questionnaires.

### Inter99 cohort

The Inter99 cohort is a non-pharmacological intervention study for the prevention of ischaemic heart disease [17]. Detailed description of the Inter99 study is given in the Additional file 1.

The present study is based on data from 2843 men and 2881 women after exclusion of participants with incomplete dietary registration ($n$ = 150), participants with missing data from the OGTT ($n$ = 359) and participants with extreme values of self-reported energy intake (< 1000 KJ/day ($n$ = 6) or > 20,000 KJ/day ($n$ = 93)). Additionally, 19 individuals had fasting serum C-peptide levels lower than 150 pmol/l and were, due to suspicion of type 1 diabetes, excluded from further analyses. Four hundred thirty-three individuals had missing information on smoking, physical activity, dietary intake or body mass index (BMI) and were thus excluded. A flowchart is given in Additional file 1: FigureS2.

Based on OGTT derived data, participants were characterised as having normal glucose tolerance (NGT) ($n$ = 4288), impaired fasting glucose (IFG) ($n$ = 474), impaired glucose tolerance (IGT) ($n$ = 655) or screen detected, treatment-naive T2D ($n$ = 214) according to the 1999 WHO criteria [18]. Additionally, a self-reported diabetes diagnosis was reported for 93 participants. In the present analytical protocol, individuals with combined IFG and IGT are presented together in the IGT group.

In the multivariate analyses of diabetes-related intermediary traits, participants with self-reported diabetes at baseline were excluded ($n = 93$) leaving 5631 participants eligible for analysis.

To assess beta cell function we used insulinogenic index and corrected insulin response as well as disposition index. To review insulin sensitivity we used Homeostatic Model Assessment of Insulin Resistance (HOMA-IR), Matsuda index of insulin sensitivity ($ISI_{Matsuda}$) and BIGTT-Si. Calculations of these indices are given in Additional file 1.

The Inter99 study participants completed, at recruitment, a validated and self-administered food frequency questionnaire (FFQ) during their visit to the Research Centre [19]. They were asked to report their dietary intake during the month before examination. The FFQ included 198 questions on food items and beverages with additional questions regarding portion sizes of selected food items. All food items in the FFQ were linked to a food item in the Danish Food Composition Databank [20]. A detailed description of the questionnaire and estimation of the dietary intake of the population has been published [19]. Smoking status and physical activities were obtained from validated questionnaires as reported [17].

### The potential renal acid load (PRAL) score

PRAL score was derived based on the estimated intake of several nutrients calculated from the FFQ used in Inter99 and DCH [6]:

$$\begin{aligned} PRAL\left(\frac{mEq}{day}\right) = {} & 0.49 \times protein\left(\frac{g}{day}\right) + 0.037 \\ & \times phosphorus\left(\frac{mg}{day}\right) - 0.021 \\ & \times potassium\left(\frac{mg}{day}\right) - 0.013 \\ & \times calcium\left(\frac{mg}{day}\right) - 0.026 \\ & \times magnesium\left(\frac{mg}{day}\right) \end{aligned}$$

### Statistical analyses

All statistical tests were performed using the R statistical package (http://cran.r-project.org/, version 3.1.3). A $p$-value of $< 0.05$ was considered statistically significant.

In the DCH cohort, Cox proportional hazards regression models with age as the time scale were used to estimate hazard ratios (HRs) of incident diabetes. Participants were censored at their date of death or emigration. PRAL score was analysed as categorised into quintiles, with the lowest category as the reference group. Two multivariate models were used: model 1 was adjusted for age (as time scale), smoking status (never-smoker/ex-smoker/current smoker), physical activity (metabolic equivalent of task (MET)) [21] and total fat, carbohydrate and energy intake, and model 2 was further adjusted for BMI. We tested the assumption of proportional hazards by visual inspection. Due to an uneven distribution of men and women across the quintiles and to address the previous diverging findings on men and women we conducted the analyses in combined datasets and stratified by sex.

In Inter99 logistic regression models were used to assess the association between PRAL score and IFG, IGT, and diabetes. Additionally, in Inter99 linear regression models were used to test whether PRAL score (as a continuous variable) was associated with diabetes-related intermediary traits in non-diabetic individuals only ($n = 5631$). Two multivariate models were used: model 1 was adjusted for age, sex, total fat, carbohydrate and energy intake, smoking status (never-smoker/ex-smoker/current smoker) and level of physical activity (0–2 h/week, 2–4 h/week, 4–7 h/week, 7–12 h/week) [22] and model 2 was further adjusted for BMI. To test whether the assumptions for linear regression analysis were fulfilled, all variables were inspected with regards to linearity as well as homogeneity of variance and normality of the residuals. Natural logarithmic transformation was used to approximate a normal distribution when needed. Test of effect modification was performed by introducing the interaction term in the linear models.

## Results

Baseline characteristics of included participants in the two cohorts are shown in Table 1 as stratified by quintiles of PRAL score. Individuals with a higher PRAL score had a higher intake of total and saturated fat, lower intake of fruits and vegetables and higher daily energy intake (see Table 1). In the subsequent analyses, we adjusted for these differences.

### Outcome from analyses of the DCH cohort

During a mean follow-up period of 15 years 7201 incident cases of diabetes occurred in the total study population. Multifactor adjusted HRs (model 1) of diabetes were 1.06 (95% CI 0.98; 1.15) ($p = 0.12$), 1.10 (95% CI 1.02; 1.19) ($p = 0.02$), 1.13 (95% CI 1.04; 1.22) ($p = 0.003$) and 1.24 (95% CI 1.14; 1.35) ($p = 7 \times 10^{-7}$), respectively, for the second, third, fourth and fifth quintile versus the first quintile of PRAL score ($p_{trend} = 6 \times 10^{-7}$) (Fig. 1). Further adjustment for BMI attenuated the HRs as HR for the 5th vs. the 1st quintile was 1.10 (95% CI 1.01; 1.20) ($p = 0.03$) (Fig. 1, model 2), but the same trend was observed across the quintiles ($p_{trend} = 0.04$). In the sex stratified analyses a similar association was observed for both men and women (Fig. 2). However, when BMI was included in the model the association with

**Table 1** Baseline characteristics of study participants in the Inter99 study and in the DCH cohort by quintiles of PRAL score

| | Quintile 1 | Quintile 2 | Quintile 3 | Quintile 4 | Quintile 5 | Total |
|---|---|---|---|---|---|---|
| Inter99 (*n* = 5631) | | | | | | |
| Participants, n | 1127 | 1126 | 1126 | 1126 | 1126 | 5631 |
| PRAL range, mEq/d | −92; − 13 | −13; − 3 | −3; 4 | 4; 12 | 12; 90 | −92; 90 |
| Men, n (%) | 469 (42) | 530 (47) | 487 (43) | 581 (52) | 722 (64) | 2789 (50) |
| Age, years | 50 (41; 55) | 50 (40; 55) | 45 (40; 50) | 45 (40; 50) | 45 (40; 50) | 45 (40; 50) |
| BMI, kg/m$^2$ | 26.2 ± 4.5 | 26.1 ± 4.4 | 26.1 ± 4.6 | 26.1 ± 4.3 | 26.3 ± 4.6 | 26.2 ± 4.5 |
| Physical activity, min/week (%) | | | | | | |
| 0–112 | 117 (10) | 136 (12) | 133 (12) | 157 (14) | 155 (14) | 698 (12) |
| 142.5–225 | 246 (22) | 248 (22) | 261 (23) | 256 (23) | 256 (23) | 1267 (23) |
| 255–420 | 601 (53) | 586 (52) | 609 (54) | 573 (51) | 571 (51) | 2940 (52) |
| 450–720 | 163 (14) | 156 (14) | 123 (11) | 140 (12) | 144 (13) | 726 (13) |
| Smoking, n (%) | | | | | | |
| Current | 539 (48) | 444 (39) | 420 (37) | 390 (35) | 396 (35) | 2189 (39) |
| Former | 283 (25) | 304 (27) | 292 (26) | 287 (25) | 267 (24) | 1433 (25) |
| Never | 305 (27) | 378 (34) | 414 (37) | 449 (40) | 463 (41) | 2009 (36) |
| Energy intake, KJ/d | 9286 ± 3082 | 9043 ± 2878 | 9049 ± 2861 | 9605 ± 2866 | 11,039 ± 3163 | 9604 ± 3064 |
| Protein, g/d | 76 ± 23 | 77 ± 23 | 79 ± 23 | 85 ± 23 | 103 ± 28 | 84 ± 26 |
| Carbohydrates, g/d | 293 ± 114 | 268 ± 96 | 263 ± 93 | 274 ± 92 | 302 ± 98 | 280 ± 100 |
| Dietary fiber, g/d | 23 ± 11 | 21 ± 8 | 20 ± 8 | 21 ± 8 | 23 ± 9 | 22 ± 9 |
| Fat intake total, g/d | 67 (51; 88) | 72 (56; 94) | 76 (59; 98) | 84 (66; 107) | 103 (79; 132) | 80 (60; 105) |
| Saturated fat, g/d | 25 (18; 35) | 28 (21; 38) | 29 (22; 39) | 33 (25; 43) | 40 (30; 53) | 31 (22; 42) |
| Diet, Cancer and Health (*n* = 54,651) | | | | | | |
| Participants, n | 10,931 | 10,930 | 10,930 | 10,930 | 10,930 | 54,651 |
| PRAL range, mEq/d | − 117; −10 | −10; −3 | −3; 4 | 4; 12 | 12; 89 | −117; 89 |
| Men, n (%) | 3564 (33) | 4215 (39) | 4838 (44) | 5789 (53) | 7402 (68) | 25,808 (47) |
| Age, years | 55 (52; 60) | 56 (52; 60) | 56 (52; 60) | 56 (52; 60) | 55 (52; 60) | 56 (52; 60) |
| BMI, kg/m$^2$ | 25.6 ± 3.9 | 25.8 ± 4.0 | 26.0 ± 3.9 | 26.1 ± 4.0 | 26.4 ± 4.1 | 26.0 ± 4.0 |
| Physical activity, MET-h/week | 59 (39; 88) | 56 (37; 84) | 56 (36; 82) | 56 (37; 83) | 57 (37; 87) | 57 (37; 85) |
| Smoking, n (%) | | | | | | |
| Current | 4551 (42) | 4203 (38) | 3723 (34) | 3615 (33) | 3605 (33) | 15,713 (29) |
| Former | 2963 (27) | 2948 (27) | 3125 (29) | 3287 (30) | 3390 (31) | 19,697 (36) |
| Never | 3417 (31) | 3779 (35) | 4082 (37) | 4028 (37) | 3935 (36) | 19,241 (35) |
| Energy intake, KJ/d | 9013 ± 2463 | 9026 ± 2405 | 9374 ± 2432 | 9948 ± 2467 | 11,384 ± 2745 | 9749 ± 2657 |
| Protein, g/d | 82 ± 23 | 86 ± 23 | 91 ± 23 | 99 ± 24 | 119 ± 29 | 95 ± 28 |
| Carbohydrates, g/d | 254 ± 78 | 240 ± 71 | 243 ± 70 | 252 ± 70 | 276 ± 75 | 253 ± 74 |
| Dietary fiber, g/d | 22 ± 8 | 20 ± 7 | 20 ± 7 | 20 ± 6 | 22 ± 7 | 21 ± 7 |
| Fat intake total, g/d | 67 (53; 83) | 73 (58; 89) | 78 (64; 96) | 86 (70; 105) | 104 (86; 126) | 81 (64; 101) |
| Saturated fat, g/d | 25 (19; 32) | 28 (22; 35) | 30 (24; 37) | 33 (27; 41) | 40 (33; 49) | 31 (24; 39) |
| Food intake, g/d | | | | | | |
| Red meat | 63 (46; 84) | 70 (52; 93) | 77 (57; 101) | 85 (63; 112) | 105 (75; 141) | 78 (56; 107) |
| Fish | 32 (21; 46) | 35 (23; 49) | 37 (25; 52) | 41 (28; 57) | 49 (33; 70) | 38 (25; 55) |
| Dairy products | 263 (121; 515) | 278 (138; 536) | 289 (152; 547) | 307 (172; 576) | 344 (206; 617) | 295 (156; 560) |
| Vegetables | 180 (113; 272) | 158 (100; 223) | 151 (99; 213) | 148 (97; 207) | 155 (104; 213) | 157 (102; 224) |
| Fruit | 202 (107; 350) | 154 (81; 254) | 141 (74; 224) | 131 (68; 204) | 117 (61; 189) | 145 (75; 240) |

Data are mean ± standard deviation or median (inter quartile range) unless otherwise specified. Descriptive data on the Inter99 cohort are on non-diabetic individuals only. *MET* Metabolic Equivalent of Task, *PRAL* Potential Renal Acid Load

**Hazard ratio of incident diabetes according to PRAL score quintiles in the DCH cohort**

| PRAL score | No. of participants | No. of events | Model 1 HR (95% CI) | Model 2 HR (95% CI) |
|---|---|---|---|---|
| (-116,-10) | 10,931 | 1.278 | 1 (reference) | 1 (reference) |
| (-10,-3) | 10,930 | 1.374 | 1.06 (0.98;1.15) | 1.03 (0.95;1.11) |
| (-3,4) | 10,930 | 1.431 | 1.10 (1.02;1.19) | 1.06 (0.98;1.14) |
| (4,12) | 10,930 | 1.486 | 1.13 (1.04;1.22) | 1.05 (0.97;1.14) |
| (12,89) | 10,930 | 1.632 | 1.24 (1.14;1.35) | 1.10 (1.01;1.20) |
| | | | p(trend)=6x10$^{-7}$ | p(trend)=0.04 |

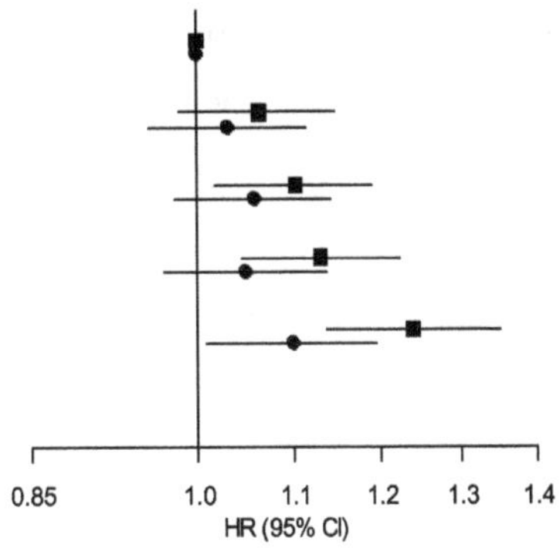


**Fig. 1** Hazard ratio (HR) of incident diabetes according to PRAL score quintiles in the full DCH cohort. Age is used as the time scale in the cox model. Model 1 is adjusted for fat, energy and carbohydrate intake, smoking and physical activity, while model 2 is adjusted for BMI, fat, energy and carbohydrate intake, smoking and physical activity. Squares indicate HR for model 1, and circles indicate HR for model 2. The *p*-value shown indicates significance of a trend test

incident diabetes disappeared for men, but remained significant for women ($p_{\text{trend}} = 0.02$).

### Outcome from analyses of the Inter99 study

The multifactor-adjusted odds ratio (OR) for a one standard deviation higher PRAL score was 1.11 (95% CI 1.01; 1.22) ($p = 0.03$) for IGT (Fig. 3). The OR diminished with further adjustment for BMI ($p = 0.11$). No significant association was observed between PRAL score and T2D (Fig. 3) and PRAL score and IFG. However, when adjusting for BMI we found an association between lowered PRAL score and IFG with an OR of 0.89 (95% CI 0.80; 0.99) ($p = 0.03$).

A higher PRAL score was associated with lower OGTT-based measures of insulin resistance (model 1) as expressed by decreased BIGTT-*Si* ($p = 4 \times 10^{-7}$) and $\text{ISI}_{\text{Matsuda}}$ ($p = 2 \times 10^{-5}$) as well as increased HOMA-IR ($p = 0.001$) (Table 2). Accordingly, a higher PRAL score was associated with higher serum insulin levels at fasting and 120 min during the OGTT ($p = 2 \times 10^{-4}$ and $p = 8 \times 10^{-16}$, respectively), and with higher plasma glucose levels at 120 min ($p = 4 \times 10^{-10}$) (Table 2). No associations were observed between PRAL score and corrected insulin response ($p = 0.2$) or insulinogenic index ($p = 0.3$), both of which are indices of beta cell function. In addition, a higher PRAL score was associated with a lower OGTT-based disposition index ($p = 0.004$). All findings remained significant after further adjustment for BMI (model 2) and with similar effect sizes.

When testing for effect modification we introduced the interaction term PRAL×sex in the linear regression models, but the interaction terms were not significant (data not shown). However; to address diverging previous findings in men and women we further stratified by sex. We found that a higher PRAL score was associated with indices of insulin sensitivity in both women and men (Table 3), but the association with increased HOMA-IR with increased PRAL score was only apparent in women. Furthermore, an association between higher PRAL score and lower HbA1c was seen in men, but only after adjustment for BMI. No associations were found between PRAL score and indices of beta cell function in the sex stratified analyses, but a higher PRAL score was associated with lower disposition index in women (Table 3).

### Sensitivity analysis

In the Inter99 cohort we further did a sensitivity analysis where we adjusted for family history of diabetes, hypertension and dietary patterns (see Additional file 1: TableS1). This information was not available to us in the DCH cohort, and so the sensitivity analysis was only conducted in the Inter99 cohort. The sensitivity analysis showed comparable associations as demonstrated in the primary analyses except the associations between PRAL score and HbA1c and disposition index. In the sensitivity analysis the two latter associations became non-significant (see Additional file 1: TableS1).

## Discussion

In the DCH cohort of more than 54,000 individuals with ~7200 incident cases of diabetes after 15 years of follow-up, we demonstrated a positive relationship between PRAL score and development of incident diabetes, substantiating previous findings [6–10]. Moreover, in baseline data from the Inter99 study of 5631 non-

**Hazard ratio of incident diabetes according to PRAL score quintiles in the DCH cohort stratified by sex**

**Men**

| PRAL score | No. of participants | No. of events | Model 1 HR (95% CI) | Model 2 HR (95% CI) |
|---|---|---|---|---|
| (-97,-7) | 5,162 | 758 | 1 (reference) | 1 (reference) |
| (-7,-1) | 5,161 | 823 | 1.10 (0.99;1.21) | 1.08 (0.97;1.19) |
| (-1,8) | 5,162 | 740 | 0.98 (0.88;1.09) | 0.96 (0.87;1.07) |
| (8,16) | 5,161 | 846 | 1.15 (1.04;1.28) | 1.07 (0.96;1.19) |
| (16,83) | 5,162 | 820 | 1.14 (1.02;1.28) | 1.03 (0.91;1.15) |
| | | | p(trend)=0.02 | p(trend)=0.7 |

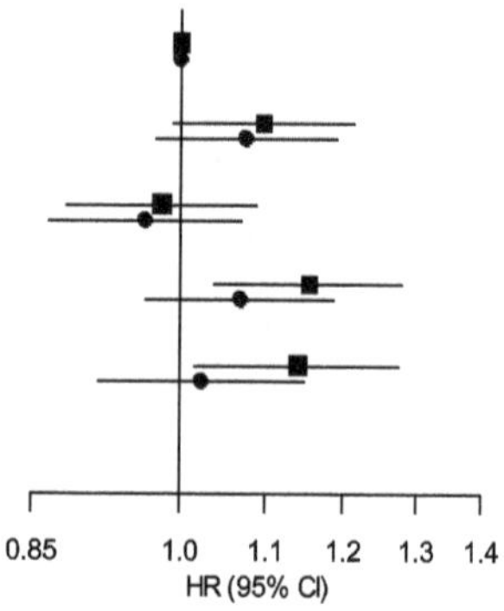


**Women**

| PRAL score | No. of participants | No. of events | Model 1 HR (95% CI) | Model 2 HR (95% CI) |
|---|---|---|---|---|
| (-116,-13) | 5,769 | 597 | 1 (reference) | 1 (reference) |
| (-13,-5) | 5,768 | 612 | 1.05 (0.93;1.18) | 1.02 (0.91;1.14) |
| (-5,1) | 5,769 | 631 | 1.10 (0.98;1.23) | 1.04 (0.93;1.17) |
| (1,8) | 5,768 | 678 | 1.22 (1.08;1.37) | 1.15 (1.02;1.29) |
| (8,89) | 5,769 | 696 | 1.30 (1.15;1.47) | 1.10 (0.98;1.25) |
| | | | p(trend)=$2 \times 10^{-6}$ | p(trend)=0.02 |

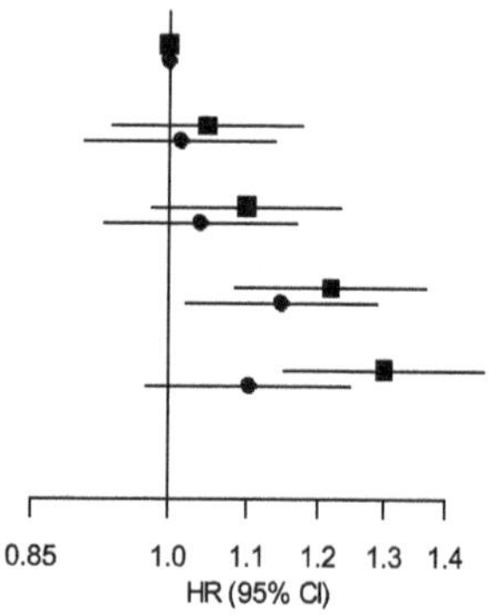


**Fig. 2** Hazard ratio (HR) of incident diabetes according to PRAL score quintiles in the DCH cohort stratified by sex. Age is used as the time scale in the cox model. Model 1 is adjusted for fat, energy and carbohydrate intake, smoking and physical activity, while model 2 is adjusted for BMI, fat, energy and carbohydrate intake, smoking and physical activity. Squares indicate HR for model 1, and circles indicate HR for model 2. The *p*-value shown indicates significance of a trend test

**Glucose tolerance status**

| Group | No. of participants | Model 1 OR (95% CI) | Model 2 OR (95% CI) |
|---|---|---|---|
| NGT | 4,288 | 1 (reference) | 1 (reference) |
| IFG | 474 | 0.91 (0.81,1.01) | 0.89 (0.80;0.99) |
| IGT | 655 | 1.11 (1.01,1.22) | 1.08 (0.98.;1.19) |
| T2D | 307 | 1.14 (0.999,1.31) | 1.12 (0.97;1.29) |

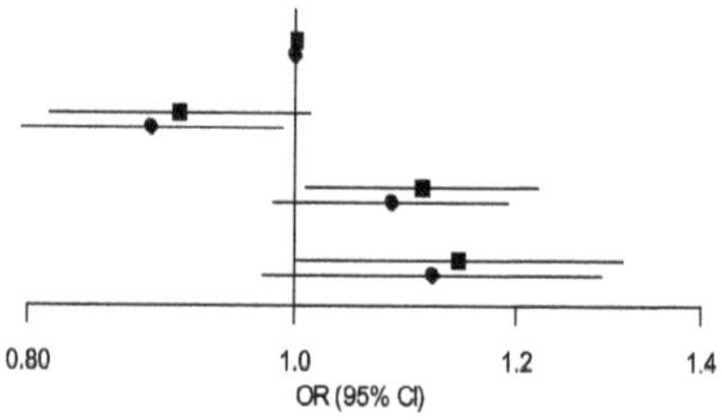


**Fig. 3** PRAL score and glucose tolerance status among participants of the Inter99 study. Odds ratios (OR) of impaired fasting glucose (IFG), impaired glucose tolerance (IGT) and type 2 diabetes (T2D) according to PRAL score as shown for one standard deviation of PRAL score in the total population (16.36 mEq/day). Model 1 is adjusted for age, sex, smoking, physical activity and fat, energy and carbohydrate intake, while model 2 is adjusted for age, sex, BMI, smoking, physical activity and fat, energy and carbohydrate intake. NGT = Normal Glucose Tolerance. Participants having combined IFG and IGT were classified as IGT. Squares indicate OR for model 1, and circles indicate OR for model 2

**Table 2** Associations between PRAL score and diabetes-related intermediary traits in the baseline part of Inter99 study as well as means and medians for the individual quintiles

| Variable | Quintile 1 | Quintile 2 | Quintile 3 | Quintile 4 | Quintile 5 | $Beta_{Model\ 1}$ (95%CI) | $P_{Model\ 1}$ | $P_{Model\ 2}$ |
|---|---|---|---|---|---|---|---|---|
| PRAL range (mEq/d) | −92; −13 | −13; −3 | −3; 4 | 4; 12 | 12; 90 | | | |
| HBA1C (%)[a] | 5.9 ± 0.5 | 5.8 ± 0.5 | 5.8 ± 0.5 | 5.8 ± 0.6 | 5.8 ± 0.5 | −0.0009 (−0.002; $-5 \times 10^{-5}$) | 0.04 | 0.01 |
| Plasma glucose (mmol/l) | | | | | | | | |
| Fasting[a] | 5.6 ± 0.8 | 5.5 ± 0.8 | 5.5 ± 0.6 | 5.6 ± 0.9 | 5.5 ± 0.9 | − 0.0003 (− 0.002; 0.001) | 0.7 | 0.2 |
| 30 min[a] | 8.7 ± 2.0 | 8.7 ± 1.9 | 8.6 ± 1.9 | 8.6 ± 1.8 | 8.7 ± 1.8 | − 0.0009 (− 0.004; 0.002) | 0.6 | 0.2 |
| 120 min | 5.7 (4.8; 6.9) | 5.9 (4.9; 6.9) | 5.9 (4.9; 6.9) | 6.0 (5.0; 7.0) | 5.9 (5.0; 7.0) | 0.2 (0.1; 0.2) | $4 \times 10^{-10}$ | $1 \times 10^{-8}$ |
| Serum insulin (pmol/l) | | | | | | | | |
| Fasting | 32 (22; 47) | 33 (23; 50) | 36 (24; 52) | 35 (25; 53) | 36 (25; 53) | 0.2 (0.09; 0.3) | $2 \times 10^{-4}$ | 0.008 |
| 30 min | 239 (171; 334) | 234 (165; 346) | 243 (181; 349) | 257 (178; 376) | 257 (183; 368) | 0.07 (− 0.03; 0.2) | 0.2 | 0.8 |
| 120 min | 145 (86; 230) | 151 (96; 246) | 164 (103; 253) | 162 (103; 273) | 162 (95; 273) | 0.6 (0.4; 0.7) | $8 \times 10^{-16}$ | $6 \times 10^{-14}$ |
| Measures of beta cell function | | | | | | | | |
| Insulinogenic index | 24.2 (16.5; 35.4) | 23.4 (15.9; 34.7) | 24.7 (17.2; 36.3) | 25.8 (17.2; 38.8) | 25.4 (17.2; 37.5) | 0.06 (−0.06; 0.2) | 0.3 | 0.8 |
| Corrected insulin response | 638 (392; 1051) | 602 (392; 1033) | 689 (413; 1107) | 691 (410; 1146) | 679 (413; 1094) | 0.09 (−0.04; 0.2) | 0.2 | 0.3 |
| Measures of insulin sensitivity | | | | | | | | |
| HOMA-IR | 1.3 (0.89; 2.0) | 1.3 (0.89; 2.1) | 1.4 (0.94; 2.2) | 1.4 (0.98; 2.2) | 1.4 (0.97; 2.2) | 0.2 (0.07; 0.3) | 0.001 | 0.04 |
| $ISI_{Matsuda}$ | 8.4 (5.6; 11.7) | 8.1 (5.3; 11.9) | 7.8 (5.1; 11.1) | 7.5 (5.1; 10.9) | 7.6 (4.9; 10.8) | −0.2 (− 0.3; − 0.1) | $2 \times 10^{-5}$ | 0.001 |
| BIGTT-Si[a] | 9.7 ± 4.1 | 9.4 ± 4.1 | 9.3 ± 4.0 | 9.0 ± 4.0 | 8.8 ± 4.0 | −0.02 (− 0.03; − 0.01) | $4 \times 10^{-7}$ | $4 \times 10^{-7}$ |
| Disposition Index | 304 (211; 447) | 291 (200; 410) | 298 (203; 419) | 297 (205; 412) | 306 (206; 415) | −0.2 (− 0.3; − 0.05) | 0.004 | 0.02 |

Data are from the Inter99 cohort ($n = 5631$) and are presented as mean ± standard deviation or median (inter quartile range) for each quintile of PRAL score as a description of the cohort. Effect sizes (95% confidence interval) are calculated using linear models with PRAL score as a continuous variable and are given as percentage increase for a one unit increase in PRAL score except for variables that have not been transformed by the natural logarithm in which case it is given as an increase per unit. The linear regression model 1 was adjusted for age, sex, smoking, physical activity and fat, energy and carbohydrate intake. The linear regression model 2 was further adjusted for BMI. BIGTT-Si was not adjusted for sex as this variable is included in the calculation of BIGTT-Si. Calculations of measures of beta cell function and insulin sensitivity were carried out as described in methods. Variables were transformed by the natural logarithm unless otherwise indicated by (a). Quintile values are raw data and are for descriptive purposes only

diabetic individuals with OGTT-derived data, we found that a higher PRAL score was associated with reduced insulin sensitivity, but not with changes in proxies of beta cell function. In addition, higher PRAL score was associated with a lower OGTT-based disposition index. We did not observe any major diverging results between the sexes, and so we cannot confirm that any specific differences exist in regards to PRAL score and sex. When adjusting for BMI in the DCH cohort, only the increased HR between the first and the fifth quintiles remained significant. Furthermore, when adjusting for BMI, the significant trend seen in males disappeared, but remained significant in women. In the Inter99 cohort, adjustment for BMI had no effect on the analyses. Since the individuals with a higher PRAL score generally had a higher overall energy intake, the increased BMI may be part of the explanation for the increased incidence of diabetes. However, since the associations persist even after adjustment for BMI, it shows that there is indeed an association between PRAL score and incident diabetes as well as diabetes intermediary traits which is independent of BMI.

Despite a lack of association with indices of beta-cell function in the Inter99 study, we did find an association with lower disposition index as an indication of a decreased beta cell secretion of insulin at the concomitant level of insulin resistance. Hence, we cannot completely discard an association between PRAL score and beta-cell function. Higher PRAL score is consistent with a generally unhealthy diet, which is reflected in our finding that individuals with a higher PRAL score also had a higher intake of total and saturated fat, lower intake of fruits and vegetables and higher daily energy intake. We have accounted for these confounders by adjusting for dietary fat, carbohydrate and total energy intake in our analyses.

The different nutrients, especially protein, embedded in the calculation of the PRAL score may come from various sources. Since the amino acid composition of plant proteins is different from the composition of animal proteins, it is possible that ingestion of plant proteins will have a different effect on the tissue acidity than animal proteins. Indeed, a previous study showed an association between incident T2D and animal protein intake, but not with plant protein intake [23]. One could therefore speculate that a type of

**Table 3** Associations in the Inter99 study between PRAL score and diabetes-related intermediary traits stratified by sex as well as means and medians for the individual quintiles

| Variable | Quintile 1 | Quintile 2 | Quintile 3 | Quintile 4 | Quintile 5 | $Beta_{Model\ 1}$ (95%CI) | $P_{Model\ 1}$ | $P_{Model\ 2}$ |
|---|---|---|---|---|---|---|---|---|
| Men | $n = 558$ | $n = 558$ | $n = 557$ | $n = 558$ | $n = 558$ | | | |
| PRAL range (mEq/d) | − 92; −11 | −11; −1 | −1; 6 | 6; 15 | 15; 90 | | | |
| HBA1C (%)[a] | 6.0 ± 0.6 | 5.9 ± 0.6 | 5.9 ± 0.4 | 5.9 ± 0.7 | 5.9 ± 0.6 | − 0.001 (− 0.003; $6 \times 10^{-5}$) | 0.06 | 0.04 |
| Plasma glucose (mmol/l) | | | | | | | | |
| Fasting[a] | 5.8 ± 1.0 | 5.7 ± 0.9 | 5.7 ± 0.7 | 5.7 ± 1.1 | 5.6 ± 0.9 | − 0.001 (− 0.004; 0.0008) | 0.2 | 0.1 |
| 30 min[a] | 9.5 ± 2.1 | 9.1 ± 1.9 | 9.2 ± 1.8 | 9.2 ± 1.8 | 9.0 ± 1.8 | −0.003 (− 0.007; 0.001) | 0.2 | 0.09 |
| 120 min | 5.6 (4.6; 7.0) | 5.9 (4.9; 6.9) | 5.9 (4.8; 6.9) | 5.7 (4.8; 6.79) | 5.9 (4.9; 7.0) | 0.2 (0.1; 0.3) | $3 \times 10^{-6}$ | $6 \times 10^{-6}$ |
| Serum insulin (pmol/l) | | | | | | | | |
| Fasting | 34 (23; 52) | 36 (24; 54) | 38 (25; 56) | 37 (25; 57) | 37 (25; 55) | 0.2 (0.02; 0.3) | 0.02 | 0.052 |
| 30 min | 244 (170; 356) | 251 (165; 368) | 255 (181; 380) | 253 (173; 382) | 264 (185; 396) | 0.06 (−0.08; 0.2) | 0.4 | 0.9 |
| 120 min | 123 (67; 223) | 141 (82; 233) | 155 (83; 255) | 143 (81; 242) | 150 (89; 275) | 0.6 (0.4; 0.8) | $4 \times 10^{-9}$ | $5 \times 10^{-9}$ |
| Measures of beta cell function | | | | | | | | |
| Insulinogenic index | 22.5 (15.0; 34.0) | 23.5 (15.2; 34.9) | 23.8 (16.2; 35.5) | 23.1 (15.5; 36.3) | 25.6 (16.6; 38.8) | 0.08 (−0.09; 0.2) | 0.3 | 0.6 |
| Corrected insulin response | 511 (306; 820) | 557 (358; 932) | 564 (353; 968) | 563 (360; 891) | 655 (384; 1008) | 0.1 (−0.04; 0.3) | 0.1 | 0.2 |
| Measures of insulin sensitivity | | | | | | | | |
| HOMA-IR | 1.5 (0.9; 2.3) | 1.5 (1.0; 2.3) | 1.6 (1.0; 2.4) | 1.6 (1.0; 2.4) | 1.5 (1.0; 2.4) | 0.1 (−0.02; 0.3) | 0.09 | 0.2 |
| $ISI_{Matsuda}$ | 7.7 (4.9; 11.5) | 7.3 (4.9; 11.1) | 7.2 (4.8; 10.6) | 7.1 (5.0; 11.0) | 7.4 (4.6; 10.6) | −0.2 (−0.3; − 0.03) | 0.02 | 0.04 |
| BIGTT-Si[a] | 8.3 ± 3.6 | 8.1 ± 3.5 | 8.0 ± 3.4 | 8.1 ± 3.5 | 8.1 ± 3.6 | −0.02 (− 0.02; − 0.007) | $3 \times 10^{-4}$ | $3 \times 10^{-4}$ |
| Disposition Index | 285 (188; 407) | 273 (185; 390) | 277 (188; 381) | 282 (186; 382) | 302 (197; 419) | −0.1 (− 0.3; 0.05) | 0.2 | 0.3 |
| Women | $n = 569$ | $n = 568$ | $n = 568$ | $n = 568$ | $n = 569$ | | | |
| PRAL range (mEq/d) | −84; −15 | −15; −5 | −5; 1 | 1; 9 | 9; 77 | | | |
| HBA1C (%)[a] | 5.8 ± 0.8 | 5.7 ± 0.4 | 5.7 ± 0.4 | 5.7 ± 0.5 | 5.7 ± 0.5 | −0.0002 (−0.001; 0.0009) | 0.7 | 0.3 |
| Plasma glucose (mmol/l) | | | | | | | | |
| Fasting[a] | 5.4 ± 0.7 | 5.3 ± 0.5 | 5.3 ± 0.5 | 5.3 ± 0.6 | 5.3 ± 0.9 | 0.001 (−0.0005; 0.003) | 0.2 | 0.4 |
| 30 min[a] | 8.1 ± 1.8 | 8.2 ± 1.7 | 8.1 ± 1.7 | 8.1 ± 1.8 | 8.2 ± 1.7 | 0.003 (− 0.002; 0.007) | 0.3 | 0.8 |
| 120 min | 5.7 (4.9; 6.7) | 5.9 (4.9; 6.9) | 6.0 (5.2; 6.9) | 6.0 (5.1; 7.0) | 6.0 (5.2; 7.1) | 0.2 (0.08; 0.2) | $3 \times 10^{-5}$ | $7 \times 10^{-4}$ |
| Serum insulin (pmol/l) | | | | | | | | |
| Fasting | 31 (22; 46) | 30 (22; 44) | 34 (23; 51) | 34 (24; 47) | 33 (24; 50) | 0.3 (0.1; 0.4) | $8 \times 10^{-4}$ | 0.03 |
| 30 min | 238 (171; 325) | 228 (168; 322) | 238 (178; 324) | 243 (179; 348) | 253 (185; 347) | 0.1 (−0.02; 0.3) | 0.08 | 0.5 |
| 120 min | 155 (104; 230) | 162 (113; 246) | 175 (114; 259) | 178 (119; 277) | 185 (123; 275) | 0.5 (0.4; 0.7) | $1 \times 10^{-8}$ | $1 \times 10^{-6}$ |
| Measures of beta cell function | | | | | | | | |
| Insulinogenic index | 25.3 (17.6; 37.4) | 24.4 (17.3; 34.4) | 24.7 (17.8; 35.9) | 26.0 (18.4; 39.5) | 27.1 (18.6; 38.7) | 0.07 (−0.09; 0.2) | 0.4 | 0.8 |
| Corrected insulin response | 736 (483; 1224) | 693 (454; 1131) | 762 (456; 1223) | 775 (494; 1278) | 827 (488; 1352) | 0.05 (−0.2; 0.3) | 0.6 | 0.7 |

**Table 3** Associations in the Inter99 study between PRAL score and diabetes-related intermediary traits stratified by sex as well as means and medians for the individual quintiles *(Continued)*

| Variable | Quintile 1 | Quintile 2 | Quintile 3 | Quintile 4 | Quintile 5 | $Beta_{Model\ 1}$ (95%CI) | $P_{Model\ 1}$ | $P_{Model\ 2}$ |
|---|---|---|---|---|---|---|---|---|
| Measures of insulin sensitivity | | | | | | | | |
| HOMA-IR | 1.2 (0.84; 1.8) | 1.2 (0.85; 1.8) | 1.3 (0.89; 2.0) | 1.3 (0.94; 1.9) | 1.3 (0.91; 2.0) | 0.3 (0.1; 0.4) | $8 \times 10^{-4}$ | 0.04 |
| $ISI_{Matsuda}$ | 8.8 (6.1; 12.1) | 8.7 (6.0; 12.3) | 8.2 (5.4; 11.7) | 8.0 (5.7; 10.9) | 7.9 (5.5; 11.0) | −0.3 (−0.5; −0.2) | $2 \times 10^{-5}$ | 0.002 |
| BIGTT-Si[a] | 10.7 ± 4.2 | 10.6 ± 4.1 | 10.3 ± 4.4 | 10.3 ± 4.1 | 10.0 ± 4.3 | −0.03 (− 0.04; − 0.02) | $8 \times 10^{-6}$ | $8 \times 10^{-6}$ |
| Disposition Index | 324 (225; 474) | 316 (217; 434) | 308 (204; 425) | 312 (227; 431) | 324 (223; 428) | −0.2 (− 0.4; − 0.08) | 0.003 | 0.02 |

Data are from the Inter99 cohort and presented as mean ± standard deviation or median (inter quartile range) for each quintile of PRAL score as a description of the cohorts. Effect sizes (95% confidence interval) are calculated using linear models with PRAL score as a continuous variable and are given as percentage increase for a one unit increase in PRAL score except for variables that have not been transformed by the natural logarithm in which case it is given as an increase per unit. The linear regression model 1 was adjusted for age, smoking, physical activity and fat, energy and carbohydrate intake. The linear regression model 2 was adjusted for age, BMI, smoking, physical activity and fat, energy and carbohydrate intake except for BIGTT-Si, which was not adjusted for BMI (as this variable is included in the calculation of BIGTT-Si). Calculations of measures of beta cell function and insulin sensitivity were carried out as described in methods. Variables were transformed by the natural logarithm unless otherwise indicated by (a). Quintile values are raw data and are for descriptive purposes only

measure where proteins were reported as of their origin or corresponding amino acids would provide useful information about the underlying theories of dietary acidity load and diabetes.

The amount of dietary fiber ingested are surprisingly similar across the quintiles. However, the food items from where the dietary fiber is obtained may vary considerably and may therefore have different impacts on the PRAL score. For instance, dietary fibers originating from vegetables and fruits will have an alkalizing effect and thus decrease the PRAL score, whereas dietary fiber originating from whole grain may have a different effect on the PRAL score [1]. As appears from the baseline table (Table 1) of the DCH cohort, the dietary fiber ingested in the lower quintiles must come from fruits and vegetables, whereas the dietary fiber in the higher quintiles originate from other food items, although we cannot say for certain which ones. Additionally, it is noteworthy that the quintiles with the highest PRAL scores are also the ones with the highest number of current smokers. This is the case in both the DCH cohort and the Inter99 cohort. It cannot be excluded that smoking status might influence food preferences. Indeed, a study by Endoh et al. shows, that the dietary patterns in Japanese men and women differ between smokers and non-smokers [24].

An intervention study conducted in American adults showed that individuals would be able to lower their PRAL score by 13 units when following a vegan diet for two to three days a week, while a reduction of almost 30 units was seen in individuals following the vegan diet every day in a week [25]. If we examine our data from the DCH cohort, we find that a reduction of 30 units would be sufficient to move an individual from Q4 to Q1. With a reduction of just 12 units an individual would step down an entire quintile. Despite the modest increased risk of diabetes between the lowest and the highest quintile, diabetes is still major burden in society today, and even slight reductions in this risk through a diet change might have considerable impact on public health.

Our study has limitations. First, in the present epidemiological studies, we did not use the hyperinsulinemic euglycemic clamp to measure insulin sensitivity, as this would not be feasible in such large cohorts; still the surrogate measures applied in the current study, HOMA-IR, $ISI_{Matsuda}$ and BIGTT-Si, have all been validated in previous studies and provide physiologically relevant proxies for insulin sensitivity [26–28]. Additionally, to overcome any uncertainties in the individual surrogate measures, we have used several different proxies of insulin sensitivity to measure the same outcome. Second, and most important, in our study of incident diabetes, information was collected at baseline only. Consequently, all conclusions based on the DCH cohort rely on the assumption that the study participants have not changed their diet or lifestyle substantially over the following 15 years of follow-up. Third, the diagnosis of diabetes was based on The Danish National Diabetes Register which does not clearly distinguish between patients with type 1 diabetes or T2D [12]. Yet, individuals in our study were at least 50 years of age at baseline, and since newly diagnosed type 1 diabetes is quite rare in Denmark above this age we do not expect this lack of diagnostic accuracy to bias our analytical outcomes. The PRAL score in our two cohorts ranged from around − 100 to 100 and with a median range of − 20.6 to 18.6 in the Inter99 cohort and − 16.3 to 18.0 in the DCH cohort, respectively. These median ranges are roughly the same as in the two studies by Kiefte-de Jong et al. (− 17.4 to 21.3) and Fagherazzi et al. (− 23.0 to 14.3). However, the PRAL score range in the study by Xu et al. was from − 40 to 323. For histograms of the PRAL scores in the two cohorts, please see Additional file 1: FigureS3 and FigureS4. We believe that these between study differences may be related to differences in dietary patterns and the demographics of the study populations. Furthermore, the variations in PRAL score may occur due to differences in how the questionnaires and food composition tables are structured between studies.

## Conclusions

We confirm the association of a high acidity load with incident T2D and suggest that the risk of T2D might be mediated partially through a decrease in insulin sensitivity. Although the present study and previous reports suggest a link between dietary acidity load and incident diabetes among middle-aged people, carefully designed and conducted dietary interventions are needed to elucidate whether a causal link exists between the two and which mechanisms might be involved.

### Abbreviations

BIGTT: Beta-cell function; Insulin sensitivity; Glucose; Tolerance; Test; BIGTT-Si: An OGTT-derived index of insulin sensitivity (Si); DCH: The Diet, Cancer and Health cohort; FFQ: Food frequency questionnaire; IFG: Impaired fasting glucose; IGT: Impaired glucose tolerance; $ISI_{Matsuda}$: Matsuda index of insulin sensitivity; MET: Metabolic equivalent of task; NEAP: Net Endogenous Acid Production; OGTT: Oral glucose tolerance test; PRAL: Potential Renal Acid Load; T2D: Type 2 diabetes

### Acknowledgements

We are indebted to the staff and participants of the Inter99 and DCH study for their important contributions. The authors wish to thank A. Forman, T. Lorentzen, B. Andreasen, G.J. Klavsen and M.J. Nielsen for technical assistance and T.F. Toldsted and G. Lademann for management assistance. The DCH study was funded by the Danish Cancer Society.

**Funding**
The Novo Nordisk Foundation Center for Basic Metabolic Research is an independent Research Center at the University of Copenhagen partially funded by an unrestricted donation from the Novo Nordisk Foundation (www.metabol.ku.dk).

**Authors' contributions**
JG: compiled and interpreted all data analyses, made tables and figures, wrote the first draft of the manuscript and delivered subsequently substantial contributions to the manuscript. TN: supported and supervised JG in analysis and interpretation of the data and delivered substantial contributions to the manuscript. MM: interpreted all data analyses and delivered substantial contributions to the manuscript. UT: took part in the execution and epidemiological analysis of the Inter99 Study. TJ: took part in the execution and epidemiological analysis of the Inter99 Study. KO: took part in the execution and epidemiological analysis of the Diet, Cancer and Health cohort. AT: took part in the execution and epidemiological analysis of the Diet, Cancer and Health cohort. TH: took part in the execution and epidemiological analysis of the Inter99 Study. KA: supported and supervised JG in analysis and interpretation of the data and delivered substantial contributions to the manuscript. OP: conceived and designed and supervised the present study and provided substantial contributions to the manuscript. All authors read and approved the final manuscript.

**Competing interests**
The authors declare that they have no competing interests.

**Author details**
[1]The Novo Nordisk Foundation Center for Basic Metabolic Research, Section of Metabolic Genetics, Faculty of Health and Medical Sciences, University of Copenhagen, Blegdamsvej 3B, DK-2200 Copenhagen, Denmark. [2]Research Centre for Prevention and Health, Copenhagen, the Capital Region of Denmark, Denmark. [3]Department of Public Health, Faculty of Health and Medical Sciences, University of Copenhagen, Copenhagen, Denmark. [4]Faculty of Medicine, Aalborg University, Aalborg, Denmark. [5]Danish Cancer Society Research Center, Copenhagen, Denmark. [6]Department of Clinical Epidemiology, Bispebjerg and Frederiksberg Hospital, Copenhagen, the Capital Region of Denmark, Denmark.

**References**
1. Adeva MM, Souto G. Diet-induced metabolic acidosis. Clin Nutr. 2011;30:416–21.
2. Engberink MF, Bakker SJ, Brink EJ, van Baak MA, van Rooij FJ, Hofman A, et al. Dietary acid load and risk of hypertension: the Rotterdam study. Am J Clin Nutr. 2012;95:1438–44.
3. Souto G, Donapetry C, Calvino J, Adeva MM. Metabolic acidosis-induced insulin resistance and cardiovascular risk. Metab Syndr Relat Disord. 2011;9:247–53.
4. Williams RS, Kozan P, Samocha-Bonet D. The role of dietary acid load and mild metabolic acidosis in insulin resistance in humans. Biochimie. 2016;124:171–7.
5. Della, Guardia L, Thomas MA, Cena H. Insulin sensitivity and glucose homeostasis can be influenced by metabolic acid load. Nutrients. 2018; 10(5):618.
6. Fagherazzi G, Vilier A, Bonnet F, Lajous M, Balkau B, Boutron-Rualt MC, et al. Dietary acid load and risk of type 2 diabetes: the E3N-EPIC cohort study. Diabetologia. 2014;57:313–20.
7. Kiefte-de Jong JC, Li Y, Chen M, Curhan GC, Mattei J, Malik VS, et al. Diet-dependent acid load and type 2 diabetes: pooled results from three prospective cohort studies. Diabetologia. 2017;60:270–9.
8. Xu H, Jia T, Huang X, Riserus U, Cederholm T, Arnlov J, et al. Dietary acid load, insulin sensitivity and risk of type 2 diabetes in community-dwelling older men. Diabetologia. 2014;57:1561–8.
9. Akter S, Kurotani K, Kashino I, Goto A, Mizoue T, Noda M, et al. High dietary acid load score is associated with increased risk of type 2 diabetes in Japanese men: the Japan public health center-based prospective study. J Nutr. 2016;146:1076–83.
10. Akter S, Eguchi M, Kuwahara K, Kochi T, Ito R, Kurotani K, et al. High dietary acid load is associated with insulin resistance: the Furukawa nutrition and health study. Clin Nutr. 2016;35:453–9.
11. Remer T, Manz F. Estimation of the renal net acid excretion by adults consuming diets containing variable amounts of protein. Am J Clin Nutr. 1994;59:1356–61.
12. Carstensen B, Kristensen JK, Marcussen MM, Borch-Johnsen K. The National Diabetes Register. Scand J Public Health. 2011;39:58–61.
13. Overvad K, Tjonneland A, Haraldsdottir J, Ewertz M, Jensen OM. Development of a semiquantitative food frequency questionnaire to assess food, energy and nutrient intake in Denmark. Int J Epidemiol. 1991;20:900–5.
14. Tjonneland A, Overvad K, Haraldsdottir J, Bang S, Ewertz M, Jensen OM. Validation of a semiquantitative food frequency questionnaire developed in Denmark. Int J Epidemiol. 1991;20:906–12.
15. Tjonneland A, Haraldsdottir J, Overvad K, Stripp C, Ewertz M, Jensen OM. Influence of individually estimated portion size data on the validity of a semiquantitative food frequency questionnaire. Int J Epidemiol. 1992;21:770–7.
16. Haraldsdottir J, Tjonneland A, Overvad K. Validity of individual portion size estimates in a food frequency questionnaire. Int J Epidemiol. 1994;23:786–96.
17. Jorgensen T, Borch-Johnsen K, Thomsen TF, Ibsen H, Glumer C, Pisinger C. A randomized non-pharmacological intervention study for prevention of ischaemic heart disease: baseline results Inter99. Eur J Cardiovasc Prev Rehabil. 2003;10:377–86.
18. WHO. Definition, diagnosis and classification of diabetes mellitus and its complications. In: Part 1: diagnosis and classification of diabetes mellitus; 1999.
19. Toft U, Kristoffersen L, Ladelund S, Bysted A, Jakobsen J, Lau C, et al. Relative validity of a food frequency questionnaire used in the Inter99 study. Eur J Clin Nutr. 2008;62:1038–46.
20. Møller A SE, Christensen A, Hartkopp H. Danish Food Composition Databank version 5.0 (Fødevaredatabanken V 5.0). Danish Institute for Food and Veterinary research, Ministry of Food, Fisheries, and AgricultureSøborg, Denmark 2002.
21. Friedenreich C, Norat T, Steindorf K, Boutron-Ruault MC, Pischon T, Mazuir M, et al. Physical activity and risk of colon and rectal cancers: the European prospective investigation into cancer and nutrition. Cancer Epidemiol Biomark Prev. 2006;15:2398–407.
22. von Huth Smith L, Borch-Johnsen K, Jorgensen T. Commuting physical activity is favourably associated with biological risk factors for cardiovascular disease. Eur J Epidemiol. 2007;22:771–9.
23. van Nielen M, Feskens EJ, Mensink M, Sluijs I, Molina E, Amiano P, et al. Dietary protein intake and incidence of type 2 diabetes in Europe: the EPIC-InterAct case-cohort study. Diabetes Care. 2014;37:1854–62.
24. Endoh K, Kuriki K, Kasezawa N, Tohyama K, Goda T. Association between smoking status and food and nutrient consumption in Japanese: a large-scale cross-sectional study. Asian Pac J Cancer Prev. 2015;16:6527–34.
25. Cosgrove K, Johnston CS. Examining the impact of adherence to a vegan diet on Acid-Base balance in healthy adults. Plant Foods Hum Nutr. 2017;72(3):308–13.
26. Gutch M, Kumar S, Razi SM, Gupta KK, Gupta A. Assessment of insulin sensitivity/resistance. Indian J Endocrinol Metab. 2015;19:160–4.
27. Hansen T, Drivsholm T, Urhammer SA, Palacios RT, Volund A, Borch-Johnsen K, et al. The BIGTT test: a novel test for simultaneous measurement of pancreatic beta-cell function, insulin sensitivity, and glucose tolerance. Diabetes Care. 2007;30:257–62.
28. Matthews DR, Hosker JP, Rudenski AS, Naylor BA, Treacher DF, Turner RC. Homeostasis model assessment: insulin resistance and beta-cell function from fasting plasma glucose and insulin concentrations in man. Diabetologia. 1985;28:412–9.
29. Tjonneland A, Olsen A, Boll K, Stripp C, Christensen J, Engholm G, et al. Study design, exposure variables, and socioeconomic determinants of participation in diet, Cancer and health: a population-based prospective cohort study of 57,053 men and women in Denmark. Scand J Public Health. 2007;35:432–41.

9

# Healthy diets ASAP – Australian Standardised Affordability and Pricing methods protocol

Amanda J Lee[1*], Sarah Kane[2], Meron Lewis[1], Elizabeth Good[3], Christina M Pollard[4,5], Timothy J Landrigan[4] and Mathew Dick[3]


## Abstract

**Background:** This paper describes the rationale, development and final protocol of the Healthy Diets Australian Standardised Affordability and Pricing (ASAP) method which aims to assess, compare and monitor the price, price differential and affordability of healthy (recommended) and current (unhealthy) diets in Australia. The protocol is consistent with the International Network for Food and Obesity / non-communicable Diseases Research, Monitoring and Action Support's (INFORMAS) optimal approach to monitor food price and affordability globally.

**Methods:** The Healthy Diets ASAP protocol was developed based on literature review, drafting, piloting and revising, with key stakeholder consultation at all stages, including at a national forum.

**Discussion:** The protocol was developed in five parts. Firstly, for the healthy (recommended) and current (unhealthy) diet pricing tools; secondly for calculation of median and low-income household incomes; thirdly for store location and sampling; fourthly for price data collection, and; finally for analysis and reporting. The Healthy Diets ASAP protocol constitutes a standardised approach to assess diet price and affordability to inform development of nutrition policy actions to reduce rates of diet-related chronic disease in Australia. It demonstrates application of the INFORMAS optimum food price and affordability methods at country level. Its wide application would enhance monitoring and utility of dietary price and affordability data from a health perspective in Australia. The protocol could be adapted in other countries to monitor the price, price differential and affordability of current and healthy diets.


**Keywords:** Diet price, Food price, Diet affordability, Food affordability, Food policy, Food environments, Healthy diets, INFORMAS, Fiscal policy, Nutrition policy, Obesity prevention, Non-communicable disease, Monitoring and surveillance

## Background

Poor diet is now the major preventable disease risk factor contributing to burden of disease, globally and in Australia [1]. Less than 4 % of the population consume diets consistent with the evidence-based Australian Dietary Guidelines [2, 3]; on average, at least 35% of the total daily energy intake of adults and at least 39% of the energy intake of children [4] are now derived from unhealthy 'discretionary' food choices, defined as foods and drinks high in saturated fat, added sugar, salt and/or alcohol that are not required for health [3]. Of particular concern is the contribution of poor diet to the rising rates of overweight and obesity. Based on measured height and weight, 25% of Australian children aged two to 17 years and 63% of Australian adults aged 18 years and over are now overweight or obese [5]. There is an urgent need for nutrition policy actions to help shift the current diet of the population towards healthy diets as recommended by the Australian Dietary Guidelines [3, 6].

The expense of healthy foods has been reported as a key barrier to consumption in Australia, particularly among low socioeconomic groups [7–11]. However, well-defined data in this area are lacking [6] as classification of 'healthy' and 'unhealthy' foods and diets varies [12, 13] and the relative price of 'healthy' and 'unhealthy' foods depends on the unit of measure (i.e. per energy unit, nutrient density, serve or weight) [14]. Comparisons can be difficult particularly in the context of the total diet and habitual dietary patterns that are the major determinant of diet-related disease [3, 15–17]. However,

* Correspondence: Amanda.Lee@saxinstitute.org.au
[1]The Australian Prevention Partnership Centre, The Sax Institute, 10 Jones Street, Ultimo, NSW 2007, Australia
Full list of author information is available at the end of the article

the relative price and affordability of current and healthy (recommended) *diets* have been assessed rarely, as opposed to the relative price of selected pairs of 'healthy' and 'less healthy' foods [6].

Various methods have been utilised to assess food prices in Australia, such as Consumer Price Indexes (CPI) [18, 19] and supermarket price surveys, however these usually tally the price of highly selected individual food items and do not necessarily relate to relative cost of the total habitual diet [6, 13]. A variety of 'food basket' diet costing tools have also been developed at state, regional and community levels [13]. These methods have the potential to measure the cost of a healthy diet. However, dissimilarity of metrics is a recognised barrier to the production of comparable data [7, 13].

A recent systematic review of food pricing methods used in Australia since 1995, identified 59 discrete surveys using five major food basket pricing tools (used in multiple survey areas and multiple time periods) and six minor food basket pricing tools (used in a single survey area or time period) [13]. No national survey had been conducted. Survey methods differed in several metrics including: type and number of foods surveyed; application of availability and/or quality measures; definition of reference households; calculation of household income; store sampling frameworks; data collection; and analysis. Hence results are not comparable across different locations or different times [13]. With exception of Queensland Health's Healthy Food Access Basket tool revised in 2015, [20] none of these fully align with a healthy diet as recommended by the Australian Dietary Guidelines [3]. Further, none accurately reflect current Australian diets [2, 4, 5, 13].

Since 1995, the vast majority of 'healthy' food pricing surveys in Australia have confirmed that: food prices in rural and remote areas are up to 40% higher than those in capital cities; lower socioeconomic households need to spend a higher proportion of their income to procure healthy diets than other Australians, and food prices generally increase over time [13, 21]. Related calls for interventions, such as for freight subsidies or food subsidies for low income groups in specific regions have gone unheeded [22, 23]. Hence, it could be asserted that these surveys have had limited utility in informing fiscal and health policy [13]. As a result, there have been several calls for the development of standardised, healthy food and diet pricing survey methods nationally in Australia [24, 25] and globally [6]. There is also a need for policy-relevant data [6, 26].

The aim of relevant nutrition policy actions is to help shift the current intake of the whole population to a healthier diet consistent with dietary recommendations. Governments can manipulate food prices through a range of complex policy approaches [6]. Three common strategies to increase the affordability of 'healthy' foods are:

- taxing 'unhealthy foods' ("fat taxes") e.g. on sugar sweetened beverages;
- exempting 'healthy foods' from goods and service tax (GST) or value added tax; and
- subsidising 'healthy foods,' such as through agricultural and transport subsidies, retail price reductions, or voucher systems targeted to vulnerable population groups [6].

Therefore, to inform relevant policy decisions, robust data are required for both current (unhealthy) and healthy (recommended) diets [6]. With respect to food price and affordability, the key health and nutrition policy relevant question to be answered by food pricing surveys is: "What is the relative price and affordability of 'current' (unhealthy) and 'healthy' (recommended) diets?"

While the potential effects of specific changes to fiscal policy have been modelled [27, 28], recent 'real life' data are lacking to inform policy decision making in Australia [29]. Assessment of the price, price differential and affordability of a healthy diet (consistent with Dietary Guidelines) and current (unhealthy) diets (based on national surveys), determined by standardised national methods, would provide more robust data to inform health and fiscal policy in Australia and monitor potential fiscal policy interventions [13].

There is a lack of such data globally; the current research helps to address this, within the food price module of the International Network for Food and Obesity/ non-communicable diseases Research, Monitoring and Action Support (INFORMAS) [6, 30]. Under the auspices of INFORMAS, the results of this study provide a potential globally-applicable stepwise food price and affordability monitoring framework that advocates 'minimal,' 'expanded' and 'optimal' approaches, to establish benchmarks and monitor the cost of healthy food, meals and diets; the level depends on availability of data and country capacity [6]. The novel INFORMAS 'optimal' approach proposes concurrent application of two food pricing tools to assess the price, price differential and affordability of a healthy diet (consistent with Dietary Guidelines) and current (unhealthy) diets (based on national surveys). It requires assessment of household income, representative sampling and, ideally, stratification by region and socio-economic status (SES).

Based on the 'optimal' approach of the INFORMAS diet price and affordability framework, we developed a standardised method to assess and compare the price and affordability of healthy and current diets in Australia, provide more robust, meaningful data to inform health and fiscal policy in Australia, and develop national data benchmarks with the potential for international comparisons [29].

This paper presents the resultant protocol for Healthy Diets ASAP methods in Australia.

## Aim

The aim of this paper is to describe the development and final protocol of the Healthy Diets ASAP methods, based on the INFORMAS optimal price and affordability approach. It details tools and methods to assist others to apply the approach in a standard manner, in order to enable comparison of the price, price differential and affordability of healthy (recommended) and current (unhealthy) diets in Australia.

## Methods

### Development of the healthy diets ASAP protocol

#### *Background: Developing and piloting the initial diet pricing tools and methods*

In November 2013, all key Australian stakeholders gave in-principle support at a national teleconference for the development of national food price and affordability monitoring methods based on the INFORMAS 'optimal' approach. The development and pilot testing of the methods using readily available dietary data for five household structures in high socio-economic (SES) and low SES areas is reported elsewhere [29]. The findings confirmed that the general approach could provide useful, meaningful data to inform potential fiscal and health policy actions. Application of the diet pricing tools accurately reflected known composite food group ratios [2] and the proportion of the mean food budget Australian households spent on discretionary foods and drinks in analysis of the Consumer Price Index (CPI) with respect to Australian Dietary Guidelines food groups [19]. However, internal validity testing suggested that construction of some of the initial diet pricing tools could be improved to enhance accuracy [29]. For example, while performance of both diet pricing tools was acceptable at household level, only the healthy diet pricing tool was acceptable at an individual level for all demographics in the sample; the unhealthy (current) diet pricing tool could be improved for the 14 year old boy and both genders aged 70 years or over [29]. Further, potential systematic errors could be minimised by the utilisation of detailed dietary survey data in the Confidentialised Unit Record Files (CURFs) from the Australian Health Survey (AHS) 2011–12 [31] and the Australian 2011–13 food composition database [32], both of which were unavailable at the time of the pilot study [29].

Development of accepted, standardised diet pricing methods also required agreement from all key stakeholders on the final approach, including accord on systematic arbitrary decisions points around application of the tools (such as whether to record the price of the next largest or smallest packet if a particular size of food was unavailable in-store). There was also a desire to simplify methods to optimise uptake and utility.

#### *Development and testing of diet pricing tools and process protocols*

The final Healthy Diets ASAP protocols were developed in two phases.

**Phase one: Revising and re-testing initial tools and methods** The food pricing tools were revised based on the pilot outcomes [29] and feedback from international food pricing experts (including at the Food Pricing Workshop convened by authors AL and CP at the 14th International Society of Behavioural Nutrition and Physical Activity (ISBNPA) conference in Edinburgh May 2015).

The revised unhealthy (current) diet pricing tools reflected dietary data at the five-digit level by age and gender groupings [4] in the CURFs of the AHS 2011–12 [31]. The most commonly available branded items and unit sizes in Australian supermarkets were identified from the pilot [29]. Other minor changes, and the reasons for these, are included in Table 1.

The revised Healthy Diets ASAP diet pricing tools and methods were applied to assess the price, price differential and affordability of current and healthy diets in six randomly selected locations in two major cities (Sydney, New South Wales and Canberra, Australian Capital Territory) in November and December 2015. The preliminary reports of these studies were provided to NSW Health and ACT Health in early 2016. Colleagues in these government departments provided feedback on the revised methods early March 2016.

**Phase 2: Development of the final protocol** At the national Healthy Diets ASAP Methods Forum (the Forum) held in Brisbane on 10 March 2016, 25 expert stakeholders from academia, government jurisdictions and non-government organisations (see Acknowledgements) worked together to finalise the Healthy Diets ASAP tools and methods for national application in Australia. De-identified preliminary data from and feedback on the reports provided to NSW Health and ACT Health were used to highlight methodological challenges and arbitrary decision points during the Forum.

Generally, the revised tools and methods applied in Sydney and Canberra were confirmed at the Forum. However, some simplifications around arbitrary decision points were recommended (Table 2).

The revised tools and methods were finalised according to the recommendations from the Forum. The resultant Healthy Diets ASAP protocol is described in detail in the results.

**Table 1** Minor revisions to the initial diet pricing tools and methods

| Improvement | Aim/rational/comment |
|---|---|
| Added bottled water, olive oil, and relatively healthy pre-made "convenience" foods, such as sandwiches and cooked chicken, to the healthy (recommended) diet pricing tools | To enhance comparability with the current (unhealthy) diet pricing tools, that include comparable, but less healthy, options |
| Further aggregated nutritionally similar products with similar utility in both diet pricing tools (for example, 'cabana' and 'bratwurst' were grouped with 'sausages') | To minimize the number of items to be priced in-store to reduce survey burden and cost |
| Included the same food groupings in the healthy food component of both current and healthy diet pricing tools | To simplify data collection, comparison between current and healthy diets and interpretation of results |
| Adjusted the diet of the 8 year old girl (who was the oldest in her age/gender group) from the base Foundation Diets levels, according to the prescribed methods of Total Diet modelling to inform the 2013 revision of the Australian Guide to Healthy Eating of the Australian Dietary Guidelines [33] | To ensure adequate energy content of the constructed healthy (recommended) diet of the 8 year old girl in the reference household |
| Adjusted median household income at Statistical Area Level 2 (SA2) level by relevant wage price index; clarified that available data sets at SA2 level provide median gross (i.e. not disposable) household income | To incorporate the effect of inflation. Median household income at sub-national (area) level is readily available from published government sources, so has been used frequently in calculation of food affordability in Australia [13]. However, published median household income data at area level reflects gross (total) income and has not been adjusted for essential expenditures such as taxation, to reflect disposable household income; results should be interpreted accordingly. |
| Included a third option for estimating median disposable household income at the national level, for use in future national diet price and affordability surveys. | To enhance comparability with low (minimum) disposable income household income, that is also calculated at the national level. Median disposable household income is available only at national level currently; however data may be available at state/territory level in the future. |

Following the Forum, the food price data collected in Sydney and Canberra in late 2015 were reanalysed according to the Healthy Diets ASAP protocol and the preliminary reports to NSW Health and ACT Health were finalised in May 2016.

## Results

### The healthy diets ASAP protocol

There are five parts to the Healthy Diets ASAP protocol.

#### *The healthy diets ASAP protocol part one: Construct of the diet pricing tools*

There are two diet pricing survey tools: the current (unhealthy) diet pricing tool; and the healthy (recommended) diet pricing tool (Table 3). The diet pricing survey tools include provision of quantities of food for a reference household consisting of four people, including an adult male 31–50 years old, an adult female 31–50 years old, a 14 year old boy and an 8 year old girl. An allowance for edible portion/as cooked, as specified in AUSNUT 2011–13 [32], is included in both diet pricing tools. Any post plate wastage was not estimated or included.

**The healthy diets ASAP current (unhealthy) diet pricing tool** The current (unhealthy) diet pricing tool constitutes the sum of the mean intake of specific foods and drinks, expressed in grams or millilitres, in each age/gender group corresponding to the four individuals comprising the reference household, as reported in the AHS 2011–12 [31]. Foods are grouped according to stakeholder recommendations (Table 2) and amounts consumed per day are derived from the CURFs at 5-digit code level [31]. The mean reported daily intake for each of the four individuals (Additional file 1) are multiplied by 14 and tallied to produce the quantities consumed per household per fortnight. The amounts of foods and drinks comprising the Healthy Diets ASAP current (unhealthy) diet for the reference household per fortnight is presented in Table 3. The total energy content of the reference household's current diet is 33,860 kJ per day. Common brands of included food and drink items are included in the data collection sheet in Table 4.

**The healthy diets ASAP healthy (recommended) diet pricing tool** The healthy diet pricing tool reflects the recommended amounts and types of foods and drinks for the reference household for a fortnight, consistent with the Australian Guide to Healthy Eating and the Australian Dietary Guidelines [3]. The amounts are calculated from the daily recommended number of servings and relevant serve size of foods for the age/gender and physical activity level (PAL) of 1.5 of the four individuals comprising the reference household in the omnivorous Foundation Diet models [33]. As the Foundation Diets were developed for the smallest adults (or in the case of children, the youngest) in each age/gender group, the amounts of foods were increased by 20% for the 8 year old

**Table 2** Arbitrary decisions made by key stakeholders at the national Healthy Diets ASAP Forum

| Decision Point | Forum decision- standard protocol | Rationale/other comments |
|---|---|---|
| Household structure | | |
| 1. Number of household structures for which results are reported? (5 different structures were developed in the pilot study) | • Report and compare results for one household structure only | • Simpler to interpret and communicate results for only one (common) household structure. Less analysis, and therefore resources, required to access diet prices, therefore the protocol is more likely to be used |
| 2. Composition of household structure? | • 2 adults and 2 children:<br>-adult male 31–50 yrs. old<br>-adult female 31–50 yrs. old<br>-boy 14 yrs. old<br>-girl 8 yrs. old<br>• Publish quantities of food to be included for a range of individuals (age/gender), in addition to those to be included in the selected household structure | • Most commonly used household structures in Australian studies are 6 and 4 person households<br>• Of these household structures, use 4 as it is closest to the median Australian household size of 3 persons<br>• Those interested in reporting results for other household structures (e.g. single parent or pensioners) could perform additional analysis post data collection |
| Data collection | | |
| 3. Which products should be included?<br>a) Branded?<br>b) Generic?<br>c) Cheapest?<br>d) Sales items?<br>e) Bulk deals?<br>f) How should any optional data collected be identified on the data collection forms? | a) Include most common market share branded products (Australia wide)<br><br>b) Include generic products only if branded items are not available (but exclude ALDI supermarket which tend to stock generic products). However, consider supporting optional inclusion of cheapest generic item, including the special/sale price (also applies to inclusion of ALDI)<br>c) Don't specifically seek to include cheapest item. However, consider supporting optional inclusion of cheapest item, including the special/ sale price (also applies to inclusion of ALDI)<br>d) Exclude sales items (as above)<br>e) Exclude bulk deals (i.e. two for the price of one deals)<br>Consider adding tick box in end column of data collection form to record if costing generic/ special/sale price items as optional extras | a) Include the most popular items reported in the Australian Health Survey (AHS) 2011–13 as current diet<br><br>b) Inclusion of generic items has potential to bias, affect comparability and distort results over time- but could be included if consumption data continues to suggest increasing intake.<br><br>c) Cheapest price could also be collected to answer an optional additional question, but inclusion of cheapest price, including of sales or generic items, has potential to bias, affect comparability and distort results over time.<br>d) As above<br>e) As above. If optionally, collecting the cheapest price, could use multi buy price by dividing to obtain single price<br>f) May need to use multiple data collection forms for each store or add additional data collection column if collecting optional prices |
| 4: Unhealthy (current) diet pricing tool | | |
| a) Adjust for known under-reporting in AHS 2011–12? | No adjustment; report as 'best case scenario' | There are no robust data on which to base adjustment factor, so could introduce error. Analysis Is not adjusted for any other reasons. |
| b) Confirm coding for five food group and discretionary foods? | • Tinned meat and vegetables- code as ½ veg and ½ meat<br>• Tinned fruit – code as fruit<br>• Ham salad sandwich- (replace with chicken salad sandwich) and code as 1/3 bread, 1/3 veg, 1/3 chicken meat<br>• Choc-chip Muesli bar – code as discretionary<br>• Flavoured milk – code as non-discretionary (decision consistent with ABS classification)<br>• Processed meats (e.g. ham) – code as discretionary<br>• Water – include ½ reported water intake as bottled water (costed) and ½ as tap water (not costed) | • Decisions should be consistent with coding used by the ABS in the AHS 2011–12<br>• Revisit decisions reassessed when the Australian Dietary Guidelines (ADGs) are reviewed (i.e. in 5 years' time) |
| 5. Healthy (recommended) diet pricing tool | | |
| Should any extra healthy foods be included? Such as more convenience options, bottled water? Is the healthy diet unrealistic without inclusion of some discretionary foods or drinks, such as alcohol? | • Water – include ½ reported water intake as bottled water<br>• Convenience items- confirmed inclusion of roasted chicken and sandwich– no further inclusions | Use the ADG Modelled Foundation diets based on rationale that:<br>–63% Australian adults are overweight/obese<br>-There was no adjustment for underreporting in current diet |

**Table 2** Arbitrary decisions made by key stakeholders at the national Healthy Diets ASAP Forum *(Continued)*

| Decision Point | Forum decision- standard protocol | Rationale/other comments |
|---|---|---|
| | • Alcohol – do not include | -Most Australians are not expending enough energy to allow for additional energy intake from any discretionary foods or drinks<br>- The healthy diet should be aspirational, and reflect that associated with optimal health outcomes |
| 6: Income data | | |
| Should mean or median income be used? What assumptions should be used to determine indicative low income? | • Include both median household (HH) income from published data and calculated low (minimum) disposable income household (HH) income (confirmed assumptions used in pilot calculations)<br>• Also consider reporting results against the Australian poverty line | • Median HH income is specific to location, but is pre-tax i.e. not disposable income<br>• Low income HH calculation is not specific to location apart from rent (which is set low so rarely changes)<br>• Poverty line is lower than 50% of the Australian median HH income<br>• Median household income and indicative low (minimum)<br>vs disposable household income are not comparable |
| 7: Sampling framework | | |
| Sampling frameworks: which areas, stores, distances (e.g. 7 km radius of centre of SA2 area) should be included? | • Sampling approach SA2 stratified by Index of Relative Socio-Economic Disadvantage for Areas (SEIFA) and including all stores within a specific radius confirmed (ALDI excluded in initial methods as above)<br>• Requested further work to determine calculating distance away from centre for inclusion of stores | • Methods of randomisation trialled is appropriate and feasible<br>• 7 km radius of inclusion may not be appropriate for all locations, particularly in rural areas |
| 8: Data collection protocols | | |
| Prioritisation of sizes and branding for pricing, as proposed on data collection sheet | • Proposed detailed methods confirmed e.g. size prescribed but if not available take next larger size first | • Detailed methods proposed are appropriate<br>• Reflect common current practice in most locations; clear and concise; easy to follow |
| 9: Definition of affordability | | |
| Should affordability level be set at 25% or 30% of disposable HH income? | • May need to assess both (post hoc) but initially use 30% pending further review of the literature and international consultation | • Based on most commonly used definition In International literature from high income countries |

girl who is the oldest in her height/age group, according to the recommendations [3].

To ensure the most commonly consumed healthy foods in Australia are used, food categories in the healthy diet pricing tool are the same as those in the current diet pricing tool (but differ in quantity). A variety of fresh, canned, frozen and dried foods is included. For example, representative categories of fresh produce reflect common fruit and vegetables available all year round in Australia. Luxury products, such as imported fruit and vegetables (particularly those out of season) and foods with very high cost per kilogram (e.g. oysters, smoked salmon) are excluded. Some 'convenience' foods are included in the healthy diet pricing tool as per stakeholder decisions (Table 2).

Consistent with Australian recommendations [3], the healthy diet pricing tool does not contain any discretionary choices. It includes: grain (cereal) foods, in the ratio 66% wholegrain and 33% refined varieties; cheese, milk, yoghurt and calcium-fortified plant based alternatives, mostly (i.e. > 50%) reduced fat, with a maximum of 2–3 serves of high fat dairy foods (cheese) per person per week; lean meat (beef, lamb, veal, pork), poultry and plant-based alternatives (with no more than 455 g red meat per person per week); a minimum of 140 g and up to 280 g fish per person per week; up to 7 eggs per person per week; a selection of different colours and varieties of vegetables (green and brassica, orange, legumes, starchy vegetables, other vegetables) with a minimum 350 g per day for adults; a variety of fruit with a minimum of 300 g per day for adults; and an allowance of unsaturated oils or spreads or the nuts/seeds from which they are derived [33]. The daily quantities of food categories recommended for each individual (age/gender) in the reference household (Additional file 2) are multiplied by 14 and tallied to provide quantities per fortnight (Table 3).

The amounts of foods and drinks comprising the Healthy Diets ASAP healthy (recommended) diet for the reference household per fortnight are presented in Table 3.

**Table 3** Composition of the current (unhealthy) and healthy (recommended) diets for the reference household[a] per fortnight

| Food or drink | Quantity |
|---|---|
| Current (unhealthy) diet | |
| *Bottled water, still (ml)* | 5296 |
| *Artificially sweetened 'diet' soft drink* | 2391 |
| *Fruit* | |
| Apples, red, loose (g) | 3497 |
| Bananas, Cavendish, loose (g) | 899 |
| Oranges, loose (g) | 1664 |
| Fruit salad, canned in juice (g) | 2046 |
| Fruit juice | 3026 |
| *Vegetables* | |
| Potato, white, loose (g) | 1460 |
| Sweetcorn, canned, no added salt (g) | 206 |
| Broccoli, loose (g) | 422 |
| White cabbage, loose (g) | 235 |
| Iceberg lettuce, whole (g) | 795 |
| Carrot, loose (g) | 753 |
| Pumpkin (g) | 240 |
| Four bean mix, canned (g) | 74 |
| Diced tomatoes, canned, in tomato juice(g) | 234 |
| Onion, brown, loose (g) | 84 |
| Tomatoes, loose (g) | 488 |
| Frozen mixed vegetables, pre-packaged (g) | 1184 |
| Frozen peas, pre-packaged (g) | 273 |
| Baked beans, canned (g) | 369 |
| Salad vegs in sandwich | 120 |
| Veg in tinned meat and vegetable casserole (g) | 646 |
| *Grain (cereal) foods* | |
| Wholegrain cereal biscuits Weet-bix™ (g) | 430 |
| Wholemeal bread, pre-packaged (g) | 1054 |
| Rolled oats, whole (g) | 870 |
| White bread, pre-packaged (g) | 3033 |
| Cornflakes (g) | 680 |
| White pasta, spaghetti (g) | 1326 |
| White rice, medium grain (g) | 1622 |
| Dry water cracker biscuit (g) | 258 |
| Bread in sandwich | 120 |
| *Meats, poultry, fish, eggs, nuts and seeds* | |
| Beef mince, lean (g) | 267 |
| Lamb loin chops (g) | 257 |
| Beef rump steak (g) | 1056 |
| Tuna, canned in vegetable oil (g) | 1052 |
| Whole barbeque chicken, cooked (g) | 1661 |
| Eggs (g) | 872 |

**Table 3** Composition of the current (unhealthy) and healthy (recommended) diets for the reference household[a] per fortnight *(Continued)*

| Food or drink | Quantity |
|---|---|
| Meat in tinned meat and vegetable casserole (g) | 646 |
| Chicken in sandwiches | 120 |
| *Milk, yoghurt, cheese and alternatives* | |
| Cheddar cheese, full fat (g) | 624 |
| Cheddar cheese, reduced fat (g) | 44 |
| Milk, full fat (ml) | 5961 |
| Milk, reduced fat (ml) | 2929 |
| Yoghurt, full fat plain (g) | 204 |
| Yoghurt, reduced fat, flavoured (vanilla) (g) | 676 |
| Flavoured milk (ml) | 2416 |
| Canola margarine (g) | 170 |
| Sunflower oil (ml) | 7 |
| Olive oil (ml) | 7 |
| *Discretionary choices* | |
| Beer, full strength (ml) | 4661 |
| White wine, sparkling (ml) | 863 |
| Whisky (ml) | 266 |
| Red wine (ml) | 1078 |
| Butter (g) | 280 |
| Muffin, commercial (g) | 1455 |
| Cream-filled sweet biscuit, pre-packaged (g) | 496 |
| Muesli bar, pre-packaged (g) | 373 |
| Peanuts, salted (g) | 255 |
| Pizza, commercial (g) | 1182 |
| Savoury flavoured biscuits (g) | 222 |
| Confectionary (g) | 418 |
| Chocolate (g) | 441 |
| Sugar sweetened beverages (Coca Cola) (ml) | 12,012 |
| Meat pie, commercial (g) | 1638 |
| Frozen lasagne, pre-packaged (g) | 4322 |
| Hamburger, commercial (g) | 2413 |
| Beef sausages (g) | 1048 |
| Ham (g) | 189 |
| Potato crisps, pre-packaged (g) | 518 |
| Potato chips, hot, commercial (g) | 670 |
| Ice cream (g) | 1830 |
| White sugar (g) | 564 |
| Salad dressing (ml) | 277 |
| Tomato sauce (ml) | 569 |
| Chicken soup, canned (g) | 1340 |
| Orange juice (ml) | 3027 |
| Fish fillet crumbed, pre-packaged (g) | 302 |

**Table 3** Composition of the current (unhealthy) and healthy (recommended) diets for the reference household[a] per fortnight *(Continued)*

| Food or drink | Quantity |
|---|---|
| Instant noodles, wheat based (g) | 381 |
| Healthy (recommended) diet | |
| *Bottled water, still (ml)* | 5296 |
| *Fruit* | |
| Apples, red, loose (g) | 5460 |
| Bananas, Cavendish, loose (g) | 5460 |
| Oranges, loose (g) | 5460 |
| *Vegetables* | |
| Potato, white, loose (g) | 2320 |
| Sweetcorn, canned, no added salt (g) | 1160 |
| Broccoli, loose (g) | 1470 |
| White cabbage, loose (g) | 1470 |
| Iceberg lettuce, whole (g) | 1470 |
| Carrot, loose (g) | 2205 |
| Pumpkin (g) | 2205 |
| Four bean mix, canned (g) | 1005 |
| Diced tomatoes, canned, in tomato juice(g) | 1638 |
| Onion, brown, loose (g) | 1638 |
| Tomatoes, loose (g) | 1638 |
| Frozen mixed vegetables, pre-packaged (g) | 1638 |
| Frozen peas, pre-packaged (g) | 1638 |
| Baked beans, canned (g) | 1005 |
| Salad vegs in sandwich | 120 |
| *Grain (cereal) foods* | |
| Wholegrain cereal biscuits Weet bix™ (g) | 2216 |
| Wholemeal bread, pre-packaged (g) | 4272 |
| Rolled oats, whole (g) | 6648 |
| White bread, pre-packaged (g) | 893 |
| Cornflakes (g) | 670 |
| White pasta, spaghetti (g) | 2042 |
| White rice, medium grain (g) | 2042 |
| Dry water cracker biscuit (g) | 781 |
| Bread in sandwich | 120 |
| *Meats, poultry, fish, eggs, nuts and seeds* | |
| Beef mince, lean (g) | 1168 |
| Lamb loin chops (g) | 1169 |
| Beef rump steak (g) | 1172 |
| Tuna, canned in vegetable oil (g) | 1841 |
| Whole barbeque chicken, cooked (g) | 1471 |
| Eggs (g) | 2208 |
| Peanuts, roasted, unsalted (g) | 780 |
| Chicken in sandwiches | 120 |

**Table 3** Composition of the current (unhealthy) and healthy (recommended) diets for the reference household[a] per fortnight *(Continued)*

| Food or drink | Quantity |
|---|---|
| *Milk, yoghurt, cheese and alternatives* | |
| Cheddar cheese, full fat (g) | 704 |
| Cheddar cheese, reduced fat (g) | 516 |
| Milk, full cream (ml) | 6438 |
| Milk, reduced fat (ml) | 12,000 |
| Yoghurt, full fat plain (g) | 2576 |
| Yoghurt, reduced fat, flavoured (vanilla) (g) | 5100 |
| Canola margarine (g) | 412 |
| Sunflower oil (ml) | 291 |
| Olive oil (ml) | 291 |

[a]The reference household comprises four people: adult male 19–50 yrs. old; adult female 19–50 yrs. old; boy 14 yrs. old; girl 8 yrs. old

The total energy content of the household's healthy diet is 33,610 kJ per day. Common brands of included food and drink items are included in the data collection sheet in Table 4.

**Diet pricing tools for additional household structures** Several stakeholders requested (Table 2) that the composition of current (unhealthy) and healthy (recommended) diets be provided for four other household compositions commonly investigated in Australia[1] (for example, for single parent or pensioner households) so that additional data analysis could be performed. These data are included in Additional file 3.

**Validity of the diet pricing survey tools** Convergent validity of the constructed healthy and current diet pricing survey tools for each age/gender group was assessed by energy and macronutrient analysis using FoodWorks 7 Professional [34] computer program installed with AUSNUT 2011–13 [32] (the food composition database used to analyse the AHS) and comparing results with Australian Nutrient Reference Values [35] and nutrient results from the AHS 2011–12 respectively [5, 31]. The results are presented in Additional file 4. As deemed acceptable for modelling outputs to develop the Australian Guide to Healthy Eating, [33] the energy content of the constructed healthy diet pricing tool is within 5% of the Foundation Diet levels and the macronutrient profiles are within the recommended ranges for more than 97% of values for all age/gender groups. Similarly, the energy content of the current diet pricing tool is within 5% of the reported energy intakes of the AHS 2011–2012 [4] for all individuals.

Internal validity indicators, such as the ratio of fruit and vegetables content between the healthy and current diet pricing tools (approximately 2:1) are consistent with

**Table 4** Healthy Diets ASAP (Australian Standardised Affordability and Price) Survey Data Collection Form

Store name ______________ Store Location: ______________ Date: __________ Collector:___

**NOTE:** Please read the methods for collection on Page 2, prior to collecting data

| Food | Specific brand | Your brand | Specific size | Your size | Your cost | Comments |
|---|---|---|---|---|---|---|
| Bottled water, still | Mt Franklin | | 600mL | | | |
| Fruit | | | | | | |
| Apples, red, loose | | | per kg | | | |
| Bananas, cavendish, loose | | | per kg | | | |
| Orange, loose | | | per kg | | | |
| Vegetables & Legumes | | | | | | |
| White potato, loose, brushed/washed | | | per kg | | | |
| Tinned sweet corn, kernels, no added salt | Edgell | | 420g | | | |
| Broccoli, loose | | | per kg | | | |
| Cabbage, white, ½ cabbage (1/2=1.5kg) (weigh if necessary) | | | 1.5kg | | | |
| Lettuce, iceberg, whole (1=0.6kg) | | | 0.6kg | | | |
| Carrot, loose | | | per kg | | | |
| Pumpkin, ½ pumpkin (1/2 av. Jap=1.5kg, 1/2 av. Butternut=1kg) (weigh if necessary) | | | per kg | | | |
| Tinned 4 bean mix | Edgell | | 420g | | | |
| Tinned diced/chopped tomatoes, in tomato juice | Ardmona | | 400g | | | |
| Brown onion, loose | | | per kg | | | |
| Tomato, loose (not vine-ripened) | | | per kg | | | |
| Frozen mixed vegetables (cheapest specified brand) | Heinz, Birdseye or McCain | | 500g | | | |
| Frozen peas (cheapest specified brand) | Edgell, Birdseye or McCain | | 500g | | | |
| Tinned baked beans, in tomato sauce | Heinz | | 420g | | | |
| Grain (Cereal) Foods | | | | | | |
| Weet-bix™ | Sanitarium | | 375g | | | |
| Wholemeal Bread | Tip Top Sunblest™ | | 650g | | | |
| Rolled oats, whole, Traditional (not quick oats) | Uncle Toby's | | 1kg | | | |
| White Bread | Tip Top Sunblest™ | | 650g | | | |
| Cornflakes | Kellogg's | | 725g | | | |
| Spaghetti (white) | San Remo | | 500g | | | |
| White rice, medium grain | SunRice™ | | 1kg | | | |
| Water Crackers, plain | Arnott's | | 125g | | | |
| Meats, Poultry, Fish & Alternatives | | | | | | |
| Lean beef mince (not heart smart) | Pre-pack (not vacuum) | | per kg | | | |
| Lamb loin chops | Pre-pack | | per kg | | | |
| Beef rump steak | Pre-pack | | per kg | | | |
| Tuna, canned in vegetable oil, unflavoured (cheapest specified brand) | John West, Greenseas or Sirena | | 185g | | | |
| Whole Barbeque Chicken, cooked - Large/ Family | Supermarket | | Each ~1.5kg | | | |
| Eggs, dozen, Free Range | Sunny Queen Farms | | 700g | | | |
| Milk, Yoghurt, Cheese & Alternatives | | | | | | |
| Cheddar cheese, regular fat | Coon | | 250g | | | |
| Cheddar cheese, reduced fat | Coon | | 250g | | | |
| Full cream milk, fresh | Paul's or Dairy Farmers | | 2L | | | |
| Reduced fat milk, fresh (not skim) | Paul's Trim or Dairy Farmers Lite | | 2L | | | |
| Plain Yoghurt, natural, Greek, regular fat (~4% fat) | Jalna | | 1kg | | | |
| Yoghurt, vanilla/flavoured, reduced fat (~1% fat) | Jalna | | 1kg | | | |
| Unsaturated Oils & Spreads | | | | | | |
| Canola Margarine, regular fat | MeadowLea | | 500g | | | |
| Sunflower oil | Crisco | | 750mL | | | |
| Olive oil, Traditional (not extra virgin) | Moro | | 1 Litre | | | |
| Other – foods not in both tools and mixed foods | | | | | | |
| Pre-made chicken & Salad Sandwich (wholemeal) (1 sandwich = ~220g) * (triangle pre-pack) | Supermarket (or Service station/garage nearby) | | 2sl bread + filling | | | |
| Fruit salad, canned in juice | Goulburn Valley | | 700g | | | |
| Peanuts – roasted, unsalted peanuts | Cheapest branded | | 250g | | | |
| Tinned steak & vegetables | Harvest | | 425g | | | |
| Discretionary Choices | | | | | | |
| Beer (Liquor store)* | VB* | | 6 x 375mL | | | |
| Sparkling white wine (Liquor store)* | Yellow* | | 750mL | | | |
| Whisky (Liquor store)* | Johnny Walker Red Label* | | 700mL | | | |
| Red wine (Liquor store)* | Penfolds Koonungara Hill Shiraz* | | 750mL | | | |
| Butter, original, salted (foil pack) | Western Star | | 250g | | | |
| Muffin, commercial, uniced | Supermarket | | $/100g | | | |
| Cream-filled biscuit | Arnott's Monte-Carlo | | 250g | | | |
| Chewy Choc Chip Muesli Bar | Uncle Toby's | | 6x30g (185g) | | | |
| Mixed nuts, (incl. peanut), salted | Nobby's | | 375g | | | |
| Supreme Pizza, thin base (1 pizza=0.55kg)* | Pizza Hut* | | 1 pizza | | | |
| Savoury flavoured biscuits | Arnott's BBQ Shapes | | 175g | | | |
| Mint confectionary | Allen's Minties | | 150g | | | |
| Dairy milk chocolate, block | Cadbury | | 200g | | | |
| Soft drink, Cola | Coca Cola™ | | 1.25L | | | |
| Artificially sweetened 'diet' soft drink, Cola | Diet Coca Cola™ | | 1.25L | | | |
| Chocolate Milk, regular fat | Breaka, Big M, Oak or Paul's | | 600mL | | | |
| Beef Pie, single serve, full pastry* | Independent Bakery* | | ~250g | | | |
| Beef lasagne, frozen | McCain | | 400g | | | |
| Beef hamburger* | McDonald's Big Mac* | | 1 burger | | | |
| Beef Sausages, pre-pack | Supermarket | | per kg | | | |
| Leg Ham, pre-pack | Don's | | 250g | | | |
| Chips/crisps, original, salted | Smith's or Thins | | 170g | | | |
| Cooked hot potato chips, 1 serve* | Independent fish and chip shop* | | ~110g | | | |
| Vanilla Ice cream, regular fat | Nestle Peters Original | | 2L | | | |
| White Sugar | CSR | | 2kg | | | |
| French Dressing, regular fat | Praise | | 330mL | | | |
| Tomato sauce, regular (not ketchup) | Heinz Big Red or Masterfoods | | 500mL | | | |
| Tinned chicken & vegetable soup, ready to eat | Campbell's Country Ladle | | 505g | | | |
| Orange Juice, Australian Grown (Fresh, chilled) | Berri | | 2L | | | |
| White crumbed fish fillet, frozen | Birds Eye | | 425g | | | |
| 2 Minute noodles, chicken (cheapest specified brand) | Maggi or Fantastic | | 70g | | | |
| * denotes non-supermarket lines | | | | | | |

available published data [2, 31] and recommendations [33]. Further, the proportion of household food expenditure on discretionary items (around 58%) [29] is similar to that described by the ABS (58.2%) using different methods based on household expenditure [19]. Hence the tools appear valid for use in estimating the cost of current and healthy diets.

### *The healthy diets ASAP protocol part two: Location and store sample selection*

A random sample of the Statistical Area Level 2 (SA2) locations in each town is selected to achieve a representative sample. SA2 locations are stratified by the Index of Relative Socio-Economic Disadvantage for Areas (SEIFA) quintile using information and maps available on the ABS website [36–38] Following sample size calculations, the required number of SA2 locations within SEIFA Quintile 1, 3 and 5 are selected randomly for participation. Food outlets within seven kilometres by car of the centre of each SA2 location are identified with Google™ Maps [39] and included in the surveys. Stores to survey include one outlet of all supermarket chains (in trials these were Coles™, Woolworths™ and Independent Grocers Australia (IGA™), Supabarn™ and ALDI™), 'fast-food'/take-away outlets (a Big Mac™ hamburger from the McDonald's™ chain; pizza from the Pizza Hut™ chain; fish and chips from independent outlets) and two alcoholic liquor outlets closest to the geographical centre of each SA2 location.

### *The healthy diets ASAP protocol part three: Collecting and entering food price data*

The Healthy Diets ASAP diet price survey data collection form (Table 4) combines the items included in the current diet and the healthy diet for convenience and utility. The agreed price data collection protocol is presented in Table 5 and is printed on each data collection form. Research assistants are trained to use the form and follow the price collection protocol strictly. Prices are collected within the same 4 week/monthly period, as prices change over time.

Permission to participate is sought from each store manager prior to data collection.

Data entry and analysis sheets have been developed using Excel™ spreadsheets [40]. Double data entry is recommended to minimise error. Data are cleaned and checked. Any missing values are imputed to ascribe the mean price of the same food item in all other relevant outlets in the same SA2 area. Data analysis tools are available from the corresponding author. As has been achieved previously for the Victorian Health Food Access Basket [41], the Healthy Diets ASAP App is under development to streamline data collection and analysis and reduce error.

**Table 5** Healthy Diets ASAP food price data collection protocol

1. Record the usual price of an item, i.e. do not collect the sale/special price unless it is the only price available (if so, note in comment column)
2. Look for the specified brand and specified size for each food item, and record the price
   - If the specified brand is not available: Choose the cheapest brand (non-generic) available in the specified size. Note this brand in the "Your brand" column
   - If the specified size is not available: Choose the nearest larger size in the specified brand. If a larger size is not available, choose the nearest smaller size. Note this size in the "Your size" column
   - If both the specified brand and specified size are not available: Choose the cheapest in the nearest larger size of another brand (non-generic). If a larger size is not available, choose the nearest smaller size
   - If multiple brands are specified, record the price of the cheapest one and note brand in the "Your brand" column
   - If the item is only available in a generic form (e.g. Home Brand, Coles, Woolworths Select, Black and Gold) choose the most expensive generic item in the specified size. If the specified size is not available, choose the nearest larger size. If a larger size is not available, choose the nearest smaller size. Note the generic name in the "Your brand" and the size in the "Your size" columns
3. Loose produce: choose the usual cheapest price per kg of the variety not on special. If the only variety available is on special, record the special price and note in comments column
4. Peanuts: choose the branded packet size closest to 250 g. If packaged, roasted, unsalted peanuts are not available, record the price of the loose 'bulk scoop & weigh' roasted, unsalted peanuts per 100 g
5. Check all data are collected and recorded as above, before leaving store

### *The healthy diets ASAP protocol part four: Determination of household income*

Household income is determined by either of three methods, depending on the purpose of the study and the granularity of available data.

**Median household gross income at area level** In Australia, national census data is the only source of SA2 level household income data and is provided only at total (gross) level. Median gross household income is determined per week (before taxation, rent and other expenses) in each SA2 area by entering relevant post codes into the Community Profile data calculator [42] that is based on the 2011 Census results [36], adjusted for the wage price index (for example, there was an increase of 11.1% from September 2011 to September 2015) and multiplying by two to derive median household income in each SA2 area per fortnight. Details and examples are provided in Additional file 5.

**Indicative low (minimum) disposable household income** Indicative low (minimum) income of the reference household (and other households of interest to specific stakeholders) is calculated based on the level of minimum wages [43] and determination of the welfare payments provided by the Department of Human Services [44] as per the methods used by the Queensland Department of Health [20]. Assumptions are made for employment, housing type, disability status, savings and investments, child support, education attendance and immunisation status of children (Table 6). As welfare policy actions can change, the most recent schedules should be used. Where it is higher than the minimum threshold, the indicative low (minimum) household income is adjusted for taxation payable [45] so also represents minimum household disposable income. Details and examples are provided in Additional file 6.

**Median household disposable income at national level** For assessment of diet affordability at the national level, median equivalised disposable household income for the reference family composition is sourced from the Survey of Income and Housing [46].

### *The healthy diets ASAP protocol part five: Data analysis and reporting*

The price of the healthy (recommended) and current diets in each store and the mean price for each SEIFA quintile is calculated for the reference household composition in each of areas surveyed in each city. Results can be presented in a range of metrics, including the cost of the total diets per household per fortnight, and the cost of purchasing specific five food group and discretionary foods and drinks (including policy relevant items such as alcohol, 'take-away foods' and sugar-sweetened beverages). The results for the current (unhealthy) diet and healthy (recommended) diet are compared to determine the differential.

Affordability of the healthy and current diets for the reference household is determined by comparing the cost of each diet with the median gross household income (Additional file 5) and also with the indicative low (minimum) disposable income of low income households (Additional file 6). Where a representative national survey of diet prices has been conducted, affordability of the healthy and current diets for the reference household is determined by comparing the cost of each diet with the median equivalised disposable income [46] and with the indicative low (minimum) disposable income of low income households. Internationally, a benchmark of 30%

**Table 6** Assumptions applied to determine the indicative low (minimum) disposable household income of the reference household

The reference household consists of an adult male, an adult female, a 14 year old boy and an 8 year old girl

- The adult male works on a permanent basis at the national minimum wage ($17.29 per hour)for 38 h a week
- The adult female works on a part-time basis at the national minimum wage ($17.29 per hour)for 6 h a week
- Both children attend school and are fully immunised
- None of the family are disabled
- The family has some emergency savings that earn negligible interest

of income has been used to indicate affordability of a diet [6, 10].

Data files can be manipulated to investigate the effects of potential fiscal policy changes on the affordability of current (unhealthy) and healthy (recommended) diets for the reference household. The price of the relevant foods and drinks can be modified readily to highlight the likely 'real-world' impacts of different scenarios, for example, to investigate the potential extension of the Goods and Services Tax (GST) on basic healthy foods [47], or the potential application of different levels of taxation on sugary drinks in Australia [29].

## Discussion

There are several methodological limitations inherent in the Healthy Diets ASAP protocols. Given that it is based on national reported mean dietary intakes, the cost of the current (unhealthy) diet is unlikely to be the same as actual expenditure on food and drinks in specific areas and among specific groups [48]. Other assumptions commonly made in similar apparent consumption and household expenditure surveys include that food is shared equitably throughout the household, that there is no home food production and minimal wastage. Nutritionally similar products were aggregated to minimise the number of items included in the diet pricing tools, but products were not necessarily homogenous in terms of price. However, similar healthy food items were included in each diet to try to minimise any unintended effects.

Ideally, the specific foods included in both diet pricing tools are culturally acceptable, commonly consumed, widely available, accessible and considered 'every day' rather than luxury items. As the foods and drinks included in the current diet pricing survey tool reflect actual consumption data, it was presumed that they were deemed by the population as a whole as meeting these requirements. No adjustments were made for costs such as transport, time, cooking equipment and utilities; as these apply to both current and healthy diets, assessment of the price differential between the two can help control for some of these hidden costs to some extent. However, these hidden costs would increase actual diet costs and decrease affordability of the diets.

No adjustments were made to account for the marked under-reporting in the AHS 2011–12 [4], reported dietary variability amongst different groups other than age/gender stratification, or the greater proportion of pre-prepared 'convenience' items in the current diet pricing tool compared with the healthy diet pricing tool. Given the high rates of overweight/obesity in Australia, the Foundation Diets were prescribed for the shortest and least active in each age group according to the modelling that informed the Australian Guide to Healthy Eating [33]; however this would under-estimate the requirements of taller, more active and healthy weight individuals.

No attempt was made to control the price of the healthy diet pricing tool or the current diet pricing tool for energy, as the diets are constructed on recommended energy levels and actual reported levels of energy respectively. Further, the energy content of each tool is a determinant variable that directly affects diet-related health outcomes [18, 49]. As most Australians are already overweight or obese, increasing recommended energy requirements in excess of Foundation Diets is not consistent with optimum health outcomes [33]. As the key exposure variable affecting the life time risk of diet-related disease is the total diet and dietary patterns, approaches such as this that compare metrics of actual current diets with recommended diets are more pertinent to the health policy debate than the more common, but limited, studies into the relative price of selected 'healthy' and 'unhealthy' foods or single 'optimised' diets [18, 50, 51].

While a benchmark of 30% of income has been used to indicate affordability of diet internationally and in Australia [6, 9, 10] it is not clear from the literature whether this income comparator is gross income or disposable income [6]. Using disposable income to estimate affordability better reflects the capacity of a household to afford food/diets [52, 53]; using gross income is a more conservative approach as it does not take taxation into account. However, in Australia currently, median disposable household income data are readily available only at national level [46]; at area level only median gross household income data are readily available. Further, the composition of the reference household does not align necessarily with that of households in the census in all areas. Comparing diet price with indicative low (minimum) disposable household more accurately estimates affordability of diets in vulnerable groups. However, the tax paid component of indicative low (minimum) disposable household income can be removed to improve comparability with estimates of affordability determined by application of gross median household income.

Arbitrary decision points occur around sampling frameworks, data collection protocols (for example, selection of cheapest comparable generic item if the branded item is unavailable in any size), analysis and presentation of results, data sources and definitions of family and household income and composition. Such methodological limitations are common to other food price studies. In order for final methods to be replicable, agreement among key stakeholders including end users on each of these decision points at the Healthy Diets ASAP Forum was invaluable. Publication of detailed protocols is essential to support uptake, replicability, fidelity and transparency of the method.

The detailed dietary survey data required to produce the current (unhealthy) diet pricing tool and the modelling data required to produce the healthy (recommended) diet pricing tool are not easily accessible in all countries and technical capacity to analyse individual records may be limited. Therefore, this optimal approach may be too complex for application to assess and monitor the price of diets from a health perspective globally. However, there is potential for the diet pricing tools to be adapted for use in other countries by substitution of food components with commonly-consumed local equivalents, dietary analysis and testing.

## Conclusion

The development of standardised Healthy Diets ASAP method protocols provides an example of how the INFORMAS optimal food price and affordability methods can be adapted at country level to help develop standardised, policy relevant diet price assessment, monitoring tools and benchmarks. The approach can be used to assess the price, price differential and relative affordability of current (unhealthy) and healthy (recommended) diets and inform scenario modelling of potential fiscal and nutrition policy actions.

The Healthy Diets ASAP method satisfies long-standing calls for the development of a nationally standardised approach to assess food prices from a health perspective, supporting comparison of results from different locations and over time, in Australia.

The protocol could be adapted in other countries to benchmark and monitor the price, price differential and affordability of current and healthy diets globally.

## Endnotes

[1]Additional data are provided for:

- Household 1($n$ = 6): adult male 31–50 yrs. old; adult female 31–50 yrs. old; older female 70+ yrs. old; boy 14 yrs. old; girl 8 yrs. old; boy 4 yrs. old
- Household 2 ($n$ = 3): single parent with 2 children: adult female 31–50 yrs. old; boy 14 yrs. old; girl 8 yrs. old
- Household 3 ($n$ = 1): single unemployed person: adult male 31–50 yrs. old
- Household 4 ($n$ = 2): older couple with no children: senior adult male 70+ yrs. old; senior adult female 70+ yrs. old: pensioners

## Additional files

**Additional file 1:** Current (unhealthy) Diets: Mean daily intake of representative categories of foods and drinks for individuals (age/gender) comprising the reference household, and other common households.

**Additional file 2:** A. Foundation diet recommended serves of foods per week for individuals (NHMRC 2011) comprising the reference household and other common households. B. Healthy (recommended) Diets: Recommended serves per day of food groups and amounts of composite foods and drinks for individuals comprising the reference household, consistent with Foundation Diets (NHMRC 2011) including commonly-consumed brands.

**Additional file 3:** Composition of the current (unhealthy) diet and healthy (recommended) diet for four additional households (HH1, HH2, HH3, HH4)[1] per fortnight.

**Additional file 4:** Energy and nutrient analysis of individual current and healthy diet baskets compared to results of the AHS and Foundation Diet modelling.

**Additional file 5:** Median income determination by SA2 Example-Median income data from the 2011 Census, ABS Community Profiles of SA2 areas for six SA2 locations in Sydney, NSW*.

**Additional file 6:** Calculations of low (minimum) disposable household income data from welfare data – Example.

### Abbreviations

ASAP: Australian Standardised Affordability and Pricing methods; CURFs: Confidential Unit Record Files

### Acknowledgements

Thank you to Research Assistants Dr. Janice Lee and Ms. Sandra Mitchell who collected food prices in two major Australian cities in November and December 2015. Thank you to all those academic, public sector and non-government organisation representatives who attended the National Healthy Diets ASAP Forum, Brisbane, March 2016 and contributed to decision-making to inform develop the final Healthy Diets ASAP methods, including Ms. Kathy Chapman, Prof Karen Charlton, Ms. Megan Cobcroft, Ms. Megan Ferguson, Prof Danielle Gallegos, Ms. Leah Galvin, Ms. Holly Jones, Dr. Carolyn Keogh, Dr. Sally McKay, Mr. Leigh Merrington, Ms. Sandra Murray, Ms. Lesley Paton, Dr. Claire Palermo, Dr. Melanie Pescud, Ms. Emma Slaytor, Ms. Beth Thomas, Ms. Carrie Turner, Ms. Julie-Anne McWhinnie together with all authors. Thank you to INFORMAS members.

### Funding

Financial support to develop the national Healthy Diets ASAP methods was provided by The Australian Prevention Partnership Centre through the NHMRC partnership centre grant scheme (Grant ID: GNT9100001) with the Australian Government Department of Health, NSW Ministry of Health, ACT Health, HCF, and the HCF Research Foundation. The funders had no role in the design, analysis or writing of this manuscript.

### Authors' contributions

AL led the project, developed concepts, constructed the current diet pricing tool, finalised the healthy diet pricing tool, developed sampling methods, convened and chaired the national stakeholders forum and drafted the manuscript; SK assisted in constructing the current diet pricing tool and finalising the healthy diet pricing tool, transposed, cleaned and analysed data and assisted with the national stakeholders forum; ML assisted with transposing and analysing food price data, finalised the household income assessment protocol and assisted with the national stakeholders forum; EG developed an early draft of the household income assessment protocol; CP provided conceptual advice; TL accessed and analysed dietary intake data from the Confidential Unit Record Files (CURFs) of the Australian Health Survey 2011–13 (ABS 2013a) to inform development of the current diet pricing tool and advised on methods to determine household income; MD developed an early draft of the healthy diet pricing tool. All co-authors reviewed drafts of the paper and contributed to the final manuscript.

**Competing interests**
The authors declare that they have no competing interests.

**Author details**
[1]The Australian Prevention Partnership Centre, The Sax Institute, 10 Jones Street, Ultimo, NSW 2007, Australia. [2]School of Public Health and Social Work, Queensland University of Technology, Brisbane, QLD, Australia. [3]Preventive Health Branch, Department of Health, Queensland Government, Brisbane, QLD, Australia. [4]School of Public Health, Curtin University, Kent Street, GPO Box U1987, Perth 6845, Western Australia. [5]Public Health Division, Department of Health, Government of Western Australia, 189 Royal Street, East Perth 6004, Western Australia.

**References**

1. Institute for Health Metrics and Evaluation. Global Burden of Disease Country Profile Australia. 2015; http://www.healthdata.org/sites/default/files/files/country_profiles/GBD/ihme_gbd_country_report_australia.pdf. Accessed 12 Nov 2017.
2. Australian Bureau of Statistics. Australian Health Survey: Consumption of food groups from the Australian dietary guidelines, 2011–12. 2016; http://www.abs.gov.au/ausstats/abs@.nsf/mf/4364.0.55.012 Accessed 12 Nov 2017.
3. National Health and Medical Research Council. Australian Dietary Guidelines - providing the scientific evidence for healthier Australian Diets. 2013; https://www.eatforhealth.gov.au/sites/default/files/content/n55_australian_dietary_guidelines.pdf. Accessed 9 Feb 2016.
4. Australian Bureau of Statistics. Australian Health Survey: Nutrition first results - foods and nutrients, 2011–12. 2014; http://www.abs.gov.au/AUSSTATS/abs@.nsf/DetailsPage/4364.0.55.0072011-12?OpenDocument. Accessed 12 Nov 2017.
5. Australian Bureau of Statistics. Australian Health Survey: Updated results, 2011–2012 - overweight and obesity. 2013; http://www.abs.gov.au/ausstats/abs@.nsf/lookup/33C64022ABB5ECD5CA257B82001794377opendocument. Accessed 12 Nov 2017.
6. Lee A, et al. Monitoring the price and affordability of foods and diets globally. Obes Rev. 2013;14(Suppl 1):82–95.
7. Kettings C, Sinclair AJ, Voevodin M. A healthy diet consistent with Australian health recommendations is too expensive for welfare-dependent families. Aust N Z J Public Health. 2009;33(6):566–72.
8. Williams PG. Can the poor in Australia afford healthy food? Nutr Diet. 2011; 68:6–7. https://doi.org/10.1111/j.1747-0080.2010.01485.x.
9. Ward PR, et al. Food stress in Adelaide: the relationship between low income and the affordability of healthy food. J Environ Public Health. 2013; 2013:10.
10. Barosh L, et al. The cost of a healthy and sustainable diet – who can afford it? Aust N Z J Public Health. 2014;38(1):7–12.
11. Landrigan TJ, et al. Removing the Australian tax exemption on healthy food adds food stress to families vulnerable to poor nutrition. Aust N Z J Public Health. 2017;41:591–7.
12. Vandevijvere S, et al. Monitoring and benchmarking population diet quality globally: a step-wise approach. Obes Rev. 2013;14(Suppl 1):135–49.
13. Lewis M, Lee A. Costing 'healthy' food baskets in Australia - a systematic review of food price and affordability monitoring tools, protocols and methods. Public Health Nutr. 2016;19(16):2872–86.
14. Carlson A, Frazao E. Are healthy foods really more expensive? It depends on how you measure the price. In: Economic information bulletin no. (EIB-96): United States Department of Agriculture Economic Research Service; 2012. https://www.ers.usda.gov/webdocs/publications/44678/19980_eib96.pdf?v=42321
15. World Health Organization and Food and Agriculture Organization of the United Nations. Diet, nutrition and the prevention of chronic diseases, Report of the joint WHO/FAO expert consultation. 2003; http://www.who.int/nutrition/publications/obesity/WHO_TRS_916/en/. Accessed 10 Nov 2017.
16. World Health Organization. Global Action Plan for the Prevention and Control of Non-communicable Diseases 2013–2020. 2013; http://www.who.int/nmh/publications/ncd-action-plan/en/. Accessed 10 Nov 2017.
17. Commission on Ending Childhood Obesity. Report of the Commission on Ending Childhood Obesity. 2016; http://www.who.int/end-childhood-obesity/publications/echo-report/en/. Accessed 10 Nov 2017.
18. Burns C, Sacks G, Gold L. Longitudinal study of consumer Price index (CPI) trends in core and non-core foods in Australia. Aust N Z J Public Health. 2008;32(5):450–3.
19. Australian Bureau of Statistics. Consumer Price Index, Australia, Dec 2015 Feature article: Australian dietary guidelines Price indexes. 2016; http://wwwabsgovau/AUSSTATS/abs@nsf/Previousproducts/6401 0Feature%20Article1Dec%202015?opendocument&tabname=Summary&prodno=64010&issue=Dec%202015&num=&view=. Accessed 12 Nov 2017.
20. Queensland Health. 2014 Healthy food access basket survey. 2015; https://wwwhealthqldgovau/research-reports/reports/public-health/food-nutrition/access/overview. Accessed 8 Feb 2016.
21. Pollard CM, et al. Geographic factors as determinants of food security: a Western Australian food pricing and quality study. Asia Pac J Clin Nutr. 2014;23(4):703–13.
22. Lee AJ, et al. Improving aboriginal and Torres Strait islander nutrition and health. Med J Aust. 2009;190(10):547–8.
23. Pollard C. Selecting interventions for food security in remote indigenous communities. In: Farmar-Bowers Q, Higgins V, Millar J, editors. Food security in Australia: challenges and prospects for the future. Boston: Springer US; 2013. p. 97–112.
24. Seal J. Monitoring the price and availability of healthy food - time for a national approach. Nutr Diet. 2004;61(4):197–8.
25. Burns C, Friel S. It's time to determine the cost of a healthy diet in Australia. Aust N Z J Public Health. 2007;31(4):363–5.
26. Hawkes C. Food taxes: what type of evidence is available to inform policy development? Nutr Bull. 2012;37(1):51–6.
27. Sacks G, et al. 'Traffic-light' nutrition labelling and 'junk-food' tax: a modelled comparison of cost-effectiveness for obesity prevention. Int J Obes. 2011;35(7): 1001–9.
28. Veerman J, Cobiac L. Removing the GST exemption for fresh fruits and vegetables could cost lives. Med J Aust. 2013;199(8):534–5.
29. Lee AJ, et al. Testing the price and affordability of healthy and current (unhealthy) diets and the potential impacts of policy change in Australia. BMC Public Health. 2016;16:315.
30. Swinburn B, et al. INFORMAS (International Network for Food and Obesity/non-communicable diseases Research, Monitoring and Action Support): overview and key principles. Obes Rev. 2013;14(Suppl 1):1–12.
31. Australian Bureau of Statistics. Microdata: Australian health survey: nutrition and physical activity, 2011–12. 2013; http://www.abs.gov.au/ausstats/abs@.nsf/PrimaryMainFeatures/4324.0.55.002?OpenDocument. Accessed 12 Nov 2017.
32. Food Standards Australia New Zealand. AUSNUT 2011–2013. 2016; http://www.foodstandards.gov.au/science/monitoringnutrients/ausnut/Pages/default.aspx. Accessed 12 Nov 2017.
33. National Health and Medical Research Council. A Modelling System to Inform the Revision of the Australian Guide To Healthy Eating. 2011; https://www.eatforhealth.gov.au/sites/default/files/files/the_guidelines/n55c_australian_dietary_guidelines_food_modelling_140121.pdf. Accessed 11 Feb 2016.
34. Xyris Software (Australia) Pty Ltd, FoodWorks Professional. 2012.
35. National Health and Medical Research Council, Australian Government Department of Health and Ageing, and New Zealand Ministry of Health. Nutrient Reference Values for Australia and New Zealand, Including Recommended Dietary Intakes 2006 Version 1.2 Updated September 2017. 2006; https://www.nhmrc.gov.au/guidelines-publications/n35-n36-n37. Accessed 12 Nov 2017.
36. Australian Bureau of Statistics. Census of Population and Housing: Socio-Economic Indexes for Areas (SEIFA), Australia. 2011; http://www.abs.gov.au/websitedbs/censushome.nsf/home/seifa. Accessed 30 Oct 2015.
37. Australian Bureau of Statistics. Census of Population and Housing: Socio-economic indexes for areas (SEIFA), Australia: Mapping Files of Statistical Area Level 2 Index of Relative Socio-economic Disadvantage, 2011. 2011; http://www.abs.gov.au/AUSSTATS/abs@.nsf/DetailsPage/2033.0.55.0012011?OpenDocument. Accessed 30 Oct 2015.
38. Australian Bureau of Statistics. Australian Statistical Geography Standard (ASGS): Volume 1 - Main structure and greater Capital City statistical areas, July 2011. 2011; http://www.abs.gov.au/AUSSTATS/abs@.nsf/DetailsPage/1270.0.55.001July%202011?OpenDocument. Accessed 20 Oct 2015.
39. Google Maps. 2017; https://maps.google.com.au/. Accessed 14 Oct 2017.
40. Microsoft Corporation, Microsoft Office 2007. 2007.
41. Palermo C, et al. Development and evaluation of an iPad app for measuring the cost of a nutritious diet. JMIR MHealth UHealth. 2014;2(4):e50.

42. Australian Bureau of Statistics. Census 2011 Community profiles. 2011; http://www.abs.gov.au/websitedbs/censushome.nsf/home/communityprofiles?opendocument&navpos=230. Accessed 1 Mar 2016.
43. Fair Work Ombudsman. Minimum Wages. https://www.fairwork.gov.au/how-we-will-help/templates-and-guides/fact-sheets/minimum-workplace-entitlements/minimum-wages. Accessed 22 Oct 2015.
44. Department of Human Services. Online Estimators. http://www.humanservices.gov.au/customer/enablers/online-estimators. Accessed 22 Oct 2015.
45. Australian Taxation Office. Simple Tax Calculator. www.ato.gov.au/calculators-and-tools/simple-tax-calculator/. Accessed 12 Nov 2017.
46. Australian Bureau of Statistics. Household Income and Wealth, Australia, 2015–16. 2017; http://abs.gov.au/household-income. Accessed 12 Nov 2017.
47. Australian Government. Re:think; better tax, better Australia. Discussion paper. 2015; http://bettertax.gov.au/publications/discussion-paper/. Accessed 15 Mar 2015.
48. Mhurchu CN, et al. Food prices and consumer demand: differences across income levels and ethnic groups. PLoS One. 2013;8(10):e75934.
49. Lee J, Ralston R, Truby H. Influence of food cost on diet quality and risk factors for chronic disease: a systematic review. Nutr Diet. 2011;68:248–61.
50. Rao M, et al. Do healthier foods and diet patterns cost more than less healthy options? A systematic review and meta-analysis. BMJ Open. 2013; 3(12):e004277.
51. Friel S, Barosh LJ, Lawrence M. Towards healthy and sustainable food consumption: an Australian case study. Public Health Nutr. 2014;17(5):1156–66.
52. Jacobs, D., Perera, D., Williams, T. Inflation and the cost of living. Reserve Bank of Australia Bulletin, March Quarter 33–46 2014; 2014. https://www.rba.gov.au/publications/bulletin/2014/mar/4.html. Accessed 12 Nov 2017.
53. Australian Council of Social Service. Minimum Wage Submission 2017. 2017; http://www.acoss.org.au/wp-content/uploads/2017/03/ACOSS-minimum-wage-submission-2017_FINAL.pdf. Accessed 10 Nov 2017.

# 10

# Dietary patterns of university students in the UK

E. F. Sprake[1], J. M. Russell[2], J. E. Cecil[3], R. J. Cooper[4], P. Grabowski[1], L. K. Pourshahidi[5] and M. E. Barker[6*]

## Abstract

**Background:** University represents a key transition into adulthood for many adolescents but there are associated concerns about health and behaviours. One important aspect relates to diet and there is emerging evidence that university students may consume poor quality diets, with potential implications for body weight and long-term health. This research aimed to characterise dietary patterns of university students in the UK and their sociodemographic and lifestyle antecedents.

**Methods:** An online, cross-sectional survey was undertaken with a convenience sample of 1448 university students from five UK universities (King's College London, Universities of St Andrews, Southampton and Sheffield, and Ulster University). The survey comprised a validated food frequency questionnaire alongside lifestyle and sociodemographic questions. Dietary patterns were generated from food frequency intake data using principal components analysis. Nutrient intakes were estimated to characterise the nutrient profile of each dietary pattern. Associations with sociodemographic variables were assessed through general linear modelling.

**Results:** Dietary analyses revealed four major dietary patterns: 'vegetarian'; 'snacking'; 'health-conscious'; and 'convenience, red meat & alcohol'. The 'health-conscious' pattern had the most favourable micronutrient profile. Students' gender, age, year of study, geographical location and cooking ability were associated with differences in pattern behaviour. Female students favoured the 'vegetarian' pattern, whilst male students preferred the 'convenience, red meat & alcohol' pattern. Less healthful dietary patterns were positively associated with lifestyle risk factors such as smoking, low physical activity and take-away consumption. The health-conscious pattern had greatest nutrient density. The 'convenience, red meat & alcohol' pattern was associated with higher weekly food spending; this pattern was also identified most consistently across universities. Students reporting greater cooking ability tended towards the 'vegetarian' and 'health-conscious' patterns.

**Conclusions:** Food intake varied amongst university students. A substantial proportion of students followed health-promoting diets, which had good nutrient profiles obviating a need for dietary intervention. However, some students consumed poor diets, incurred greater food costs and practised unfavourable lifestyle behaviours, which may have long-term health effects. University policy to improve students' diets should incorporate efforts to promote student engagement in cooking and food preparation, and increased availability of low cost healthier food items.

**Keywords:** Food consumption, Principal components analysis, Survey, University students

* Correspondence: Margo.Barker@shu.ac.uk
[6]Food & Nutrition Group, Business School, Sheffield Hallam University, Sheffield S1 1WB, UK
Full list of author information is available at the end of the article

## Background

University students represent a substantial proportion (50%) of the UK young adult population [1] and an individual's university career may be influential in the establishment of long-term eating patterns and thus chronic disease risk. This population also represents a group of young adults with a set of unique factors driving dietary intake: the transition to university life may be associated with increased autonomy over food choice, small food budgets, and exposure to new social groups and food cultures.

A limited body of data indicates that the dietary behaviours of UK university students are not conducive to either short- or long-term health. Alcohol consumption has received most research attention revealing that binge drinking is endemic [2, 3]. There are also indications of high intakes of confectionery and fast foods, and low consumption of fruit and vegetables [3, 4]. Although there is some evidence that dietary behaviours track from adolescence to adulthood [5, 6], the transition from home to university life has been associated with unfavourable changes to food intake: increases in alcohol and sugar intake, and decreases in fruit and vegetable consumption have been reported [7].

Additionally, the first year of university life has been identified as a period associated with body weight gain in both North American [8] and UK students [9, 10] Such weight gain may have long-term repercussions, since overweight during young adulthood has been identified as a significant predictor of obesity later in life [11]. Furthermore, high rates of body dissatisfaction and dieting behaviours have been noted, particularly amongst female students [12, 13]. Such engagement in dieting behaviour and dysfunctional relationships with food not only impact on dietary adequacy [14, 15], but may also create tension and conflict for young people as they develop relationships with new peer groups [16].

Dietary studies of British university students are constrained by crude dietary assessment, small sample size and generally focus on a single university [3, 4]. Furthermore, their analytical approach has been on single foods and/or nutrients, which has allowed assessment of intake relative to dietary recommendations. Using multivariate statistical techniques to identify dietary patterns through intake of multiple interrelated food groups captures the complexity and multidimensional nature of diet, which is representative of real life food consumption [17]. This approach also allows greater insight into the different patterns of food consumption that naturally occur within a population and facilitates identification of sub-groups who may be most in need of health promotion efforts. Universities in particular may represent a setting in which dietary behaviours are open to change and large groups of young adults can be reached, representing an appropriate target for health promotion efforts. A dietary patterns approach has been used widely in various UK population groups, but has not been employed to characterise the diets of university students.

This study aimed to identify dietary patterns that exist within a UK university student population, to assess the nutritional profile of these patterns, and to examine socio-demographic and lifestyle variables underpinning these patterns.

## Methods

### Study design

This cross-sectional study involved a convenience sample of five regionally and socio-economically diverse universities throughout the UK (Universities of: Sheffield, Ulster, King's College London (KCL), Southampton and St Andrews). These universities had responded positively to an invitation to participate in the research study; contact was made via university Human Nutrition or Health Sciences departments. A web-survey, comprising a validated food frequency questionnaire (FFQ) (Tinuviel Software Ltd., Warrington, UK) was used to assess dietary intake. Socio-demographic and lifestyle data were also collected. The survey was conducted between Autumn 2013 and Spring 2015. Data collection was preceded by a pilot study, which was used to refine the web-survey.

Ethical approval was obtained from each participating university. Informed consent for participation was obtained on the first page of the web-survey.

### Subjects & recruitment

All British and European Union students less than 30 years of age at the five participating universities represented eligible participants. A cut-off of 30 years was chosen in order to focus on the dietary behaviours of young adults. International students (non-Home or non-EU) were not included because of possible heterogeneity in food choice (this issue was identified in the pilot study), and the dietary assessment instrument used was Euro-centric. Students identifying as international students on the first page of the online survey could not proceed. Only health sciences students were recruited at the University of Southampton, because of logistical issues in distribution of the survey. All students were recruited through university email distribution lists. This email provided study details and emphasised that students did not have to be eating a healthy diet to participate. Participants were required to recall their habitual diet over the most recent university semester (three months). This was the autumn semester 2013 for students at Sheffield, the autumn semester 2014 for students at Ulster and KCL, and the spring semester 2014 for students at Southampton and St Andrews. Participants who provided their contact details were entered into a prize draw; each person could win one of 40 £20 high street vouchers.

### Participant eligibility

A total of 1683 students across the five universities responded to the survey. Figure 1 shows numbers of students excluded based on fulfilment of various eligibility criteria. The cut-offs for implausible energy intakes in the Nurses' Health Study (< 500 Kcal/day and > 3500 Kcal/day) and Healthcare Professionals' Follow-up Study (< 800 Kcal/day or > 4200 Kcal/day) were used to identify and exclude participants reporting implausible energy intakes the current study. Using this method, 24 participants were identified as over-reporters (8 males; 16 females) and three participants were identified as under-reporters (1 male; 2 females). A total of 1448 students comprised the final sample.

### Dietary data

A validated 111-item FFQ originally developed by the Medical Research Council was employed to assess dietary intake (DietQ; Tinuviel Software Ltd., Warrington, UK; [18, 19]. The FFQ was piloted among 40 students at the University of Sheffield. Feedback from the pilot study led to three further items being incorporated into the questionnaire (consumption of hummus; tofu; water).

Frequencies of consumption in the questionnaire were expressed as follows: every day = 7/week, through to once per week = 1/week; once every 2–3 weeks (F) = 0.5/week; rarely/never (R) = 0. Where absolute quantities of consumption were given, these were converted into number of portions consumed per day. Food and nutrient intakes were generated directly from these FFQ data using the nutritional analysis software QBuilder (Tinuviel Software, Warrington, UK). The original 111 foods/food groups listed in the FFQ were condensed into 55 broader foods/food groups for dietary patterns analysis. These 55 foods/food groups are detailed in Additional file 1: Table S1.

### Socio-demographic, anthropometric and lifestyle data

The following socio-demographic information was collected: age; gender; degree programme and year of study; full/part-time study; nature of term-time residence; ethnicity; religion; socioeconomic status (SES); maternal education; and university attended. Information on dieting/weight loss behaviour, supplement use, cooking ability (four response options from 'able to cook wide range of meals from raw ingredients' through to 'unable to cook at all'), smoking status (students were asked to self-identify as a never smoker, ex-smoker, social smoker or regular smoker), self-reported physical activity levels (students were required to self-identify as not very active, moderately active or very active), body weight (kg) and height (m) (for calculation of body mass index (BMI), kg/m$^2$), cooking behaviours (consumption of: meals made from raw ingredients; pre-prepared foods; ready meals and take-aways; and meals from university cafeteria) and weekly food expenditure (£) was also collected.

### Identification of dietary patterns

To generate dietary patterns, the 55 food/food group intake variables were entered into a principal component analysis (PCA) and a varimax (orthogonal) rotation was performed. The number of components retained was determined by the scree plot, parallel analysis and component interpretability [20]. Food/food groups with factor loadings > 0.32 were used to interpret each dietary pattern.

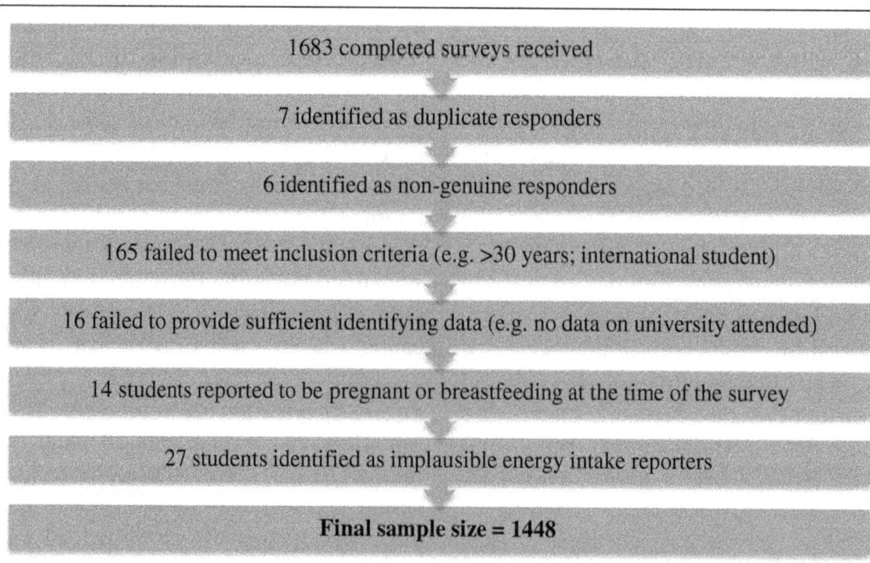


**Fig. 1** Numbers of students excluded based on fulfilment of various eligibility criteria

### Statistical analysis

Pearson's product moment correlation coefficients were calculated between pattern scores and absolute nutrient intakes. Partial correlation coefficients were also calculated, which adjusted for energy intake. Correlation coefficients ≥0.5 and ≤ − 0.5 were considered strong. Examination of scatter plots revealed no evidence of non-linear relationships between component scores and nutrient intakes.

General linear models (GLMs) were firstly fitted for demographic variables alone (model 1) and then with additional eating factors (model 2). Maternal education was not included in the models, since data were not available for all students. Religion was also not included due to confounding with ethnic background.

Variables were categorised into two groups for entry into a GLM: 1) demographic variables: gender, age, leisure-time physical activity, BMI, smoking, ethnicity, year of study, term-time accommodation, university attended, and full-time/part-time status 2) cooking- and eating-related variables: cooking ability, animal food consumption, frequency of consumption of meals prepared using raw ingredients, frequency of consumption of meals using pre-prepared foods, frequency of consumption of ready-meals and take-aways, frequency of consumption of meals from university cafeteria, frequency of skipping breakfast, frequency of skipping lunch, and amount spent on food.

For each retained dietary component a GLM was fitted with demographic variables only (Group 1). A second GLM was then fitted, which included significant demographic variables and variables from Group 2. Multi-comparison post-hoc tests with Sidak correction were carried out to aid interpretation of significant factors in the GLM. The Statistical Package for the Social Sciences (SPSS) Version 20 was used for all statistical analyses. A $p$ value of < 0.05 was considered significant.

## Results

### Participant characteristics

The sociodemographic characteristics of the sample are shown in Table 1. The sample comprised 1064 (73.5%) women and 384 (26.5%) men. The majority of students were White British ($n$ = 911; 62.9%) and registered for full-time study ($n$ = 1394; 96.3%). The mean age of the sample was 21.5 years (SD 2.63 years). The majority of respondents were from the University of Sheffield ($n$ = 567; 39.2%), Ulster University in Northern Ireland ($n$ = 443; 30.6%) and KCL ($n$ = 305; 21.1%). The remaining students were from the Universities of Southampton ($n$ = 79; 5.5%) and St Andrews, Scotland ($n$ = 54; 3.7%). Just over one-third of students were studying a health-related degree. The majority of students ($n$ = 1000; 69.1%) reported a healthy BMI (18.5–24.99 kg/m$^2$); mean BMI was 22.8 kg/m$^2$ (SD 4.64 kg/m$^2$).

In terms of eating behaviours of the sample, just under two-thirds of students described themselves as regular meat-eaters, whilst approximately 10% of students identified themselves as vegetarian. Just over half (55%) of students reported that they were able to cook a wide range of meals from raw ingredients, and 73% consumed self-cooked meals from raw ingredients 'every' or 'most' days. One in four students reported that they consumed meals cooked from pre-prepared foods, which could be assumed to represent convenience foods, 'most days' or 'everyday'. Approximately 30% of students reported that they skipped breakfast at least most days. Just less than one quarter of students spent less than £20 on food each week; a weekly food budget of £20–29 was most common. Almost one in five students spent over £40 on food each week. Full details are provided in tabular form in Additional file 1: Table S2).

### Dietary patterns

Four principal components were retained, which explained 21.7% of the total variance in food intake. The first component explained 8.4% variance; the three remaining components explained 5.7%, 4.2% and 3.4% of the variance in food intake respectively. Table 2 shows the factor loadings of each of the food groups in the four dietary components retained.

The first dietary component had high positive factor loadings (≥ 0.32) for pulses, beans and lentils, tofu, meat alternatives, hummus, nuts, and other green vegetables and salad items. It had high negative factor loadings for poultry, processed meat, and red meat and offal. This dietary pattern was labelled 'vegetarian', because there was a clear tendency towards consumption of non-meat protein sources and avoidance of all meat and fish products. The second dietary component had high positive factor loadings for biscuits, cakes and sweet pastries, milk- and cream-based desserts, confectionery, crisps and savoury snacks, fruit juice, other bread, pizza and fizzy drinks. This component was labelled 'snacking', because it was mainly characterised by snack-type foods that generally did not represent components of main meals, require no preparation and offered many options for mobile consumption. The third component had high positive factor loadings for fatty fish and canned tuna, white- and shellfish, nuts, eggs, fresh fruit, other green vegetables and salad items, oat- and bran-based breakfast cereals, herbal and green tea, and low fat/low calorie yogurts. This dietary pattern was labelled 'health-conscious', because it was characterised by foods typically associated with improved health, and was congruent with dietary components labelled 'health-conscious' or 'prudent' in other dietary pattern studies [21]. Finally, the

**Table 1** Socio-demographic characteristics of the sample

| | Number | Percentage (%)[a] |
|---|---|---|
| Gender | | |
| Male | 384 | 26.5 |
| Female | 1064 | 73.5 |
| Age (years) | | |
| 17–21 | 873 | 60.3 |
| 22–25 | 412 | 28.5 |
| 26–30 | 163 | 11.3 |
| BMI (kg.m$^{-2}$) | | |
| < 18.5 | 112 | 7.7 |
| 18.5–24.9 | 1000 | 69.1 |
| 25–29.9 | 220 | 15.2 |
| ≥30 | 76 | 5.2 |
| Leisure-time physical activity | | |
| Not very active | 473 | 32.7 |
| Moderately active | 748 | 51.7 |
| Very active | 227 | 15.7 |
| University attended | | |
| University of Sheffield | 567 | 39.2 |
| Ulster University | 443 | 30.6 |
| KCL | 305 | 21.1 |
| University of Southampton | 79 | 5.5 |
| University of St Andrews | 54 | 3.7 |
| Faculty of study | | |
| Arts | 252 | 17.4 |
| Social science | 285 | 19.7 |
| Engineering | 109 | 7.5 |
| Science | 212 | 14.6 |
| Medicine and health | 521 | 36.0 |
| Full or part time status | | |
| Full time | 1394 | 96.3 |
| Part time | 54 | 3.7 |
| Year of study | | |
| 1st year undergraduate | 489 | 33.8 |
| 2nd year undergraduate | 301 | 20.8 |
| 3rd year undergraduate | 264 | 18.2 |
| 4th or higher year undergraduate | 136 | 9.4 |
| Postgraduate | 245 | 16.9 |
| Other | 13 | 0.9 |
| Term-time residence | | |
| University catered accommodation | 58 | 4.0 |
| University self-catered accommodation | 340 | 23.5 |
| Private accommodation with other friends/students | 610 | 42.1 |
| Private accommodation on own | 63 | 4.4 |
| With parents/relatives | 205 | 14.2 |
| With partner | 107 | 7.4 |
| With parents/partner & children | 48 | 3.3 |
| With children only | 9 | 0.6 |
| Other | 8 | 0.6 |
| Ethnic background | | |
| White British | 911 | 62.9 |
| White Irish | 235 | 16.2 |
| Other White ethnicity | 139 | 9.6 |
| Mixed ethnicity | 45 | 3.1 |
| Asian/Asian British | 69 | 4.8 |
| Black/African/Caribbean/Black British | 15 | 1.0 |
| Other | 16 | 1.1 |
| Would rather not say | 18 | 1.2 |
| Mother's level of education | | |
| CSE | 80 | 5.5 |
| Vocational | 59 | 4.1 |
| O Level | 184 | 12.7 |
| A Level | 96 | 6.6 |
| Degree | 342 | 23.6 |
| Would rather not say | 120 | 8.3 |
| Not asked[b] | 567 | 39.2 |
| Smoking habits | | |
| Never smoker | 1090 | 75.3 |
| Ex-smoker | 72 | 5.0 |
| Social smoker | 192 | 13.3 |
| Regular smoker | 94 | 6.5 |

[a]where percentages do not total 100% this is due to missing data
[b]This question was not available for University of Sheffield students

fourth component was labelled 'convenience, red meat & alcohol', because it had high factor loadings for red meat and savoury foods requiring little or no preparation, and it was the only component with a positive loading on alcoholic drinks. There were also high factor loadings for fried food, pasta and rice, ready-made sauces, pizza, chips, alcoholic drinks, processed meat, red meat and offal, and eggs; there was a strong negative factor loading for low fat/low calorie yogurts.

### Correlational analyses

Pearson's correlation coefficients between dietary pattern scores and energy intake were calculated. These are displayed in Table 3. There was a weak negative correlation between the 'vegetarian' pattern and energy intake ($r = -0.096$; $p < 0.01$), but a weak positive correlation between the 'health-conscious' pattern and energy

**Table 2** Factor loadings of the 55 food groups in the four principal components extracted from the PCA of frequency of food intake data of 1448 university students

| Food group (% variance) | Vegetarian (8.4%) | Snacking (5.7%) | Health-conscious (4.2%) | Convenience, red meat & alcohol (3.4%) |
|---|---|---|---|---|
| Pulses, beans & lentils | **0.642** | − 0.113 | 0.216 | |
| Tofu | **0.627** | | | 0.105 |
| Meat alternatives | **0.586** | 0.126 | − 0.109 | 0.121 |
| Hummus | **0.585** | | 0.147 | |
| Chicken/poultry | *−0.456* | | 0.106 | 0.277 |
| Processed meat | *−0.453* | 0.277 | | **0.354** |
| Red meat & offal | *−0.439* | 0.163 | 0.134 | **0.332** |
| Biscuits, cakes & sweets | | **0.623** | | − 0.106 |
| Milk & cream-based desserts | | **0.531** | 0.160 | |
| Confectionery | − 0.174 | **0.524** | | |
| Crisps & savoury snacks | | **0.413** | −0.170 | 0.253 |
| White bread | −0.141 | **0.393** | −0.209 | 0.214 |
| Fruit juice | | **0.354** | | |
| Other bread | 0.104 | **0.342** | | |
| Canned fruit | 0.101 | **0.320** | 0.100 | −0.124 |
| Fruit squash (not low calorie) | | 0.293 | −0.182 | |
| Other yogurts | | 0.276 | 0.216 | −0.105 |
| Other spread | | 0.251 | | |
| Added sugar in tea, coffee & cereal | | 0.239 | | 0.128 |
| Quiche | 0.201 | 0.218 | | 0.124 |
| Fatty fish & canned tuna | −0.120 | | **0.616** | |
| White fish & shell fish | −0.157 | | **0.531** | |
| Nuts | **0.324** | | **0.491** | |
| Eggs | −0.151 | − 0.120 | **0.477** | **0.350** |
| Fresh fruit | 0.174 | | **0.443** | −0.108 |
| Other green vegetables, onions & salad items | **0.369** | −0.258 | **0.376** | 0.127 |
| Oat- & bran-based breakfast cereals | | −0.172 | **0.372** | −0.170 |
| Herbal & green tea | 0.313 | −0.153 | **0.365** | |
| Low fat & low-calorie yogurts | | | **0.334** | −0.308 |
| Tea & coffee | | 0.122 | 0.251 | |
| Fried food | | | | **0.503** |
| Pasta & rice | 0.135 | | | **0.451** |
| Ready-made sauces | | | | **0.396** |
| Pizza | | **0.327** | −0.171 | **0.392** |
| Chips | − 0.160 | 0.301 | − 0.221 | **0.379** |
| Alcoholic drinks | | | | **0.328** |
| Butter | −0.166 | 0.137 | | 0.312 |
| Mayonnaise, salad cream & other dressings | −0.115 | 0.249 | 0.225 | 0.277 |
| Cream | | 0.128 | 0.198 | 0.209 |
| Crispbread | 0.144 | | 0.132 | −0.179 |
| Peas | | | 0.115 | |
| Boiled, mashed, roast & jacket potatoes | −0.211 | 0.261 | | 0.113 |
| Root vegetables & sweetcorn | 0.237 | | 0.300 | |

**Table 2** Factor loadings of the 55 food groups in the four principal components extracted from the PCA of frequency of food intake data of 1448 university students *(Continued)*

| Food group (% variance) | Vegetarian (8.4%) | Snacking (5.7%) | Health-conscious (4.2%) | Convenience, red meat & alcohol (3.4%) |
|---|---|---|---|---|
| Baked beans | | 0.112 | | 0.112 |
| Wheat bran | | | 0.124 | −0.136 |
| Low calorie squash & fizzy drinks | | 0.115 | | |
| Non-white bread | | | | |
| Low fat, olive & pufa spread | | | −0.124 | |
| Fizzy drinks (not low calorie) | −0.180 | **0.332** | −0.204 | 0.282 |
| Jam, marmalade & honey | | 0.255 | | −0.125 |
| Cheese | 0.214 | 0.145 | | 0.218 |
| Water | | −0.253 | 0.292 | |
| Milk | −0.162 | 0.107 | 0.120 | 0.106 |
| Other breakfast cereals | −0.150 | 0.168 | −0.194 | |
| Soups | 0.209 | 0.125 | 0.215 | |

Food groups with factor loadings ≥0.10 & ≤ − 0.10 are displayed; those ≥0.32 are highlighted in bold and those ≤ − 0.32 are italicised

intake ($r = 0.271$; $P < 0.01$). The 'snacking' and 'convenience, red meat and alcohol' dietary patterns exhibited the strongest correlations with energy intake ($r = 0.582$ and $r = 0.547$ respectively). Owing to these significant associations, energy-adjusted nutrient intakes were used to explore relationships with dietary patterns scores. There were strong positive correlations ($0.5 \geq r < 0.6$; $p < 0.01$) between the 'vegetarian' pattern and energy-adjusted intakes of fibre, copper and thiamin. The 'health-conscious' pattern was the most nutrient dense, with significant, positive, strong correlations ($0.5 \geq r < 0.7$; $p < 0.01$) for energy-adjusted intakes of selenium, vitamin D, vitamin B12, and biotin. The 'snacking' pattern was strongly positively correlated with energy-adjusted non-milk extrinsic sugars (NMES) ($r = 0.524$; $P < 0.01$). Alcohol intake (energy-adjusted) was negatively correlated with scores on the 'snacking' pattern ($r = -0.317$; $P < 0.01$). Only intake of total sugars (energy-adjusted) was strongly and negatively correlated with the 'convenience, red meat & alcohol' pattern ($r = -0.577$; $P < 0.01$).

### General linear models

Adjusted mean pattern scores by demographic and cooking/eating behaviour variables from the GLMs are provided in Table 4 (Model 1) and Table 5 (Model 2). The text that follows summarises the key findings.

#### *Pattern 1 – Vegetarian*

In Model 1 (demographic variables only) female gender ($p < 0.001$), middle age group ($p = 0.020$), moderate leisure-time activity levels ($p = 0.045$) and ex-smoker status ($p = 0.025$) were independently associated with higher scores on the vegetarian dietary pattern. Attendance at Ulster University was independently associated with lower 'vegetarian' pattern scores ($p < 0.001$).

In Model 2 (demographic variables & food/eating related variables), female gender ($p < 0.001$), middle age group ($p = 0.020$), greatest self-reported cooking ability ($p = 0.036$), least frequent consumption of pre-prepared foods ($p = 0.047$) and lower consumption of animal products ($p = 0.036$) were independently associated with higher 'vegetarian' pattern scores. Attendance at Ulster University ($p < 0.001$) was independently associated with lower scores.

#### *Pattern 2 – Snacking*

In Model 1, low leisure-time physical activity ($p < 0.001$), attendance at Ulster University ($p = 0.003$), full time student status ($p = 0.001$) and living with parents/other relatives ($p < 0.001$) were independently associated with higher 'snacking' pattern scores.

In Model 2, lower leisure-time physical activity participation ($p = 0.012$), attendance at Ulster University ($p = 0.029$), living with parents/other relatives or in university catered accommodation ($p = 0.033$), and full-time student status ($p < 0.001$) were independently associated with greater pattern score. Infrequent consumption of meals prepared from raw ingredients ($p < 0.001$), and frequent consumption of pre-prepared foods ($p < 0.001$) and ready meals/take-aways ($p < 0.001$) were also independently associated with high 'snacking' pattern scores.

#### *Pattern 3 – Health-conscious*

In Model 1, 'very active' physical activity levels ($p < 0.001$), 'White Other' ethnicity ($p = 0.004$) and third year of undergraduate study ($p = 0.041$) were independently

**Table 3** Pearson's correlations between dietary pattern scores and estimated average daily nutrient intakes from frequency of food intake data

| | Vegetarian | | Snacking | | Health-conscious | | Convenience, red meat & alcohol | |
|---|---|---|---|---|---|---|---|---|
| Nutrient | Absolute | Adjusted | Absolute | Adjusted | Absolute | Adjusted | Absolute | Adjusted |
| Energy (kcal) | −0.096 $^{Y}$ | | **0.582** $^{Y}$ | | 0.271 $^{Y}$ | | **0.547** $^{Y}$ | |
| Protein (g) | −0.304 $^{Y}$ | − 0.389 $^{Y}$ | 0.309 $^{Y}$ | − 0.343 $^{Y}$ | 0.483 $^{Y}$ | 0.469 $^{Y}$ | 0.491 $^{Y}$ | 0.334 $^{Y}$ |
| Total fat (g) | − 0.171 $^{Y}$ | − 0.183 $^{Y}$ | **0.602** $^{Y}$ | 0.232 $^{Y}$ | 0.291 $^{Y}$ | 0.116 $^{Y}$ | **0.535** $^{Y}$ | 0.134 $^{Y}$ |
| Total carbohydrate (g) | 0.073 $^{Y}$ | 0.322 $^{Y}$ | **0.633** $^{Y}$ | 0.316 $^{Y}$ | 0.101 $^{Y}$ | − 0.287 $^{Y}$ | 0.330 $^{Y}$ | − 0.358 $^{Y}$ |
| NMES (g) | −0.163 $^{Y}$ | − 0.110 $^{Y}$ | **0.696** $^{Y}$ | **0.524** $^{Y}$ | − 0.124 $^{Y}$ | − 0.393 $^{Y}$ | 0.234 $^{Y}$ | − 0.174 $^{Y}$ |
| Saturated fat (g) | − 0.266 $^{Y}$ | − 0.326 $^{Y}$ | **0.638** $^{Y}$ | 0.347 $^{Y}$ | 0.166 $^{Y}$ | − 0.098 $^{Y}$ | 0.485 $^{Y}$ | 0.080 $^{Y}$ |
| Monounsaturated fat (g) | − 0.241 $^{Y}$ | − 0.306 $^{Y}$ | **0.558** $^{Y}$ | 0.144 $^{Y}$ | 0.302 $^{Y}$ | 0.142 $^{Y}$ | **0.507** $^{Y}$ | 0.091 $^{Y}$ |
| Polyunsaturated fat (g) | 0.018 $^{Y}$ | 0.143 $^{Y}$ | 0.430 $^{Y}$ | −0.026 | 0.336 $^{Y}$ | 0.209 $^{Y}$ | 0.492 $^{Y}$ | 0.137 |
| Total sugars (g) | 0.019 | 0.123 $^{Y}$ | **0.602** $^{Y}$ | 0.333 $^{Y}$ | 0.295 $^{Y}$ | 0.154 $^{Y}$ | 0.043 | **−0.577** $^{Y}$ |
| Fibre (g) | 0.443 $^{Y}$ | **0.551** $^{Y}$ | 0.080 $^{Y}$ | −0.259 $^{Y}$ | 0.386 $^{Y}$ | 0.306 $^{Y}$ | 0.096 $^{Y}$ | −0.207 $^{Y}$ |
| Sodium (mg) | 0.113 $^{Y}$ | 0.286 $^{Y}$ | 0.439 $^{Y}$ | −0.002 $^{Y}$ | 0.313 $^{Y}$ | 0.172 $^{Y}$ | 0.436 $^{Y}$ | 0.040 $^{Y}$ |
| Potassium (mg) | 0.035 | 0.196 $^{Y}$ | 0.360 $^{Y}$ | −0.240 $^{Y}$ | 0.472 $^{Y}$ | 0.451 $^{Y}$ | 0.352 $^{Y}$ | −0.212 $^{Y}$ |
| Calcium (mg) | 0.073 $^{Y}$ | 0.183 $^{Y}$ | 0.449 $^{Y}$ | 0.106 $^{Y}$ | 0.315 $^{Y}$ | 0.189 $^{Y}$ | 0.199 $^{Y}$ | −0.258 $^{Y}$ |
| Magnesium (mg) | 0.229 $^{Y}$ | 0.461 $^{Y}$ | 0.253 $^{Y}$ | −0.347 $^{Y}$ | **0.509** $^{Y}$ | 0.482 $^{Y}$ | 0.304 $^{Y}$ | − 0.197 $^{Y}$ |
| Iron (mg) | 0.147 $^{Y}$ | 0.332 $^{Y}$ | 0.247 $^{Y}$ | −0.350 | 0.339 $^{Y}$ | 0.214 | 0.400 $^{Y}$ | − 0.017 |
| Copper (mg) | 0.343 $^{Y}$ | **0.545** $^{Y}$ | 0.229 $^{Y}$ | −0.256 $^{Y}$ | 0.458 $^{Y}$ | 0.387 $^{Y}$ | 0.340 $^{Y}$ | − 0.035 |
| Zinc (mg) | −0.264 $^{Y}$ | −0.318 $^{Y}$ | 0.289 $^{Y}$ | − 0.382 $^{Y}$ | 0.391 $^{Y}$ | 0.304 $^{Y}$ | 0.483 $^{Y}$ | 0.080 $^{Y}$ |
| Selenium (mg) | −0.221 $^{Y}$ | − 0.208 $^{Y}$ | 0.208 $^{Y}$ | − 0.259 $^{Y}$ | **0.584** $^{Y}$ | **0.555** $^{Y}$ | 0.423 $^{Y}$ | 0.115 $^{Y}$ |
| Iodine (μg) | − 0.260 $^{Y}$ | − 0.247 $^{Y}$ | 0.259 $^{Y}$ | − 0.065 | **0.524** $^{Y}$ | 0.488 $^{Y}$ | 0.126 $^{Y}$ | −0.224 $^{Y}$ |
| Vitamin A (μg) | 0.132 $^{Y}$ | 0.163 $^{Y}$ | 0.050 | − 0.129 $^{Y}$ | 0.362 $^{Y}$ | 0.314 $^{Y}$ | 0.065 | − 0.095 $^{Y}$ |
| Vitamin E (mg) | 0.163 $^{Y}$ | 0.286 $^{Y}$ | 0.347 $^{Y}$ | −0.022 | **0.505** $^{Y}$ | 0.447 $^{Y}$ | 0.244 $^{Y}$ | − 0.145 $^{Y}$ |
| Vitamin D (μg) | −0.136 $^{Y}$ | − 0.113 $^{Y}$ | 0.015 | − 0.209 $^{Y}$ | **0.645** $^{Y}$ | **0.613** $^{Y}$ | 0.159 $^{Y}$ | −0.009 |
| Thiamin (mg) | 0.484 $^{Y}$ | **0.558** $^{Y}$ | 0.217 $^{Y}$ | 0.010 | 0.044 | −0.059 | 0.200 $^{Y}$ | 0.004 |
| Riboflavin (mg) | −0.223 $^{Y}$ | − 0.216 $^{Y}$ | 0.338 $^{Y}$ | − 0.090 $^{Y}$ | 0.394 $^{Y}$ | 0.298 $^{Y}$ | 0.210 $^{Y}$ | −0.258 $^{Y}$ |
| Niacin (mg) | −0.359 $^{Y}$ | −0.429 $^{Y}$ | 0.221 $^{Y}$ | − 0.377 $^{Y}$ | 0.465 $^{Y}$ | 0.408 $^{Y}$ | 0.408 $^{Y}$ | 0.008 |
| Vitamin $B_6$ (mg) | −0.210 $^{Y}$ | − 0.226 $^{Y}$ | 0.266 $^{Y}$ | − 0.435 $^{Y}$ | 0.332 $^{Y}$ | 0.199 $^{Y}$ | 0.439 $^{Y}$ | − 0.011 |
| Vitamin $B_{12}$ (mg) | − 0.315 $^{Y}$ | − 0.311 $^{Y}$ | 0.180 $^{Y}$ | − 0.163 $^{Y}$ | **0.583** $^{Y}$ | **0.537** $^{Y}$ | 0.230 $^{Y}$ | − 0.065 |
| Folate (μg) | 0.177 $^{Y}$ | 0.313 $^{Y}$ | 0.191 $^{Y}$ | − 0.294 $^{Y}$ | 0.416 $^{Y}$ | 0.329 $^{Y}$ | 0.253 $^{Y}$ | − 0.155 $^{Y}$ |
| Biotin (μg) | 0.088 $^{Y}$ | 0.169 $^{Y}$ | 0.100 $^{Y}$ | −0.319 $^{Y}$ | **0.690** $^{Y}$ | **0.673** $^{Y}$ | 0.212 $^{Y}$ | − 0.123 $^{Y}$ |
| Vitamin C (mg) | 0.202 $^{Y}$ | 0.244 $^{Y}$ | 0.163 $^{Y}$ | −0.017 $^{Y}$ | 0.299 $^{Y}$ | 0.237 $^{Y}$ | 0.009 | − 0.197 $^{Y}$ |
| Alcohol (g) | 0.023 | 0.064 | −0.020 | − 0.317 $^{Y}$ | 0.026 | − 0.086 $^{Y}$ | 0.345 $^{Y}$ | 0.180 $^{Y}$ |

$^{Y}P < 0.01$

Correlation coefficients between absolute nutrient intakes and relative nutrient intakes adjusted for energy intakes are both shown. Correlation coefficients ≥0.5 are highlighted in bold

associated with higher scores on the 'health-conscious' pattern. Youngest age group ($p = 0.015$) and attendance at University of Sheffield were independently associated with lower scores ($p < 0.001$).

In Model 2, the five significant demographic factors identified in Model 1 remained independently associated with 'health-conscious' pattern scores. Additionally, reporting being 'able to cook a wide range of meals from raw ingredients' ($p = 0.002$), daily consumption of meals made from raw ingredients ($p < 0.001$) and pre-prepared foods ($p = 0.002$), greatest amount of money spent on food (≥50/week) ($p < 0.001$), at least occasional consumption of animal products ($p < 0.001$) and infrequent skipping of breakfast ($p < 0.001$) were independently associated with higher health-conscious pattern scores. Rare – compared to occasional or almost daily - consumption of take-aways/ready meals was associated with lower scores ($p = 0.042$).

**Table 4** General Linear Model 1 – Demographic Variables

| | Vegetarian | | Snacking | | Health-conscious | | Convenience, red meat & alcohol | |
|---|---|---|---|---|---|---|---|---|
| Lack of fit | $p = 0.612$ | | $p = 0.330$ | | $p = 0.280$ | | $p = 0.012$ | |
| Demographic variable | Adjusted mean pattern score | *p* value | Adjusted mean pattern score | *p* value | Adjusted mean pattern score | *p* value | Adjusted mean pattern score | *p* value |
| Gender | | | | | | | | |
| Male | **0.082** | **< 0.001** | −0.315 | 0.074 | 0.378 | 0.132 | **0.475** | **< 0.001** |
| Female | **0.304** | | −0.428 | | 0.469 | | **−0.117** | |
| Age | | | | | | | | |
| 17–21 | **0.133[a]** | **0.020** | −0.326 | 0.424 | **0.262[b]** | **0.015** | 0.228 | 0.496 |
| 22–25 | **0.339[a]** | | −0.429 | | **0.434[a]** | | 0.210 | |
| 26–29 | **0.197** | | −0.361 | | **0.574[b]** | | 0.100 | |
| Leisure-time physical activity | | | | | | | | |
| Not very active | **0.184[a]** | **0.045** | **−0.171[ab]** | **< 0.001** | **0.029[ab]** | **< 0.001** | **0.250[a]** | **0.032** |
| Moderately active | **0.308[a]** | | **−0.356[ac]** | | **0.383[ac]** | | **0.097[a]** | |
| Very active | **0.177** | | **−0.588[bc]** | | **0.857[bc]** | | **0.191** | |
| BMI | | | | | | | | |
| < 18.5 | 0.292 | 0.221 | −0.281 | 0.391 | 0.437 | 0.055 | 0.139 | 0.092 |
| 18.5–24.9 | 0.289 | | −0.436 | | 0.407 | | 0.073 | |
| 25–29.9 | 0.154 | | −0.432 | | 0.574 | | 0.144 | |
| ≥ 30 | 0.156 | | −0.339 | | 0.275 | | 0.361 | |
| Smoking status | | | | | | | | |
| Never | **0.086[a]** | **0.025** | −0.333 | 0.270 | 0.404 | 0.173 | **−0.026[ab]** | **< 0.001** |
| Ex | **0.421[a]** | | −0.393 | | 0.387 | | **0.121[c]** | |
| Social | **0.159** | | −0.254 | | 0.562 | | **0.311[ac]** | |
| Regular | **0.225** | | −0.507 | | 0.340 | | **0.310[b]** | |
| Ethnicity | | | | | | | | |
| White British | 0.214 | 0.441 | −0.299 | 0.810 | **0.263[a]** | **0.004** | 0.206 | 0.585 |
| White Irish | 0.364 | | −0.381 | | **0.276[b]** | | 0.254 | |
| White Other | 0.182 | | −0.322 | | **0.545[ab]** | | 0.140 | |
| Mixed | 0.105 | | −0.352 | | **0.627** | | 0.297 | |
| Asian/Asian British | 0.281 | | −0.272 | | **0.309** | | 0.211 | |
| Black/Black British | 0.003 | | −0.274 | | **0.048** | | −0.041 | |
| Other | 0.103 | | −0.705 | | **0.882** | | 0.489 | |
| Rather not say | 0.531 | | −0.370 | | **0.437** | | −0.123 | |
| Year of study | | | | | | | | |
| 1st year UG | 0.212 | 0.194 | −0.240 | 0.154 | **0.477[a]** | **0.041** | 0.179 | 0.134 |
| 2nd year UG | 0.080 | | −0.439 | | **0.503** | | 0.203 | |
| 3rd year UG | 0.090 | | −0.475 | | **0.614[a]** | | 0.139 | |
| ≥ 4th year UG | 0.091 | | −0.431 | | **0.480** | | 0.410 | |
| Postgraduate | 0.177 | | −0.374 | | **0.282** | | 0.309 | |
| Other | 0.687 | | −0.272 | | **0.182** | | −0.166 | |
| Term-time accommodation | | | | | | | | |
| Uni catered | 0.129 | 0.963 | **−0.104[a]** | **< 0.001** | 0.176 | 0.068 | 0.374 | 0.053 |
| Uni self-catered | 0.245 | | **−0.517[b]** | | 0.236 | | 0.219 | |
| Private with friends | 0.242 | | **−0.397[a]** | | 0.341 | | 0.201 | |

**Table 4** General Linear Model 1 – Demographic Variables *(Continued)*

| | Vegetarian | | Snacking | | Health-conscious | | Convenience, red meat & alcohol | |
|---|---|---|---|---|---|---|---|---|
| Lack of fit | $p = 0.612$ | | $p = 0.330$ | | $p = 0.280$ | | $p = 0.012$ | |
| Demographic variable | Adjusted mean pattern score | *p* value | Adjusted mean pattern score | *p* value | Adjusted mean pattern score | *p* value | Adjusted mean pattern score | *p* value |
| Private on own | 0.324 | | **−0.265** | | 0.450 | | −0.275 | |
| Parents/relatives | 0.173 | | **−0.076[bc]** | | 0.524 | | 0.175 | |
| Partner | 0.269 | | **− 0.306[c]** | | 0.456 | | 0.187 | |
| Parents/partner + children | 0.138 | | **−0.247** | | 0.290 | | 0.074 | |
| Children only | 0.218 | | **−0.555** | | 0.344 | | 0.254 | |
| Other | 0.268 | | **−0.879** | | 0.992 | | 0.402 | |
| University | | | | | | | | |
| Sheffield | **0.146[abc]** | **< 0.001** | **−0.370[a]** | **0.003** | **0.098[abcd]** | **< 0.001** | 0.166 | 0.270 |
| Ulster | **−0.376[adef]** | | **−0.214[ab]** | | **0.318[aef]** | | 0.299 | |
| KCL | **0.398[bd]** | | **−0.569[b]** | | **0.541[be]** | | 0.237 | |
| Southampton | **0.227[e]** | | **−0.264** | | **0.584[cf]** | | 0.221 | |
| St Andrews | **0.719[cf]** | | **−0.442** | | **0.576[d]** | | −0.027 | |
| Faculty | | | | | | | | |
| Arts | 0.334 | 0.234 | −0.308 | 0.527 | 0.456 | 0.766 | 0.275 | 0.277 |
| Social science | 0.180 | | −0.357 | | 0.464 | | 0.191 | |
| Engineering | 0.123 | | −0.416 | | 0.400 | | 0.153 | |
| Science | 0.216 | | −0.453 | | 0.357 | | 0.177 | |
| Medicine & health | 0.261 | | −0.324 | | 0.410 | | 0.099 | |
| Full-time vs. part-time student status | | | | | | | | |
| Full-time | 0.183 | 0.582 | **−0.109** | **0.001** | 0.381 | 0.560 | 0.246 | 0.378 |
| Part-time | 0.263 | | **−0.634** | | 0.466 | | 0.113 | |

Independent associations between dietary pattern scores and non-nutrient variables. *p* values < 0.05 are highlighted in bold. Common superscript letters indicate significant post-hoc differences between categories within each variable

### *Pattern 4 – Convenience, red meat & alcohol*

In Model 1, male gender ($p < 0.001$), lowest leisure-time physical activity levels ($p = 0.032$), and regular/social smoking status ($p < 0.001$) were independently associated with higher scores on the 'convenience, red meat & alcohol' diet pattern. An independent inverse association between living alone in private accommodation and score on this pattern approached significance ($p = 0.053$).

In Model 2, higher pattern scores were independently associated with male gender ($p < 0.001$), regular/social smoking status ($p < 0.001$), most frequent consumption pre-prepared foods ($p = 0.040$), frequent consumption of ready-meals/take-aways ($p < 0.001$), frequent breakfast skipping ($p < 0.001$), regular consumption of animal products ($p < 0.001$) and greater amounts of money spent on food ($p < 0.001$). Lower scores were independently associated with living alone ($p = 0.026$) and spending less money on food ($p < 0.001$).

## Discussion

This study aimed to identify dietary patterns within a UK university student population and to delineate the socio-demographic, lifestyle and other behavioural characteristics of students favouring these patterns. Dietary patterns analysis unveiled heterogeneity in food choice with students following four major dietary patterns: 'vegetarian', 'snacking', 'health-conscious' and 'convenience, red meat & alcohol'. These patterns explained approximately one fifth of the variance in food intake. Students' gender, age, geographical location and cooking ability were associated with differences in pattern behaviour. Clustering of lifestyle risk factors with dietary patterns was also evident, with less healthful dietary patterns associated with smoking, low physical activity and take-away consumption. Students tending to the 'convenience, red meat & alcohol' pattern reported spending more money on food each week.

The 'vegetarian', 'snacking' and 'health-conscious' patterns identified here are analogous to those previously reported

**Table 5** General Linear Model 2 – Demographic + Eating related variables

| | Vegetarian | | Snacking | | Health-conscious | | Convenience, red meat & alcohol | |
|---|---|---|---|---|---|---|---|---|
| Lack of fit | $p = 0.001$ | | $p = 0.748$ | | $p = 0.426$ | | $p = 0.017$ | |
| Demographic variable (n) | Adjusted mean pattern score | *p* value | Adjusted mean pattern score | *p* value | Adjusted mean pattern score | *p* value | Adjusted mean pattern score | *p* value |
| Gender | | | | | | | | |
| Male | **1.119** | **< 0.001** | *Not entered into model* | | *Not entered into model* | *N/A* | **0.645** | **< 0.001** |
| Female | **1.304** | | | | | | **0.129** | |
| Age | | | | | | | | |
| 17–21 | **1.140**$^{a}$ | **0.020** | *Not entered into model* | *N/A* | **−0.047** | **0.049** | *Not entered into model* | *N/A* |
| 22–25 | **1.301**$^{a}$ | | | | **0.113**$^{a}$ | | | |
| 26–29 | **1.314** | | | | **0.161**$^{b}$ | | | |
| Leisure-time physical activity | | | | | | | | |
| Not very active | 1.258 | 0.183 | **0.270**$^{ab}$ | **0.012** | **−0.187**$^{ab}$ | **< 0.001** | 0.436 | 0.117 |
| Moderately active | 1.297 | | **0.208**$^{ac}$ | | **0.064**$^{ac}$ | | 0.327 | |
| Very active | 1.199 | | **0.034**$^{bc}$ | | **0.350**$^{bc}$ | | 0.399 | |
| BMI | | | | | | | | |
| < 18.5 | *Not entered into model* | *N/A* | *Not entered into model* | *N/A* | 0.110 | 0.215 | *Not entered into model* | *N/A* |
| 18.5–24.9 | | | | | 0.057 | | | |
| 25–29.9 | | | | | 0.173 | | | |
| ≥ 30 | | | | | −0.037 | | | |
| Smoking status | | | | | | | | |
| Never | 1.190 | 0.292 | *Not entered into model* | *N/A* | *Not entered into model* | *N/A* | **0.224**$^{ab}$ | **< 0.001** |
| Ex | 1.321 | | | | | | **0.272**$^{c}$ | |
| Social | 1.264 | | | | | | **0.520**$^{ac}$ | |
| Regular | 1.230 | | | | | | **0.532**$^{b}$ | |
| Ethnicity | | | | | | | | |
| White British | *Not entered into model* | *N/A* | *Not entered into model* | *N/A* | **−0.107**$^{ab}$ | **0.016** | *Not entered into model* | *N/A* |
| White Irish | | | | | **−0.080**$^{c}$ | | | |
| White Other | | | | | **0.123**$^{ac}$ | | | |
| Mixed | | | | | **0.243** | | | |
| Asian/Asian British | | | | | **0.033** | | | |
| Black/Black British | | | | | **− 0.081** | | | |
| Other | | | | | **0.370**$^{b}$ | | | |
| Rather not say | | | | | **0.106** | | | |
| Year of study | | | | | | | | |
| 1st year UG | *Not entered into model* | *N/A* | *Not entered into model* | *N/A* | **0.048**$^{a}$ | **0.004** | *Not entered into model* | *N/A* |
| 2nd year UG | | | | | **0.069** | | | |
| 3rd year UG | | | | | **0.200**$^{a}$ | | | |
| ≥ 4th year UG | | | | | **−0.008** | | | |
| Postgraduate | | | | | **− 0.158** | | | |
| Other | | | | | **0.304** | | | |
| Term-time accommodation | | | | | | | | |
| Uni catered | *Not entered into model* | *N/A* | **0.427**$^{ab}$ | **0.033** | *Not entered into model* | *N/A* | **0.595** | **0.026** |
| Uni self-catered | | | **0.159**$^{ac}$ | | | | **0.495** | |
| Private with friends | | | **0.149**$^{bd}$ | | | | **0.469** | |

**Table 5** General Linear Model 2 – Demographic + Eating related variables *(Continued)*

| | Vegetarian | | Snacking | | Health-conscious | | Convenience, red meat & alcohol | |
|---|---|---|---|---|---|---|---|---|
| Lack of fit | *p* = 0.001 | | *p* = 0.748 | | *p* = 0.426 | | *p* = 0.017 | |
| Demographic variable (n) | Adjusted mean pattern score | *p* value | Adjusted mean pattern score | *p* value | Adjusted mean pattern score | *p* value | Adjusted mean pattern score | *p* value |
| Private on own | | | **0.218** | | | | **0.030[a]** | |
| Parents/relatives | | | **0.390[cde]** | | | | **0.431[a]** | |
| Partner | | | **0.248[e]** | | | | **0.378** | |
| Parents/partner + children | | | **0.378** | | | | **0.293** | |
| Children only | | | **– 0.178** | | | | **0.430** | |
| Other | | | **–0.256** | | | | **0.364** | |
| University | | | | | | | | |
| Sheffield | **1.218[abc]** | **< 0.001** | **0.136[a]** | **0.029** | **–0.270[abcd]** | **< 0.001** | *Not entered into model* | *N/A* |
| Ulster | **0.894[adef]** | | **0.242[abc]** | | **0.069[aef]** | | | |
| KCL | **1.424[bd]** | | **0.036[b]** | | **0.196[be]** | | | |
| Southampton | **1.298[eg]** | | **0.337** | | **0.187[cf]** | | | |
| St Andrews | **1.424[cfg]** | | **0.103[c]** | | **0.197[d]** | | | |
| Full-time vs. part-time student status | | | | | | | | |
| Full-time | *Not entered into model* | *N/A* | **0.442** | **< 0.001** | *Not entered into model* | *N/A* | *Not entered into model* | *N/A* |
| Part-time | | | **–0.101** | | | | | |
| Cooking/eating-related variables | | | | | | | | |
| Cooking ability | | | | | | | | |
| Wide range | **1.350[ab]** | **0.036** | 0.024 | 0.190 | **0.257[ab]** | **0.002** | 0.261 | 0.297 |
| Limited range | **1.239[ac]** | | 0.015 | | **0.065[ac]** | | 0.301 | |
| Pre-prepared only | **1.125[bc]** | | 0.151 | | **–0.101[bc]** | | 0.527 | |
| Unable to cook at all | **1.292** | | 0.492 | | **0.082** | | 0.459 | |
| Animal food consumption | | | | | | | | |
| Regular meat-eater | **–0.171[abcd]** | **< 0.001** | 0.187 | 0.080 | **0.445[a]** | **< 0.001** | **0.500[ab]** | **< 0.001** |
| Flexitarian | **0.291[aefg]** | | 0.199 | | **0.488[b]** | | **0.185[ac]** | |
| Lacto-ovo | **1.635[beh]** | | 0.314 | | **0.101** | | **0.534[c]** | |
| Ovo | **1.707[chi]** | | 0.319 | | **–0.459[ab]** | | **0.201[b]** | |
| Vegan | **2.795[dghi]** | | –0.238 | | **–0.196** | | **0.517** | |
| Meals made from scratch | | | | | | | | |
| Every day | 1.322 | 0.136 | **–0.060[abc]** | **0.001** | **0.339[abc]** | **< 0.001** | **0.622** | **< 0.001** |
| Most days | 1.272 | | **0.146[ade]** | | **0.198[ade]** | | **0.495** | |
| Occasionally | 1.172 | | **0.246[bd]** | | **–0.034[bd]** | | **0.345** | |
| Rarely/never | 1.240 | | **0.350[ce]** | | **–0.200[ce]** | | **0.088** | |
| Meals made from pre-prepared foods | | | | | | | | |
| Every day | **1.302[a]** | **0.047** | **0.338[a]** | **< 0.001** | **0.178[ab]** | **0.002** | **0.591[abc]** | **0.040** |
| Most days | **1.151[bc]** | | **0.304[bc]** | | **0.046[acd]** | | **0.336[a]** | |
| Occasionally | **1.231[bd]** | | **0.143[bd]** | | **–0.069[bce]** | | **0.265[b]** | |
| Rarely/never | **1.321[acd]** | | **–0.102[acd]** | | **0.148[de]** | | **0.356[c]** | |
| Ready-meals/take-aways | | | | | | | | |
| Every day | 1.511 | 0.257 | **0.584[ab]** | **< 0.001** | **0.273** | **0.042** | **0.552[a]** | **< 0.001** |
| Most days | 1.222 | | **0.290[cd]** | | **0.025[a]** | | **0.570[bc]** | |
| Occasionally | 1.130 | | **–0.036[bd]** | | **–0.068[b]** | | **0.302[cd]** | |

**Table 5** General Linear Model 2 – Demographic + Eating related variables *(Continued)*

| | Vegetarian | | Snacking | | Health-conscious | | Convenience, red meat & alcohol | |
|---|---|---|---|---|---|---|---|---|
| Lack of fit | $p = 0.001$ | | $p = 0.748$ | | $p = 0.426$ | | $p = 0.017$ | |
| Demographic variable (n) | Adjusted mean pattern score | *p* value | Adjusted mean pattern score | *p* value | Adjusted mean pattern score | *p* value | Adjusted mean pattern score | *p* value |
| Rarely/never | 1.143 | | **−0.155$^{acd}$** | | **0.073$^{ab}$** | | **0.125$^{abd}$** | |
| Meals in university cafeteria | | | | | | | | |
| Every day | 1.156 | 0.062 | 0.153 | 0.547 | 0.141 | 0.922 | 0.375 | 0.336 |
| Most days | 1.253 | | 0.245 | | 0.047 | | 0.485 | |
| Occasionally | 1.311 | | 0.170 | | 0.069 | | 0.372 | |
| Rarely/never | 1.286 | | 0.115 | | 0.046 | | 0.317 | |
| Skipped breakfast | | | | | | | | |
| Every day | 1.358 | 0.062 | 0.221 | 0.101 | **−0.179$^{ab}$** | **< 0.001** | **0.514$^{ab}$** | **< 0.001** |
| Most days | 1.276 | | 0.257 | | **0.066$^{c}$** | | **0.609$^{cd}$** | |
| Occasionally | 1.193 | | 0.114 | | **0.126$^{ad}$** | | **0.307$^{ace}$** | |
| Rarely/never | 1.179 | | 0.091 | | **0.290$^{bcd}$** | | **0.119$^{bde}$** | |
| Skipped lunch/dinner | | | | | | | | |
| Every day | 1.245 | 0.991 | 0.089 | 0.131 | 0.284 | 0.404 | **0.001** | **0.012** |
| Most days | 1.252 | | 0.236 | | 0.066 | | **0.443** | |
| Occasionally | 1.261 | | 0.116 | | −0.031 | | **0.503** | |
| Rarely/never | 1.248 | | 0.241 | | −0.016 | | **0.602** | |
| Amount spent on food | | | | | | | | |
| < £20 | 1.278 | 0.268 | 0.101 | 0.534 | **−0.171$^{abcd}$** | **< 0.001** | **0.162$^{abcd}$** | **< 0.001** |
| £20–29 | 1.269 | | 0.146 | | **−0.005$^{aef}$** | | **0.344$^{aef}$** | |
| £30–39 | 1.251 | | 0.150 | | **0.138$^{beg}$** | | **0.385$^{b}$** | |
| £40–49 | 1.333 | | 0.264 | | **0.096$^{eh}$** | | **0.481$^{ce}$** | |
| ≥ £50 | 1.127 | | 0.192 | | **0.320$^{dfgh}$** | | **0.564$^{df}$** | |

Independent associations between dietary pattern scores and non-nutrient variables. *p* values < 0.05 are highlighted in bold. Common superscript letters indicate significant post-hoc differences between categories within each variable

in adult and adolescent UK populations [22, 23]. The 'convenience, red meat & alcohol' pattern shares features (positive factor loadings for red meat, chips, alcohol) with a major dietary pattern (labelled drinker/social) reported among approximately 480 20–25 year olds in Northern Ireland, derived from 7-day diet history data [24].

The 'snacking' and 'convenience, red meat and alcohol' patterns have common features with published data on the food preferences of British university students [2, 4]. Existing studies allude to non-prudent consumption patterns, reporting low consumption of fruit and vegetables alongside high intakes of confectionery, alcohol, and fried, ready-made and convenience foods [2–4].

We have shown that both the 'snacking' and 'convenience, red meat and alcohol' patterns were least nutrient-dense. Indeed it is noteworthy that these two patterns were additionally positively correlated with energy intake and did not feature fruit and vegetables; dependence on such a pattern may increase risk of positive energy balance and hence weight gain. The 'health-conscious' pattern, which had a favourable nutrient profile - being particularly dense in micronutrients such as biotin, vitamin B12, vitamin D and selenium - is at odds with the stereotype of student eating patterns, but concurs with published research on dietary patterns among UK adults [21, 22] and a small-scale study of university students in Birmingham, UK [4].

It is of note that a vegetarian diet was the predominant pattern identified in the current study, and indeed 10% of students described themselves as vegetarian. The latter figure is less than that reported in a survey of over 3000 university students studying in Northern Ireland, which reported that 22% of students did not eat meat [3]. Although a vegetarian pattern has been described in the wider UK diet pattern literature [21–23], it was a minor component, in keeping with the low prevalence of vegetarianism among British adults nationally (3%) [25].

Whilst high rates of binge drinking have previously been documented among student populations [3, 26], and there is a popular stereotype of students as heavy drinkers, only one pattern ('convenience, red meat &

alcohol') was high in alcoholic beverages. Furthermore students following this pattern were also more likely to smoke, have frequent consumption of take-aways and pre-prepared foods and engage in lower levels of physical activity. This clustering of behaviours is important, since the negative health outcomes associated with multiple lifestyle risk factors are greater than the sum of individual health risk behaviours [27]. Conversely students favouring more healthful dietary patterns reported greater engagement in other health-promoting lifestyle choices, including not smoking, greater participation in physical activity. Aggregation of lifestyle behaviours has previously been reported in both university student and adult populations [26–28].

Gendered food preferences were also evident, especially in relation to meat consumption. Specifically, female students favoured a 'vegetarian' diet, whilst male students scored highly on the 'convenience, red meat & alcohol' pattern. Greater meat and fast food consumption among male students has previously been reported, and vegetarianism is more prevalent amongst female students [3, 24]. Although a recent British student study observed no gender differences between eating patterns [4], this study lacked detailed dietary assessment.

Dietary preferences also varied between participating universities. Generally, students at Ulster University favoured less healthful patterns, whilst those at the Universities of Southampton, St Andrews and KCL tended towards more healthful diets. Students attending the University of Sheffield were least likely to adopt a 'health-conscious' dietary pattern. This gradient is congruent with national data, which indicates that the population of Northern Ireland consumes a diet of poorer quality than the UK as a whole [29]. Dietary gradients were also evident in relation to geography in a comparative study of university students from seven universities across the UK, although absence of information on specific university location limits comparison [2].

It is also possible that dietary differences observed between universities may arise because of socioeconomic gradients across universities. Missing data on social class for students at the University of Sheffield precluded adjustment for this possibility. However information from the Higher Education Statistics Agency (HESA) indicates an SES gradient between universities: a greater proportion of students at Ulster University are from manual occupational backgrounds than from KCL, Sheffield and Southampton (no data available for St Andrews) [30]. Maternal education data for Ulster, KCL, St Andrews & Southampton corroborated these differences (data for University of Sheffield not available). The wider literature consistently reports a positive association between socioeconomic status and diet quality across UK population groups [21, 23, 28]. However, the tendency for students at the University of Sheffield to score lowest on a 'health-conscious' diet is not in line with this explanation.

The possibility of selection bias should be considered. There were differences in recruitment method between the University of Sheffield and Ulster University (recruitment email distributed directly to all students via a global mailing list), and the other three participating sites (e.g. study advertisement on student volunteers webpage). These recruitment differences may have biased the sample towards health-motivated students at KCL, St Andrews and Southampton.

The lack of association between university attended and consumption of the 'convenience, red meat & alcohol' diet also deserves attention. This homogeneity suggests that this pattern is pervasive across all universities studied, substantiating popular beliefs that the diet of UK university students is one of poor quality.

This study also revealed that older students favoured more healthful dietary patterns and there was evidence of a positive linear relationship between age and scores on the 'health-conscious' pattern. It is possible that as students mature they become increasingly aware of the impact of dietary choices on health and well-being, and health thus becomes an increasingly important determinant of food choice. Studies among the general UK adult population report similar age effects [21, 22]. A student survey conducted in Northern Ireland reported a positive gradient in diet quality by year of study [3]. In contrast, other student-specific research has failed to detect an association between eating habits and age (or year of study), although most of these studies have not collected detailed dietary data [2, 4, 10, 26].

Finally, 45% of the current sample reported limited (or non-existent) cooking ability, being at best only able to cook a limited range of meals from raw ingredients. Students with poor cooking ability were less likely to adopt healthier (vegetarian; health-conscious) diets than their more skilled counterparts. This association has not been documented among a university student population, but corroborates associations found in several adult studies [31, 32]. No association, however, was identified between cooking ability and scores on the less healthful dietary patterns (snacking; convenience, red meat & alcohol). Whilst it is likely that students who lack culinary skills may be forced to rely on convenience foods to ensure meal provision, other factors such as time pressures and (lack of) cooking enjoyment may be more salient in determining students' decisions around consumption of these foods [33, 34] .

### Study strengths and limitations

The current study had a number of strengths and limitations that should be acknowledged. FFQs are not optimal for the measurement of absolute dietary intake, but the use of a dietary pattern approach permitted ranking according to food group intake and so was considered appropriate. Furthermore, use of an FFQ allowed dietary intake to be captured over a 3-month semester and facilitated recruitment of a large, geographically diverse sample, albeit a convenience one. Ideally, the sampling frame would have included a greater number of universities and involved stratification by year of study, subject group and socioeconomic indices in order to give a nationally representative profile of student eating patterns. Moreover, only health-sciences students were recruited at Southampton, which may represent a source of bias.

The small number of students recruited from St Andrews may been seen as an under-representation of students from a Scottish university, but it should be noted that the total student population at St Andrews (population of around 8000 students) is much smaller than that of Sheffield, Ulster and KCL (between 25,000 and 30,000 students). It should also be noted that all dietary studies suffer from selection bias, in which more health- or diet-aware individuals choose to participate. Consequently, the prominence of the vegetarian and health-conscious dietary patterns may have been over-estimated in this study. Indeed, the BMI distributions were also biased towards healthy, in keeping with other student surveys [4, 26].

There was lack of fit in statistical models for 'convenience, red meat and alcohol', and 'vegetarian' dietary patterns. It should be noted that these models are developmental and clearly only cover some of the potential antecedents of following such patterns. Convenience, red meat, alcohol and vegetarian dietary choices are likely to be influenced by a raft of social, cultural and political factors, which have not been included in the model. For example, it is recognised that adoption of a vegetarian diet is related to concern about the environment and animal welfare, as well as for health reasons and weight management [35, 36]. Similarly, there is enormous heterogeneity in motives for drinking alcohol including coping, enhancement of social status, religious practice, personality type and alcohol availability [37, 38].

### Implications for policy and future research directions

Importantly, policy makers must recognise not all students consume poor diets at university: a large group of students consumed nutritionally favourable and health-promoting diets and do not appear in need of dietary intervention. However, students who consumed poor diets and practised unfavourable lifestyle behaviours were also identified, which may have long-term health effects. Targeted interventions towards these students are necessary. Furthermore, contemporary policy to limit red meat and alcohol consumption has greatest relevance to male students. University policy to improve students' diets should also incorporate efforts to promote student engagement in cooking and food preparation, and increased availability of low cost healthier food items.

This study also highlights a number of future research needs. Replication of this research among a large representative sample of UK university students would be pertinent. Secondly, in light of the association between cooking ability and dietary consumption patterns, investigation of the potential for a cooking skills intervention to improve dietary intake is warranted. Finally, the public health impact of dietary patterns and other lifestyle risk factors established during university become most important if these behaviours track forward into working adult life and represent a blueprint for long-term dietary preferences. Longitudinal research is now needed to investigate this possibility.

## Conclusion

This study provides a unique insight into the dietary patterns of UK university students along with associated nutritional content. It has identified a number of antecedents of both healthful and unhealthful dietary practices. Four patterns emerged, with evidence of more healthful dietary practices amongst female and older students, and those with greater self-reported cooking ability. Students in Northern Ireland appeared to favour less healthful dietary patterns than those in Great Britain. Male students tended towards a diet founded on convenience food, red meat and alcohol; this pattern was germane to all participating universities. These findings are relevant to future health promotion interventions and behaviour change in this important population.

#### Acknowledgments

The authors gratefully acknowledge Professor Peter Emery at King's College London and Dr. Penelope Nestel at The University of Southampton for their assistance in administration of the survey. We would also like to acknowledge Anthony Johns from Tinuviel Software for his assistance in setting up the online survey.

#### Funding

This study was conducted as part of EFS's PhD project. The University of Sheffield was its sponsor.

#### Authors' contributions

This manuscript represents original work, which has not been published previously and is not being considered by another Journal. The authors' responsibilities were as follows: EFS, JMR & MEB conceived and designed the study. EFS was primarily responsible for data collection and analysis, with advice from JMR. EFS wrote the first draft of the manuscript, with help from MEB. JC & LKP facilitated recruitment of students from the University of St Andrews and Ulster University, respectively. All authors contributed to revisions and approval of the final manuscript.

## Competing interests

The authors declare that they have no competing interest.

## Author details

[1]Human Nutrition Unit, Department of Oncology & Metabolism, The Medical School, University of Sheffield, Sheffield S10 2RX, UK. [2]Corporate Information & Computing Service, University of Sheffield, Sheffield S10 2GU, UK. [3]Medical & Biological Sciences Building, University of St Andrews, St Andrews KY16 9TF, UK. [4]School of Health and Related Research, University of Sheffield, Sheffield S1 4DA, UK. [5]Nutrition Innovation Centre for Food & Health (NICHE), Ulster University, Coleraine BT52 1SA, UK. [6]Food & Nutrition Group, Business School, Sheffield Hallam University, Sheffield S1 1WB, UK.

## References

1. British Government. Participation Rates in Higher Education: Academic Years 2006/2007–2013/2014. London: British Government; 2015.
2. El AW, Stock C, John J, Deeny P, Phillips C, Snelgrove S, et al. Health promoting behaviours and lifestyle characteristics of students at seven universities in the UK. Cent Eur J Public Health. 2011;19:197–204.
3. Devine P, Lloyd K, Gray AM. University student food attitudes and behaviour survey. Belfast: University of Ulster; 2006.
4. Tanton J, Dodd LJ, Woodfield L, Mabhala M. Eating Behaviours of British University Students: A Cluster Analysis on a Neglected Issue. Adv Prev Med. 2015;2015:639239 Available from: http://www.hindawi.com/journals/apm/2015/639239/. [cited 2018 Aug 29].
5. Lake AA, Adamson AJ, Craigie AM, Rugg-Gunn AJ, Mathers JC. Tracking of dietary intake and factors associated with dietary change from early adolescence to adulthood: the ASH30 study. Obes Facts. 2009;2:157–65 Available from: http://www.ncbi.nlm.nih.gov/pubmed/20054220. [cited 2018 Aug 29].
6. Mikkilä V, Räsänen L, Raitakari OT, Pietinen P, Viikari J. Consistent dietary patterns identified from childhood to adulthood: the cardiovascular risk in young Finns study. Br J Nutr. 2005;93:923–31 Available from: http://www.ncbi.nlm.nih.gov/pubmed/16022763. [cited 2018 Aug 29].
7. Papadaki A, Hondros G, Scott J, Kapsokefalou M. Eating habits of university students living at, or away from home in Greece. Appetite. 2007;49:169–76.
8. Crombie AP, Ilich JZ, Dutton GR, Panton LB, Abood DA. The freshman weight gain phenomenon revisited. Nutr Rev. 2009;67:83–94.
9. Finlayson G, Cecil J, Higgs S, Hill A, Hetherington M. Susceptibility to weight gain. Eating behaviour traits and physical activity as predictors of weight gain during the first year of university. Appetite. 2012;58:1091–8 Available from: http://www.ncbi.nlm.nih.gov/pubmed/22407132. [cited 2012 Nov 29].
10. Nikolaou CK, Hankey CR, Lean MEJ. Weight changes in young adults : a mixed-methods study. Int J Obes. 2014;39:508–13.
11. Guo SS, Huang C, Maynard LM, Demerath E, Towne B, Chumlea WC, et al. Body mass index during childhood , adolescence and young adulthood in relation to adult overweight and adiposity: the Fels longitudinal study. Int J Obes. 2000;24:1628–35.
12. Neumark-Sztainer D, Wall M, Larson N, Eisenberg M, Loth K. Dieting and disordered eating behaviors from adolescence to young adulthood: findings from a 10-year longitudinal study. J Am Diet Assoc. 2011;111:1004–11.
13. Fayet F, Petocz P, Samman S. Prevalence and correlates of dieting in college women: a cross sectional study. Int J Womens Health. 2012;13:405–11.
14. Larson NI, Neumark-Sztainer D, Story M. Weight control behaviors and dietary intake among adolescents and young adults: longitudinal findings from project EAT. J Am Diet Assoc. 2009;109:1869–77.
15. Woodruff SJ, Hanning RM, Lambraki I, Storey KE, McCargar L. Healthy eating index-C is compromised among adolescents with body weight concerns, weight loss dieting, and meal skipping. Body Image. 2008;5:404–8.
16. Schutz HK, Paxton SJ. Friendship quality, body dissatisfaction, dieting & disordered eating in adolescent girls. Br J Clin Psychol. 2007;46:67–83.
17. Slattery ML. Defining dietary consumption: is the sum greater than its parts? Am J Clin Nutr. 2008;88:14–5.
18. Yarnell JW, Fehily AM, Milbank J, Sweetnam P, Walker C. A short dietary questionnaire for use in an epidemiological survey: comparison with weight dietary records. Hum Nutr Appl Nutr. 1983;37:103–12.
19. Tinuviel Software Ltd. DIETQ Validation. 1999.
20. Tabachnick BG, Fidell LS. Using multivariate statistics. 6th ed. New York: Harper Row; 2012.
21. Northstone K, Emmett P, Rogers I. Dietary patterns in pregnancy and associations with socio-demographic and lifestyle factors. Eur J Clin Nutr. 2008;62:471–9.
22. Northstone K, Emmett PM. Dietary patterns of men in the ALSPAC: associations with socio-demographic and lifestyle characteristics, nutrient intakes and comparison with women's dietary patterns. Eur J Clin Nutr. 2010;64:978–86.
23. Northstone K, Smith AD, Cribb VL, Emmett PM. Dietary patterns in UK adolescents obtained from a dual-source FFQ and their associations with socio-economic position, nutrient intake and modes of eating. Public Health Nutr. 2013;17:1476–85.
24. Mccourt HJ, Draffin CR, Woodside JV, Cardwell CR, Young IS, Hunter SJ, et al. Dietary patterns and cardiovascular risk factors in adolescents and young adults: the Northern Ireland young hearts project. Br J Nutr. 2014;112:1685–98.
25. Pigott S, Bates B, Nass L. Socio-demographic characteristics of the NDNS RP sample - National Diet and Nutrition Survey. Results from Years 1–4 (combined) of the Rolling Programme (2008/2009–2011/12); 2014. p. 55–60.
26. Dodd LJ, Al-Nakeeb Y, Nevill A, Forshaw MJ. Lifestyle risk factors of students: a cluster analytical approach. Prev Med (Baltim). 2010;51:73–7 Available from: https://doi.org/10.1016/j.ypmed.2010.04.005.
27. Buck D, Frosini F. Clustering of unhealthy behaviours over time - Implications for policy and practice. Kings Fund. 2012;1–24. Available from: http://www.kingsfund.org.uk/publications/clustering-unhealthy-behaviours-over-time. Cited 29 Aug 2018.
28. Barker ME, McClean SI, Thompson KA, Reid NG. Dietary behaviours and sociocultural demographics in Northern Ireland. Br J Nutr. 1990;64:319–29 Available from: http://www.ncbi.nlm.nih.gov/pubmed/2223737.
29. Lennox A, Prynne C, Swan G, Roberts C, Steer T, Pell D, et al. Dietary intakes - National Diet and Nutrition Survey. Results from Years 1–4 (combined) of the Rolling Programme (2008/2009–2011/12). Northern Ireland: Public Health England; 2014. p. 61–84.
30. Higher Education Statistics Agency Ltd. Working class students at university, 2008/09. 2010.
31. Bamia C, Trichopoulos D, Ferrari P, Overvad K, Bjerregaard L, Tjønneland A, et al. Dietary patterns and survival of older Europeans: the EPIC-elderly study (European prospective investigation into Cancer and nutrition). Public Health Nutr. 2007;10:590–8.
32. Wrieden WL, Anderson AS, Longbottom PJ, Valentine K, Stead M, Caraher M, et al. The impact of a community-based food skills intervention on cooking confidence, food preparation methods and dietary choices – an exploratory trial. Public Health Nutr. 2007;10:203–11.
33. Brunner TA, van der Horst K, Siegrist M. Convenience food products. Drivers for consumption. Appetite. 2010;55:498–506.
34. Larson NI, Perry CL, Story M, Neumark-Sztainer D. Food preparation by young adults is associated with better diet quality. J Am Diet Assoc. 2006;106:2001–7.
35. Ruby MB. Vegetarianism. A blossoming field of study. Appetite. 2012;58:141–50 Available from: http://www.ncbi.nlm.nih.gov/pubmed/22001025. [cited 2012 Mar 13].
36. Kenyon PM, Barker ME. Attitudes towards meat-eating in vegetarian and non-vegetarian teenage girls in England--an ethnographic approach. Appetite. 1998;30:185–98 Available from: http://www.ncbi.nlm.nih.gov/pubmed/9573452.
37. Lac A, Donaldson CD. Alcohol attitudes, motives, norms, and personality traits longitudinally classify nondrinkers, moderate drinkers, and binge drinkers using discriminant function analysis. Addict. Behav. 2016;61:91–8 Available from: https://doi.org/10.1016/j.addbeh.2016.05.006.
38. Kuntsche E, Knibbe R, Gmel G, Engels R. Why do young people drink? A review of drinking motives. Clin Psychol Rev. 2005;25:841–61.

11

# Pessimism, diet and the ability to improve dietary habits: a three-year follow-up study among middle-aged and older Finnish men and women

Mikko Pänkäläinen[1*], Mikael Fogelholm[2], Raisa Valve[2], Olli Kampman[3,4], Markku Kauppi[4,5], Erja Lappalainen[1] and Jukka Hintikka[1,4]

## Abstract

**Background:** Dietary habits have a great influence on physiological health. Even though this fact is generally recognized, people do not eat as healthily as they know they should. The factors that support a healthy diet, on the other hand, are not well known. It is supposed that there is a link between personal traits and dietary habits. Personal traits may also partially explain why some people manage to make healthy dietary changes while some fail to do so or are not able to try to make changes even when they desire to do so. There is some information suggesting that dispositional optimism plays a role in succeeding in improving dietary habits. The aim of this study was to determine the role of optimism and pessimism in the process of dietary changes.

**Methods:** Dispositional optimism and pessimism were determined using the revised Life Orientation Test in 2815 individuals (aged 52–76 years) participating in the GOAL study in the region of Lahti, Finland. The dietary habits of the study subjects were analysed. After 3 years, the subjects' dietary habits and their possible improvements were registered. The associations between dispositional optimism and pessimism, dietary habits at baseline, and possible changes in dietary habits during the follow-up were studied with logistic regression. We also studied if the dietary habits or certain lifestyle factors (e.g. physical exercising and smoking) at baseline predicted success in improving the diet.

**Results:** Pessimism seemed to correlate clearly negatively with the healthiness of the dietary habits at baseline – i.e. the higher the level of pessimism, the unhealthier the diet. Optimism also showed a correlation with dietary habits at baseline, although to a lesser extent. Those who managed to improve their dietary habits during follow-up or regarded their dietary habits as healthy enough even without a change were less pessimistic at baseline than those who failed in their attempts to improve their diet or did not even try, even when they recognized the need for a change.

**Conclusions:** Pessimistic people are more likely to eat an unhealthy diet than others. Pessimism reduces independently the possibilities to improve dietary patterns.

**Keywords:** Pessimism, Optimism, Life orientation test – revised, Dietary habits

* Correspondence: mikko.pankalainen@phsotey.fi
[1]Department of Psychiatry, Päijät-Häme Central Hospital, Keskussairaalankatu 7, FI-15850 Lahti, Finland
Full list of author information is available at the end of the article

## Background

Despite the well-known connection between dietary habits and health, many people do not eat what is recommended as a healthy diet [1]. Dietary habits are related e.g. to the risk of coronary heart disease (CHD) [2] and improving dietary habits has showed significant cardioprotective effects in a secondary prevention program among women with CHD [3].

While the intention to prevent diseases is usually thought to be an important reason for a healthier diet, psychosocial and lifestyle related factors seem to be one of the major causes for not eating healthily. The most common factors mentioned in preventing a healthy diet are a lack of time, a reluctance to give up favourite foods, and a lack of motivation and willpower [4–6]. A healthy diet is also thought to be more expensive than unhealthy one, even if this belief seems to be false [7, 8].

The terms optimism and its antonym pessimism derive from Latin words 'optimus' and 'pessimus', respectively (the first meaning 'the best' and the latter meaning 'the worst' [9]) and they are used in describing people's outlook and expectations concerning their future. Persons who have a feeling or belief that good things will happen in the future are called optimists and they are said to see "the glass as half-full rather than half-empty". Pessimists in turn generally feel that bad things are more likely to happen than good things [10]. Optimism is regarded in psychology as a cognitive, affective and motivational construct [11]. On other words, optimists not only think, but also feel positively about the future. Like other personal trait, also optimism and pessimism develop during the childhood and early adulthood influenced by both heritage and environment [12, 13], and unlike e.g. mood, the construct of optimism (including both optimistic and pessimistic properties) is thought to be quite stable after it has evolved, regardless of negative or positive incidents [14, 15].

People are often categorized as optimists or pessimists. This can lead to the conclusion that optimism and pessimism are the two extremities of the same unidimensional continuum (dispositional optimism). Nevertheless, the concept of optimism itself has long been controversial: there is debate over whether the optimism construct should be seen as one bipolar dimension or if optimism and pessimism should be seen as two separate dimensions that exist simultaneously and may be unattached to each other.

Optimism is sometimes confused with other concepts, e.g. features like the sense of control [16], self-efficacy [17] and hope [18]. There are still differences with these terms. Unlike the concept of optimism, these properties include also how the desired outcomes are expected to happen. For example, a person with high self-efficacy believes that his/her personal efforts or skills are what will determine the positive outcome while an optimist does not rely on his/her own abilities.

Numerous psychosocial factors have been noted to influence dietary behaviour. A connection seems to exist between psychosocial features and current diet, and also between psychosocial features and the ability to improve the diet. Psychosocial features of interest include e.g. socio-economic status, willpower, self-efficacy, and satisfaction with life. There are many studies on the associations between these psychosocial factors and healthy eating [4, 19–24], but the number of studies concerning the optimism construct and dietary habits is quite small. The findings of these few studies suggest that there might be a positive connection between optimism and the willingness and capability to eat in a healthier way [25–29]. In all of these studies on the connection between the optimism construct and dietary habits, optimism has been associated with healthier diet and/or pessimism vice versa. In a study on young Finnish adults, unipolarly measured optimism had an influence on dietary habits, and pessimism was linked to an unhealthy diet [25]. In a study on elderly men, a low level of optimism was associated with an unhealthy lifestyle, including unhealthy dietary habits [29]. In the large Women's Health Initiative study, high optimism was strongly related to healthier eating habits and greater levels of success in improving dietary habits [26, 27]. In a study on Polish menopausal women, optimism was positively correlated with a healthier diet [28]. However, we did not find any previous studies with general population samples focusing on the dietary habits and the optimism construct that would handle optimism and pessimism as independent factors. We conducted this 3-year follow-up study on middle-aged and older Finnish men and women to determine whether optimism and pessimism are factors that associate with dietary habits and predict success in improving those habits.

## Methods

The GOAL study (Good Ageing in Lahti Region) started in 2002. Its aim was to determine and improve the health and well-being of the ageing population of the region of Lahti, a city in southern Finland. The entire project consisted of a cohort study and several community-based interventions and it lasted for 10 years. In the present study, data from baseline (year 2002) and 3-year follow-up (year 2005) of the cohort study were used.

The cohort study group consisted of a stratified (age, sex, municipality) random sample of men and women born in 1926–30, 1936–40, and 1946–50. The study participants were drawn from the population registry of all 14 municipalities in the Lahti region. A total of 4272 subjects were invited, and 2815 (66%) participated.

At the beginning of the GOAL study, cross-sectional data on the dietary habits, current health, and lifestyles of the study subjects were gathered by using questionnaires. The study subjects were asked about their recent dietary habits with a food frequency questionnaire (FFQ) where different foods were divided into 24 categories. The respondents were asked how often they had consumed the foods in each category during the last 7 days. The answers were scaled from 1 (not at all) to 4 (on 6 or 7 days). Study subjects were measured for height and weight and their body mass indexes (BMI) were calculated. According to their smoking habits, the study subjects were divided into two groups, 'daily smokers' (i.e. those who smoked every day, regardless of the amount) and 'non-daily smokers'. Study subjects who used five or more units of alcohol (one unit = 12 g EtOH) in one sitting formed the 'heavy drinkers' group, while the rest were 'non-heavy drinkers'. The study subjects were asked if they had been diagnosed with CHD by a doctor. Finally, the subgroup 'regular physical exercise' was formed to include those who exercised for 30 min at least twice a week. In addition to the questionnaires, several blood tests were taken. The samples were measured for the levels of blood glucose and cholesterol, among other things.

Levels of dispositional optimism and pessimism were measured by using the revised version of the Life Orientation Test (LOT-R). The test was initially developed in the mid-1980s to assess the beneficial effects of optimism on psychological and physiological health (Life Orientation Test (LOT)) [30]. The scale was re-evaluated and revised (LOT-R) later to focus its item content more closely on the subject's expectations of the future [31].

LOT-R includes six statements, three worded positively for optimism (e.g. 'In uncertain times, I usually expect the best') and three worded negatively to indicate pessimism (e.g. 'If something can go wrong for me, it will'). The respondents are asked to indicate how much they agree with the statements in general, as expressed on a scale from 0 ('I disagree a lot') to 4 ('I agree a lot'). A higher score refers to greater optimism or greater pessimism depending on the statement. Originally, both LOT and LOT-R were thought to be unidimensional scales, but later studies have suggested that they may have two separate independent dimensions, namely optimism and pessimism [32–36]. In the one-dimensional bipolar model with optimism and pessimism as opposites, the optimism scores and pessimism scores are calculated together and they might cancel out and hide each other's results. Our previous study showed clearly that in this study sample, LOT-R has two separate subscales: optimism and pessimism [37]. Thus, in the final analyses, we used the independent scores separately for optimism and pessimism.

After 3 years, in 2005, the study subjects were examined again. A total of 2625 subjects (93% of the original sample) had adequate responses in both 2002 and 2005, and could therefore be included in the final analyses. In 2005, the study subjects were asked if they had tried to improve or were about to improve their dietary habits, and if they had tried to improve their diet, how had they managed to achieve their goals. The possible improving styles in the diet were divided into five subgroups: reducing the consumption of fat, changing to low-fat products, reducing the consumption of sugar, increasing the consumption of vegetables, and increasing the consumption of berries and fruits.

We divided the study subjects in these five subgroups of different improving styles into four categories according to the possible changes in their diets: 1) those who had not tried to change their eating habits to a healthier diet, even when they thought it would have been beneficial, 2) those who thought their dietary habits were healthy enough even without an improvement, 3) those who had succeeded in improving of their diet, and 4) those who had tried to improve their diet but had failed to do so.

In the statistical analyses, we created dietary pattern models for grouping of the sample by using principal component analysis (PCA) with Varimax rotation and Kaiser normalization. Factor loadings with $> 0.35$ were considered as significant. Student's t-test was used to study the associations between optimism, pessimism, and the different dietary patterns. When studying the differences in levels of optimism and pessimism, according to the success in the improvement of dietary habits in four categories, we used the Kruskal–Wallis test due to skewed distributions.

Finally, we calculated logistic regression models to discover the fully adjusted odds ratios for different variables for the risk of not succeeding in improving dietary habits.

## Results

Using the data from the food frequency questionnaire in 2002, we divided the study subjects into different dietary pattern groups by using principal component analysis. The analysis resulted in four nearly independent dietary patterns, which we named as 'healthy', 'sweet unhealthy', 'fatty unhealthy' and 'traditional' diets (Table 1). In further analyses, principal component analysis scores were used as independent variables to describe the amount of each different dietary pattern in the study subjects. We used the medians of the LOT-R optimism and pessimism subscale scores to classify the study subjects into low and high optimism and pessimism groups. Principal component analysis scores were compared between these groups (Table 2).

At baseline, higher optimism and lower pessimism were associated with a 'healthy' dietary pattern. Optimism and pessimism did not seem to play any role in

**Table 1** Rotated factor matrix for dietary patterns created by using principal component analysis. Factor loadings with absolute values of > 0.35 have been presented in bold. Negative loadings indicate the lack of foodstuff in question belonging to certain dietary patterns

| Foodstuff | Dietary pattern | | | |
|---|---|---|---|---|
| | Healthy | Sweet unhealthy | Fatty unhealthy | Traditional |
| Porridge, cereals | **0.382** | −0.001 | −0.152 | 0.249 |
| Fish | **0.397** | −0.109 | 0.060 | −0.097 |
| Lunch meats, cold cuts | **0.359** | 0.214 | 0.055 | 0.142 |
| Fresh vegetables/root vegetables | **0.664** | −0.018 | −0.131 | 0.005 |
| Cooked vegetables | **0.646** | −0.049 | −0.032 | − 0.098 |
| Berries and fruits | **0.589** | 0.076 | −0.171 | 0.181 |
| Fruit or berry juice | **0.378** | 0.081 | 0.189 | 0.037 |
| Sweet pastries | 0.109 | **0.597** | −0.031 | 0.256 |
| Ice cream | 0.088 | **0.495** | 0.085 | −0.131 |
| Candies | −0.043 | **0.701** | 0.033 | 0.078 |
| Chocolate | 0.035 | **0.677** | 0.098 | −0.032 |
| Salty snacks | −0.024 | **0.352** | 0.195 | −0.221 |
| Fried potatoes, French fries | −0.005 | 0.026 | **0.489** | −0.059 |
| Low-fat cheese | **0.411** | 0.142 | **−0.368** | −0.066 |
| Other cheese | −0.004 | 0.025 | **0.609** | 0.108 |
| Sausages | −0.147 | 0.240 | **0.493** | 0.065 |
| Sliced sausages | −0.111 | 0.139 | **0.558** | 0.053 |
| Eggs | 0.151 | 0.013 | **0.475** | −0.057 |
| Soft drinks | −0.103 | 0.305 | **0.352** | −0.125 |
| Meat dishes | 0.028 | 0.132 | **0.366** | **0.552** |
| Chicken, turkey | **0.443** | 0.003 | −0.048 | **0.415** |
| Boiled or mashed potatoes | 0.230 | 0.002 | 0.101 | **0.658** |
| Rice, pasta | 0.294 | 0.088 | 0.115 | **−0.409** |
| Pizza, hamburgers | −0.021 | 0.263 | 0.169 | −0.302 |

the 'sweet unhealthy' and 'traditional' dietary patterns, but high pessimism and the 'fatty unhealthy' dietary pattern associated significantly (Table 2).

The association between changes in dietary habits during the 3-year follow-up and pessimism was quite clear (Table 3). There was a strong trend that those who managed to change to a healthier diet were less pessimistic compared to others. The differences were statistically significant in four dietary categories: reducing fat, changing to low-fat products, increasing vegetables, and increasing berries and fruits. The higher the level of pessimism, the less likely was the improvement of diet. Nevertheless, those who had tried but failed reducing sugar were not more pessimistic than others. Optimism was associated with only one dietary change; those who had tried but failed to increase consumption of berries and fruits were less optimistic than others.

**Table 2** Comparisons of principal component analysis scores of dietary patterns between groups with low or high pessimism, and low or high optimism

| | Principal component analysis scores (mean) | | | | | | | |
|---|---|---|---|---|---|---|---|---|
| | Healthy dietary pattern | p [1] | Sweet unhealthy dietary pattern | p [1] | Fatty unhealthy dietary pattern | p [1] | Traditional dietary pattern | p [1] |
| Low pessimism ($N = 1274$) [2] | 0.071 | | 0.029 | | −0.048 | | −0.006 | |
| High pessimism ($N = 1351$) [3] | −0.066 | **< 0.001** | − 0.027 | 0.153 | 0.046 | **0.016** | 0.006 | 0.762 |
| Low optimism ($N = 1210$) [2] | −0.085 | | 0.000 | | −0.019 | | 0.026 | |
| High optimism ($N = 1415$) [3] | 0.073 | **< 0.001** | −0.000 | 0.995 | 0.016 | 0.365 | −0.022 | 0.213 |

[1] Student's t-test; [2] Below the median; [3] Median or higher
p[1]-scores indicating statistical significance are bolded

**Table 3** The association between optimism and pessimism, and the change in dietary habits

| | Has not changed | No need to change | Has changed | Tried to change, but failed | p[1] |
|---|---|---|---|---|---|
| Reducing fat | N = 82 | N = 1059 | N = 1280 | N = 204 | |
| Optimism (Mean (SD)) | 8.60 (2.02) | 8.26 (2.24) | 8.39 (2.08) | 8.18 (2.14) | 0.385 |
| Pessimism (SD) | 4.59 (2.60) | 4.19 (2.79) | 3.62 (2.58) | 4.44 (2.81) | **< 0.001** |
| Changing to low-fat products | N = 155 | N = 1098 | N = 1266 | N = 106 | |
| Optimism (Mean (SD)) | 8.37 (2.20) | 8.28 (2.21) | 8.39 (2.09) | 8.18 (2.15) | 0.674 |
| Pessimism (Mean (SD)) | 4.46 (2.74) | 4.15 (2.77) | 3.65 (2.60) | 4.47 (2.76) | **< 0.001** |
| Increasing vegetables | N = 198 | N = 1141 | N = 1090 | N = 196 | |
| Optimism (Mean (SD)) | 8.46 (2.16) | 8.25 (2.28) | 8.43 (2.01) | 8.10 (2.06) | 0.058 |
| Pessimism (Mean (SD)) | 4.10 (2.69) | 4.09 (2.77) | 3.69 (2.59) | 4.43 (2.79) | **< 0.001** |
| Reducing sugar | N = 110 | N = 1287 | N = 986 | N = 242 | |
| Optimism (Mean (SD)) | 8.23 (2.13) | 8.29 (2.23) | 8.42 (2.04) | 8.17 (2.18) | 0.520 |
| Pessimism (Mean (SD)) | 4.16 (2.54) | 4.04 (2.75) | 3.78 (2.69) | 3.95 (2.54) | 0.145 |
| Increasing berries and fruits | N = 128 | N = 1520 | N = 859 | N = 118 | |
| Optimism (Mean (SD)) | 8.38 (2.05) | 8.39 (2.20) | 8.32 (2.05) | 7.81 (2.22) | **0.041** |
| Pessimism (Mean (SD)) | 4.43 (2.77) | 4.02 (2.78) | 3.68 (2.51) | 4.35 (2.72) | **0.002** |

[1] Kruskal–Wallis test
p[1]-scores indicating statistical significance are bolded

Finally, we calculated multivariate logistic regression models including several predicting variables for the risk of failure in improving dietary habits (Table 4). Because of the relatively small subgroups, we combined those who had failed in their dietary changes with those who had not even tried to improve their diet even when they recognized the need to do so into one group. We also combined those who saw no need to improve their diets with those who had managed to make healthy changes into another group.

The models included different dietary patterns, age, sex smoking and alcohol consumption habits, physical exercise, the levels of blood glucose and cholesterol, body mass index, the possible existence of CHD, and pessimism as explaining variables. A fatty unhealthy dietary pattern associated with the risk of failure in changing to low-fat products and in increasing vegetables. Sweet unhealthy dietary pattern associated with the risk of failure in increasing vegetables, in reducing sugar and in increasing berries and fruits. Finally, the effect of pessimism seemed clear in three out of five subgroups. Pessimism increased the probability of failure in reducing fat, changing to low-fat products, and increasing the consumption of berries and fruits.

To emphasize the association between pessimism and failures in changing dietary habits, we compared the highest and the lowest quarters of pessimism in logistic regression models which were fully adjusted for age, sex,

**Table 4** Odds ratios of different dietary pattern groups, coronary heart disease and pessimism (rows) on the risk of failure in change to more healthy dietary habits (columns) analysed by logistic regression models[a]

| | Dietary change | | | | | | | | | |
|---|---|---|---|---|---|---|---|---|---|---|
| | No change and fail in reducing fat | | No change and fail in changing to low-fat products | | No change and fail in increasing vegetables | | No change and fail in reducing sugar | | No change and fail in increasing berries and fruits | |
| | OR | 95% CI | OR | 95% CI | OR | 95% CI | OR | 95% CI | OR | 95% CI |
| Healthy dietary pattern | 0.87 | 0.76–1.00 | 0.88 | 0.76–1.01 | 0.79 | 0.70–0.89 | 0.92 | 0.82–1.04 | 0.75 | 0.65–0.86 |
| Sweet unhealthy dietary pattern | 1.13 | 0.99–1.29 | 1.07 | 0.94–1.23 | **1.26** | **1.13–1.40** | **1.30** | **1.16–1.45** | **1.23** | **1.08–1.40** |
| Fatty unhealthy dietary pattern | 1.10 | 0.96–1.26 | **1.14** | **1.00–1.31** | **1.17** | **1.05–1.32** | 1.03 | 0.92–1.16 | 1.13 | 0.98–1.30 |
| Traditional dietary pattern | 1.12 | 0.98–1.27 | 1.02 | 0.90–1.17 | 0.97 | 0.87–1.08 | 1.01 | 0.90–1.14 | 0.89 | 0.78–1.02 |
| Coronary heart disease | 1.07 | 0.66–1.73 | 0.91 | 0.54–1.54 | 1.20 | 0.81–1.80 | **1.52** | **1.00–2.31** | 1.41 | 0.87–2.28 |
| Pessimism | **1.07** | **1.02–1.12** | **1.07** | **1.02–1.13** | 1.03 | 0.99–1.07 | 1.02 | 0.98–1.07 | **1.05** | **1.00–1.11** |

*OR* Odds ratio, *CI* Confidence interval
[a]Models are fully adjusted for age, sex, smoking and alcohol consumption habits, physical exercise, the levels of glucose, cholesterol and body mass index
p[1]-scores indicating statistical significance are bolded

smoking and alcohol consumption habits, physical exercise, the levels of glucose, cholesterol, body mass index and the possible existence of CHD. Those who belonged to the highest quarter of pessimism had a 1.4-fold risk of not succeeding in reducing their consumption of fat (adjusted OR 1.44, 95% CI 1.00–2.08, $p = 0.05$), a 1.5-fold risk of not succeeding in changing to low-fat products (adjusted OR 1.51, 95% CI 1.03–2.21, $p = 0.03$), and a 1.5-fold risk of failing to increase the consumption of berries and fruits in their diet (adjusted OR 1.46, 95% CI 1.01–2.12, $p = 0.02$) compared to the study subjects in the lowest quarter of pessimism.

## Discussion

Our main findings were that the dietary habits of study subjects with a higher level of pessimism were unhealthier compared to the dietary habits of others, and that the high level of pessimism was associated with greater difficulties in improving dietary habits. High levels of pessimism have been linked independently with an elevated risk of CHD [37–39]. While pessimism seems to be an independent risk factor for CHD, our results suggest that it may also be related to increased risk of CHD via an unhealthier diet.

There seemed to be no association between sweet unhealthy dietary pattern as well as fail in reducing sugar and optimism/pessimism. It has been speculated that the physiological and psychological mechanisms concerning sugar consumption might be different compared to the mechanism of other dietary habits. For example, when trying to eat healthily, the lack of sweet foods is often seen as the most difficult task [40] and when treating binge eating with baclofen, the medication seems to suppress binge eating of pure fat but not a sugar-rich diet [41].

It can be discussed whether the test subjects had proper information about good dietary habits, but it has been stated that the factor preventing people from eating healthy is not a lack of knowledge but rather the fact that people do not eat as healthily they know they should [1, 42, 43]. While there are many different recommendations about healthy diets which can make it challenging to know how to eat healthily it also seems that the correlation between nutrition knowledge and healthy dietary intake is quite weak [44].

Our study also strengthens the idea of optimism and pessimism as two different and independent variables. The statistical power of the optimism subscale was very small, while pessimism had stronger associations with several outcomes.

Improving the diet has a role in both prevention and treatment of several chronic diseases. The result of our study – pessimism being associated with difficulties in improving one's diet – is parallel with earlier studies on psychosocial factors and adherence to various treatments. For example, adherence to treatment of asthma patients, hypertensive patients, cardiac patients, and rehabilitation patients after surgery seemed to relate to psychosocial factors, including dispositional optimism [45–48]. A higher level of optimism has also been associated, for example, with greater success in achieving good results in health changes among cardiac patients [49, 50] and in dental health [51]. Optimism and good compliance to treatment might also be connected in HIV patients [52].

An earlier study suggested that optimistic people exert greater efforts at goal attainment than pessimists do, for example, in alcoholism treatment [53]. In cross-sectional analyses, optimists have been shown to choose healthier foods when no preceding instructions are given [54, 55]. According to these studies, it seems that dispositional optimism and pessimism relate to the motivation in the treatment compliance, overall health behaviour, and the ability to make changes in lifestyle in order to improve physical well-being. The results of our study strengthen this claim.

As mentioned, there are some previous studies on associations between optimism/pessimism and dietary patterns [25–29]. However, there are some shortcomings in these studies. In these studies optimism and pessimism were dealt as a bipolar, single variable, and except for one study, the study participants were all of the same gender. It has been recognized in many other studies that optimism and pessimism are probably two independent variables that are present at same the time – i.e. one has both pessimistic and optimistic traits simultaneously [35]. The method of using optimism and pessimism as two different dimensions rather than one bipolar single variable may reveal much more information when the opposite ends of the bipolar variable do not cancel each other [32–36]. Separating optimism from pessimism turned out to be beneficial also in our study; optimism and pessimism seemed to be two different and independent factors as optimism seemed to have a connection with only one type of change in diet, while pessimism was associated much more strongly with many dietary behaviour changes. This endorses the need to separate optimism and pessimism to achieve more accurate results. Analysing optimism and pessimism as a unidimensional variable in this study would probably have covered some of the current results.

It has also been suggested that dispositional optimism might be a unidimensional continuum, but questions oriented pessimistically are better in determining this variable [54], thus diminishing the statistical power of optimistically oriented questions.

Even if it seems that people with high levels of pessimism have an unhealthier diet than others do and they are less likely to be able to change their dietary habits, it has been found that after proper education and monitoring, the association between pessimism and the ability to improve diet disappears. This conclusion was drawn following a trial derived from the GOAL study [56]. In the study, the subjects with higher pessimism levels had unhealthier lifestyles, including unhealthier dietary habits. However, after the pessimists had received education concerning healthier lifestyles and were subjected to close monitoring, they managed to improve their lifestyles equally to other subjects. Keeping this in mind, it would seem only natural that determining pessimism could help in finding those who probably have unhealthier diets and are in greater risk in failing to improve them. Those subjects could then be targeted with proper education about healthy diets, and the monitoring of dietary changes could lower the risk of various diseases. Naturally, the independent risk of pessimism in developing those illnesses – for example, CHD – is still unlikely to diminish. Determining the level of dispositional pessimism is quick to assess and practically cost free, so it can be expected to be very cost-effective.

There are some strengths and weaknesses in our study and methods. The population was drawn as a random sample and it is representative of Lahti Region with 200,000 inhabitants. However, it seems that poorly functioning and institutionalized persons had a lower participation rate than community-dwelling subjects [57]. The design is longitudinal and observational, but it can obviously not detect any causality between the assessed variables. We have measured a great number of variables, hence the possibility to adjust for a number of confounders was good. However, and typical of cohort studies, the methods were mostly simple and we were unable to describe the diet by, e.g., an extensive food-frequency questionnaire. In the analyses, we classified reduction of fat as an indication of a healthy change. This may of course be debated, since more recent studies indicate that fat quality (shift from saturated towards unsaturated fats) is more important than the intake of total fat per se [58]. In early 2000's, reductions in dietary fat and in fatty foods were generally - at least among many lay individuals - regarded as healthy. Hence, we chose to use fat reduction as an indication of a choice to improve dietary quality.

Much of the data used in this study is based on self-rated questionnaires, so there might be some inconsistency between the answers and the reality in the questions concerning, for example, smoking habits and use of alcohol.

## Conclusions

Dietary habits play an important role in the development of many diseases, and improving the diet reduces the risk for developing many severe illnesses. Pessimism and to some extent optimism seem to play a role in current dietary habits and in the ability to change these habits. By determining optimism and particularly pessimism, it is possible to detect individuals in greater need of guidance and support in ameliorating their dietary habits. Separating optimism and pessimism seems to make a clearer connection between the optimism construct and dietary habits as well as between the optimism construct and the ability to make healthy dietary changes.

#### Abbreviations

BMI: Body mass index; CHD: Coronary heart disease; FFQ: Food frequency questionnaire; GOAL: Good Ageing in Lahti Region study; LOT: Life orientation test; LOT-R: Revised version of the life orientation test; PCA: Principal component analysis

#### Acknowledgements

We thank all the participants in the GOAL Project.

#### Funding

This study was supported with an EVO (special state funding) grant from Päijät-Häme Central Hospital.

#### Authors' contributions

Authors MP and JH designed the study. RV, MF, OK, MK and EL participated in the conception of the study. JH managed and conducted the statistical analyses and interpreted the data. MP wrote the first draft and MP, JH, RV, MF, OK, MK and EL revised it to make the final manuscript. All authors have approved the final manuscript.

#### Competing interests

The authors declare that they have no competing interests.

#### Author details

[1]Department of Psychiatry, Päijät-Häme Central Hospital, Keskussairaalankatu 7, FI-15850 Lahti, Finland. [2]Department of Food and Environmental Sciences, University of Helsinki, Helsinki, Finland. [3]Department of Psychiatry, Seinäjoki Hospital District, Seinäjoki, Finland. [4]School of Medicine, University of Tampere, Tampere, Finland. [5]Department of Internal Medicine, Päijät-Häme Central Hospital, Lahti, Finland.

#### References

1. Guenther PM, Casavale KO, Kirkpatrick SI, Reedy J, Hiza HAB, Kuczynski KJ, Kahle LL, Krebs-Smith SM. Diet quality of Americans in 2001-02 and 2007-08 as measured by the healthy eating Index-2010. Nutrition Insight. 2013;51.
2. Schwingshackl L, Hoffmann G. Diet quality as assessed by the healthy eating index, the alternate healthy eating index, the dietary approaches to stop hypertension score, and health outcomes: a systematic review and meta-analysis of cohort studies. J Acad Nutr Diet. 2015;5:780–800.
3. de Lorgeril M, Patricia S, Martin J-L, Monjaud I, Delaye J, Mamelle N. Mediterranean diet, traditional risk factors, and the rate of cardiovascular complications after myocardial infarction: final report of the Lyon diet heart study. Circulation. 1999;6:779–85.

4. Lappalainen R, Saba A, Holm L, Mykkänen H, Gibney MJ. Difficulties in trying to eat healthier: descriptive analysis of perceived barriers for healthy eating. Eur J Clin Nutr. 1997;51:36–40.
5. López-Azpiazu I, Martínez-González MA, Kearney J, Gibney M, Martínez JA. Perceived barriers of, and benefits to, healthy eating reported by a Spanish national sample. Public Health Nutr. 1998;2:209–15.
6. Andajani-Sutjahjo S, Ball K, Warren N, Inglis V, Crawford D. Perceived personal, social and environmental barriers to weight maintenance among young women: a community survey. Int J Behav Nutr Phys Act. 2004;1:7.
7. Mitchell DC, Shannon BM, Mckenzie J, Smiciklas-Wright H, Miller BM, Tershakovec AM. Lower fat diets for children did not increase food costs. J Nutr Educ. 2000;32:100–3.
8. Goulet J, Lamarche B, Lemieux S. A nutritional intervention promoting a Mediterranean food pattern does not affect total daily dietary cost in north American women in free-living conditions. J Nutr. 2008;138:54–9.
9. Lewis CT, Short C. A Latin dictionary. Oxford: Oxford Press; 1879.
10. Cambridge Free English Dictionary and Thesaurus. Cambridge University Press. http://dictionary.cambridge.org/. Accessed 8 June 2018.
11. Peterson C. The future of optimism. Am Psychol. 2000;55:44–55.
12. Schulman P, Keith D. Seligman MEP. Is optimism heritable (a study of twins). Behav Res Ther. 1993;6:569–74.
13. Mosing MA, Medland SE, McRae A, Landers JG, Wright MJ, Martin NG. Genetic influences on life span and its relationship to personality: a 16-year follow-up study of a sample of aging twins. Psychosom Med. 2012;74:16–22.
14. Billingsley KD, Waehler CA, Hardin SI. Stability of optimism and choice of coping strategy. Percept Mot Skills. 1993;76:91–7.
15. Schou I, Ekeberg O, Sandvik L, Ruland CM. Stability in optimism-pessimism in relation to bad news: a study of women with breast cancer. J Pers Assess. 2005;2:148–54.
16. Thompson SC. The role of personal control in adaptive functioning. In: Snyder CR, Lopez SJ, editors. Handbook of positive psychology. New York: Oxford University Press; 2002. p. 202–13.
17. Bandura A. Self-efficacy: the exercise of control. New York: Freeman; 1997.
18. Snyder CR. The psychology of hope: you can get there from here. New York: Free Press; 1994.
19. de Ridder D, Kroese F, Evers C, Adriaanse M, Gillebaart M. Healthy diet: health impact, prevalence, correlates. and interventions Psychology & Health. 2017;32:907–41.
20. Brownell KD, Cohen LR. Adherence to dietary regimen 2: components of effective intervention. Behav Med. 1995;20:155.
21. Strachan SM, Brawley LR. Healthy-eater identity and self-efficacy predict healthy eating behavior. J Health Psychol. 2009;14:684–95.
22. van de Rest O, de Goede J, Sytsma F, Oude Griep LM, Geleijnse JM, Kromhout D, Giltay EJ. Association of n-3 long chain PUFA and fish intake with depressive symptoms an low dispositional optimism in older subjects with a history of myocardial infarction. Br J Nutr. 2010;103:1381–7.
23. Kumanyika SK, Bowen D, Rolls BJ, Von Horn L, Perri MG, Czajkowski SM, Schron E. Maintenance of dietary behavior change. Health Psychol. 2000; 19:42–56.
24. Steptoe A, Doherty S, Kerry S, Rink E, Hilton S. Sociodemographic and psychological predictors of changes in dietary fat consumption in adults with high blood cholesterol following counselling in primary care. Health Psychol. 2000;19:411–9.
25. Kelloniemi H, Ek E, Laitinen J. Optimism, dietary habits, body mass index and smoking among young Finnish adults. Appetite. 2005;45:169–76.
26. Tinker LF, Rosal MC, Young AF, Perri MG, Patterson RE, Van Horn L, Assaf AR, Bowen DJ, Ockene J, Hays J. Wu L. predictors of dietary change and maintenance in the women's health initiative dietary modification trail. J Am Diet Assoc. 2007;107:1155–65.
27. Hingle MD, Wertheim BC, Tindle HA, Tinker L, Seguin RA, Rosal MC, Thomson CA. Optimism and diet quality in the women's health initiative. Journal of academy of nutrition and dietetics. 2014,114.1036–45.
28. Gacek M. Individual differences as predictors of dietary patterns among menopausal women with arterial hypertension. Prz Menopauzalny. 2014; 13:101–8.
29. Giltay EJ, Geleijnse JM, Zitman FG, Buijsse B, Kromhout D. Lifestyle and dietary correlates of dispositional optimism in men: the Zutphen elderly study. J Psychosom Res. 2007;63:483–90.
30. Scheier MF, Carver CS. Optimism, coping and health: assessment and implications of generalized outcome expectancies. Health Psychol. 1985; 4:219–47.
31. Scheier MF, Carver CS, Bridges MW. Distinguishing optimism from neuroticism (and trait anxiety, self-mastery, and self-esteem): a re-evaluation of the life orientation test. J Pers Soc Psychol. 1994;6:1063–78.
32. Chang EC, Maydeu-Olivares A, D'Zurilla TJ. Optimism and pessimism as partially independent constructs: relationship to positive and negative affectivity and physiological well-being. Pers Indiv Differ. 1997;3:433–40.
33. Robinson-Whelen S, Kim C, MacCallum RC, Kiecolt-Glaser JK. Distinguishing optimism from pessimism in older adults: is it more important to be optimistic or not to be pessimistic? J Pers Soc Psychol. 1997;6:1345–53.
34. Kubzansky LD, Kubzansky PE, Maselko J. Optimism and pessimism in the context of health: bipolar opposites or separate constructs? Personal Soc Psychol Bull. 2004;30:943–56.
35. Herzberg PY, Glaesmer H, Hoyer J. Separating optimism and pessimism: a robust psychometric analysis of the revised life orientation test (LOT-R). Psychol Assessment. 2006;18:433–8.
36. Glaesmer H, Rief W, Martin A, Mewes R, Brahler E, Zenger M, Hinz A. Psychometric properties and population-based norms of the life orientation test revised (LOT-R). Br J Health Psychol. 2012;17:432–45.
37. Pänkäläinen M, Kerola T, Hintikka J. Pessimism and the risk for coronary heart disease among middle-aged and older Finnish men and women: a ten-year follow-up study. BMC Cardiovasc Disord. 2015;15:113.
38. Kubzansky LD, Sparrow D, Vokonas P. Kawachi I. is the glass half empty or half full? A prospective study of optimism and coronary heart disease in the normative aging study. Psychosom Med. 2001;63:910–6.
39. Tindle HA, Chang YF, Kuller LH, Manson JE, Robinson JG, Rosal MC, Siegle GJ, Matthews KA. Optimism, cynical hostility, and incident coronary heart disease and mortality in the Women's Health Initiative. Circulation. 2009;120:656–62.
40. Macdiarmid JI, Loe J, Kyle J, McNeill G. "It was an education in portion size". Experience of eating a healthy diet and barriers to long term dietary change. Appetite. 2013;71:411–9.
41. Bernera LA, Bocarslya ME, Hoebela BG, Avena NM. Baclofen suppresses binge eating of pure fat but not a sugar-rich or sweet-fat diet. Behav Pharmacol. 2009;20:631–4.
42. Lappalainen R, Kearneyc J, Gibneyc MA. Pan EU survey of consumer attitudes to food, nutrition and health: an overview. Food Qual Prefer. 1998; 9:467–78.
43. Paquette MC. Perceptions of healthy eating: state of knowledge and research gaps. Canadian Journal of Public Health. 2005;96:15–9.
44. Spronk I, Kullen C, Burdon C, O'Connor H. Relationship between nutrition knowledge and dietary intake. Br J Nutr. 2014;111:1713–26.
45. Bruzzese JM, Carcone AI, Lam P, Ellis DA, Naar-King S. Adherence to asthma medication regimens in urban African American adolescents: application of self-determination theory. Health Psychol. 2014;33:461–4.
46. Nabi H, Vahtera J, Singh-Manoux A, Pentti J, Oksanen T, Gimeno D, Elovainio M, Virtanen M, Klaukka T, Kivimäki M. Do psychological attributes matter for adherence to antihypertensive medication? The Finnish public sector cohort study. J Hypertens. 2008;26:2236–43.
47. Schroder KEE, Schwarzer R. Habitual self-control and management of health behavior among heart patients. Soc Sci Med. 2005;60:859–75.
48. Brewer BW, Cornelius AE, Van Raalte JL, Tennen H, Armeli S. Predictors of adherence to home rehabilitation exercises following anterior cruciate ligament reconstruction. Rehabilitation Psychology. 2013;58:64–72.
49. Shepperd JA, Maroto JJ, Pbert LA. Dispositional optimism as a predictor of health changes among cardiac patients. J Res Pers. 1996;30:517–34.
50. O'Brien LA, Thow MK, Rafferty D. Predicting adherence to phase III cardiac rehabilitation: should we be more optimistic? Br J Cardiol. 2009;16:250–3.
51. Ylöstalo PV, Ek E, Knuuttila MLE. Coping and optimism in relation to dental health behaviour – a study among Finnish young adults. Eur J Oral Sci. 2003;111:477–82.
52. Godin G, Côté J, Naccache H, Lambert LD, Trottier S. Prediction of adherence to antiretroviral therapy: a one-year longitudinal study. AIDS Care. 2005;17:493–504.
53. Strack S, Carver CS, Blaney PH. Predicting successful completion of an aftercare program following treatment for alcoholism: the role of dispositional optimism. J Pers Soc Psychol. 1987;53:579–84.
54. Roy B, Diez-Roux AV, Seeman T, Ranjit N, Shea S, Cushman M. Association of Optimism and Pessimism with Inflammation and hemostasis in the multi-ethnic study of atherosclerosis (MESA). Psychosom Med. 2010;72:134–40.
55. Boehm JK, William DR, Rimm EB, Ryff C, Kubzansky LD. Association between optimism and serum antioxidants in the midlife in the United States study. Psychosom Med. 2013;75:2–10.

56. Hankonen N, Vollmann M, Renner B, Absetz P. What is setting the stage for abdominal obesity reduction? A comparison between personality and health-related social cognitions. J Behav Med. 2010:415–22.
57. Nummela O, Sulander T, Helakorpi S, Haapola I, Uutela A, Heinonen H, Valve R, Fogelholm M. Register-based data indicated nonparticipation bias in a health study among aging people. J Clin Epidemiol. 2011;64:1418–25.
58. Schwab U, Uusitupa M. Diet heart controversies – quality of fat matters. Nutrition, Metabolism & Cardiovascular Diseases. 2015;25:617–22.

# 12

# Association of dietary patterns, anthropometric measurements and metabolic parameters with C-reactive protein and neutrophil-to-lymphocyte ratio in middle-aged and older adults with metabolic syndrome in Taiwan

Ahmad Syauqy[1,2], Chien-Yeh Hsu[3,4], Hsiao-Hsien Rau[5] and Jane C.-J. Chao[1,4,6*]


## Abstract

**Background:** Metabolic syndrome is commonly associated with inflammation. The underlying factors of inflammation in metabolic syndrome are not fully understood. The objective of the study was to determine the association of dietary patterns, anthropometric measurements, and metabolic parameters with inflammatory markers in middle-aged and older adults with metabolic syndrome in Taiwan.

**Methods:** A total of 26,016 subjects aged ≥35 y with metabolic syndrome were recruited from Mei Jau institution between 2004 and 2013 for a cross sectional study. Metabolic syndrome was defined by the International Diabetes Federation. Multivariate logistic regression was performed to evaluate the association of dietary patterns, anthropometric measurements, and metabolic parameters with C-reactive protein (CRP) and neutrophil-to-lymphocyte ratio (NLR) in men and women with metabolic syndrome. Crude and adjusted models were analyzed by gender.

**Results:** The western dietary pattern, obesity, high body fat, high waist or hip circumference, and high waist-to-hip ratio were significantly associated with increased odds ratios of high CRP and NLR in both genders. High systolic or diastolic blood pressure (BP), low high-density lipoprotein-cholesterol (HDL-C), high low-density lipoprotein-cholesterol (LDL-C), high total cholesterol (TC), high serum triglycerides (TG), and high fasting blood glucose (FBG) were significantly correlated with increased odds ratios of high CRP in both genders. Low HDL-C, high LDL-C, high serum TG, and high FBG were significantly associated with increased odds ratios of high NLR in both genders. However, high systolic (OR = 1.124, 95% CI 1.047–1.206, $P < 0.01$) or diastolic BP (OR = 1.176, 95% CI 1.087–1.273, $P < 0.001$) and high TC (OR = 1.138, 95% CI 1.062–1.220, $P < 0.001$) were significantly correlated with increased odds ratios of high NLR only in men.


(Continued on next page)


* Correspondence: chenjui@tmu.edu.tw
[1]School of Nutrition and Health Sciences, College of Nutrition, Taipei Medical University, 250 Wu-Hsing Street, Taipei 110, Taiwan
[4]Master Program in Global Health and Development, College of Public Health, Taipei Medical University, Taipei, Taiwan
Full list of author information is available at the end of the article

(Continued from previous page)
**Conclusions:** The western dietary pattern, obese-related anthropometric parameters, and most components of metabolic syndrome are positively associated with CRP levels and NLR in men and women with metabolic syndrome.

**Keywords:** Dietary patterns, Anthropometric measurements, Metabolic parameters, C-reactive protein, Neutrophil-to-lymphocyte ratio, Inflammation, Metabolic syndrome

## Background

Metabolic syndrome is defined by central obesity, increased systolic and diastolic blood pressure (BP), decreased high-density lipoprotein cholesterol (HDL-C), increased serum triglycerides (TG), and elevated fasting blood glucose (FBG). The International Diabetes Federation (IDF) declared that central obesity was strongly associated with metabolic syndrome and its components [1]. The prevalence of metabolic syndrome has been increased obviously throughout the world [2–4], and it has become a main public health issue in recent years. Moreover, metabolic syndrome is one of the risk factors of cardiovascular disease (CVD). The prevalence of metabolic syndrome and central obesity increased with age, with the highest rates seen among middle-aged and older adults [5]. Additionally, metabolic syndrome was associated with inflammation which may exacerbate the development of CVD [6]. The increased levels of inflammatory markers have also been strongly correlated with both central obesity and metabolic syndrome. However, the underlying factors of inflammation in metabolic syndrome are not fully understood.

Dietary patterns are associated with inflammation. The previous study revealed that high intake of trans fatty acids had a positive correlation with inflammation [7]. Additionally, a diet high in meat and processed food was positively correlated with inflammation [8, 9]. In contrast, higher intake of vegetables was inversely associated with C-reactive protein (CRP) concentrations [10, 11]. Anthropometric parameters were also correlated with inflammation. Obesity defined by body mass index (BMI) and waist circumference was associated with inflammation [12]. Body fat, skinfold thickness, and other measures of abdominal adiposity were also positively correlated with inflammation [13, 14]. Furthermore, metabolic disorders might interfere with inflammatory status. Components of metabolic syndrome were significantly increased with both CRP and neutrophil-to-lymphocyte ratio (NLR) levels [15, 16]. Dyslipidemia, which is characterized by high levels of total cholesterol (TC), serum TG, low-density lipoprotein-cholesterol (LDL-C) levels, or low HDL-C levels, has also been positively correlated with elevated plasma CRP levels, soluble intracellular adhesion molecule (sICAM)-1, and soluble endothelial selectin [17].

Several studies have investigated the effect of dietary patterns, anthropometric measurements, or metabolic parameters on inflammatory markers [18, 19]. However, the study investigated all these factors in metabolic syndrome population using CRP and NLR as the indicators of inflammation was still rare. Both CRP and NLR serve as inflammatory indicators that can be easily measured and serve as independent predictors for both the development of metabolic syndrome and CVD [20]. Thus, the objective of the study was to determine the association of dietary patterns, anthropometric measurements, and metabolic parameters with inflammatory markers using CRP and NLR among middle-aged and older adults with metabolic syndrome in Taiwan.

## Methods

### Subjects and study design

The cross-sectional study was performed to examine data collected from a Mei Jau (MJ) Group, a private health management screening institution in Taiwan, from 2004 to 2013. The MJ Group's four health screening centers in Taiwan in Taipei, Taoyuan, Taichung, and Kaohsiung (listed from north to south) were used to collect pertinent information for the study. Data collected included demographic data, lifestyle, diet, anthropometric data, biochemical parameters, and other health related data from the individuals who came to their health screening centers for a regular health check-up [9]. A total of 60,769 individuals with age ≥ 35 y met criteria of metabolic syndrome from the MJ database between 2004 and 2013. After excluding the individuals ($n = 23{,}377$) who had renal dysfunction, liver problems, or all types of cancer, and those who ($n = 11{,}376$) with missing data on food frequency questionnaire (FFQ), anthropometric measurements, or biochemical parameters, a total of 26,016 subjects were finally recruited for analysis in this study.

### Definition of metabolic syndrome and inflammation

The components of metabolic syndrome were proposed by the IDF in 2005 and defined as individuals who had central obesity (waist circumference ≥ 90 cm for men or ≥ 80 cm for women in Taiwan) with two of four factors: (1) systolic BP ≥ 130 mmHg, diastolic BP ≥ 85 mmHg or history of the therapy of hypertension, (2) HDL-C < 1.03 mmol/L for men, < 1.29 mmol/L for women or specific therapy for lipid abnormality, (3) serum TG ≥ 1.70 mmol/L or specific therapy for lipid abnormality, and (4) FBG ≥ 5.60 mmol/L or previously diagnosed type 2 diabetes mellitus [1]. The definition of metabolic syndrome with central obesity was selected due to the growing prevalence of central obesity in Taiwan in recent years [9]. The definition of inflammation in this study was CRP ≥ 28.6 nmol/L [21] or NLR ≥ 3.0 [22]. Ethical approval for this study was granted by Taipei Medical University-Joint Institutional Review Board (N201706051). Written informed consents were obtained from all subjects prior to the health check-up when they visited each MJ Group health screening center. The data were de-identified and used for academic study only.

### Assessment of dietary patterns

Dietary intake was analyzed using a validated FFQ collected by the MJ Group. All subjects were requested to complete the FFQ before they had health check-up. The FFQ included 22 food groups or food items referred to the characteristics of Taiwanese dietary patterns. The FFQ collected intake frequency data with the information of portion size and the corresponding pictures of measuring tools in each question. For instance, the description for milk consumption was "How much milk do you drink? (1 cup is equivalent to 240 mL of fresh milk, 240 mL of yogurt, or 4 tablespoons of powdered milk)", and the options for intake frequency were "none or < 1 cup a week, 1-3 cups a week, 4-6 cups a week, 1 cup a day, or ≥ 2 cups a day". Each question had 5 options for intake frequency from the lowest to the highest. Food intake scores of 1 to 5 were assigned from the lowest to the highest frequency. Principal component analysis was performed to derive dietary patterns. We used the eigenvalues ≥2 in the orthogonal rotation to derive dietary patterns, and factor loading ≥0.30 to classify dietary patterns. The eigenvalues ≥2 have been used in the previous studies, and represented a strong correlation between each component and smaller variance compared with the eigenvalue < 2 [23, 24]. The factor scores of dietary patterns were calculated using the sum of food intake scores divided by factor loadings [9], and were classified into tertiles for each dietary pattern.

### Anthropometric measurements

The assessments of anthropometric data were carried out by the medical staff in the MJ health screening centers. Weight (kg), height (cm), and body fat (%) were measured by using a bioelectrical impedance analysis instrument (InBody Co., Ltd., Seoul, South Korea). BMI was computed as weight (kg) divided by the square of height ($m^2$), and classified as underweight, normal weight, overweight, or obesity (BMI < 18.5 kg/$m^2$, 18.5 kg/$m^2$ ≤ BMI < 24 kg/$m^2$, 24 kg/$m^2$ ≤ BMI < 27 kg/$m^2$, and BMI ≥ 27 kg/$m^2$, respectively) [25]. Body fat was defined as low (< 25% for men and < 30% for women) and high (≥ 25% for men and ≥ 30% for women) [26–28]. Waist circumference was assessed at the mid-point between the lowest rib and the iliac crest on standing position, while hip circumference was assessed at the point generating the maximum circumference in the buttocks using a measuring tape. We used the mean of waist or hip circumference as the cut-off point to dichotomize these two variables into low (waist circumference < 95.8 cm for men and < 85.2 cm for women, hip circumference < 100.5 cm for men and < 101.1 cm for women) and high (waist circumference ≥ 95.8 cm for men and ≥ 85.2 cm for women, hip circumference ≥ 100.5 cm for men and ≥ 101.1 cm for women). Waist-to-hip ratio was calculated and defined as low (< 0.90 for men and < 0.85 for women) and high (≥ 0.90 for men and ≥ 0.85 for women) [29].

### Blood pressure and biochemical measurements

Blood samples were collected after overnight fasting for 12–14 h. BP was measured in a sitting position using a sphygmomanometer. Blood HDL-C, TC, TG, FBG, and CRP levels were analyzed using the commercial reagents or kits, and LDL-C levels were calculated using Friedewald's formula: LDL-C (mg/dL) = TC-(HDL-C + TG/5). The number of neutrophils and lymphocytes was determined, and NLR was calculated using the absolute neutrophil count divided by the absolute lymphocyte count. The IDF definition was used to define metabolic syndrome to categorize systolic BP (low < 130 mmHg and high ≥130 mmHg), diastolic BP (low < 85 mmHg and high ≥85 mmHg), HDL-C (low < 1.03 mmol/L and high ≥1.03 mmol/L for men, low < 1.29 mmol/L and high ≥1.29 mmol/L for women), TG (low < 1.70 mmol/L and high ≥1.70 mmol/L), and FBG (low < 5.60 mmol/L and high ≥5.60 mmol/L) [1]. Whereas TC and LDL-C levels were defined as low (< 6.2 mmol/L for TC and < 4.1 mmol/L for LDL-C) and high (≥ 6.2 mmol/L for TC and ≥ 4.1 mmol/L for LDL-C) [30].

### Covariates

Demographic and lifestyle characteristics such as sex, age, marital status, education, occupation, current smoking or drinking status, and physical activity were collected using an administered questionnaire from the MJ Group. Education level was dichotomized as low (high school and below) and high (above high school). Physical activity was categorized as low (< 1 h a week), moderate (1–2 h a week), and high (> 2 h a week).

### Statistical analysis

Chi-square test and general linear model test were used to determine the differences of categorical and continuous variables, respectively, in the characteristics of the subjects with low or high CRP and NLR levels. Odds ratios (OR) with 95% confidence interval were derived using multivariate logistic regression analysis to compare the association of dietary patterns, anthropometric status, and metabolic parameters with CRP and NLR levels in men and women. Model 1 was unadjusted and model 2 was adjusted for age, marital status, education, occupation, smoking, drinking status, and physical activity. A significance level of $P \leq 0.05$ was used for all analyses, and SPSS 24 (IBM Corp., Armonk, NY, USA) software was used to analyze the data.

## Results

Among 26,016 subjects with metabolic syndrome, 4639 (27.5%), 6650 (39.4%), 4089 (24.2%), 5687 (33.7%), 8933 (52.9%), and 11,903 (70.5%) subjects had high waist circumference (≥ 95.8 cm), high systolic BP, high diastolic BP, low HDL-C, high TG, and high FBG levels, respectively, among men, and 5131 (56.2%), 4139 (46.4%), 1658 (18.2%), 2785 (30.5%), 4155 (45%), and 6333 (69.4%) subjects had high waist circumference (≥ 85.2 cm), high systolic BP, high diastolic BP, low HDL-C, high TG, and high FBG levels, respectively, among women (data not shown).

### Dietary patterns

Two dietary patterns were derived from principal component analysis (Table 1) and defined as the western and prudent dietary patterns. The western and prudent dietary patterns had 12 and 9 food groups or food items, respectively. Legumes or soy products and seafood had factor loading ≥0.30 in both factors, and had higher factor loadings in the prudent dietary pattern. Therefore, we classified both food groups in the prudent dietary pattern. The western dietary pattern was reflected as high intake of deep-fried food, processed food (e.g. sausage, ham, and canned food), sugary drinks, meat (e.g. beef, lamb, pork, veal, chicken and duck), sauce (e.g. pepper salt, ketchup, vinegar, hot sauce and soy sauce), eggs (e.g. chicken, duck and quail eggs), organ meats (e.g. kidneys, intestines, liver and heart), rice or flour cooked in oil (e.g. fried noodle and rice noodle), instant noodle, jam or honey, rice or flour products (e.g. rice, plain bread, noodle and cruller), and refined desert; while the prudent dietary pattern was reflected by high intake of dark-colored vegetables (e.g. spinach, squash, carrot and tomato), light-colored vegetables (e.g. cabbage, pechay, cucumber and radish), vegetables with oil or dressing, fruit, legumes or soy products (e.g. soybean milk, tofu and dried bean curd), milk (e.g. powdered and fresh milk), dairy products (e.g. cheese and yoghurt), root crops (e.g. corn, potato and taro), and seafood (e.g. fish, shells, oysters and shrimps). The western and prudent dietary patterns had a total variance of 26.3% (16.9 and 9.4%, respectively) and eigenvalues > 2. The two dietary patterns were similar to the unhealthy and healthy dietary patterns, respectively.

**Table 1** Factor loadings and dietary patterns derived from principal component analysis of food frequency questionnaire data

| Food Groups | Factor I Western dietary pattern | Factor II Prudent dietary pattern |
|---|---|---|
| Milk | −0.045 | 0.380 |
| Dairy products | 0.166 | 0.377 |
| Eggs | 0.502 | 0.112 |
| Meat | 0.531 | 0.131 |
| Organ meats | 0.500 | 0.110 |
| Legumes/soy products | 0.306 | 0.390 |
| Seafood | 0.316 | 0.363 |
| Light-colored vegetables | −0.039 | 0.799 |
| Dark-colored vegetables | −0.057 | 0.831 |
| Fruit | −0.014 | 0.521 |
| Vegetables with oil/dressing | 0.261 | 0.524 |
| Rice/flour products | 0.381 | 0.143 |
| Whole grains | 0.071 | 0.228 |
| Root crops | 0.201 | 0.369 |
| Refined dessert | 0.319 | 0.131 |
| Jam/honey | 0.382 | 0.108 |
| Sugary drinks | 0.542 | −0.098 |
| Rice/flour cooked in oil | 0.436 | 0.066 |
| Deep-fried food | 0.619 | 0.044 |
| Instant noodle | 0.392 | −0.083 |
| Processed food | 0.586 | 0.036 |
| Sauce | 0.526 | 0.071 |

### Characteristics of subjects

The characteristics of subjects with low or high CRP and NLR in both genders are summarized in Table 2. There were 10,096 (38.8%) and 7857 (30.2%) subjects with high CRP and NLR, respectively. Among those who had high CRP or NLR, the proportion of men was 59.6 and 65.6%, respectively. The majority of the subjects with high CRP or NLR were between the ages of 46 and 60 years (55.6 and 55.6%), were married (84.3 and 85.5%), had education level of high school and below (54.1 and 52.9%), had professional jobs (43.6 and 45.2%), did not smoke (95.0 and 95.5%), did not drink alcohol (94.0 and 94.2%), and had low physical activity (51.2 and 49.6%). The results also showed that subjects with high

**Table 2** Characteristics of subjects across values of C-reactive protein and neutrophil-to-lymphocyte ratio ($n = 26{,}016$) [a]

| Variables | C-reactive protein | | $P^b$ | Neutrophil-to-lymphocyte ratio | | $P^b$ |
|---|---|---|---|---|---|---|
| | < 28.6 nmol/L | ≥ 28.6 nmol/L | | < 3.0 | ≥ 3.0 | |
| Sex, % | | | 0.000 | | | 0.049 |
| Men | 68.2 | 59.6 | | 64.6 | 65.6 | |
| Women | 31.8 | 40.4 | | 35.4 | 34.4 | |
| Age, % | | | 0.205 | | | 0.973 |
| 35–45 y | 15.8 | 15.0 | | 15.4 | 15.5 | |
| 46–60 y | 55.4 | 55.6 | | 55.4 | 55.6 | |
| > 60 y | 28.9 | 29.4 | | 29.2 | 28.9 | |
| Marital status, % | | | 0.043 | | | 0.009 |
| Not married | 3.0 | 3.5 | | 3.2 | 3.0 | |
| Married | 84.6 | 84.3 | | 84.0 | 85.5 | |
| Divorced | 12.4 | 12.2 | | 12.7 | 11.5 | |
| Education, % | | | 0.000 | | | 0.247 |
| Low | 51.7 | 54.1 | | 52.5 | 52.9 | |
| High | 48.3 | 45.9 | | 47.5 | 47.1 | |
| Occupation, % | | | 0.000 | | | 0.004 |
| Professional | 48.3 | 43.6 | | 47.0 | 45.2 | |
| Not professional | 31.2 | 35.7 | | 32.9 | 33.0 | |
| Unemployed/retired | 20.5 | 20.7 | | 20.1 | 21.8 | |
| Current smoking, % | | | 0.000 | | | 0.000 |
| No | 96.9 | 95.0 | | 96.4 | 95.5 | |
| Yes | 3.1 | 5.0 | | 3.6 | 4.5 | |
| Current drinking status, % | | | 0.000 | | | 0.000 |
| No | 96.4 | 94.0 | | 95.9 | 94.2 | |
| Yes | 3.6 | 6.0 | | 4.1 | 5.8 | |
| Physical activity, % | | | 0.000 | | | 0.000 |
| Low | 48.8 | 51.2 | | 41.3 | 49.6 | |
| Moderate | 45.5 | 42.3 | | 52.8 | 43.9 | |
| High | 5.8 | 6.5 | | 5.9 | 6.4 | |
| Western dietary pattern, % | | | 0.000 | | | 0.000 |
| T1, *n* | 34.4 | 31.7 | | 34.7 | 30.2 | |
| T2, *n* | 33.5 | 33.1 | | 32.9 | 34.2 | |
| T3, *n* | 32.1 | 35.2 | | 32.4 | 35.6 | |
| Prudent dietary patterns, % | | | 0.000 | | | 0.000 |
| T1, *n* | 31.7 | 36.0 | | 32.9 | 34.4 | |
| T2, *n* | 31.4 | 36.2 | | 32.8 | 34.5 | |
| T3, *n* | 36.9 | 27.8 | | 34.3 | 31.1 | |
| Body mass index, kg/m$^2$ | 26.9 ± 2.3 | 27.6 ± 2.8 | 0.000 | 27.0 ± 2.4 | 27.4 ± 2.6 | 0.000 |
| Body fat, % | 26.7 ± 4.3 | 28.0 ± 4.7 | 0.000 | 27.0 ± 4.4 | 27.6 ± 4.6 | 0.000 |
| Waist circumference, cm | 92.0 ± 6.5 | 94.4 ± 8.6 | 0.000 | 92.1 ± 6.9 | 94.6 ± 8.1 | 0.000 |
| Hip circumference, cm | 100.0 ± 5.9 | 101.5 ± 6.7 | 0.000 | 100.2 ± 6.1 | 101.3 ± 6.3 | 0.000 |
| Waist-to-hip ratio | 0.92 ± 0.07 | 0.93 ± 0.07 | 0.000 | 0.92 ± 0.06 | 0.94 ± 8.13 | 0.000 |
| Systolic blood pressure, mmHg | 120 ± 30 | 124 ± 33 | 0.000 | 120 ± 31 | 125 ± 32 | 0.000 |

**Table 2** Characteristics of subjects across values of C-reactive protein and neutrophil-to-lymphocyte ratio ($n = 26{,}016$) [a] *(Continued)*

| Variables | C-reactive protein | | $P^b$ | Neutrophil-to-lymphocyte ratio | | $P^b$ |
|---|---|---|---|---|---|---|
| | < 28.6 nmol/L | ≥ 28.6 nmol/L | | < 3.0 | ≥ 3.0 | |
| Diastolic blood pressure, mmHg | 74 ± 20 | 75 ± 19 | 0.000 | 74 ± 20 | 75 ± 19 | 0.000 |
| High-density lipoprotein-cholesterol, mmol/L | 1.19 ± 0.34 | 1.12 ± 0.31 | 0.000 | 1.17 ± 0.34 | 1.15 ± 0.07 | 0.026 |
| Low-density lipoprotein-cholesterol, mmol/L | 3.61 ± 0.83 | 3.75 ± 0.87 | 0.000 | 3.62 ± 0.83 | 3.73 ± 0.89 | 0.000 |
| Total cholesterol, mmol/L | 5.19 ± 0.87 | 5.29 ± 0.89 | 0.000 | 5.20 ± 0.86 | 5.30 ± 0.92 | 0.000 |
| Triglycerides, mmol/L | 1.96 ± .37 | 2.17 ± 1.34 | 0.000 | 2.01 ± 1.39 | 2.09 ± 1.30 | 0.000 |
| Fasting blood glucose, mmol/L | 6.11 ± 1.54 | 6.76 ± 2.43 | 0.000 | 6.20 ± 1.73 | 6.67 ± 2.29 | 0.000 |

[a]Data are presented as % for categorical variables and mean ± SD for continuous variables
[b]*P*-values were derived from chi-square test for categorical variables and general linear regression for continuous variables

CRP or NLR were more likely to consume the highest tertile in the western dietary pattern (35.2 and 35.6%) and the lowest tertile in the prudent dietary pattern (36.0 and 34.4%). Subjects with high CRP or NLR had significantly higher BMI (27.6 ± 2.8 and 27.4 ± 2.6 kg/m$^2$), body fat (28.0 ± 4.7% and 27.6 ± 4.6%), waist circumference (94.4 ± 8.6 and 94.6 ± 8.1 cm), hip circumference (101.5 ± 6.7 and 101.3 ± 6.3 cm), and waist-to-hip ratio (0.93 ± 0.07 and 0.94 ± 8.13) than those who with low CRP or NLR. Additionally, subjects with high CRP or NLR had significantly higher systolic BP (124 ± 33 and 125 ± 32 mmHg), diastolic BP (75 ± 19 and 75 ± 19 mmHg), LDL-C (3.75 ± 0.87 and 3.73 ± 0.89 mmol/L), TC (5.29 ± 0.89 and 5.30 ± 0.92 mmol/L), TG (2.17 ± 1.34 and 2.09 ± 1.30 mmol/L), and FBG (6.76 ± 2.43 and 6.67 ± 2.29 mmol/L) but lower HDL-C (1.12 ± 0.31 and 1.15 ± 0.07 mmol/L) than those who with low CRP or NLR.

### Dietary patterns, nutritional status and levels of CRP and NLR in men and women

The results showed that regardless of gender, subjects who had higher tertiles (T2 and T3) of the western dietary pattern, overweight or obesity, high body fat, high waist or hip circumference, high waist-to-hip ratio, high systolic or diastolic BP, low HDL-C, high LDL-C, high TC, high TG, or high FBG had significantly increased odds ratios of high CRP (≥ 28.6 nmol/L) in both models (Table 3). However, higher tertiles (T2 and T3) of the prudent dietary pattern were significantly associated with decreased odds ratios of high CRP in men and women in both models.

Furthermore, subjects who had the highest tertile (T3) of the western dietary pattern, obesity, high body fat, high waist or hip circumference, high waist-to-hip ratio, low HDL-C, high LDL-C, high TG, or high FBG had significantly increased odds ratios of high NLR (≥ 3.0) in men and women in both models (Table 4). However, the highest tertile (T3) of the prudent dietary pattern was significantly correlated with reduced odds ratios of high NLR (≥ 3.0) in men and women in both models. Only men with high systolic or diastolic BP or high TC had increased odds ratios of high NLR (≥ 3.0) in both models.

## Discussion

Our main findings are that dietary patterns, anthropometric measurements, and metabolic parameters were directly associated with CRP and NLR among Taiwanese men and women aged 35 and above with metabolic syndrome. Subjects who consumed more western dietary pattern were positively correlated with inflammation, while subjects who consumed more prudent dietary pattern were inversely associated with inflammation in both genders. Moreover, anthropometric measurements and metabolic parameters were strongly associated with CRP and NLR in both genders.

The present study revealed that subjects with the high levels of inflammatory markers were more frequent in men and less active physically compared with those with low levels of inflammatory markers. The findings were consistent with the results in the previous studies [16, 31]. The western dietary pattern in this study was similar to the unhealthy dietary pattern that included a high relative amount of red meat, processed food, high-fat food, sweets, salts, and food additives [8]. This dietary pattern was significantly correlated with increased CRP and NLR levels in the subjects with metabolic syndrome. The previous study found that an unhealthy dietary pattern was positively associated with the levels of inflammatory markers such as CRP, interleukin-6 and sICAM-1 [32]. Additionally, there was a positive association between western dietary pattern and CRP concentration [9, 33]. An animal study also revealed that neutrophil counts were increased in mice fed a high-fat diet [34]. In contrast with the unhealthy dietary pattern, the prudent dietary pattern in this study was defined by foods high in complex carbohydrate, unsaturated fat, fiber, antioxidants, vitamins, and minerals. Moreover, a healthy dietary pattern had beneficial effects on inflammation [35]. The prudent breakfast high in dietary fiber and β-glucan for 12 weeks improved plasma CRP in overweight and mildly hypercholesterolemic adults aged of 25–67 years compared with

**Table 3** Odds ratios for high C-reactive protein by different dietary patterns, anthropometric measurements, and metabolic parameters

| Variables | Odds ratio (95% Confidence interval) | | | |
|---|---|---|---|---|
| | Men ($n = 6021$) | | Women ($n = 4075$) | |
| | Model 1[1] | Model 2[2] | Model 1[1] | Model 2[2] |
| Western dietary pattern | | | | |
| T1 | 1 | 1 | 1 | 1 |
| T2 | 0.892 (0.843–0.944) *** | 0.903 (0.853–0.956) *** | 0.843 (0.778–0.913) *** | 0.855 (0.788–0.927) *** |
| T3 | 1.116 (1.053–1.184) *** | 1.108 (1.044–1.176) ** | 1.162 (1.070–1.263) *** | 1.181 (1.086–1.284) *** |
| Prudent dietary pattern | | | | |
| T1 | 1 | 1 | 1 | 1 |
| T2 | 0.810 (0.765–0.857) *** | 0.815 (0.770–0.863) *** | 0.886 (0.824–0.954) ** | 0.891 (0.827–0.959) ** |
| T3 | 0.693 (0.654–0.735) *** | 0.696 (0.656–0.738) *** | 0.814 (0.756–0.877) *** | 0.806 (0.748–0.869) *** |
| Body mass index | | | | |
| Normal | 1 | 1 | 1 | 1 |
| Overweight | 1.230 (1.147–1.320) *** | 1.225 (1.141–1.315) *** | 1.149 (1.036–1.275) ** | 1.182 (1.065–1.313) ** |
| Obese | 1.315 (1.190–1.454) *** | 1.328 (1.199–1.470) *** | 1.961 (1.702–2.260) *** | 1.971 (1.709–2.273) *** |
| Body fat | | | | |
| Low | 1 | 1 | 1 | 1 |
| High | 1.734 (1.613–1.864) *** | 1.749 (1.624–1.884) *** | 1.454 (1.023–2.068) * | 1.413 (0.981–2.028) * |
| Waist circumference | | | | |
| Low | 1 | 1 | 1 | 1 |
| High | 1.963 (1.826–2.110) *** | 1.916 (1.782–2.061) *** | 1.986 (1.820–2.168) *** | 2.003 (1.834–2.188) *** |
| Hip circumference | | | | |
| Low | 1 | 1 | 1 | 1 |
| High | 1.422 (1.264–1.599) *** | 1.406 (1.247–1.587) *** | 1.637 (1.499–1.787) *** | 1.651 (1.510–1.805) *** |
| Waist-to-hip ratio | | | | |
| Low | 1 | 1 | 1 | 1 |
| High | 1.487 (1.384–1.598) *** | 1.488 (1.383–1.601) *** | 1.298 (1.184–1.423) *** | 1.307 (1.190–1.436) *** |
| Systolic blood pressure | | | | |
| Low | 1 | 1 | 1 | 1 |
| High | 1.258 (1.176–1.345) *** | 1.280 (1.195–1.371) *** | 1.294 (1.188–1.409) *** | 1.306 (1.196–1.425) *** |
| Diastolic blood pressure | | | | |
| Low | 1 | 1 | 1 | 1 |
| High | 1.303 (1.208–1.405) *** | 1.303 (1.208–1.406) *** | 1.306 (1.170–1.457) *** | 1.313 (1.175–1.467) *** |
| High-density lipoprotein-cholesterol | | | | |
| High | 1 | 1 | 1 | 1 |
| Low | 1.625 (1.517–1.740) *** | 1.635 (1.525–1.753) *** | 1.379 (1.257–1.512) *** | 1.419 (1.292–1.558) *** |
| Low-density lipoprotein-cholesterol | | | | |
| Low | 1 | 1 | 1 | 1 |
| High | 1.278 (1.191–1.373) *** | 1.276 (1.188–1.371) *** | 1.239 (1.132–1.356) *** | 1.250 (1.141–1.369) *** |

**Table 3** Odds ratios for high C-reactive protein by different dietary patterns, anthropometric measurements, and metabolic parameters *(Continued)*

| Variables | Odds ratio (95% Confidence interval) | | | |
|---|---|---|---|---|
| | Men ($n$ = 6021) | | Women ($n$ = 4075) | |
| | Model 1[1] | Model 2[2] | Model 1[1] | Model 2[2] |
| Total cholesterol | | | | |
| Low | 1 | 1 | 1 | 1 |
| High | 1.157 (1.083–1.237) *** | 1.148 (1.074–1.227) *** | 1.228 (1.123–1.342) *** | 1.225 (1.118–1.342) *** |
| Triglycerides | | | | |
| Low | 1 | 1 | 1 | 1 |
| High | 1.493 (1.397–1.595) *** | 1.475 (1.379–1.578) *** | 1.717 (1.576–1.871) *** | 1.694 (1.553–1.847) *** |
| Fasting blood glucose | | | | |
| Low | 1 | 1 | 1 | 1 |
| High | 1.366 (1.270–1.470) *** | 1.398 (1.297–1.506) *** | 1.257 (1.146–1.380) *** | 1.245 (1.133–1.368) *** |

[1]Unadjusted. [2]Adjusted for age, marital status, education, occupation, smoking, drinking status, and physical activity. *$P < 0.05$, **$P < 0.01$, ***$P < 0.001$. The variables were defined as the following: CRP: low < 28.6 nmol/L and high ≥28.6 nmol/L, normal BMI: 18.5 kg/m$^2$ ≤ BMI < 24 kg/m$^2$; overweight BMI: 24 kg/m$^2$ ≤ BMI < 27 kg/m$^2$; obesity BMI: ≥ 27 kg/m$^2$, body fat: low < 25% and high ≥25% for men; low < 30% and high ≥30% for women, waist circumference: low < 95.8 cm and high ≥95.8 cm for men; low < 85.2 cm and high ≥85.2 cm for women, hip circumference: low < 100.5 cm and high ≥100.5 cm for men; low < 101.1 cm and high ≥101.1 cm for women, waist-to-hip ratio: low < 0.90 and high ≥0.90 for men; low < 0.85 and high ≥0.85 for women, systolic BP: low < 130 mmHg and high ≥130 mmHg, diastolic BP: low < 85 mmHg and high ≥85 mmHg, HDL-C: low < 1.03 mmol/L and high ≥1.03 mmol/L for men; low < 1.29 mmol/L and high ≥1.29 mmol/L for women, LDL-C: low < 4.1 mmol/L and high ≥4.1 mmol/L, TC: low < 6.2 mmol/L and high ≥6.2 mmol/L, TG: low < 1.70 mmol/L and high ≥1.70 mmol/L, FBG: low < 5.60 mmol/L and high ≥5.60 mmol/L

the usual breakfast [36]. Furthermore, the Mediterranean diet characterized as high in fiber, antioxidants, and unsaturated and polyunsaturated fatty acids [37] was correlated with decreases in platelet count, white blood cells (WBC) count and CRP [38, 39]. Our findings showed that there were no differences between men and women in the effects of the western or prudent dietary pattern on CRP and NLR levels. Similar to our results, following the Mediterranean diet for 4 weeks, had similar effects on high-sensitivity CRP levels in mildly hypercholesterolemic men and women aged of 24–53 years with CVD risk factors [40], indicating there were no differences between men and women in the effects of the Mediterranean diet on systemic inflammation.

Our results reported that the anthropometric measures such as BMI, body fat, waist or hip circumference, and waist-to-hip ratio were associated with inflammation in both men and women with metabolic syndrome. Some evidences supported our findings. BMI was independently correlated with certain markers related to inflammatory responses, including CRP, amylin, C-peptide, insulin, leptin, WBC, and NLR [41, 42]. The indicators of central obesity such as waist or hip circumference and waist-to-hip ratio showed a strong positive correlation with CRP not only in healthy population, but also in the population with metabolic syndrome [43, 44]. Moreover, waist circumference was increased with elevated WBC and NLR, suggesting that waist circumference might be used as a parameter of evaluating WBC or NLR [45]. Body fat and BMI were also significantly associated with CRP in obese males and females with metabolic syndrome and heart failure [46]. Additionally, obese subjects had higher NLR compared with healthy subjects, and elevated NLR considered as an inflammatory marker was an independent predictor of type 2 diabetes in obese subjects [47]. Furthermore, this study found that more than 30% of subjects with metabolic syndrome had higher levels of CRP (38.8%) or NLR (30.2%). The previous studies also revealed that the components of metabolic syndrome influenced the levels of CRP and NLR [48, 49]. Subjects with metabolic syndrome had significantly increased neutrophil counts, but reduced lymphocyte counts [50]. Hypercholesterolemia was one of the major risk factors of elevated pro-inflammatory cytokines. Hyperlipidemia had effects on homeostasis of immune cells and was associated with increased neutrophil counts [51]. The levels of CRP were positively correlated with fasting and 2-h post-load glucose concentrations in individuals with impaired glucose tolerance [52], and individuals with prediabetes also had higher CRP levels [53]. The potential interaction among obesity, metabolic disorder, and activated inflammation in subjects with metabolic syndrome has been reported. The association between chronic inflammation and metabolic syndrome was linked to central adiposity, which was accompanied by a decrease of adiponectin formed in adipose tissue and increased secretion of inflammatory markers such as CRP [54].

Our results found that both men and women with high consumption of the western dietary pattern, low consumption of the prudent dietary pattern, high values of anthropometric parameters or metabolic disorder

**Table 4** Odds ratios for high neutrophil-to-lymphocyte ratio by different dietary patterns, anthropometric measurements, and metabolic parameters

| Variables | Men ($n = 5155$) | | Women ($n = 2702$) | |
|---|---|---|---|---|
| | Model 1[1] | Model 2[2] | Model 1[1] | Model 2[2] |
| Western dietary pattern | | | | |
| T1 | 1 | 1 | 1 | 1 |
| T2 | 0.955 (0.900–1.013) | 0.963 (0.908–1.022) | 0.941 (0.867–1.021) | 0.945 (0.871–1.026) |
| T3 | 1.189 (1.118–1.264) *** | 1.199 (1.126–1.275) *** | 1.100 (1.012–1.195) * | 1.108 (1.019–1.204) * |
| Prudent dietary pattern | | | | |
| T1 | 1 | 1 | 1 | 1 |
| T2 | 0.916 (0.864–0.972) ** | 0.921 (0.868–0.977) ** | 1.134 (1.046–1.228) | 1.111 (1.023–1.205) |
| T3 | 0.881 (0.830–0.935) *** | 0.883 (0.832–0.938) *** | 0.961 (0.873–1.056) * | 0.963 (0.874–1.059) * |
| Body mass index | | | | |
| Normal | 1 | 1 | 1 | 1 |
| Overweight | 1.154 (1.073–1.241) *** | 1.141 (1.061–1.227) *** | 1.081 (0.978–1.195) | 1.096 (0.998–1.212) |
| Obese | 1.162 (1.049–1.288) ** | 1.188 (1.070–1.319) ** | 1.575 (1.375–1.804) *** | 1.576 (1.375–1.806) *** |
| Body fat | | | | |
| Low | 1 | 1 | 1 | 1 |
| High | 1.276 (1.186–1.374) *** | 1.286 (1.192–1.386) *** | 1.301 (1.143–1.480) *** | 1.158 (1.015–1.323) * |
| Waist circumference | | | | |
| Low | 1 | 1 | 1 | 1 |
| High | 1.711 (1.588–1.843) *** | 1.690 (1.568–1.822) *** | 1.468 (1.335–1.614) *** | 1.475 (1.341–1.623) *** |
| Hip circumference | | | | |
| Low | 1 | 1 | 1 | 1 |
| High | 1.185 (1.052–1.334) ** | 1.201 (1.063–1.358) ** | 1.259 (1.145–1.386) *** | 1.275 (1.157–1.404) *** |
| Waist-to-hip ratio | | | | |
| Low | 1 | 1 | 1 | 1 |
| High | 1.626 (1.506–1.754) *** | 1.630 (1.509–1.761) *** | 1.336 (1.211–1.474) *** | 1.331 (1.204–1.472) *** |
| Systolic blood pressure | | | | |
| Low | 1 | 1 | 1 | 1 |
| High | 1.122 (1.047–1.203) ** | 1.124 (1.047–1.206) ** | 1.037 (0.946–1.138) | 1.038 (0.944–1.142) |
| Diastolic blood pressure | | | | |
| Low | 1 | 1 | 1 | 1 |
| High | 1.182 (1.092–1.278) *** | 1.176 (1.087–1.273) *** | 0.946 (0.839–1.067) | 0.928 (0.821–1.049) |
| High-density lipoprotein-cholesterol | | | | |
| High | 1 | 1 | 1 | 1 |
| Low | 1.197 (1.114–1.286) *** | 1.203 (1.119–1.294) *** | 1.138 (1.031–1.257) * | 1.162 (1.051–1.286) ** |
| Low-density lipoprotein-cholesterol | | | | |
| Low | 1 | 1 | 1 | 1 |
| High | 1.197 (1.112–1.289) *** | 1.200 (1.114–1.293) *** | 1.105 (1.002–1.219) * | 1.113 (1.008–1.229) * |

**Table 4** Odds ratios for high neutrophil-to-lymphocyte ratio by different dietary patterns, anthropometric measurements, and metabolic parameters *(Continued)*

| Variables | Men ($n = 5155$) | | Women ($n = 2702$) | |
|---|---|---|---|---|
| | Model 1[1] | Model 2[2] | Model 1[1] | Model 2[2] |
| Total cholesterol | | | | |
| Low | 1 | 1 | 1 | 1 |
| High | 1.138 (1.063–1.219) *** | 1.138 (1.062–1.220) *** | 1.070 (0.971–1.179) | 1.069 (0.968–1.180) |
| Triglycerides | | | | |
| Low | 1 | 1 | 1 | 1 |
| High | 1.262 (1.179–1.352) *** | 1.251 (1.167–1.342) *** | 1.157 (1.055–1.269) ** | 1.140 (1.039–1.252) ** |
| Fasting blood glucose | | | | |
| Low | 1 | 1 | 1 | 1 |
| High | 1.294 (1.199–1.396) *** | 1.300 (1.203–1.405) *** | 1.199 (1.083–1.328) *** | 1.180 (1.064–1.308) ** |

[1]Unadjusted. [2] Adjusted for age, marital status, education, occupation, smoking, drinking status and physical activity. *$P < 0.05$, **$P < 0.01$, ***$P < 0.001$. The variables were defined as the following: NLR: low < 3.0 and normal ≥3.0; normal BMI: 18.5 kg/m$^2$ ≤ BMI < 24 kg/m$^2$; overweight BMI: 24 kg/m$^2$ ≤ BMI < 27 kg/m$^2$; obesity BMI: ≥ 27 kg/m$^2$, body fat: low < 25% and high ≥25% for men; low < 30% and high ≥30% for women, waist circumference: low < 95.8 cm and high ≥95.8 cm for men; low < 85.2 cm and high ≥85.2 cm for women, hip circumference: low < 100.5 cm and high ≥100.5 cm for men; low < 101.1 cm and high ≥101.1 cm for women, waist-to-hip ratio: low < 0.90 and high ≥0.90 for men; low < 0.85 and high ≥0.85 for women, systolic BP: low < 130 mmHg and high ≥130 mmHg, diastolic BP: low < 85 mmHg and high ≥85 mmHg, HDL-C: low < 1.03 mmol/L and high ≥1.03 mmol/L for men; low < 1.29 mmol/L and high ≥1.29 mmol/L for women, LDL-C: low < 4.1 mmol/L and high ≥4.1 mmol/L, TC: low < 6.2 mmol/L and high ≥6.2 mmol/L, TG: low < 1.70 mmol/L and high ≥1.70 mmol/L, FBG: low < 5.60 mmol/L and high ≥5.60 mmol/L

increased the likelihood of being high CRP or NLR. However, there were gender differences in the effects of BP or TC on NLR values. Higher systolic or diastolic BP or TC was significantly associated with increased odds ratios of high NLR in men, but not in women. There is still a conflicting evidence regarding whether NLR is a good indicator of inflammation in a metabolic syndrome population. Neutrophil-to-lymphocyte ratio was not a better indicator of inflammation compared with CRP in obese subjects with metabolic syndrome [55], although both CRP and NLR were simple and effective predictors of inflammation in subjects with metabolic syndrome. CRP as an acute phase protein is a sensitive biomarker for systemic inflammation and correlated significantly with metabolic abnormality [56]. Contrarily, high neutrophil counts play an important role in atherogenesis and atherothrombosis, and low lymphocyte counts have been observed in patients with acute coronary syndrome and its complication [57]. Use of the neutrophil-to-lymphocyte ratio has recently emerged as an alternate potential biomarker for both metabolic syndrome and CVD events [49, 58].

### Strengths and limitations

This study has some strengths. This is the first study to discuss the association of dietary patterns, anthropometric measures and metabolic parameters with inflammatory markers in Taiwanese middle-aged and older adults with metabolic syndrome. In addition, the sample size was large from the population of interest. We defined metabolic syndrome by using the IDF definition, which uses central obesity as an essential component followed by other components of metabolic syndrome. This parameter was appropriate because the prevalence of central obesity or metabolic syndrome increases with age in both genders in Taiwan [5] and was expected to adequately represent the health issues most prevalent among middle-aged and older adults in Taiwan. Some limitations of the study included the cross-sectional study design that limits the applicability of the findings in establishing causality between the variables. Furthermore, there may be some potential confounders in this study that could not be controlled for due to the inherent limitations of nutrition research; such as the intake of energy, protein, and other specific nutrients. The conclusion may not be applied to the whole Taiwanese population with metabolic syndrome, since we only analyzed the subjects aged 35 years and older, and the data from one private health management screening institution with multi-centers in Taiwan.

## Conclusions

Men and women have a similar association of dietary patterns and anthropometric measurements with inflammatory markers. The western dietary pattern is positively correlated with CRP and NLR. In contrast, the prudent dietary pattern is inversely associated with CRP and NLR. Furthermore, better BMI, body fat, waist or hip circumference, and waist-to-hip ratio improve CRP and NLR. Men and women have similar associations between metabolic parameters (systolic and diastolic BP, HDL-C, LDL-C, TC, TG, and FBG) and CRP. However, systolic or diastolic BP and TC show significantly positive correlations with NLR only in men.

**Abbreviations**

BMI: Body mass index; BP: Blood pressure; CRP: C-reactive protein; CVD: Cardiovascular disease; FBG: Fasting blood glucose; FFQ: Food frequency questionnaire; HDL-C: High-density lipoprotein-cholesterol; IDF: International Diabetes Federation; LDL-C: Low-density lipoprotein-cholesterol; MJ: Mei Jau; NLR: Neutrophil-to-lymphocyte ratio; OR: Odds ratios; sICAM: Soluble intracellular adhesion molecule; TC: Total cholesterol; TG: Triglycerides; WBC: White blood cells

**Acknowledgements**

The authors would like to thank the Indonesia Endowment Fund for Education (LPDP-BUDI LN) offered by the Ministry of Finance and the Ministry of Research Technology Higher Education, Republic of Indonesia to support AS for his PhD degree.

**Funding**

AS is supported by Indonesia Endowment Fund for Education (LPDP-BUDI LN) scholarship offered by the Ministry of Finance and the Ministry of Research Technology Higher Education, Republic of Indonesia.

**Authors' contributions**

JCJC was the principal investigator. AS and JCJC designed the research. CYH and HHR managed and retrieved the data. AS, JCJC, CYH and HHR contributed to data analysis and interpretation of data. AS and JCJC wrote the manuscript. All authors participated in critical revision of the manuscript for important intellectual content, and have read and approved the final manuscript.

**Competing interests**

The authors declare that they have no competing interests.

**Author details**

[1]School of Nutrition and Health Sciences, College of Nutrition, Taipei Medical University, 250 Wu-Hsing Street, Taipei 110, Taiwan. [2]Department of Nutrition Science, Faculty of Medicine, Diponegoro University, Semarang, Indonesia. [3]Department of Information Management, National Taipei University of Nursing and Health Sciences, Taipei, Taiwan. [4]Master Program in Global Health and Development, College of Public Health, Taipei Medical University, Taipei, Taiwan. [5]Joint Commission of Taiwan, New Taipei City, Taiwan. [6]Nutrition Research Center, Taipei Medical University Hospital, Taipei, Taiwan.

**References**

1. Alberti KG, Zimmet P, Shaw J. The metabolic syndrome-a new worldwide definition. Lancet. 2005;366:1059–62. https://doi.org/10.1016/s0140-6736(05)67402-8.
2. Beltran-Sanchez H, Harhay MO, Harhay MM, McElligott S. Prevalence and trends of metabolic syndrome in the adult U.S. population, 1999-2010. J Am Coll Cardiol. 2013;62:697–703. https://doi.org/10.1016/j.jacc.2013.05.064.
3. Gundogan K, Bayram F, Capak M, Tanriverdi F, Karaman A, Ozturk A, et al. Prevalence of metabolic syndrome in the Mediterranean region of Turkey: evaluation of hypertension, diabetes mellitus, obesity, and dyslipidemia. Metab Syndr Relat Disord. 2009;7:427–34. https://doi.org/10.1089/met.2008.0068.
4. Scuteri A, Laurent S, Cucca F, Cockcroft J, Cunha PG, Manas LR, et al. Metabolic syndrome across Europe: different clusters of risk factors. Eur J Prev Cardiol. 2015;22:486–91. https://doi.org/10.1177/2047487314525529.
5. Yeh CJ, Chang HY, Pan WH. Time trend of obesity, the metabolic syndrome and related dietary pattern in Taiwan: from NAHSIT 1993-1996 to NAHSIT 2005-2008. Asia Pac J Clin Nutr. 2011;20:292–300.
6. Ridker PM, Buring JE, Cook NR, Rifai N. C-reactive protein, the metabolic syndrome, and risk of incident cardiovascular events: an 8-year follow-up of 14719 initially healthy American women. Circulation. 2003;107:391–7.
7. Lopez-Garcia E, Schulze MB, Meigs JB, Manson JE, Rifai N, Stampfer MJ, et al. Consumption of trans fatty acids is related to plasma biomarkers of inflammation and endothelial dysfunction. J Nutr. 2005;135:562–6. https://doi.org/10.1093/jn/135.3.562.
8. Esmaillzadeh A, Kimiagar M, Mehrabi Y, Azadbakht L, Hu FB, Willett WC. Dietary patterns and markers of systemic inflammation among Iranian women. J Nutr. 2007;137:992–8. https://doi.org/10.1093/jn/137.4.992.
9. Syauqy A, Hsu C-Y, Rau H-H, JC-J C. Association of dietary patterns with components of metabolic syndrome and inflammation among middle-aged and older adults with metabolic syndrome in Taiwan. Nutrients. 2018;10:143. https://doi.org/10.3390/nu10020143.
10. Esmaillzadeh A, Kimiagar M, Mehrabi Y, Azadbakht L, Hu FB, Willett WC. Fruit and vegetable intakes, C-reactive protein, and the metabolic syndrome. Am J Clin Nutr. 2006;84:1489–97. https://doi.org/10.1093/ajcn/84.6.1489.
11. Lee Y, Kang D, Lee SA. Effect of dietary patterns on serum C-reactive protein level. Nutr Metab Cardiovasc Dis. 2014;24:1004–11. https://doi.org/10.1016/j.numecd.2014.05.001.
12. DeLoach S, Keith SW, Gidding SS, Falkner B. Obesity associated inflammation in African American adolescents and adults. Am J Med Sci. 2014;347:357–63. https://doi.org/10.1097/MAJ.0b013e31829555f0.
13. Menke A, Muntner P, Wildman RP, Reynolds K, He J. Measures of adiposity and cardiovascular disease risk factors. Obesity (Silver Spring). 2007;15:785–95. https://doi.org/10.1038/oby.2007.593.
14. Vikram NK, Misra A, Dwivedi M, Sharma R, Pandey RM, Luthra K, et al. Correlations of C-reactive protein levels with anthropometric profile, percentage of body fat and lipids in healthy adolescents and young adults in urban North India. Atherosclerosis. 2003;168:305–13.
15. Yasar Z, Buyuksirin M, Ucsular FD, Kargi A, Erdem F, Talay F, et al. Is an elevated neutrophil-to-lymphocyte ratio a predictor of metabolic syndrome in patients with chronic obstructive pulmonary disease? Eur Rev Med Pharmacol Sci. 2015;19:956–62.
16. Sun M, Zhang L, Chen S, Liu X, Shao X, Zou H. Association of C-reactive protein and metabolic disorder in a Chinese population. Int J Environ Res Public Health. 2015;12:8228–42. https://doi.org/10.3390/ijerph120708228.
17. Tang L, Peng H, Xu T, Wang A, Wang G, Tong W, et al. Association of biomarkers of inflammation with dyslipidemia and its components among Mongolians in China. PLoS One. 2014;9:e89023. https://doi.org/10.1371/journal.pone.0089023.
18. Gouda M, Moustafa A, Hussein L, Hamza M. Three week dietary intervention using apricots, pomegranate juice or/and fermented sour sobya and impact on biomarkers of antioxidative activity, oxidative stress and erythrocytic glutathione transferase activity among adults. Nutr J. 2016;15:52. https://doi.org/10.1186/s12937-016-0173-x.
19. Zaki M, Hussein L, Gouda M, Bassuoni R, Hassanein A. Nutritional epidemiological study to estimate usual intake and to define optimum nutrient profiling choice in the diet of Egyptian youths. Food Nutr Sci. 2015;6:1422–36.
20. Ridker PM, Hennekens CH, Buring JE, Rifai N. C-reactive protein and other markers of inflammation in the prediction of cardiovascular disease in women. N Engl J Med. 2000;342:836–43. https://doi.org/10.1056/nejm200003233421202.
21. Pearson TA, Mensah GA, Alexander RW, Anderson JL, Cannon RO 3rd, Criqui M, et al. Markers of inflammation and cardiovascular disease: application to clinical and public health practice: a statement for healthcare professionals from the Centers for Disease Control and Prevention and the American Heart Association. Circulation. 2003;107:499–511. https://doi.org/10.1161/01.CIR.0000052939.59093.45.
22. Arbel Y, Finkelstein A, Halkin A, Birati EY, Revivo M, Zuzut M, et al. Neutrophil/lymphocyte ratio is related to the severity of coronary artery disease and clinical outcome in patients undergoing angiography. Atherosclerosis. 2012;225:456–60. https://doi.org/10.1016/j.atherosclerosis.2012.09.009.
23. Osler M, Heitmann BL, Gerdes LU, Jorgensen LM, Schroll M. Dietary patterns and mortality in Danish men and women: a prospective observational study. Br J Nutr. 2001;85:219–25.
24. Newby PK, Tucker KL. Empirically derived eating patterns using factor or cluster analysis: a review. Nutr Rev. 2004;62:177–203.

25. Muga MA, Owili PO, Hsu CY, Rau HH, Chao JC. Dietary patterns, gender, and weight status among middle-aged and older adults in Taiwan: a cross-sectional study. BMC Geriatr. 2017;17:268. https://doi.org/10.1186/s12877-017-0664-4.
26. Lee O-G, Hur Y-I, Kang J-H, Park H-A, Kim K-W, Cho Y-G, et al. The cutoff value of waist circumference for predicting metabolic risks in pre- and post-menopausal Korean women: analysis of 2010 Korean National Health and nutrition examination survey data. Korean J Fam Med. 2013;34:307–18. https://doi.org/10.4082/kjfm.2013.34.5.307.
27. Cho YG, Song HJ, Kim JM, Park KH, Paek YJ, Cho JJ, et al. The estimation of cardiovascular risk factors by body mass index and body fat percentage in Korean male adults. Metabolism. 2009;58:765–71. https://doi.org/10.1016/j.metabol.2009.01.004.
28. Kim JY, Han SH, Yang BM. Implication of high-body-fat percentage on cardiometabolic risk in middle-aged, healthy, normal-weight adults. Obesity (Silver Spring). 2013;21:1571–7. https://doi.org/10.1002/oby.20020.
29. Jaeschke L, Steinbrecher A, Pischon T. Measurement of waist and hip circumference with a body surface scanner: feasibility, validity, reliability, and correlations with markers of the metabolic syndrome. PLoS One. 2015;10:e0119430. https://doi.org/10.1371/journal.pone.0119430.
30. Grundy SM, Cleeman JI, Bairey Merz CN, Brewer HB, Clark LT, Hunninghake DB, et al. Implications of recent clinical trials for the National Cholesterol Education Program Adult Treatment Panel III guidelines. J Am Coll Cardiol. 2004;44:720–32. https://doi.org/10.1016/j.jacc.2004.07.001.
31. Svensson E, Mor A, Rungby J, Berencsi K, Nielsen JS, Stidsen JV, et al. Lifestyle and clinical factors associated with elevated C-reactive protein among newly diagnosed type 2 diabetes mellitus patients: a cross-sectional study from the nationwide DD2 cohort. BMC Endocr Disord. 2014;14:74. https://doi.org/10.1186/1472-6823-14-74.
32. Fung TT, Rimm EB, Spiegelman D, Rifai N, Tofler GH, Willett WC, et al. Association between dietary patterns and plasma biomarkers of obesity and cardiovascular disease risk. Am J Clin Nutr. 2001;73:61–7. https://doi.org/10.1093/ajcn/73.1.61.
33. Lopez-Garcia E, Schulze MB, Fung TT, Meigs JB, Rifai N, Manson JE, et al. Major dietary patterns are related to plasma concentrations of markers of inflammation and endothelial dysfunction. Am J Clin Nutr. 2004;80:1029–35. https://doi.org/10.1093/ajcn/80.4.1029.
34. Maysami S, Haley MJ, Gorenkova N, Krishnan S, McColl BW, Lawrence CB. Prolonged diet-induced obesity in mice modifies the inflammatory response and leads to worse outcome after stroke. J Neuroinflammation. 2015;12:140. https://doi.org/10.1186/s12974-015-0359-8.
35. Root MM, McGinn MC, Nieman DC, Henson DA, Heinz SA, Shanely RA, et al. Combined fruit and vegetable intake is correlated with improved inflammatory and oxidant status from a cross-sectional study in a community setting. Nutrients. 2012;4:29–41. https://doi.org/10.3390/nu4010029.
36. Adamsson V, Reumark A, Marklund M, Larsson A, Riserus U. Role of a prudent breakfast in improving cardiometabolic risk factors in subjects with hypercholesterolemia: a randomized controlled trial. Clin Nutr. 2015;34:20–6. https://doi.org/10.1016/j.clnu.2014.04.009.
37. Bonaccio M, Di Castelnuovo A, Bonanni A, Costanzo S, De Lucia F, Pounis G, et al. Adherence to a Mediterranean diet is associated with a better health-related quality of life: a possible role of high dietary antioxidant content. BMJ Open. 2013;3. https://doi.org/10.1136/bmjopen-2013-003003.
38. Arouca A, Michels N, Moreno LA, Gonzalez-Gil EM, Marcos A, Gomez S, et al. Associations between a Mediterranean diet pattern and inflammatory biomarkers in European adolescents. Eur J Nutr. 2017. https://doi.org/10.1007/s00394-017-1457-4.
39. Bonaccio M, Di Castelnuovo A, De Curtis A, Costanzo S, Persichillo M, Donati MB, et al. Adherence to the Mediterranean diet is associated with lower platelet and leukocyte counts: results from the Moli-sani study. Blood. 2014;123:3037–44. https://doi.org/10.1182/blood-2013-12-541672.
40. Bédard A, Lamarche B, Corneau L, Dodin S, Lemieux S. Sex differences in the impact of the Mediterranean diet on systemic inflammation. Nutr J. 2015;14:46. https://doi.org/10.1186/s12937-015-0035-y.
41. Furuncuoglu Y, Tulgar S, Dogan AN, Cakar S, Tulgar YK, Cakiroglu B. How obesity affects the neutrophil/lymphocyte and platelet/lymphocyte ratio, systemic immune-inflammatory index and platelet indices: a retrospective study. Eur Rev Med Pharmacol Sci. 2016;20:1300–6.
42. Kitahara CM, Trabert B, Katki HA, Chaturvedi AK, Kemp TJ, Pinto LA, et al. Body mass index, physical activity, and serum markers of inflammation, immunity, and insulin resistance. Cancer Epidemiol Biomark Prev. 2014;23:2840–9. https://doi.org/10.1158/1055-9965.epi-14-0699-t.
43. Nakamura H, Ito H, Egami Y, Kaji Y, Maruyama T, Koike G, et al. Waist circumference is the main determinant of elevated C-reactive protein in metabolic syndrome. Diabetes Res Clin Pract. 2008;79:330–6. https://doi.org/10.1016/j.diabres.2007.09.004.
44. Santos AC, Lopes C, Guimaraes JT, Barros H. Central obesity as a major determinant of increased high-sensitivity C-reactive protein in metabolic syndrome. Int J Obes. 2005;29:1452–6. https://doi.org/10.1038/sj.ijo.0803035.
45. Vuong J, Qiu Y, La M, Clarke G, Swinkels DW, Cembrowski G. Reference intervals of complete blood count constituents are highly correlated to waist circumference: should obese patients have their own "normal values"? Am J Hematol. 2014;89:671–7. https://doi.org/10.1002/ajh.23713.
46. Motie M, Evangelista LS, Horwich T, Lombardo D, Zaldivar F, Hamilton M, et al. Association between inflammatory biomarkers and adiposity in obese patients with heart failure and metabolic syndrome. Exp Ther Med. 2014;8:181–6. https://doi.org/10.3892/etm.2014.1673.
47. Yilmaz H, Ucan B, Sayki M, Unsal I, Sahin M, Ozbek M, et al. Usefulness of the neutrophil-to-lymphocyte ratio to prediction of type 2 diabetes mellitus in morbid obesity. Diabetes Metab Syndr. 2015;9:299–304. https://doi.org/10.1016/j.dsx.2014.04.009.
48. Sur G, Floca E, Kudor-Szabadi L, Sur ML, Sur D, Samasca G. The relevance of inflammatory markers in metabolic syndrome. Maedica (Buchar). 2014;9:15–8.
49. Surendar J, Indulekha K, Mohan V, Pradeepa R. Association of neutrophil-lymphocyte ratio with metabolic syndrome and its components in Asian Indians (CURES-143). J Diabetes Complicat. 2016;30:1525–9. https://doi.org/10.1016/j.jdiacomp.2016.08.006.
50. Buyukkaya E, Karakas MF, Karakas E, Akcay AB, Tanboga IH, Kurt M, et al. Correlation of neutrophil to lymphocyte ratio with the presence and severity of metabolic syndrome. Clin Appl Thromb Hemost. 2014;20:159–63. https://doi.org/10.1177/1076029612459675.
51. Soehnlein O, Drechsler M, Hristov M, Weber C. Functional alterations of myeloid cell subsets in hyperlipidaemia: relevance for atherosclerosis. J Cell Mol Med. 2009;13:4293–303. https://doi.org/10.1111/j.1582-4934.2009.00965.x.
52. Guerrero-Romero F, Simental-Mendía LE, Rodríguez-Morán M. Association of C-reactive protein levels with fasting and postload glucose levels according to glucose tolerance status. Arch Med Res. 2014;45:70–5. https://doi.org/10.1016/j.arcmed.2013.11.004.
53. Jaiswal A, Tabassum R, Podder A, Ghosh S, Tandon N, Bharadwaj D. Elevated level of C-reactive protein is associated with risk of prediabetes in Indians. Atherosclerosis. 2012;222:495–501. https://doi.org/10.1016/j.atherosclerosis.2012.02.034.
54. Brooks GC, Blaha MJ, Blumenthal RS. Relation of C-reactive protein to abdominal adiposity. Am J Cardiol. 2010;106:56–61. https://doi.org/10.1016/j.amjcard.2010.02.017.
55. Bahadir A, Baltaci D, Turker Y, Turker Y, Iliev D, Ozturk S, et al. Is the neutrophil-to-lymphocyte ratio indicative of inflammatory state in patients with obesity and metabolic syndrome? Anatol J Cardiol. 2015;15:816–22. https://doi.org/10.5152/akd.2014.5787.
56. Lin CC, Kardia SL, Li CI, Liu CS, Lai MM, Lin WY, et al. The relationship of high sensitivity C-reactive protein to percent body fat mass, body mass index, waist-to-hip ratio, and waist circumference in a Taiwanese population. BMC Public Health. 2010;10:579. https://doi.org/10.1186/1471-2458-10-579.
57. Duffy BK, Gurm HS, Rajagopal V, Gupta R, Ellis SG, Bhatt DL. Usefulness of an elevated neutrophil to lymphocyte ratio in predicting long-term mortality after percutaneous coronary intervention. Am J Cardiol. 2006;97:993–6. https://doi.org/10.1016/j.amjcard.2005.10.034.
58. Uthamalingam S, Patvardhan EA, Subramanian S, Ahmed W, Martin W, Daley M, et al. Utility of the neutrophil to lymphocyte ratio in predicting long-term outcomes in acute decompensated heart failure. Am J Cardiol. 2011;107:433–8. https://doi.org/10.1016/j.amjcard.2010.09.039.

# 13

# Association between eating behaviour and diet quality: eating alone vs. eating with others

Wonjeong Chae[1,2], Yeong Jun Ju[1,2], Jaeyong Shin[2,3], Sung-In Jang[2,3] and Eun-Cheol Park[2,3*]

**Abstract**

**Background:** To discover the association between eating alone and diet quality among Korean adults who eat alone measured by the mean adequacy ratio (MAR),

**Methods:** The cross-sectional study in diet quality which was measured by nutrient intakes, indicated as MAR and nutrient adequacy ratio (NAR) with the Korean National Health and Nutrition Examination Survey (KNHANES) VI 2013–2015 data. Study population was 8523 Korean adults. Multiple linear regression was performed to identify the association between eating behaviour and MAR and further study analysed how socioeconomic factors influence the diet quality of those who eat alone.

**Results:** We found that the diet quality of people who eat alone was lower than that of people who eat together in both male (β: − 0.110, $p = 0.002$) and female participants (β: − 0.069, $p = 0.005$). Among who eats alone, the socioeconomic factors that negatively influenced MAR with the living arrangement, education level, income levels, and various occupation classifications.

**Conclusions:** People who eat alone have nutrition intake below the recommended amount. This could lead to serious health problems not only to those who are socially disadvantaged but also those who are in a higher social stratum. Policy-makers should develop strategies to enhance diet quality to prevent potential risk factors.

**Keywords:** MAR, NAR, Eating alone, Diet quality, Socioeconomic status

## Background

Food intake is an essential factor related to health status [1–4]. Adequate nutrients must be consumed through diet in order to survive. These days, people who care about what they eat think about how it will affect their well-being and lifestyle rather than how it can help to survive day-to-day life [5, 6]. When we observe how food is produced and consumed, there is no significant difference compared to the past [7]. However, the range of nutrients consumed has expanded widely and eating behaviours have changed with economic growth. Diet quality is described in nutritional epidemiology literature in a variety of ways, including a healthy diet, balanced diet, nutritious foods, functional foods, and nutrient-rich diet [8]. Those terms point to the bottom-line idea of achieving an optimal level of health via a balanced nutrient intake.

Academic research to investigate the relationship between diet quality and diseases are increasing. There are studies that show effects of healthy eating and a reduction in risk for chronic diseases [1, 9, 10] and mortality [9, 11, 12]. Studies among elderly Japanese population demonstrated that solitary eating negatively influenced meal quality, which is consistent with our theory [10, 12, 13]. Eating alone discourages people from having a well-balanced meal. Some even see eating alone as an efficient way of having a meal, and as a new trend is being adopted, we might have to face a socially isolated generation [13, 14]. Poor eating quality will become a new public health issue. Eating alone can cause vulnerability in nutrition among elderly population [15] yet commensality

* Correspondence: ECPARK@yuhs.ac
[2]Institute of Health Services Research, Yonsei University, 50 Yonsei-ro, Seodaemun-gu, Seoul 120-752, Republic of Korea
[3]Department of Preventive Medicine, College of Medicine, Yonsei University, 50 Yonsei-ro, Seodaemun-gu, Seoul 120-752, Republic of Korea
Full list of author information is available at the end of the article

can influence positively to elder population [16]. In contrast, eating together, such as in a family, promotes the healthy eating habits to lead a healthy lifestyle [17]. Also the study on middle and high school students on the frequency of family meals, breakfast and dinner, shows the students who had a higher frequency of family meals had better dietary intake and quality than who did not have family meals [18].

With an increase in the interest in diet quality, eating behaviour has also evolved in modern society. The traditional definition of a meal includes companions such as family or friends [13]. The new form of living style brought the concept of eating alone (solitary eating), and it became a new trend in some generations. Selecting foods for a day is easily influenced by the social environment and eating together or alone plays a big role in that decision [2, 13, 19, 20]. When people plan to eat alone, the meal will not take long; usually they pick a simple and quick meal rather than a nutritionally balanced meal [13, 20, 21]. Regardless of this new trend, solitary eating causes dietary problems such as modern malnutrition [2, 11]. For people who eat alone, it is hard to consume adequate nutrients, especially for micronutrients due to the limited consumption of fruits and vegetables [2]. In fact, it leads not only to modern malnutrition, it could also cause clinical malnutrition due to insufficient nutrient intake [11]. Eating alone puts people at risk of potential illness, as has been reported in earlier studies [11, 12].

Previous studies were conducted to search for causative factors of illness due to nutrition. There are studies that found health status resulted from imbalanced nutrition [12, 22]. Also, some studies assessed the impact of socioeconomic status on nutritional health and eating patterns [20, 23]. Research on eating alone and quality of meals is comparatively new yet expected to increase in our society. By looking at the increasing prevalence of the elderly population and one-person households [24] and rapid changes in environmental factors [2, 25], we expect to see an increase in the prevalence of people who eat alone. Our study aims to evaluate the association between diet quality of the modern Korean adult population based on the eating behaviour and the socioeconomic factors that influence their diet quality.

## Methods

### Study subjects

This study was conducted with data from the sixth Korea National Health and Nutrition Examination Survey (KNHANES VI-3) by the Korea Centers for Disease Control and Prevention, which contains survey data for the cross-sectional study from the health interview survey, the health examination survey, and the nutrition survey from 2013 through 2015. The 2015 Dietary Reference Intakes for Koreans by the Korean Nutrition Society and Ministry of Health and Welfare, Korea were used to reference data for the recommended nutrient intakes [26]. The final population for this study is 3365 men and 5158 women who are age 19 to 64 years old.

### Dependent variable

The dependent variable of mean adequacy ratio (MAR) was used to measure the quality of the meal. In order to compute MAR, the nutrient adequacy ratio (NAR) of each nutrient was calculated by the formula below. In 1972, Madden and Yoder [27] first used MAR and NAR to evaluate food stamp efficiency and commodity distribution. NAR shows the ratio of each nutrient intake relative to the recommended dietary intake or recommended dietary allowance [27, 28]. For this study, we applied the Dietary Reference Intakes for Korean 2015 as the reference value of RDA and collected nutrients are protein, calcium, phosphate, iron, vitamin A, vitamin B1, vitamin B2, Niacin, and Vitamin C through the nutrition survey for assessment. The formulae for MAR and NAR are below [22]:

$$\text{MAR} = \text{Sum of NAR of nutrients/the number of nutrients}$$

$$\text{NAR} = \text{Nutrient intake/recommended nutrient intake}$$

NAR, which is obtained from the recommended nutrient intake, refers to sex and age-specific 0references for daily intakes. A NAR close to 1 indicates the consumed meal is near the recommended amount of that specific nutrient for the day; when it is $>1$, it means the consumed meal exceeded the recommended amount of the nutrient [22, 27]. This study included various foods and beverages since both of them could be significant sources of nutrients.

### Independent variable of main interest

The variable of main interest was eating behaviour, which represents whether they have company during the meal. The variable was described using categorical data based on participants responding in "yes" or "no" format. The questions were asked by each meal, breakfast, lunch, and dinner. The final grouping was designed after considering the frequency of the meal and the existence of company during the meal (Box 1). The population was separated by gender, and then categorized them into three groups: 'alone' for those who ate all meals alone, 'some together' for those who ate some meals with others, and 'together' for those who ate with others for every meal.

### Covariates

This study included demographic, socioeconomic, and health behaviour factors as covariates. Demographic factors used to assess general characteristics of the study population included living arrangement, age group, and residential area. The socioeconomic factors reviewed were marital status, education level, income level, and occupation status in four categories (white collar: administrative and management role, blue collar: manual labour industry and pick collar: service industry). For the health behaviour factors, body mass index (BMI: underweight: BMI < 18.5, normal: 18.5 ≤ BMI < 25.0, and overweight: BMI > 25.0) weight changes in the past 1 year, alcohol consumption, smoking status, and stress level were assessed. We also added nutrition behaviour-related factors such as nutritional education, nutrition supplement intake more than 2 weeks per year, and nutritional fact usage to evaluate whether or not there are associations with MAR.

### Statistical analysis

To compare the proportion of variables by MAR, independent t-test and ANOVA were used and a univariate analysis was performed. Multiple linear regression analysis was used to determine an association between MAR and eating behaviour using a generalized linear model (GLM). We performed further analysis to discover an association between socioeconomic status and eating behaviour with diet quality measured by MAR.

## Results

The characteristics of the study population ($N = 8523$) are presented in Table 1. The participants were grouped by sex; there were 3365 (39.48%) men and 5158 (60.52%) women. The mean MAR for male and female populations was the same at 1.03 ± 0.48. Participants were also grouped into three categories based on their eating behaviour. In the male group, 256 (7.61%) ate every meal alone, 1199 (35.63%) ate some meals together, and 1910 (56.76%) ate every meal together. In the female group, 502 (9.73%) ate very meal alone, 2255 (43.72%) ate some meals together, and 2401 (46.55%) ate every meal together. Male participants' MAR was not influenced by whether or not they were living together, while female participants' MAR was influenced by their living arrangement ($p < 0.001$) (Table 1).

The results of regression analyses of the association between eating behaviour and MAR are presented in Table 2. Demographic and socioeconomic information, health status, and nutrition-related variables were adjusted for the analysis. The comparison between 'some together' and 'alone' showed that the 'alone' group's diet quality was lower than the 'together' group as measured by MAR (male: β: − 0.110, $p = 0.002$; female: β: − 0.069, $p = 0.005$). The association between age groups and MAR results are different by gender that male participants have higher MAR than female participants. In male participants, age group and MAR shows positive correlation with statistically significant values while in female participants the negative correlation is detected (male age group 19–29: β: 0.305, $p < 0.001$; male age group 30–39: β: 0.259, $p <$ 0.001; male age group 40–49: β: 0.137, $p < 0.001$; male age group 50–59: β: − 0.052, p:0.086; female age group 19–29: β: − 0.035, $p = 0.346$; female age group 30–39: β: − 0.010, $p = 0.725$; male age group 40–49: β: − 0.074, $p = 0.006$; male age group 50–59: β: 0.001 p: 0.981). The living arrangement did not influence the MAR, neither before nor after adjustment. As per stress level, MAR and stress level shows positive correlation among male participants and negative correlation among female participants (male high: β: 0.023, p: 0.423; male medium: β: 0.003, $p = 0.901$; female high: β: − 0.044, $p = 0.053$; female medium: β: − 0.040, $p = 0.053$). People who take nutritional supplement more than 2 weeks per year show higher MAR then who does not take supplements (male: β: − 0.021, $p = 0.643$; female: β: − 0.019, $p = 0.567$) but the value is not statistically significant. Participants who does not use nutritional facts appear to have lower MAR in both gender with significant value (male: β: − 0.087, $p < 0.001$; female: β: − 0.056, $p < 0.001$). (Table 2). In addition to Tables 1 and 2, the general characteristics of the study population according to eating behabiour and the analysis of unadjusted model is presented in Additional file 1: Appendix 1 and 2.

Table 3 shows the result of subgroup analysis based on socioeconomic factors living arrangement, income level, education level, and occupation by eating behaviour. For male participants, when they live with others (β: − 0.134, $p = 0.001$); completed with tertiary education (β: − 0.212, $p < 0.001$); earns the lowest (β: − 0.216, $p = 0.002$) or highest income (β: − 0.167, $p = 0.040$); categorize as 'others' (β: − 0.193, $p = 0.006$) for occupational status which means not currently working with the eating alone behaviour shows inadequate diet with lower MAR than those who eat together within the same categories. The results of female study are as followed. Similar to male's results when they live with others (β: − 0.081, $p = 0.002$); completed primary education (β: − 0.163, $p = 0.003$) or secondary education (β: − 0.146, $p = 0.040$); work in pink-collar industry (β: − 0.125, $p = 0.035$) or blue-collar industry (β: − 0.178, $p = 0.004$) have insufficient nutrient intake with they eat alone (Table 3).

Nutrient intake was measured from the dietary survey and was used to assess patterns of food consumption in the previous year. Figure 1 shows the MAR and NAR of individual nutrients by eating behaviour and sex. Regardless of sex, participants consumed inadequate nutrients when they ate alone (Fig. 1). Detailed results on individual 9 nutrients are presented in Additional file 1: Appendix 3. Also, additional analysis such as MAR with the cutoff value of 0.5, different models related to socioeconomic factors, and interactions are included in Additional file 2: Appendix 4, 5 and 6.

**Table 1** General characteristics of the study population

| Variables | General characteristics | | | | | | | | | |
|---|---|---|---|---|---|---|---|---|---|---|
| | Male | | | | | Female | | | | |
| | Subject | | MAR | | | Subject | | MAR | | |
| | N | % | MEAN | SD | *p*-value | N | % | MEAN | SD | *p*-value |
| Eating Type | | | | | <.001 | | | | | <.001 |
| Alone | 256 | 7.61 | 1.033 | 0.483 | | 502 | 9.73 | 1.035 | 0.476 | |
| Some Together | 1199 | 35.63 | 1.187 | 0.497 | | 2255 | 43.72 | 1.143 | 0.473 | |
| Together | 1910 | 56.76 | 1.200 | 0.505 | | 2401 | 46.55 | 1.148 | 0.472 | |
| One person household | | | | | 0.103 | | | | | <.001 |
| Yes | 245 | 7.28 | 1.133 | 0.563 | | 283 | 5.49 | 1.006 | 0.471 | |
| No | 3120 | 92.72 | 1.187 | 0.497 | | 4875 | 94.51 | 1.142 | 0.473 | |
| Age Group | | | | | <.001 | | | | | <.001 |
| 19–29 | 614 | 18.25 | 1.292 | 0.553 | | 764 | 14.81 | 1.125 | 0.499 | |
| 30–39 | 715 | 21.25 | 1.313 | 0.539 | | 1120 | 21.71 | 1.186 | 0.491 | |
| 40–49 | 796 | 23.66 | 1.187 | 0.491 | | 1293 | 25.07 | 1.115 | 0.448 | |
| 50–59 | 832 | 24.73 | 1.075 | 0.438 | | 1370 | 26.56 | 1.139 | 0.466 | |
| 60 above | 408 | 12.12 | 1.002 | 0.385 | | 611 | 11.85 | 1.085 | 0.474 | |
| Residential Area | | | | | 0.064 | | | | | 0.370 |
| Urban | 2771 | 82.35 | 1.190 | 0.507 | | 4364 | 84.61 | 1.137 | 0.474 | |
| Rural | 594 | 17.65 | 1.148 | 0.476 | | 794 | 15.39 | 1.121 | 0.474 | |
| BMI | | | | | 0.013 | | | | | 0.901 |
| Underweight | 71 | 2.11 | 1.126 | 0.475 | | 314 | 6.09 | 1.126 | 0.509 | |
| Overweight | 1341 | 39.85 | 1.213 | 0.507 | | 1335 | 25.88 | 1.132 | 0.494 | |
| Normal | 1953 | 58.04 | 1.164 | 0.499 | | 3509 | 68.03 | 1.137 | 0.463 | |
| Weight Changes | | | | | <.001 | | | | | <.001 |
| Same | 464 | 13.79 | 1.137 | 0.519 | | 616 | 11.94 | 1.071 | 0.462 | |
| Decreased | 726 | 21.58 | 1.259 | 0.522 | | 1554 | 30.13 | 1.167 | 0.512 | |
| Increased | 2175 | 64.64 | 1.167 | 0.489 | | 2988 | 57.93 | 1.131 | 0.454 | |
| Marital Status | | | | | <.001 | | | | | <.001 |
| Married | 2365 | 70.28 | 1.170 | 0.481 | | 3813 | 73.92 | 1.151 | 0.461 | |
| Separated | 144 | 4.28 | 0.936 | 0.409 | | 504 | 9.77 | 1.023 | 0.462 | |
| Single | 856 | 25.44 | 1.260 | 0.556 | | 841 | 16.30 | 1.127 | 0.529 | |
| Education Level | | | | | <.001 | | | | | <.001 |
| Primary | 247 | 7.34 | 0.950 | 0.431 | | 654 | 12.68 | 0.991 | 0.431 | |
| Secondary | 273 | 8.11 | 1.047 | 0.454 | | 532 | 10.31 | 1.093 | 0.471 | |
| Upper Secondary | 1355 | 40.27 | 1.213 | 0.521 | | 2000 | 38.77 | 1.149 | 0.476 | |
| Tertiary | 1490 | 44.28 | 1.219 | 0.489 | | 1972 | 38.23 | 1.180 | 0.476 | |
| Income Level | | | | | <.001 | | | | | <.001 |
| Lowest | 776 | 23.06 | 1.123 | 0.527 | | 1243 | 24.10 | 1.052 | 0.473 | |
| Lower-Middle | 893 | 26.54 | 1.136 | 0.468 | | 1283 | 24.87 | 1.094 | 0.451 | |
| Upper-Middle | 823 | 24.46 | 1.222 | 0.505 | | 1320 | 25.59 | 1.168 | 0.473 | |
| Highest | 873 | 25.94 | 1.247 | 0.501 | | 1312 | 25.44 | 1.220 | 0.481 | |
| Occupation | | | | | <.001 | | | | | <.001 |
| White | 1155 | 34.32 | 1.229 | 0.498 | | 1254 | 24.31 | 1.160 | 0.460 | |
| Pink | 431 | 12.81 | 1.251 | 0.478 | | 848 | 16.44 | 1.155 | 0.491 | |

**Table 1** General characteristics of the study population *(Continued)*

| Variables | General characteristics | | | | | | | | | |
|---|---|---|---|---|---|---|---|---|---|---|
| | Male | | | | | Female | | | | |
| | Subject | | MAR | | | Subject | | MAR | | |
| | N | % | MEAN | SD | *p*-value | N | % | MEAN | SD | *p*-value |
| Blue | 1186 | 35.25 | 1.144 | 0.489 | | 762 | 14.77 | 1.071 | 0.441 | |
| Others | 593 | 17.62 | 1.121 | 0.539 | | 2294 | 44.47 | 1.135 | 0.484 | |
| Alcohol Consumption | | | | | 0.202 | | | | | 0.222 |
| Yes | 3261 | 96.91 | 1.185 | 0.502 | | 4568 | 88.56 | 1.138 | 0.474 | |
| No | 104 | 3.09 | 1.121 | 0.513 | | 590 | 11.44 | 1.112 | 0.475 | |
| Cigarettes | | | | | 0.055 | | | | | 0.557 |
| Smoker | 1382 | 41.07 | 1.180 | 0.524 | | 273 | 5.29 | 1.123 | 0.538 | |
| Ex-Smoker | 1158 | 34.41 | 1.163 | 0.486 | | 288 | 5.58 | 1.109 | 0.478 | |
| Non-Smoker | 825 | 24.52 | 1.217 | 0.486 | | 4597 | 89.12 | 1.137 | 0.470 | |
| Stress Level | | | | | 0.016 | | | | | 0.247 |
| High | 836 | 24.84 | 1.219 | 0.522 | | 1360 | 26.37 | 1.120 | 0.501 | |
| Medium | 2048 | 60.86 | 1.178 | 0.501 | | 3170 | 61.46 | 1.137 | 0.460 | |
| Low | 481 | 14.29 | 1.139 | 0.468 | | 628 | 12.18 | 1.157 | 0.483 | |
| Nutritional Education | | | | | 0.741 | | | | | 0.124 |
| No | 3247 | 96.49 | 1.182 | 0.501 | | 4947 | 95.91 | 1.133 | 0.474 | |
| Yes | 118 | 3.51 | 1.198 | 0.526 | | 211 | 4.09 | 1.184 | 0.480 | |
| Nutrition Supplement Intake (more than2 weeks/year) | | | | | <.001 | | | | | <.001 |
| No | 2065 | 61.37 | 1.145 | 0.487 | | 2540 | 49.24 | 1.091 | 0.461 | |
| Yes | 1300 | 38.63 | 1.242 | 0.520 | | 2618 | 50.76 | 1.178 | 0.482 | |
| Nutritional Fact Usage | | 0.00 | | | <.001 | | | | | <.001 |
| No | 2770 | 82.32 | 1.157 | 0.485 | | 3225 | 62.52 | 1.102 | 0.472 | |
| Yes | 595 | 17.68 | 1.305 | 0.558 | | 1933 | 37.48 | 1.189 | 0.471 | |
| Total | 3365 | 100.00 | 1.182 | 0.501 | | 5158 | 100.00 | 1.133 | 0.471 | |

## Discussion

The results from this study show that diet quality is influenced by eating behaviour, as indicated by the association between MAR and eating alone. We observed that when Korean adults ate without a companion, their MAR was significantly lower than those who consistently ate with others. Poor quality meals in Korean adults could possibly lead to "modern malnutrition" that not receiving adequate nutrients yet reached the recommended total calories per day. This could result in further health-related problems [5, 10]. When MAR is equal to 1 or above it means that in average the individual consumed the recommended amount of nutrients. However, since it is the average value, further observation of nutrient intake should be performed to decide the quality of the diet. Especially, modern days, there are people who exceed the recommended food intake amount through high-calorie foods and unbalanced diet which lead to poor diet quality.

For socioeconomic element covariates, we chose education level, income level, and occupation variables to identify the vulnerable class to provide social support. Also, those factors could be related to the nutrient intake. After reviewing the interaction between education level, income level, and occupation, we have performed analyses to find the interaction between those variables. As the results, the interactions existed therefore, we used a stratified variable.

After the main analysis, we studied in more depth the association between socioeconomic factors of Korean adults and their diets. We performed subgroup analyses for living arrangement, education level, income level, and occupation status to investigate what other factors could influence diet quality beyond demographic factors [2]. The outcomes of the analyses conflicted with social norms and common beliefs, [19, 23, 25] yet they represent a current social phenomenon in Korea [29]. These results could be applicable as a version of modern society in other countries as well. Our findings indicate that Korean male adults who eat alone have a poor diet with inadequate nutrient intake compared to when they live

**Table 2** Factors associated with MAR

| Variables | MAR | | | | | |
|---|---|---|---|---|---|---|
| | Male | | | Female | | |
| | β | S.E | *p*-value | β | S.E | *p*-value |
| Eating Style | | | | | | |
| Alone | −0.110 | 0.035 | 0.002 | − 0.069 | 0.024 | 0.005 |
| Some Together | −0.001 | 0.018 | 0.936 | −0.010 | 0.014 | 0.474 |
| Together | Ref. | | | Ref. | | |
| One person household | | | | | | |
| Yes | 0.042 | 0.037 | 0.262 | −0.040 | 0.032 | 0.221 |
| No | Ref. | | | Ref. | | |
| Age Group | | | | | | |
| 19–29 | 0.305 | 0.045 | <.001 | −0.035 | 0.037 | 0.346 |
| 30–39 | 0.259 | 0.036 | <.001 | −0.010 | 0.029 | 0.725 |
| 40–49 | 0.137 | 0.033 | <.001 | −0.074 | 0.027 | 0.006 |
| 50–59 | 0.052 | 0.030 | 0.086 | 0.001 | 0.024 | 0.981 |
| 60 above | Ref. | | | Ref. | | |
| Residential Area | | | | | | |
| Urban | 0.001 | 0.023 | 0.975 | − 0.013 | 0.019 | 0.469 |
| Rural | Ref. | | | Ref. | | |
| BMI | | | | | | |
| Underweight | − 0.030 | 0.025 | 0.610 | −0.011 | 0.028 | 0.707 |
| Overweight | 0.024 | 0.018 | 0.015 | 0.024 | 0.016 | 0.125 |
| Normal | Ref. | | | Ref. | | |
| Weight Changes | | | | | | |
| Decreased | −0.035 | 0.025 | 0.161 | − 0.048 | 0.021 | 0.021 |
| Increased | −0.035 | 0.022 | 0.274 | 0.030 | 0.015 | 0.047 |
| Same | Ref. | | | Ref. | | |
| Marital Status | | | | | | |
| Married | 0.043 | 0.032 | 0.178 | 0.021 | 0.027 | 0.435 |
| Once Married | −0.063 | 0.051 | 0.219 | −0.023 | 0.035 | 0.522 |
| Single | Ref. | | | Ref. | | |
| Education Level | | | | | | |
| Primary | −0.048 | 0.039 | 0.223 | −0.162 | 0.028 | <.001 |
| Secondary | −0.018 | 0.036 | 0.614 | −0.077 | 0.027 | 0.005 |
| Upper Secondary | 0.032 | 0.021 | 0.124 | −0.019 | 0.017 | 0.248 |
| Tertiary | Ref. | | | Ref. | | |
| Income Level | | | | | | |
| Lowest | −0.091 | 0.026 | <.001 | −0.113 | 0.020 | <.001 |
| Lower-Middle | −0.103 | 0.024 | <.001 | −0.097 | 0.019 | <.001 |
| Upper-Middle | −0.027 | 0.024 | 0.249 | −0.038 | 0.018 | 0.040 |
| Highest | Ref. | | | Ref. | | |
| Occupation | | | | | | |
| White Collar | 0.049 | 0.029 | 0.095 | −0.013 | 0.018 | 0.478 |
| Pink Collar | 0.091 | 0.032 | 0.005 | 0.032 | 0.019 | 0.098 |
| Blue Collar | 0.065 | 0.027 | 0.018 | −0.013 | 0.021 | 0.528 |
| Others | Ref. | | | Ref. | | |
| Alcohol Consumption | | | | | | |
| Yes | −0.001 | 0.049 | 0.977 | 0.009 | 0.021 | 0.679 |
| No | Ref. | | | Ref. | | |
| Cigarettes | | | | | | |
| Smoker | 0.002 | 0.022 | 0.931 | 0.034 | 0.030 | 0.258 |
| Once Smoked | 0.011 | 0.023 | 0.628 | −0.019 | 0.029 | 0.501 |
| Non-Smoker | Ref. | | | Ref. | | |
| Stress Level | | | | | | |
| High | 0.023 | 0.028 | 0.423 | −0.044 | 0.023 | 0.053 |
| Medium | 0.003 | 0.025 | 0.901 | −0.040 | 0.020 | 0.053 |
| Low | Ref. | | | Ref. | | |
| Nutritional Education | | | | | | |
| No | −0.021 | 0.046 | 0.643 | −0.019 | 0.033 | 0.567 |
| Yes | Ref. | | | Ref. | | |
| Nutrition Supplement Intake (more than2 weeks/year) | | | | | | |
| No | −0.089 | 0.018 | <.001 | −0.072 | 0.013 | <.001 |
| Yes | Ref. | | | Ref. | | |
| Nutritional Fact Usage | | | | | | |
| No | −0.087 | 0.022 | <.001 | −0.056 | 0.014 | <.001 |
| Yes | Ref. | | | Ref. | | |

Adjusted for living arrangement, residential area, BMI, weight changes, marital status, educational level, income level, occupation, alcohol consumption, smoking, stress level, nutritional education, nutrient supplement intake, and nutrition facts usage

with others; this finding is consistent in subgroups who have a tertiary education, have the lowest or highest income level, and are part of the 'others' group in occupation classification, which includes those who are not currently working. From our study, we also found the result showing gender difference. Men were showing positive correlation to MAR while women were showing negative in age group and stress level. We interpreted the results that it is possible that gender difference could be related to the result. We reviewed previous studies and found that that men and women have different patterns and choices related to food consumption that men choose more toward meat products while women are more in vegetables [30–32]. Like their findings, our study shows vitamins such as Vitamin A, Vitamin B1and Vitamin C intakes were higher in women. Regarding the stress level related to MAR, there are many discussions that men and women have a different stress coping mechanism [33–35]. Also, stress and diet quality has an association that stress can influence eating patterns [36, 37]. Due to the stress, some people changes their eating

**Table 3** Eating style and MAR by socioeconomic status

| Variables | Eating Style | | | | | | |
|---|---|---|---|---|---|---|---|
| | Together | Alone | | | Some Together | | |
| | β | β | S.E | *p*-value | β | S.E | *p*-value |
| Male | | | | | | | |
| One person household | | | | | | | |
| Yes | Ref. | −0.072 | 0.105 | 0.495 | 0.030 | 0.090 | 0.742 |
| No | Ref. | −0.134 | 0.039 | 0.001 | −0.002 | 0.018 | 0.919 |
| Education Level | | | | | | | |
| Primary | Ref. | −0.141 | 0.091 | 0.124 | 0.022 | 0.062 | 0.725 |
| Secondary | Ref. | 0.019 | 0.114 | 0.867 | −0.039 | 0.499 | 0.499 |
| Upper Secondary | Ref. | −0.036 | 0.056 | 0.520 | 0.000 | 0.030 | 0.999 |
| Tertiary | Ref. | −0.212 | 0.059 | <.001 | −0.002 | 0.027 | 0.934 |
| Income Level | | | | | | | |
| Lowest | Ref. | −0.216 | 0.068 | 0.002 | 0.024 | 0.040 | 0.539 |
| Lower-Middle | Ref. | −0.045 | 0.063 | 0.479 | 0.010 | 0.033 | 0.752 |
| Upper-Middle | Ref. | −0.058 | 0.079 | 0.462 | −0.008 | 0.037 | 0.827 |
| Highest | Ref. | −0.167 | 0.081 | 0.040 | −0.032 | 0.036 | 0.367 |
| Occupation | | | | | | | |
| White Collar | Ref. | −0.003 | 0.085 | 0.970 | 0.030 | 0.031 | 0.343 |
| Pink Collar | Ref. | −0.067 | 0.085 | 0.435 | −0.123 | 0.050 | 0.015 |
| Blue Collar | Ref. | −0.112 | 0.059 | 0.057 | 0.015 | 0.029 | 0.595 |
| Others | Ref. | −0.193 | 0.070 | 0.006 | −0.007 | 0.046 | 0.887 |
| Female | | | | | | | |
| One person household | | | | | | | |
| Yes | Ref. | 0.059 | 0.092 | 0.519 | 0.103 | 0.086 | 0.234 |
| No | Ref. | −0.081 | 0.026 | 0.002 | −0.010 | 0.014 | 0.475 |
| Education Level | | | | | | | |
| Primary | Ref. | −0.163 | 0.055 | 0.003 | −0.040 | 0.039 | 0.309 |
| Secondary | Ref. | −0.146 | 0.071 | 0.040 | −0.068 | 0.045 | 0.128 |
| Upper Secondary | Ref. | −0.048 | 0.042 | 0.252 | 0.009 | 0.022 | 0.695 |
| Tertiary | Ref. | −0.024 | 0.043 | 0.578 | −0.008 | 0.023 | 0.710 |
| Income Level | | | | | | | |
| Lowest | Ref. | −0.077 | 0.046 | 0.096 | −0.020 | 0.030 | 0.501 |
| Lower-Middle | Ref. | −0.083 | 0.048 | 0.086 | −0.010 | 0.027 | 0.702 |
| Upper-Middle | Ref. | −0.086 | 0.051 | 0.092 | −0.041 | 0.028 | 0.135 |
| Highest | Ref. | −0.044 | 0.052 | 0.400 | 0.031 | 0.028 | 0.271 |
| Occupation | | | | | | | |
| White Collar | Ref. | −0.026 | 0.052 | 0.622 | −0.002 | 0.027 | 0.950 |
| Pink Collar | Ref. | −0.125 | 0.059 | 0.035 | −0.016 | 0.036 | 0.669 |
| Blue Collar | Ref. | −0.178 | 0.062 | 0.004 | −0.055 | 0.034 | 0.107 |
| Others | Ref. | −0.038 | 0.037 | 0.306 | −0.006 | 0.021 | 0.795 |

Adjusted for living arrangement, residential area, BMI, weight changes, marital status, educational level, income level, occupation, alcohol consumption, smoking, stress level, nutritional education, nutrient supplement intake, and nutrition facts usage

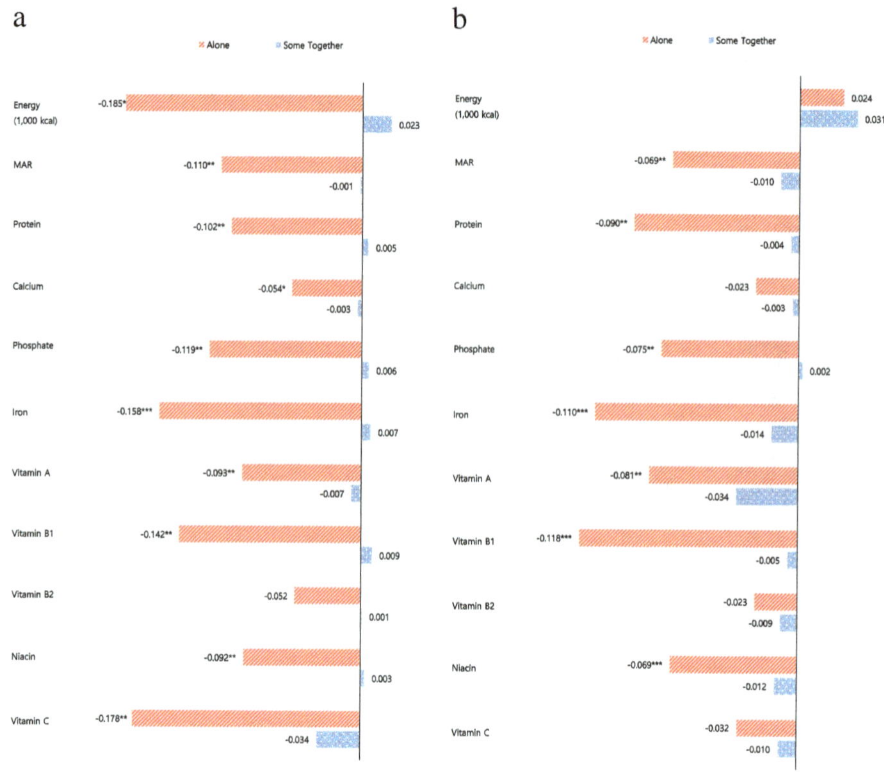


- Adjusted for living arrangement, residential area, BMI, weight changes, marital status, educational level, income level, occupation, alcohol consumption, smoking, stress level, nutritional education, nutrient supplement intake, and nutrition facts usage; Reference: With Others

*p<0.05 **p<0.01 ***p<0.001

**Fig. 1 a** Energy, MAR, and NAR per day in men. **b** Energy, MAR, and NAR per day in women. Alone, Some together, Energy (1000 kcal), MAR Protein, Protein, Calcium, Phosphate, Iron, Vitamin A, Vitamin B1, Vitamin B2, Niacin, Vitamin

habits and eat more and some eat less and even develop an eating disorder [38]. Therefore, our results could be led by gender differences in stress coping strategies by eating patterns.

With the result of the subgroup analysis, we discovered that the living arrangement for male and female does not influence the diet quality. As per socioeconomic factors, occupation status shows an association between diet qualities. Compared to men who have an office job, men in the service industry, manual work, and others show a gradual decline in diet quality when they eat alone. In the female population, education level expressed a similar trend. From the higher education level to lower education level, the diet quality declined when they eat alone. In the occupational status, women who are in manual work or service industry showed a significant low diet quality.

MAR which is the mean adequacy ratio is one of the indicators to evaluate the individual's nutrient intake. To obtain the value of MAR, the nutrient adequacy ratio, NAR is needed. NAR is the measure of a nutrient intake that is corresponding to the recommended dietary allowance (RDA) for the specific gender and age group [27, 28]. Unlike other nutrition indicators, it does not include total individual energy intake. However, it is allowed to express the comprehensiveness of the dietary quality. In measuring individual's dietary quality, MAR has been considered as a valid indicator as it references to the recommended dietary allowance [39, 40]. Therefore, we used the Korean Recommended Allowance for Nutrients as the reference to calculate NAR. When the NAR or MAR is 1 or above 1, it indicates that the individual has consumed the adequate amount of nutrient that reached RDA. Compared to previous studies, some of our outcomes were similar [20, 23] in men with low income levels. Additionally, related to income, a previous study concluded that people with higher education and income levels will have a better diet because they can afford diet costs [2, 20]. Our results provide another point of view different from the conventional idea of most previous studies; people who have higher socioeconomic status have better meals [2, 20, 41, 42] yet, their diet quality at the individual nutrient level shows insufficient in a certain nutrient.

Our study was conducted with a national survey and the sample is representative of the general Korean population. In addition, previous studies on nutrition were heavily focused on specific generation, while our study population is adults [19, 21, 43]. The volume of research on eating alone has increased as it has become a social issue that is very relevant in today's society. However, there are hardly any studies evaluating an association between eating behaviour and diet quality through MAR, so this is one of the advantages of this study. The outcomes from our study provide another perspective on the association between socioeconomic status and diet quality. To determine overall diet quality we used MAR, which was calculated by the NAR for each of nine nutrients. This allowed us to view specific details about diet quality as the NAR indicates the exact amount of each nutrient in the diet. In addition, the simple calculation of MAR is composed of micronutrients that provide more detailed nutrient intake and quality information than categorized food groups such as Healthy Eating Index [44].

While there are advantages compared to other studies, there are also several limitations that require investigation through further study. First, there are limitations inherent in a cross-sectional study design and use of survey data. A causal relationship between variables cannot be determined, unlike a study conducted through cohort data [25] in health survey data and nutrition survey data. Therefore, the cause and effect could be vice versa. Also, we might not include all the possible cofounders for the study. In addition, from the nutrition survey, we cannot ensure participants answered with an exact awareness of their food consumption history. The survey was designed to answer for the past 1 year of dietary data rather than 24-h recall data. This would lead to recall bias. Also, the question, by asking for the average of 1 week of the past 1 year to provide supportive evidence to lower the potential bias. This allowed the survey to get general information regarding dietary habits. In this study, carbohydrate and fat did not calculate for NAR and MAR. Based on the methods of KNHANES data on nutrients intake, it was not able to measure NAR for fat and carbohydrates. To calculate NAR, the measurement of units of denominator and numerator should be comparable. In this study, the unit of denominator value is the Recommended Dietary Allowance (RDA) which is reported by The Korean Nutrition Society and The Ministry of Health and Welfare of Korea announce the RDA for the Korean population. In the report, the fat and carbohydrate are given in the Acceptable Macronutrient Distribution Range (AMDR) while the survey, the numerator is collected in the unit of a gram per day. Therefore, matching those two different units of measure to calculate the NAR or MAR was limited when NAR and MAR require to measure the amount of consumed nutrient. Therefore, we reviewed the adequate nutrient intake of nine nutrients and level of energy [26, 29]. Many studies using MAR and NAR as the outcome values, they do not have the exact same nutrients or all macronutrients to evaluate the level of MAR. Previous investigations [22, 45, 46] in the Korean population, they also excluded carbohydrates and fats measures. Those studies included protein, calcium, phosphorus, iron vitamin A, vitamin B, vitamin B1, vitamin B2, niacin, Vitamin C which was the same as our nutrients. In addition, the recent study done by Donna B. Johnson et al. [47] to assess the nutritional quality of adolescents in US Washington State. In that study, they included calcium, vitamin C, vitamin A, iron, fibre, and protein to measure MAR. As the MAR is the mean value of adequacy of nutrients, the choice of nutrients is dependent on the researchers. Also, due to the data source, we were able to collect nine nutrients and energy to be studied. Therefore, we suggest conducting comprehensive studies with other nutrients such as carbohydrates, fats, fibre, sodium, and other minerals. We measured diet quality with MAR, which is the average nutrient intake. Since it represents the average amount of adequate nutrient intake ratio, it might be misinterpreted that when the MAR equal to 1. There is a possibility that some of the nutrients are compensating for each other in the MAR. Therefore, the investigation of each nutrient would be helpful. To overcome this type of error, we prepared supplementary tables (Additional file 1: Appendix 3) to see the NAR for each nutrient and noticed certain nutrients are below the recommendations such as calcium, vitamin A, and niacin.

In 2015, the one-person household was reported at 27.2% of the total population of Korea, compared to 15.2% in 2000. It is reasonable to expect that the prevalence of persons eating alone will also increase [24]. The Korea Statistics projects that, in 2045, one-person households will make up 36.6% of the total population. It has also been forecasted that the elderly population will expand as well [14, 24]. Based on these numbers, it is not hard to expect that solitary eating will become a common way of eating. Many studies warn that a poor diet could lead to serious health problems [10–12] and emphasize the importance of quality meals [9, 23]. People today experience "modern malnutrition", which is caused by modern diet habits such as high intakes of sugar, fat, fast food, and soda [8, 11, 48–50]. This type of diet is typically found in solitary eating. If people continue to eat alone, they will have potential risks of developing obesity and metabolic syndromes [11, 45].

The new social phenomena of an increase in one-person households creates public isolation, which can affect public health [14], but at the same time, we need to acknowledge that we have been ignoring the potential risk that another party could have. We were able to infer that, along with changes in our daily lifestyle, products that supplement diet balance for people who live alone may be beneficial. However, people who live together, mostly with family [25] consider their meals better than others even when they eat alone. Similar to that idea, people who are in a higher social stratum are considered more able to maintain their health by themselves. As we discovered from our analyses, poor meal quality does not appear only among the socially disadvantaged or those who live alone. The results indicate that we should promote nutritional health awareness to the lower socioeconomic class yet we should discriminate to improve diet quality for the entire population as the result of subgroup analysis shown.

## Conclusions

This study provides evidence to promote interventions to improve the quality of the diet of the public. Many Korean adults are experiencing low diet quality when they eat alone. The number of people who eat alone is increasing along with the changes of lifestyle. Also, the people who were considered as upper socio-economic status, such as who have high income, education level and white collar occupation status, are also experiencing issues in diet quality. Our study is highly recommended to policy-makers to utilize it as evidence to develop and improve social welfare services for the general population.

### Abbreviations

BMI: Body mass index; GLM: Generalized linear model; KNHANES: Korean National Health and Nutrition Examination Survey; MAR: Mean adequacy ratio; NAR: The nutrient adequacy ratio; RDA: Recommended dietary allowance

### Acknowledgements

The authors appreciate the Yonsei University Institute of Health Services Research for its administrative support. Also, they thank Korea Centers for Disease Control and Prevention that provided meaningful data.

### Funding

This research received no specific grant from any funding agency, commercial or not-for-profit sectors.

### Authors' contributions

WJC, JS, YJJ and SIJ designed the research and developed the overall research plan. WJC analysed the data and wrote the manuscript. JS and YJJ contributed to perform the statistical analysis. JS and SIJ provided intellectual input for the manuscript. ECP supervised the study. All members read and approved the final manuscript for quality assurance of the study.

### Competing interests

The authors declare that they have no competing interests.

### Author details

[1]Department of Public Health, College of Medicine, Yonsei University, Seoul, Republic of Korea. [2]Institute of Health Services Research, Yonsei University, 50 Yonsei-ro, Seodaemun-gu, Seoul 120-752, Republic of Korea. [3]Department of Preventive Medicine, College of Medicine, Yonsei University, 50 Yonsei-ro, Seodaemun-gu, Seoul 120-752, Republic of Korea.

### References

1. Becker EM, Nissen LR, Skibsted LH. Antioxidant evaluation protocols: food quality or health effects. Eur Food Res Technol. 2004;219(6):561–71. https://doi.org/10.1007/s00217-004-1012-4.
2. Darmon N, Drewnowski A. Does social class predict diet quality? Am J Clin Nutr. 2008;87(5):1107–17. https://doi.org/10.1093/ajcn/87.5.1107.
3. Zaki M, Hussein L, Gouda M, Bassuoni R, Hassanein A. Nutritional epidemiological study to estimate usual intake and to define optimum nutrient profiling choice in the diet of Egyptian youths. Food Nutr Sci. 2015; 06(15):15. https://doi.org/10.4236/fns.2015.615147.
4. Gouda M, Moustafa A, Hussein L, Hamza M. Three week dietary intervention using apricots, pomegranate juice or/and fermented sour sobya and impact on biomarkers of antioxidative activity, oxidative stress and erythrocytic glutathione transferase activity among adults. Nutr J. 2016;15:52. https://doi.org/10.1186/s12937-016-0173-x.
5. Rozin P. The meaning of food in our lives: a cross-cultural perspective on eating and well-being. J Nutr Educ Behav. 2005;37:S107–S12. https://doi.org/10.1016/S1499-4046(06)60209-1.
6. Rozin P, Fischler C, Imada S, Sarubin A, Wrzesniewski A. Attitudes to food and the role of food in life in the USA, Japan, Flemish Belgium and France: possible implications for the diet–health debate. Appetite. 1999;33(2):163–80. https://doi.org/10.1006/appe.1999.0244.
7. Lásztity RR. Food quality and standard. In: Encyclopedia of life support systems. Oxford: Eolss Publishers; 2009. p. 1–41.
8. Alkerwi AA. Diet quality concept. Nutrition. 2014;30(6):613–8. https://doi.org/10.1016/j.nut.2013.10.001.
9. Wirt A, Collins CE. Diet quality--what is it and does it matter? Public Health Nutr. 2009;12(12):2473–92. https://doi.org/10.1017/s136898000900531x.
10. Lee Y, Mitchell DC, Smiciklas-Wright H, Birch LL. Diet quality, nutrient intake, weight status, and feeding environments of girls meeting or exceeding recommendations for total dietary fat of the American Academy of Pediatrics. Pediatrics. 2001;107(6):e95-e. https://doi.org/10.1542/peds.107.6.e95.
11. Mwatsama M, Stewart L. Food poverty and health food poverty and health. London: Royal Colleges of Physicians of the United Kingdom; 2005.
12. McCullough ML, Feskanich D, Stampfer MJ, Giovannucci EL, Rimm EB, Hu FB, et al. Diet quality and major chronic disease risk in men and women: moving toward improved dietary guidance. Am J Clin Nutr. 2002;76(6): 1261–71. https://doi.org/10.1093/ajcn/76.6.1261.
13. Kimura Y, Wada T, Okumiya K, Ishimoto Y, Fukutomi E, Kasahara Y, et al. Eating alone among community-dwelling Japanese elderly: association with depression and food diversity. J Nutr Health Aging. 2012;16(8):728–31. https://doi.org/10.1007/s12603-012-0067-3.
14. Victor C, Scambler S, Bond J, Bowling A. Being alone in later life: loneliness, social isolation and living alone. Rev Clin Gerontol. 2000;10(04):407–17. https://doi.org/10.1017/S0959259800104101.
15. Hays NP, Roberts SB. The anorexia of aging in humans. Physiol Behav. 2006; 88(3):257–66. https://doi.org/10.1016/j.physbeh.2006.05.029.
16. Vesnaver E, Keller HH, Sutherland O, Maitland SB, Locher JL. Alone at the table: food behavior and the loss of commensality in widowhood. J Gerontol B. 2016;71(6):1059–69. https://doi.org/10.1093/geronb/gbv103.
17. Woodruff SJ, Hanning RM. Family Meals and Diet Quality. In: Preedy VR, Hunter L-A, Patel VB, editors. Diet Quality: an evidence-based approach, vol. 2. New York: Springer New York; 2013. p. 89–100.
18. Larson N, MacLehose R, Fulkerson JA, Berge JM, Story M, Neumark-Sztainer D. Eating breakfast and dinner together as a family: associations with sociodemographic characteristics and implications for diet quality and weight status. J Acad Nutr Diet. 2013;113(12):1601–9. https://doi.org/10.1016/j.jand.2013.08.011.
19. Larson NI, Neumark-Sztainer D, Hannan PJ, Story M. Family meals during adolescence are associated with higher diet quality and healthful meal patterns during young adulthood. J Am Diet Assoc. 2007;107(9):1502–10. https://doi.org/10.1016/j.jada.2007.06.012.

20. Aggarwal A, Monsivais P, Cook AJ, Drewnowski A. Does diet cost mediate the relation between socioeconomic position and diet quality? Eur J Clin Nutr. 2011;65(9):1059–66. https://doi.org/10.1038/ejcn.2011.72.
21. Hughes G, Bennett KM, Hetherington MM. Old and alone: barriers to healthy eating in older men living on their own. Appetite. 2004;43(3):269–76. https://doi.org/10.1016/j.appet.2004.06.002.
22. Moon H-K, Kong J-E. Assessment of nutrient intake for middle aged with and without metabolic syndrome using 2005 and 2007 Korean National Health and nutrition survey. Kor J Nutr. 2010;43(1):69–78. https://doi.org/10.4163/kjn.2010.43.1.69.
23. Patrick H, Nicklas TA. A review of family and social determinants of children's eating patterns and diet quality. J Am Coll Nutr. 2005;24(2):83–92. https://doi.org/10.1080/07315724.2005.10719448.
24. Lee EJ. Estimated future population 2015–2045. Korea Statistics; 2017. http://kostat.go.kr/portal/korea/kor_nw/2/2/1/index.board?bmode=read&bSeq=&aSeq=359963&pageNo=1&rowNum=10&navCount=10&currPg=&sTarget=title&sTxt=2045. Accessed 7 Apr 2017.
25. Conklin AI, Forouhi NG, Surtees P, Khaw KT, Wareham NJ, Monsivais P. Social relationships and healthful dietary behaviour: evidence from over-50s in the EPIC cohort, UK. Soc Sci Med. 2014;100:167–75. https://doi.org/10.1016/j.socscimed.2013.08.018.
26. Ministry of Health & Welfare, The Korean Nutrition Society. Dietary reference intakes for Koreans 2015. Seoul: The Korean Nutrition Society; 2015.
27. Kant AK. Indexes of overall diet quality: a review. J Am Diet Assoc. 1996;96(8):785–91. https://doi.org/10.1016/s0002-8223(96)00217-9.
28. Hatløy A, Torheim L, Oshaug A. Food Variety - A Good Indicator of Nutritional Adequacy of the Diet? A Case Study from an Urban Area in Mali, West Africa; 1998.
29. Yoon JS. Evaluation of nutritional status of adults by food guide and food composition group score. J Liv Sci Res. 2002;28:1–10.
30. Wardle J, Haase AM, Steptoe A, Nillapun M, Jonwutiwes K, Bellisie F. Gender differences in food choice: the contribution of health beliefs and dieting. Ann Behav Med. 2004;27(2):107–16. https://doi.org/10.1207/s15324796abm2702_5.
31. Fraser GE, Welch A, Luben R, Bingham SA, Day NE. The effect of age, sex, and education on food consumption of a middle-aged English cohort—EPIC in East Anglia. Prev Med. 2000;30(1):26–34. https://doi.org/10.1006/pmed.1999.0598.
32. Morse KL, Driskell JA. Observed sex differences in fast-food consumption and nutrition self-assessments and beliefs of college students. Nutr Res 2009;29(3):173–9. https://doi.org/10.1016/j.nutres.2009.02.004.
33. Narayanan L, Menon S, Spector PE. Stress in the workplace: a comparison of gender and occupations. J Organ Behav. 1999;20(1):63–73. https://doi.org/10.1002/(SICI)1099-1379(199901)20:1<63::AID-JOB873>3.0.CO;2-J.
34. Assari S, Lankarani MM. Association between stressful life events and depression; intersection of race and gender. J Racial Ethn Health Disparities. 2016;3(2):349–56. https://doi.org/10.1007/s40615-015-0160-5.
35. Matud MP. Gender differences in stress and coping styles. Personal Individ Differ. 2004;37(7):1401–15. https://doi.org/10.1016/j.paid.2004.01.010.
36. Tryon MS, Carter CS, DeCant R, Laugero KD. Chronic stress exposure may affect the brain's response to high calorie food cues and predispose to obesogenic eating habits. Physiol Behav. 2013;120:233–42. https://doi.org/10.1016/j.physbeh.2013.08.010.
37. Michels N, Sioen I, Braet C, Eiben G, Hebestreit A, Huybrechts I, et al. Stress, emotional eating behaviour and dietary patterns in children. Appetite. 2012;59(3):762–9. https://doi.org/10.1016/j.appet.2012.08.010.
38. Harrison A, Sullivan S, Tchanturia K, Treasure J. Emotional functioning in eating disorders: attentional bias, emotion recognition and emotion regulation. Psychol Med. 2010;40(11):1887–97. https://doi.org/10.1017/S0033291710000036.
39. Acham H, Wilna O-T, Egal A. Dietary diversity, micronutrient intake and their variation among black women in informal settlements in South Africa: a cross-sectional study; 2012.
40. Steyn NP, Nel J, Labadarios D, Maunder EMW, Kruger HS. Which dietary diversity indicator is best to assess micronutrient adequacy in children 1 to 9 y? Nutrition. 2014;30(1):55–60. https://doi.org/10.1016/j.nut.2013.06.002.
41. Ahmed FE, Gouda MM, Hussein LA, Ahmed NC, Vos PW, Mohammad MA. Role of melt curve analysis in interpretation of Nutrigenomics' MicroRNA expression data. Cancer Genomics Proteomics. 2017;14(6):469–81. https://doi.org/10.21873/cgp.20057.
42. Shankar V, Gouda M, Moncivaiz J, Gordon A, Reo NV, Hussein L, et al. Differences in gut metabolites and microbial composition and functions between Egyptian and U.S. children are consistent with their diets. mSystems. 2017;2:1. https://doi.org/10.1128/mSystems.00169-16.
43. Larson N, Fulkerson J, Story M, Neumark-Sztainer D. Shared meals among young adults are associated with better diet quality and predicted by family meal patterns during adolescence. Public Health Nutr. 2013;16(5):883–93. https://doi.org/10.1017/s1368980012003539.
44. Torheim LE, Ouattara F, Diarra MM, Thiam FD, Barikmo I, Hatløy A, et al. Nutrient adequacy and dietary diversity in rural Mali: association and determinants. Eur J Clin Nutr. 2004;58:594. https://doi.org/10.1038/sj.ejcn.1601853.
45. Kim MH. Characteristics of nutrient intake according to metabolic syndrome in Korean elderly - using data from the Korea National Health and nutrition examination survey 2010 Korean J. Food Nutr. 2013;26(3):515–25. https://doi.org/10.9799/ksfan.2013.26.3.515.
46. H-s L, Cho G, Kim S. Evaluation of nutrient intake and diet quality of gastric cancer patients in Korea. Nutr Res Pract. 2012;6:213–20. https://doi.org/10.4162/nrp.2012.6.3.213.
47. Johnson DB, Podrabsky M, Rocha A, Otten JJ. Effect of the healthy hunger-free kids act on the nutritional quality of meals selected by students and school lunch participation rates. JAMA Pediatr. 2016;170(1):e153918. https://doi.org/10.1001/jamapediatrics.2015.3918.
48. Gouda M, Zu L, Ma S, Sheng L, Ma M. Influence of bio-active terpenes on the characteristics and functional properties of egg yolk. Food Hydrocoll. 2018;80:222–30. https://doi.org/10.1016/j.foodhyd.2018.02.009.
49. Fouad MT, Moustafa A, Hussein L, Romeilah R, Gouda M. In-vitro antioxidant and antimicrobial activities of selected fruit and vegetable juices and fermented dairy products commonly consumed in Egypt; 2015.
50. Gouda M, Shisi Z, Yuanyuan L, Sheng L, Ma M. Effects of four natural antioxidant phenyl terpenes on emulsifying and rheological properties of egg yolk. 2017.

14

# Greenhouse gas emissions of self-selected diets in the UK and their association with diet quality: is energy under-reporting a problem?

Kentaro Murakami[1*] and M. Barbara E. Livingstone[2]

**Abstract**

**Background:** While the admittedly limited number of epidemiological findings on the association between diet-related greenhouse gas emissions (GHGE) and diet quality are not always consistent, potential influence of bias in the estimation of diet-related GHGE caused by misreporting of energy intake (EI) has not been investigated. This cross-sectional study evaluated diet-related GHGE in the UK and their association with diet quality, taking account of EI under-reporting.

**Methods:** Dietary data used were from the National Diet and Nutrition Survey rolling programme 2008/2009–2013/2014, in which 4-day food diaries were collected from 3502 adults aged ≥19 years. Diet-related GHGE were estimated based on 133 food groups, using GHGE values from various secondary sources. Diet quality was assessed by the healthy diet indicator (HDI), Mediterranean diet score (MDS) and Dietary Approaches to Stop Hypertension (DASH) score. EI misreporting was assessed as reported EI divided by estimated energy requirement (EI:EER).

**Results:** Mean value of daily GHGE was 5.7 kg carbon dioxide equivalents ($CO_2eq$), which is consistent with those reported from a number of national representative samples in other European countries. Mean EI:EER was 0.74. Assuming that all the dietary variables were misreported in proportion to the misreporting of EI, the mean value of the misreporting-adjusted diet-related GHGE was 8.2 kg $CO_2eq$/d. In the entire population, after adjustment for potential confounders (i.e., age, sex, ethnicity, socioeconomic classification, smoking status and physical activity), diet-related GHGE were inversely associated with HDI and DASH score but not with MDS. However, with further adjustment for EI:EER, diet-related GHGE showed inverse associations with all three measures of diet quality. Similar associations were observed when only under-reporters (EI:EER < 0.70; $n = 1578$) were analysed. Conversely, in the analysis including only plausible reporters (EI:EER 0.70–1.43; $n = 1895$), diet-related GHGE showed inverse associations with all diet quality measures irrespective of adjustment.

**Conclusions:** With taking account of EI under-reporting, this study showed inverse associations between diet related GHGE and diet quality not only in the entire sample but also in the separate analyses of plausible reporters and under-reporters, as well as potential underreporting of diet-related GHGE.

**Keywords:** Sustainable diets, Healthy diets, Food consumption, Misreporting

* Correspondence: kenmrkm@m.u-tokyo.ac.jp
[1]Interfaculty Initiative in Information Studies, University of Tokyo, Tokyo 113 0033, Japan
Full list of author information is available at the end of the article

## Background

Rising concerns about climate change led the UK Government to pass the 2008 Climate Change Act, which mandates a reduction in greenhouse gas emissions (GHGE) by 80% by 2050 against the 1990 level [1]. The food supply chain is a major source of GHGE, and the food sector has been estimated to account for 15 to 30% of total GHGE in developed countries [2–4]. Reducing this burden of contemporary food consumption practices on the environment while also improving human health concerns is thus a major challenge of the twenty-first century [5]. While red meat is the top contributor to diet-related GHGE in high-income countries [6–9], higher consumption of red meat has been associated with an increasing risk of total, CVD and cancer mortality [10–12]. Conversely, higher intakes of plant-based foods with lower GHGE such as vegetables, fruits, whole grains and nuts have been associated with lower mortality [11, 13].

Nevertheless, the admittedly limited number of epidemiological findings derived using self-selected diets are not always consistent [14]. Some have reported inverse associations between diet-related GHGE and measures of diet quality [15, 16] while others report positive associations [6]. These heterogeneous results might reflect differences in the types of data sources used, system boundaries in the emission factors adopted, participant characteristics and food and nutrient intake patterns associated with diet-related GHGE [7, 9, 17, 18], in addition to different measures of diet quality. Alternatively, because diet related GHGE are directly correlated with energy intake (EI) [8, 15, 19], these associations might be confounded by misreporting of EI, particularly under-reporting, which remains an ongoing problem with all self-reported dietary surveys. Although several researchers have raised concerns about the potential influence of this bias in this research field [7, 9, 20, 21], no comprehensive evaluation of its putative impact has yet been made.

A simple and easy way to account for EI under-reporting is to exclude individuals with implausible EI from the analysis, as conducted in several previous studies [7, 9, 20, 21]. However, because EI under-reporting is associated with certain characteristics, particularly overweight and obesity [22–24], this procedure is likely to introduce a selection bias (in addition to reducing sample size) [22, 25]. Another way to account for EI under-reporting is to incorporate the ratio of EI to estimated energy requirement (EER) as a covariate in statistical models [26–29]. Here, we conducted a cross-sectional study to evaluate the GHGE of self-selected diets in the UK and their association with measures of diet quality, while taking account of EI under-reporting.

## Methods

### Data source and analytic sample

The study was conducted under a cross-sectional design using data obtained between 2008/2009 and 2013/2014 as part of the National Diet and Nutrition Survey (NDNS) rolling programme. Details of that study are provided elsewhere [30, 31]. In brief, a nationally representative sample (approximately 500 adults aged ≥19 years and 500 children aged 1.5–18 years) is selected each year via a multi-stage random probability design using a selection of post codes throughout the UK. Further, additional recruitment is carried out in Scotland, Wales and Northern Ireland to obtain country-specific representative data (up to 600 participants per year) [32, 33]. Households are then selected, followed finally by individuals (up to one adult and one child) in participating households. Data collection is conducted throughout the year. The overall response rate ranged from 53% to 56%, depending on survey year [30, 31]. The number of participants aged ≥19 years in the 2008/2009–2013/2014 NDNS rolling programme was 4738. After excluding individuals with missing or invalid information on the variables of interest ($n = 330$ for height and weight; $n = 1$ for smoking status; $n = 814$ for physical activity (PA)) and those without 4-day dietary data ($n = 91$), the final analytic sample comprised 3502 adults. None of the women included in the analysis were pregnant or breastfeeding during the survey period. The NDNS rolling programme is conducted according to the guidelines laid down in the Declaration of Helsinki and all procedures involving human subjects are approved by the Oxfordshire Research Ethics Committee. Written informed consent is obtained from all participants. Data for the present study were obtained from the UK Data Archive.

### Assessment of basic characteristics

Body height (to the nearest 0.1 cm) and weight (to the nearest 0.1 kg) were measured while the participant was wearing light clothes only, without shoes. Body mass index (BMI; kg/m$^2$) was calculated as weight (kg) divided by height (m) squared. Self-reported information was collected on the following variables. Socioeconomic status was determined by the National Statistics socioeconomic classification [34], and categorized as higher and managerial occupation, intermediate occupation, routine and manual occupation or other. Ethnicity was categorized as white or nonwhite. Smoking status was categorized as current, former or never smoker.

PA was assessed by a validated questionnaire (i.e., Recent Physical Activity Questionnaire) [35]. In brief, this questionnaire is designed to assess a wide range of PA in the past month in four domains (home, work, commuting and leisure activities). As described elsewhere [36], the time per day spent in moderate-to-vigorous physical activity (MVPA) was calculated. Descriptions on PA categories (i.e., sedentary, low active, active and very active) and the amount of time spent in MVPA are available in the US Dietary Reference Intakes (DRI) [37]. Specifically, the guidelines state that participation in an additional 30 min of moderate activity raises an individual from the sedentary to the low-active PA category, and about 60 min of moderate activity raises an individual from the sedentary to the active PA category [38, 39]. Thus, the following four categories on PA were created and used in the present analysis: sedentary (< 30 min of MVPA), low active (≥30 to < 60 min of MPVA), active (≥60 to < 120 min of MVPA) and very active (≥120 min of MVPA).

#### Dietary assessment

Dietary data were collected using a 4-consecutive-day estimated food diary. A detailed description of the procedure has been published elsewhere [40]. In brief, the participants were requested to maintain a record of all items eaten or drunk for four consecutive days. The recording schedule was designed so that all days of the week were evenly represented. Each participant was supplied with a recording diary and a set of photographs of 15 major foods in small, median and large portion sizes, as well as written and verbal instructions by trained interviewers on how the diary should be maintained. The participants used the photographs to describe the portion sizes of foods they consumed. For other foods, portion sizes were described in household measures (e.g., one tablespoon of baked beans) or as the weight indicated on the food package. Trained interviewers visited the household once during the recording period and once within three days after it to check on the completeness of food recording, and whenever necessary sought additional information or modification of the record. The collected diaries were checked by trained coders and editors for coding of food items and for portion sizes. Estimates of daily intake for foods, energy and selected nutrients were calculated based on the Department of Health's NDNS nutrient data bank, which itself is based on McCance and Widdowson's Composition of Foods series [41]. For all dietary variables, mean values over the 4 recording days were used in the analysis.

#### Assessment of diet quality

Overall diet quality was assessed using the healthy diet indicator (HDI) [42, 43], Mediterranean diet score (MDS) [43, 44] and Dietary Approaches to Stop Hypertension (DASH) score [45, 46] (see Additional file 1: Table S1). These diet quality measures have been prospectively associated with certain desired health outcomes, including lower mortality [16, 42, 44, 47, 48]. The HDI was chosen as a diet quality measure for its primary focus on nutrient intake, while the MDS and DASH score were selected for their primary focus on intake of food group/type.

The HDI incorporates six nutrients and one food group (saturated fat; polyunsaturated fat; protein; dietary fibre; cholesterol; and non-milk extrinsic sugar; and fruits and vegetables) [42, 43]. If intake remained within the recommended WHO guideline range, that component was assigned a score of one; if not, it was assigned a score of zero, giving a total score range of zero to seven, with a higher score reflecting a healthier dietary pattern.

The MDS represents the Mediterranean diet type, based on the consumption of nine components (vegetables; legumes; fruits, nuts and seeds; cereals; fish; unsaturated to saturated fat ratio; dairy products; meat; and alcohol) [43, 44]. Regarding alcohol, moderate intake (i.e., 10–50 g/d for men and 5–25 g/d for women) was assigned a score of one. For dairy products and meat, a score of one was assigned to intake below or equal to the sex-specific median. For other components, a score of one was assigned to intake above or equal to the sex-specific median. Scores for the nine components were summed to give a total possible range of zero to nine, with a higher score reflecting better consistency with a Mediterranean-type diet.

The Fung's DASH score, originally developed for the US Nurse's Health Study [45], was used with the slight modification of Penney et al., which considered UK dietary habits [46]. Components considered in this measure are vegetables, fruits, whole grain foods, nuts and legumes, low fat dairy products, red and processed meats, non-milk extrinsic sugar, and sodium. Participants were classified for each component into sex-specific quintiles by intake. Scores ranged from 1 to 5 for each quintile; for vegetables, fruits, whole grain foods, nuts and legumes, and low fat dairy products, higher intakes were given higher scores, while for red and processed meats, non-milk extrinsic sugar and sodium, higher intakes were given lower scores. Scores for the eight components were summed, giving a total possible score range of 8, indicating lowest adherence, to 40, for maximum adherence.

#### Estimation of diet-related greenhouse gas emissions

Diet-related GHGE, expressed as kg of carbon dioxide equivalent ($CO_2$eq), were calculated as the sum of the product of GHGE value of food group and intake of food group. GHGE values of each food group were taken from Green et al. [49], where values were calculated using life cycle analysis data from the literature, mainly from the UK and Europe, based on all stages from food production, packing, distribution, storage/refrigeration, transportation (farm-to-outlet and retailer-to-home), food handling/preparation (including trimmings and cooking losses) to consumer waste (including spoilage and plate waste). The GHGE value of each food group ($n = 133$) used in this study is shown in Additional file 1: Table S2. GHGE for the following four food groups were not included in the analysis because of a lack of information in Green et al. [49]: tap water only; beverages dry weight; nutrition powders and drinks; and savoury sauces pickles gravies and condiments.

### Evaluation of the accuracy of energy intake misreporting

Misreporting of EI was evaluated based on the ratio of EI to EER, namely, the procedure proposed by Huang et al. [50]. Participants were identified as plausible reporters, under-reporters or over-reporters of EI according to whether the individual's ratio was within, below or above the 95% confidence limits of the expected EI:EER of 1.0. We calculated each subject's EER, based on the information on age, weight, height and PA category (i.e., sedentary, low-active, active or very active, as mentioned above), with the use of equations published from the US DRI [37]. The sex- and age-specific equations for use in populations with a range of weight statuses [37] were used. The 95% confidence limits of the expected EI:EER ratio of 0 on the natural log scale were calculated, taking into account CV in intakes and other components of energy balance (i.e., the within-subject variation in EI: 23%; the error in the EER equations: 11%; and the day-to-day variation in total energy expenditure: 8.2%) [37, 50, 51] as well as the number of diet recording days (4 d). Consequently, under-reporters, plausible reporters and over-reporters were defined as having an EI:EER < 0.70, 0.70–1.43 and > 1.43, respectively.

### Statistical analysis

Statistical analyses were performed using SAS statistical software (version 9.4, SAS Institute). All reported $P$ values are two-tailed, and $P < 0{\cdot}05$ was considered to be statistically significant. Initially, analyses were conducted separately for men and women, but the results were essentially the same, albeit that mean value of diet-related GHGE and the percentage of under-reporters were higher in men than women, as shown in the Results section. We therefore present the results for men and women combined.

Descriptive data are presented as means and SD for continuous variables and percentages of participants for categorical variables. Differences in diet-related GHGE across categories of each of the selected characteristics were examined by the independent $t$ test or ANOVA. When the overall $P$ value from ANOVA was < 0.05, Bonferroni's post hoc test was performed. Differences in plausible reporters and under-reporters (but not over-reporters, because of their small number) were tested by the independent $t$ test for continuous variables and the chi-square test for categorical variables. Correlations of diet-related GHGE and measures of diet quality (HDI, MDS and DASH score) with EI and EI:EER were investigated using Pearson correlation analyses.

Associations between diet-related GHGE and measures of diet quality were investigated by linear regression analyses using the PROC REG procedure. Potential confounding factors considered were age, sex, ethnicity, socioeconomic classification, smoking status and physical activity (model 1). Further adjustment was made for EI:EER (model 2). All analyses were conducted for the entire population, and also for plausible reporters only and for under-reporters only. It should be noted that adjustment for EI:EER in the analysis of plausible reporters was made because they are just those whose EI values are not extreme enough to be labelled as under- or over-reporters, and thus relatively small misreporting may still occur in plausible reporters.

Data used in the present analysis were weighted to account for the survey's complex sampling structure and non-response bias, using the published weights for combining data from the NDNS rolling programme 2008/2009 to 2013/2014, which has been described elsewhere [33, 52].

## Results

This analysis included 1429 men and 2073 women with a mean age of 48 years (Table 1). The mean value of crude diet-related GHGE was 5.7 kg $CO_2$eq/d (1st, 5th, 95th and 99th percentiles: 2.1, 3.0, 9.5 and 11.6 kg $CO_2$eq/d, respectively). Compared with EER, EI was under-reported by an average of 26%. Assuming that all the dietary variables were misreported in proportion to the misreporting of EI, the mean value of the misreporting-adjusted diet-related GHGE was 8.2 kg $CO_2$eq/d (1st, 5th, 95th and 99th percentiles: 3.4, 4.2, 14.1 and 17.0 kg $CO_2$eq/d, respectively). There were significant associations between diet-related GHGE and all of the potential confounding factors considered (Additional file 1: Table S3).

The percentages of plausible reporters and under-reporters of EI were 54 and 45%, respectively (only 29 participants (0.8%) were classified as over-reporters) (Table 1). Compared with plausible reporters, under-reporters were more likely to be younger, male, employed in routine and manual occupations, current smokers and physically active. They also had higher means of BMI, EER, HDI and DASH score and lower means of diet-related GHGE, EI and MDS.

In the entire population, red meat contributed about one-quarter of diet-related GHGE (24.4%), followed by dairy products, which contributed about one-eighth

**Table 1** Characteristics of participants [a]

| | All ($n$ = 3502) [b] | | Plausible reporters ($n$ = 1895) | | Under-reporters ($n$ = 1578) | | |
|---|---|---|---|---|---|---|---|
| | Mean | SD | Mean | SD | Mean | SD | $P$ [c] |
| Age (years) | 47.6 | 17.7 | 49.9 | 18.4 | 45.0 | 16.2 | < 0.0001 |
| Sex (% male) | 49.2 | | 44.3 | | 55.3 | | < 0.0001 |
| Ethnicity (% white) | 89.4 | | 90.0 | | 88.4 | | 0.13 |
| Socioeconomic classification (%) | | | | | | | < 0.0001 |
| Higher and managerial occupation | 44.3 | | 46.9 | | 41.4 | | |
| Intermediate occupation | 19.7 | | 20.4 | | 18.7 | | |
| Routine and manual occupation | 31.7 | | 27.9 | | 36.1 | | |
| Other | 4.4 | | 4.8 | | 3.9 | | |
| Smoking status (%) | | | | | | | < 0.0001 |
| Current | 21.5 | | 17.9 | | 24.9 | | |
| Former | 23.9 | | 23.6 | | 24.6 | | |
| Never | 54.7 | | 58.5 | | 50.5 | | |
| Physical activity (%) | | | | | | | < 0.0001 |
| Sedentary | 39.1 | | 50.4 | | 25.0 | | |
| Low active | 19.4 | | 21.9 | | 16.8 | | |
| Active | 19.6 | | 16.9 | | 23.1 | | |
| Very active | 21.8 | | 10.7 | | 35.1 | | |
| BMI (kg/m$^2$) | 27.4 | 5.4 | 26.4 | 4.9 | 28.6 | 5.6 | < 0.0001 |
| EI (kJ/d) | 7653 | 2375 | 8611 | 2119 | 6410 | 1847 | < 0.0001 |
| EER (kJ/d) | 10,699 | 2673 | 9788 | 2340 | 11,821 | 2803 | < 0.0001 |
| EI:EER | 0.74 | 0.23 | 0.89 | 0.14 | 0.55 | 0.11 | < 0.0001 |
| Diet-related GHGE (kg $CO_2$eq/d) | 5.7 | 2.1 | 6.3 | 2.1 | 5.0 | 1.8 | < 0.0001 |
| HDI | 2.3 | 1.1 | 2.2 | 1.2 | 2.4 | 1.1 | < 0.0001 |
| MDS | 4.5 | 1.7 | 4.6 | 1.7 | 4.3 | 1.7 | < 0.0001 |
| DASH score | 24.3 | 5.2 | 23.9 | 5.2 | 24.7 | 5.2 | < 0.0001 |

*BMI* body mass index, *$CO_2$eq* carbon dioxide equivalents, *DASH* Dietary Approaches to Stop Hypertension, *EER* estimated energy requirement, *EI* energy intake, *GHGE* greenhouse gas emissions, *HDI* healthy diet indicator, *MDS* Mediterranean diet score

[a] Plausible reporters were defined as participants with an EI:EER 0.70–1.43; under-reporters were defined as participants with an EI:EER < 0.70

[b] Including over-reporters ($n$ = 29), defined as participants with an EI:EER > 1.43

[c] $P$ values for differences between plausible reporters and under-reporters based on the independent $t$ test for continuous variables and the chi-square test for categorical variables

(13.6%) (Table 2). Other important contributors (≥5%) were soft drinks (7.3%), cereals (6.9%), sugar and confectioneries (6.0%), fish (6.0%), white meat (5.9%), fat and oils (5.5%) and vegetables (5.3%). Similar results were observed in the analysis of plausible reporters only and of under-reporters only.

Diet-related GHGE were strongly positively correlated with both EI and EI:EER in the entire population (Additional file 1: Table S4). While HDI and DASH score showed weak inverse correlations with EI and EI:EER, MDS was weakly and positively correlated with these measures. The correlations became somewhat weak (or nonsignificant) when analysed for plausible reporters and under-reporters separately, except for inverse correlations for HDI and positive correlations for MDS in under-reporters.

Table 3 shows associations between diet-related GHGE and diet quality measures. In the entire population, after adjustment for potential confounding factors (i.e., age, sex, ethnicity, socioeconomic classification, smoking status and physical activity; model 1), diet-related GHGE were inversely associated with HDI and DASH score but not with MDS. However, with further adjustment for EI:EER (model 2), diet-related GHGE showed inverse associations with all three measures of diet quality. Similar associations were observed when only under-reporters were analysed (albeit that the inverse association for MDS did not reach statistical significance). Conversely, in the analysis including only plausible reporters, diet-related GHGE showed inverse associations with all diet quality measures irrespective of adjustment.

**Table 2** Food group intake and percentage contribution of each food group to diet-related GHGE [a]

| | All ($n = 3502$) [b] | | | | Plausible reporters ($n = 1895$) | | | | Under-reporters ($n = 1578$) | | | |
|---|---|---|---|---|---|---|---|---|---|---|---|---|
| | Intake (g/d) | | Contribution to GHGE (%) | | Intake (g/d) | | Contribution to GHGE (%) | | Intake (g/d) | | Contribution to GHGE (%) | |
| | Mean | SD | Mean | SD | Mean | SD | Mean | SD | Mean | SD | Mean | SD |
| Red meat | 85.2 | 67.1 | 24.4 | 16.9 | 90.5 | 69.8 | 24.2 | 16.2 | 77.9 | 61.3 | 24.8 | 17.8 |
| White meat | 44.3 | 55.4 | 5.9 | 6.8 | 44.9 | 59.3 | 5.4 | 6.3 | 42.6 | 47.9 | 6.5 | 7.3 |
| Fish | 30.8 | 37.3 | 6.0 | 7.5 | 35.1 | 39.3 | 6.4 | 7.4 | 25.5 | 33.9 | 5.5 | 7.5 |
| Dairy products | 223.0 | 150.3 | 13.6 | 8.6 | 247.6 | 155.4 | 14.3 | 8.7 | 191.8 | 134.6 | 12.7 | 8.4 |
| Eggs | 20.5 | 33.9 | 1.8 | 2.5 | 22.9 | 40.5 | 1.8 | 2.5 | 17.4 | 23.3 | 1.8 | 2.5 |
| Cereals | 185.5 | 96.8 | 6.9 | 5.1 | 198.8 | 99.9 | 6.8 | 4.9 | 168.9 | 89.3 | 7.1 | 5.3 |
| Potatoes | 90.1 | 67.1 | 2.8 | 2.2 | 96.6 | 68.8 | 2.8 | 2.0 | 82.2 | 64.3 | 2.9 | 2.4 |
| Vegetables | 139.2 | 93.3 | 5.3 | 4.0 | 148.3 | 91.2 | 5.1 | 3.6 | 127.8 | 94.3 | 5.5 | 4.5 |
| Beans and pulses | 24.4 | 35.8 | 0.7 | 1.2 | 25.4 | 35.7 | 0.7 | 1.0 | 23.2 | 36.1 | 0.8 | 1.5 |
| Nuts and seeds | 3.6 | 11.6 | 0.2 | 0.6 | 4.4 | 11.6 | 0.2 | 0.4 | 2.8 | 11.6 | 0.1 | 0.7 |
| Fruit | 101.2 | 105.5 | 2.8 | 3.0 | 111.3 | 108.5 | 2.8 | 2.8 | 88.8 | 99.4 | 2.8 | 3.2 |
| Fats and oils | 13.8 | 11.1 | 5.5 | 4.9 | 16.0 | 11.6 | 5.8 | 5.0 | 11.0 | 9.1 | 5.0 | 4.6 |
| Sugar and confectioneries | 97.7 | 78.4 | 6.0 | 5.8 | 112.7 | 78.3 | 6.2 | 5.2 | 77.1 | 70.2 | 5.6 | 6.4 |
| Soft drinks | 222.6 | 347.1 | 7.3 | 10.0 | 223.6 | 354.4 | 6.6 | 8.9 | 216.4 | 322.0 | 8.1 | 10.9 |
| Fruit juice | 50.1 | 101.9 | 2.1 | 4.0 | 59.6 | 110.5 | 2.3 | 4.0 | 37.4 | 78.6 | 1.8 | 3.8 |
| Alcoholic beverages | 212.2 | 401.5 | 4.8 | 8.0 | 252.2 | 452.0 | 5.2 | 8.0 | 165.0 | 318.8 | 4.4 | 8.0 |
| Tea, coffee and water | 783.8 | 494.3 | 3.9 | 4.5 | 828.3 | 492.2 | 3.5 | 3.7 | 733.0 | 492.6 | 4.5 | 5.3 |

*GHGE* greenhouse gas emissions

[a] Plausible reporters were defined as participants with a ratio of reported energy intake (EI) to estimated energy requirement (EER) 0.70–1.43; under-reporters were defined as participants with an EI:EER < 0.70

[b] Including over-reporters ($n = 29$), defined as participants with an EI:EER > 1.43

## Discussion

To our knowledge, this is the first study to examine diet-related GHGE in relation to measures of diet quality, taking account of EI under-reporting. Assuming that all the dietary variables were misreported in proportion to the misreporting of EI, diet-related GHGE were underestimated by 30% in this cross-sectional study based on the UK NDNS rolling programme. In the entire population, diet-related GHGE were inversely associated with HDI and DASH score but not with MDS after adjustment for potential confounders. However, with further adjustment for EI:EER, diet-related GHGE showed inverse associations with all three diet quality measures. Similar associations were observed when only under-reporters were analysed, while in the analysis including only plausible reporters, diet-related GHGE showed inverse associations with all diet quality measures irrespective of adjustment. These findings highlight the importance of taking account of EI misreporting in the entire sample, rather than just excluding EI misreporters.

Our mean estimate of diet-related GHGE was 5.7 kg $CO_2$eq/d, which is consistent with those reported from a number of national representative samples in other European countries, such as France (4.1 kg $CO_2$eq/d) [6], Ireland (6.5 kg $CO_2$eq/d) [9], Sweden (women: 4.1 kg $CO_2$eq/d; men: 5.5 kg $CO_2$eq/d) [18] and the Netherlands (women: 3.7 kg $CO_2$eq/d; men: 4.8 kg $CO_2$eq/d) [7]. These differences may be due to differences in the types of data sources used and in system boundaries in the emission factors adopted, in addition to differences in dietary assessment methods and participant characteristics (such as age range and dietary habits). However, we observed that the mean value of diet-related GHGE increased by 30% (8.2 kg $CO_2$eq/d) with an assumption that all the dietary variables were misreported in proportion to the misreporting of EI. Under-reporting of EI was on average 26% in this study, which is quite similar to that in a subsample of the NDNS rolling programme as assessed against total energy expenditure by the doubly labelled water method (34% in individuals aged 16–64 years and 29% in those aged ≥65 years) [30]. Indeed, this degree of under-reporting is quite common in dietary surveys [53]. It is therefore highly likely that diet-related GHGE will be underestimated to a certain degree if EI misreporting is not taken into account.

In this study, red meat was the top contributor to diet-related GHGE, followed by dairy products. This is

**Table 3** Associations between diet-related GHGE and diet quality measures [a]

| | Model 1 [b] | | | Model 2 [c] | | |
|---|---|---|---|---|---|---|
| | β [d] | SE [d] | *P* | β [d] | SE [d] | *P* |
| All (*n* = 3502) [e] | | | | | | |
| HDI | −0.12 | 0.01 | < 0.0001 | −0.14 | 0.01 | < 0.0001 |
| MDS | 0.002 | 0.01 | 0.86 | −0.07 | 0.02 | < 0.0001 |
| DASH score | −0.51 | 0.04 | < 0.0001 | −0.42 | 0.05 | < 0.0001 |
| Plausible reporters (*n* = 1895) | | | | | | |
| HDI | −0.12 | 0.01 | < 0.0001 | −0.14 | 0.02 | < 0.0001 |
| MDS | −0.08 | 0.02 | 0.0003 | −0.10 | 0.02 | < 0.0001 |
| DASH score | −0.51 | 0.06 | < 0.0001 | −0.47 | 0.06 | < 0.0001 |
| Under-reporters (*n* = 1578) | | | | | | |
| HDI | −0.15 | 0.02 | < 0.0001 | −0.15 | 0.02 | < 0.0001 |
| MDS | 0.01 | 0.03 | 0.70 | −0.05 | 0.03 | 0.06 |
| DASH score | −0.42 | 0.07 | < 0.0001 | −0.35 | 0.08 | < 0.0001 |

*DASH* Dietary Approaches to Stop Hypertension, *EER* estimated energy requirement, *EI* energy intake, *GHGE* greenhouse gas emissions, *HDI* healthy diet indicator, *MDS* Mediterranean diet score
[a] Plausible reporters were defined as participants with an EI:EER 0.70–1.43; under-reporters were defined as participants with an EI:EER < 0.70
[b] Adjustment was made for age (years, continuous), sex (male or female), ethnicity (white or nonwhite), socioeconomic classification (higher and managerial occupation, intermediate occupation, routine and manual occupation or other), smoking status (current, former or never), and physical activity (sedentary, low active, active or very active)
[c] Adjustment was made for variables used in model 1 and EI:EER (continuous)
[d] Indicating the change of diet quality measures with a 1-kg of carbon dioxide equivalents increase of diet-related GHGE (per day)
[e] Including over-reporters (*n* = 29), defined as participants with an EI:EER > 1.43

consistent with previous studies in Ireland [9], the Netherlands [7] and France [8]. Thus, this study provides further evidence based on self-selected diet that reducing meat consumption is likely to contribute to lower diet-related GHGE [2], as indicated in modeling studies [49, 54, 55]. Nevertheless, avoidance or lower intake of animal foods such as red meat may also contribute to nutritional inadequacy of several micronutrients such as iron, zinc and vitamin B-12 [56]. In any case, further research is required to determine the amount of meat consumption (particularly red meat) which is optimum for not only human health but also for the health of the planet.

Misreporting of dietary intake is a common phenomenon. It appears to arise non-randomly [24, 53] and be selective for different kinds of foods, and accordingly nutrients [57–60]. Misreporting has the potential to cause differential errors in dietary data, which in turn hampers the interpretation of studies concerning diet and health. In the worst case it can lead to spurious diet-health relationships [22, 25, 58]. In our present study, EI misreporter (i.e., under-reporters and over-reporters) prevalence was 46%, which is similar to that in previous studies based on similar dietary assessment methods (37% [61] and 38% [62]). The present findings are similarly consistent with many other studies [22–24, 53, 61] showing that under-reporters differ considerably from plausible reporters, such as with regard to higher body fatness, higher PA, lower socio-economic status and rate of current tobacco use. These differences notwithstanding, the associations of diet-related GHGE with diet quality (in addition to the contribution of food groups to GHGE) seen in under-reporters were reasonably similar to those seen in plausible reporters, after taking into account EI:EER. Nevertheless, misreporting (particularly under-reporting) of EI appeared to confound the inverse associations with diet quality (i.e., MDS), suggesting the importance of taking into account of EI misreporting. The reason for this observation is not precisely known, but one speculation is that even though foods are differentially misreported, these reporting errors are correlated with EI misreporting, to some extent at least (Pearson correlations between EI and food group intakes ranged from 0.08 to 0.46 in this study). This does not conflict with observations based on biomarkers of protein, potassium and sodium (24-h urinary excretion) [57, 60, 63].

After taking account of EI misreporting, we identified inverse associations between diet-related GHGE and all three measures of diet quality (i.e., HDI, MDS and DASH score). An inverse association with DASH score was similarly observed in British [15] and Dutch [16] populations. An inverse association with HDI was also observed in the Dutch study [16]. Conversely, a study in France showed a positive association between diet-related GHGE and diet quality assessed as a composite measure of three different indices, namely mean adequacy ratio, mean excess ratio and energy density [6]. These heterogeneous findings may be at least partly explained by the use of different measures for diet quality, given that different diet scores have conceptual differences. Given the improbability of identifying a diet quality index which is able to capture all aspects of healthy diets, the use of different measures of diet quality, as conducted in this study, may be an important approach to ensuring the robustness of the findings.

The strengths of this study include its detailed dietary information obtained from a 4-d food diary, measured anthropometric data, and use of an individualized measure of EER to assess EI misreporting in a representative sample in the UK. However, several limitations also warrant mention. First, because of the limited availability of food-level GHGE data, we obtained the estimates of diet-related GHGE from GHGE values for 133 food groups, rather than those assigned to individual food items (> 2000 in the NDNS). Accordingly, we have likely underestimated variation in diet-related GHGE. Nevertheless, this strategy is currently the only feasible approach in many epidemiological studies given the challenges of building a standardised comprehensive food database [64]. Further, our estimate of diet-related GHGE is of a comparable magnitude to those provided in studies in Europe [6, 7, 9, 18]. Second, environmental impact was indicated using GHGE only, rather than such criteria as land and water use or biodiversity. As highlighted in a recent systematic review [65], these should be simultaneously taken into consideration in future studies.

At present, the use of doubly labelled water as a biomarker is the only way to secure unbiased information on energy requirements in free-living settings [53]. Nevertheless, this technique is expensive and cannot be practically applied to large-scale dietary surveys like the NDNS. As a replacement, we determined EER with the use of published equations [37]. In the absence of measured total energy expenditure, these equations with high $R^2$ values (0.82 for men and 0.79 for women) [37] would serve as the best proxy, although the selection of PA category was based on self-report (i.e. a validated questionnaire), which may be susceptible to reporting bias. This notion is evidenced, at the population level at least, by the finding of under-reporting in this study, and of under-reporting observed in comparison with total energy expenditure using doubly labelled water in a subsample of the NDNS rolling programme [30], as mentioned above.

Another limitation of this study is its relatively low response rate (53 to 56% among survey years). However, an analysis based on the previous NDNS, which had a response rate for dietary recording of 47%, concluded that there was no evidence to suggest confounding by a serious non-response bias in the NDNS [66]. Finally, although we adjusted for a variety of potential confounding variables, residual confounding could not be ruled out.

## Conclusion

This cross-sectional study, based on self-selected diets in the UK, revealed that consistent inverse associations between diet-related GHGE and measures of diet quality were observed when misreporting of EI was taken into account, as well as potential underestimation of diet-related GHGE. Thus, misreporting (particularly under-reporting) of EI appeared to confound the inverse associations with diet quality. However, because these associations were observed not only in the entire population but also in both plausible reporters and under-reporters separately, simple exclusion of individuals with implausible EI was not justified. Given the widespread presence of misreporting in dietary surveys [24, 53], and the fact that reporting errors in the intake of individual foods and nutrients appear to correlate with reporting errors in EI to some extent at least [57, 60, 63], routine utilization of procedures to take account of EI misreporting [26] would likely improve the accuracy of studies of diet-related GHGE.

### Abbreviations

BMI: Body mass index; $CO_2$eq: Carbon dioxide equivalents; DASH: Dietary Approaches to Stop Hypertension; DRI: Dietary Reference Intakes; EER: Estimated energy requirement; EI: Energy intake; GHGE: Greenhouse gas emissions; HDI: Healthy diet indicator; MDS: Mediterranean diet score; MVPA: Moderate-to-vigorous physical activity; NDNS: National Diet and Nutrition Survey; PA: Physical activity

### Funding

This work was supported in part by Grants-in-Aid for Young Scientists (B) from the Ministry of Education, Culture, Sports, Science and Technology of Japan (to KM; grant number 15K16213). The Ministry of Education, Culture, Sports, Science and Technology of Japan had no role in the design, analysis or writing of this article.

### Authors' contributions

KM formulated the hypothesis, designed the study, analysed and interpreted the data and wrote the manuscript. MBEL helped in the writing of the manuscript. Both authors read and approved the final manuscript.

### Competing interests

Both authors declare that they have no competing interests.

### Author details

[1]Interfaculty Initiative in Information Studies, University of Tokyo, Tokyo 113 0033, Japan. [2]Northern Ireland Centre for Food and Health, Ulster University, Coleraine BT52 1SA, UK.

### References

1. UK Government. Climate change act 2008. http://www.legislation.gov.uk/ukpga/2008/27/contents (Accessed 17 Oct 2017).
2. Garnett T. Where are the best opportunities for reducing greenhouse gas emissions in the food system (including the food chain)? Food Policy. 2011; 36:S23–32.
3. Tukker A, Goldbohm RA, De Koning A, Verheijden M, Kleijn R, Wolf O, et al. Environmental impacts of changes to healthier diets in Europe. Ecol Econ. 2011;70:1776–88.
4. Kim B, Neff R. Measurement and communication of greenhouse gas emissions from U.S. food consumption via carbon calculators. Ecol Econ. 2009;69:186–96.
5. Macdiarmid JI, Kyle J, Horgan GW, Loe J, Fyfe C, Johnstone A, et al. Sustainable diets for the future: can we contribute to reducing greenhouse gas emissions by eating a healthy diet? Am J Clin Nutr. 2012;96:632–9.
6. Vieux F, Soler LG, Touazi D, Darmon N. High nutritional quality is not associated with low greenhouse gas emissions in self-selected diets of French adults. Am J Clin Nutr. 2013;97:569–83.
7. Temme EH, Toxopeus IB, Kramer GF, Brosens MC, Drijvers JM, Tyszler M, et al. Greenhouse gas emission of diets in the Netherlands and associations with food, energy and macronutrient intakes. Public Health Nutr. 2015;18: 2433–45.

8. Vieux F, Darmon N, Touazi D, Soler LG. Greenhouse gas emissions of self-selected individual diets in France: changing the diet structure or consuming less? Ecol Econ. 2012;75:91–101.
9. Hyland JJ, Henchion M, McCarthy M, McCarthy SN. The climatic impact of food consumption in a representative sample of Irish adults and implications for food and nutrition policy. Public Health Nutr. 2017;20:726–38.
10. Pan A, Sun Q, Bernstein AM, Schulze MB, Manson JE, Stampfer MJ, et al. Red meat consumption and mortality: results from 2 prospective cohort studies. Arch Intern Med. 2012;172:555–63.
11. Schwingshackl L, Schwedhelm C, Hoffmann G, Lampousi AM, Knuppel S, Iqbal K, et al. Food groups and risk of all-cause mortality: a systematic review and meta-analysis of prospective studies. Am J Clin Nutr. 2017;105:1462–73.
12. Sinha R, Cross AJ, Graubard BI, Leitzmann MF, Schatzkin A. Meat intake and mortality: a prospective study of over half a million people. Arch Intern Med. 2009;169:562–71.
13. Wang X, Ouyang Y, Liu J, Zhu M, Zhao G, Bao W, et al. Fruit and vegetable consumption and mortality from all causes, cardiovascular disease, and cancer: systematic review and dose-response meta-analysis of prospective cohort studies. BMJ. 2014;349:g4490.
14. Perignon M, Vieux F, Soler LG, Masset G, Darmon N. Improving diet sustainability through evolution of food choices: review of epidemiological studies on the environmental impact of diets. Nutr Rev. 2017;75:2–17.
15. Monsivais P, Scarborough P, Lloyd T, Mizdrak A, Luben R, Mulligan AA, et al. Greater accordance with the dietary approaches to stop hypertension dietary pattern is associated with lower diet-related greenhouse gas production but higher dietary costs in the United Kingdom. Am J Clin Nutr. 2015;102:138–45.
16. Biesbroek S, Verschuren WMM, Boer JMA, van de Kamp ME, van der Schouw YT, Geelen A, et al. Does a better adherence to dietary guidelines reduce mortality risk and environmental impact in the Dutch sub-cohort of the European prospective investigation into cancer and nutrition? Br J Nutr. 2017;118:69–80.
17. Balter K, Sjors C, Sjolander A, Gardner C, Hedenus F, Tillander A. Is a diet low in greenhouse gas emissions a nutritious diet? - analyses of self-selected diets in the LifeGene study. Arch Public Health. 2017;75:17.
18. Sjors C, Hedenus F, Sjolander A, Tillander A, Balter K. Adherence to dietary recommendations for Swedish adults across categories of greenhouse gas emissions from food. Public Health Nutr. 2017;20:3381–93.
19. Masset G, Vieux F, Verger EO, Soler LG, Touazi D, Darmon N. Reducing energy intake and energy density for a sustainable diet: a study based on self-selected diets in French adults. Am J Clin Nutr. 2014;99:1460–9.
20. Berners-Lee M, Hoolohan C, Cammack H, Hewitt CN. The relative greenhouse gas impacts of realistic dietary choices. Energy Policy. 2012;43:184–90.
21. Hoolohan C, Berners-Lee M, McKinstry-West J, Hewitt CN. Mitigating the greenhouse gas emissions embodied in food through realistic consumer choices. Energy Policy. 2013;63:1065–74.
22. Jessri M, Lou WY, L'Abbe MR. Evaluation of different methods to handle misreporting in obesity research: evidence from the Canadian national nutrition survey. Br J Nutr. 2016;115:147–59.
23. Murakami K, McCaffrey TA, Livingstone MB. Associations of dietary glycaemic index and glycaemic load with food and nutrient intake and general and central obesity in British adults. Br J Nutr. 2013;110:2047–57.
24. Murakami K, Livingstone MB. Prevalence and characteristics of misreporting of energy intake in US adults: NHANES 2003-2012. Br J Nutr. 2015;114:1294–303.
25. Mendez MA, Popkin BM, Buckland G, Schroder H, Amiano P, Barricarte A, et al. Alternative methods of accounting for underreporting and overreporting when measuring dietary intake-obesity relations. Am J Epidemiol. 2011;173:448–58.
26. Banna JC, McCrory MA, Fialkowski MK, Boushey C. Examining plausibility of self-reported energy intake data: considerations for method selection. Front Nutr. 2017;4:45.
27. Murakami K, Livingstone MB. Eating frequency in relation to body mass index and waist circumference in British adults. Int J Obes. 2014;38:1200–6.
28. Murakami K, Livingstone MB. Eating frequency is positively associated with overweight and central obesity in US adults. J Nutr. 2015;145:2715–24.
29. Leech RM, Timperio A, Livingstone KM, Worsley A, McNaughton SA. Temporal eating patterns: associations with nutrient intakes, diet quality, and measures of adiposity. Am J Clin Nutr. 2017;106:1121–30.
30. Public Health England and Food Standards Agency. National Diet and Nutrition Survey. Results from Years 1, 2, 3 and 4 (combined) of the Rolling Programme (2008/2009 – 2011/2012). https://www.google.co.jp/url?sa=t&rct=j&q=&esrc=s&source=web&cd=1&cad=rja&uact=8&ved=0ahUKEwjlpPTM6s3KAhXI46YKHcYTDpEQFggdMAA&url=https%3A%2F%2Fwww.gov.uk%2Fgovernment%2Fuploads%2Fsystem%2Fuploads%2Fattachment_data%2Ffile%2F310995%2FNDNS_Y1_to_4_UK_report.pdf&usg=AFQjCNGXhDQZVyuauuF80F7rFBEUKfcSEQ. Accessed 17 Oct 2017.
31. Public Health England and Food Standards Agency. National Diet and Nutrition Survey. Results from Years 5 and 6 (combined) of the Rolling Programme (2012/2013 – 2013/2014). https://www.gov.uk/government/uploads/system/uploads/attachment_data/file/551352/NDNS_Y5_6_UK_Main_Text.pdf . Accessed 17 Oct 2017.
32. NatCen Social Research. National Diet and Nutrition Survey Years 1–4 2008/09–2011/12. User Guide for UK Data (core & country boost data). http://doc.ukdataservice.ac.uk/doc/6533/mrdoc/pdf/6533_ndns_yrs1-4_uk_user_guide.pdf. Accessed 26 Dec 2017.
33. NatCen Social Research. National Diet and Nutrition Survey Years 5–6 2012/13–2013/14. User Guide for UK Data. http://doc.ukdataservice.ac.uk/doc/6533/mrdoc/pdf/6533_ndns_yrs5-6_uk_user_guide.pdf. Accessed 26 Dec 2017.
34. Rose D, Pevalin D, O'Reilly K. The National Statistics Socio-Economic Classification: origins, development and use. Hampshire: Palgrave Macmillan; 2005.
35. Besson H, Brage S, Jakes RW, Ekelund U, Wareham NJ. Estimating physical activity energy expenditure, sedentary time, and physical activity intensity by self-report in adults. Am J Clin Nutr. 2010;91:106–14.
36. Mindell J. Appendix V to National Diet and Nutrition Survey. Results from Years 1-4 (combined) of the Rolling Programme (2008/2009-2011/12). Measuring physical activity in adults using the Recent Physical Activity Questionnaire (RPAQ). London: Public Health England. https://www.food.gov.uk/sites/default/files/ndns-appendix-v.pdf. Accessed 17 Oct 2017.
37. Institute of Medicine. Dietary reference intakes for energy, carbohydrate, fiber, fat, fatty acids, cholesterol, protein and amino acids. Washington, DC: National Academy Press; 2002.
38. Brooks GA, Butte NF, Rand WM, Flatt JP, Caballero B. Chronicle of the Institute of medicine physical activity recommendation: how a physical activity recommendation came to be among dietary recommendations. Am J Clin Nutr. 2004;79:921S–30S.
39. Noel SE, Mattocks C, Emmett P, Riddoch CJ, Ness AR, Newby P. Use of accelerometer data in prediction equations for capturing implausible dietary intakes in adolescents. Am J Clin Nutr. 2010;92:1436–45.
40. Berners-Lee M, Hoolohan C, Cammack H, Hewitt CN. Appendix A to National Diet and Nutrition Survey. Results from Years 1-4 (combined) of the Rolling Programme (2008/2009-2011/12). Dietary data collection and editing. London: Public Health England. https://www.food.gov.uk/sites/default/files/ndns-appendix-a.pdf. Accessed 17 Oct 2017.
41. Food Standards Agency. McCance and Widdowson's the composition of foods. 6th ed. Cambridge: Royal Society of Chemistry; 2002.
42. Huijbregts P, Feskens E, Rasanen L, Fidanza F, Nissinen A, Menotti A, et al. Dietary pattern and 20 year mortality in elderly men in Finland, Italy, and The Netherlands: longitudinal cohort study. BMJ. 1997;315:13–7.
43. Struijk EA, Beulens JW, May AM, Fransen HP, Boer JM, de Wit GA, et al. Dietary patterns in relation to disease burden expressed in disability-adjusted life years. Am J Clin Nutr. 2014;100:1158–65.
44. Trichopoulou A, Orfanos P, Norat T, Bueno-de-Mesquita B, Ocke MC, Peeters PH, et al. Modified Mediterranean diet and survival: EPIC-elderly prospective cohort study. BMJ. 2005;330:991.
45. Fung TT, Chiuve SE, McCullough ML, Rexrode KM, Logroscino G, Hu FB. Adherence to a DASH-style diet and risk of coronary heart disease and stroke in women. Arch Intern Med. 2008;168:713–20.
46. Penney TL, Jones NRV, Adams J, Maguire ER, Burgoine T, Monsivais P. Utilization of away-from-home food establishments, dietary approaches to stop hypertension dietary pattern, and obesity. Am J Prev Med. 2017;53:e155–63.
47. Reedy J, Krebs-Smith SM, Miller PE, Liese AD, Kahle LL, Park Y, et al. Higher diet quality is associated with decreased risk of all-cause, cardiovascular disease, and cancer mortality among older adults. J Nutr. 2014;144:881–9.
48. Jankovic N, Geelen A, Streppel MT, de Groot LC, Orfanos P, van den Hooven EH, et al. Adherence to a healthy diet according to the World Health Organization guidelines and all-cause mortality in elderly adults from

Europe and the United States. Am J Epidemiol. 2014;180:978–88.
49. Green R, Milner J, Dangour AD, Haines A, Chalabi Z, Markandya A, et al. The potential to reduce greenhouse gas emissions in the UK through healthy and realistic dietary change. Clim Chang. 2015;129:253–65.
50. Huang TT, Roberts SB, Howarth NC, McCrory MA. Effect of screening out implausible energy intake reports on relationships between diet and BMI. Obes Res. 2005;13:1205–17.
51. Black AE. Critical evaluation of energy intake using the Goldberg cut-off for energy intake:basal metabolic rate. A practical guide to its calculation, use and limitations. Int J Obes Relat Metab Disord. 2000;24:1119–30.
52. NatCen Social Research. National Diet and Nutrition Survey Years 1–6, 2008/09–2013/14. Combining Years 1–4 and Years 5 and 6 data - Advice for users. https://www.google.co.jp/url?sa=t&rct=j&q=&esrc=s&source=web&cd=1&cad=rja&uact=8&ved=0ahUKEwjm8-bEwJXZAhVGWbwKHZXpCXwQFggnMAA&url=http%3A%2F%2Fdoc.ukdataservice.ac.uk%2Fdoc%2F6533%2Fmrdoc%2Fpdf%2F6533_combining_the_y1-4_and_y56_datasets_on_the_archive_final_version.pdf&usg=AOvVaw36XsNPUN6ZDVHgZkbrdu0o . Accessed 8 Feb 2018.
53. Livingstone MB, Black AE. Markers of the validity of reported energy intake. J Nutr. 2003;133:895S–920S.
54. Seves SM, Verkaik-Kloosterman J, Biesbroek S, Temme EH. Are more environmentally sustainable diets with less meat and dairy nutritionally adequate? Public Health Nutr. 2017;20:2050–62.
55. Perignon M, Masset G, Ferrari G, Barré T, Vieux F, Maillot M, et al. How low can dietary greenhouse gas emissions be reduced without impairing nutritional adequacy, affordability and acceptability of the diet? A modelling study to guide sustainable food choices. Public Health Nutr. 2016;19:2662–74.
56. Derbyshire E. Associations between red meat intakes and the micronutrient intake and status of UK females: a secondary analysis of the UK National Diet and nutrition survey. Nutrients. 2017;9:E768.
57. Subar AF, Kipnis V, Troiano RP, Midthune D, Schoeller DA, Bingham S, et al. Using intake biomarkers to evaluate the extent of dietary misreporting in a large sample of adults: the OPEN study. Am J Epidemiol. 2003;158:1–13.
58. Rosell MS, Hellenius MLB, De Faire UH, Johansson GK. Associations between diet and the metabolic syndrome vary with the validity of dietary intake data. Am J Clin Nutr. 2003;78:84–90.
59. Heitmann BL, Lissner L. Dietary underreporting by obese individuals: is it specific or non-specific? BMJ. 1995;311:986–9.
60. Murakami K, Sasaki S, Uenishi K. The degree of misreporting of the energy-adjusted intake of protein, potassium, and sodium does not differ among under-, acceptable, and over-reporters of energy intake. Nutr Res. 2012;32:741–50.
61. Nielsen BM, Nielsen MM, Toubro S, Pedersen O, Astrup A, Sorensen TI, et al. Past and current body size affect validity of reported energy intake among middle-aged Danish men. J Nutr. 2009;139:2337–43.
62. Black AE. The sensitivity and specificity of the Goldberg cut-off for EI:BMR for identifying diet reports of poor validity. Eur J Clin Nutr. 2000;54:395–404.
63. Freedman LS, Commins JM, Moler JE, Willett W, Tinker LF, Subar AF, et al. Pooled results from 5 validation studies of dietary self-report instruments using recovery biomarkers for potassium and sodium intake. Am J Epidemiol. 2015;181:473–87.
64. Bertoluci G, Masset G, Gomy C, Mottet J, Darmon N. How to build a standardized country-specific environmental food database for nutritional epidemiology studies. PLoS One. 2016;11:e0150617.
65. Aleksandrowicz L, Green R, Joy EJ, Smith P, Haines A. The impacts of dietary change on greenhouse gas emissions, land use, water use, and health: a systematic review. PLoS One. 2016;11:e0165797.
66. Food Standards Agency. NDNS Previous Survey Reports. http://webarchive.nationalarchives.gov.uk/20100406130654/food.gov.uk/science/dietarysurveys/ndnsdocuments/ndnspreviousssurveyreports/ . Accessed 17 Oct 2017.

# Adherence to Mediterranean and low-fat diets among heart and lung transplant recipients: a randomized feasibility study

Timothy R. Entwistle[1], Adèle C. Green[2,3], James E. Fildes[1,4] and Kyoko Miura[2*]

**Abstract**

**Background:** Heart and lung transplant recipients are at a substantially increased risk of cardiovascular disease (CVD). Since both low-fat and Mediterranean diets can reduce CVD in immunocompetent people at high risk, we assessed adherence among thoracic transplant recipients allocated to one or other of these diets for 12 months.

**Methods:** Forty-one transplant recipients (20 heart; 21 lung) randomized to a Mediterranean or a low-fat diet for 12 months received diet-specific education at baseline. Adherence was primarily assessed by questionnaire: 14-point Mediterranean diet (score 0–14) and 9-point low-fat diet (score 0–16) respectively, high scores indicating greater adherence. Median scores at baseline, 6 months, 12 months, and 6-weeks post-intervention were compared by dietary group. We further assessed changes in weight, body mass index (BMI) and serum triglycerides from baseline to 12 months as an additional indicator of adherence.

**Results:** In those randomized to a Mediterranean diet, median scores increased from 4 (range 1–9) at baseline, to 10 (range 6–14) at 6-months and were maintained at 12 months, and also at 6-weeks post-intervention (median 10, range 6–14). Body weight, BMI and serum triglycerides decreased over the 12-month intervention period (mean weight − 1.8 kg, BMI −0.5 kg/m$^2$, triglycerides − 0.17 mmol/L). In the low-fat diet group, median scores were 11 (range 9–14) at baseline; slightly increased to 12 (range 9–16) at 6 months, and maintained at 12 months and 6 weeks post-intervention (median 12, range 8–15). Mean changes in weight, BMI and triglycerides were − 0.2 kg, 0.0 kg/m$^2$ and − 0.44 mmol/L, respectively.

**Conclusions:** Thoracic transplant recipients adhered to Mediterranean and low-fat dietary interventions. The change from baseline eating habits was notable at 6 months; and this change was maintained at 12 months and 6 weeks post-intervention in both Mediterranean diet and low-fat diet groups. Dietary interventions based on comprehensive, well-supported education sessions targeted to both patients and their family members are crucial to success. Such nutritional strategies can help in the management of their substantial CVD risk.

**Keywords:** Mediterranean diet, Low fat diet, Dietary compliance, Randomized study, Pilot projects, Organ transplant recipients

* Correspondence: Kyoko.Miura@qimrberghofer.edu.au
[2]Cancer and Population Studies Group, QIMR Berghofer Medical Research Institute, 300 Herston Road, Herston, QLD 4006, Australia
Full list of author information is available at the end of the article

## Background

Cardio-metabolic disturbance is common in heart and lung transplant recipients and is associated with cardiovascular disease (CVD)-related morbidity and mortality [1, 2]. Despite careful patient management, blood pressure and blood lipids tend to rise after transplantation such that 5 years after heart transplantation, the cumulative incidence rates of hypertension and hyperlipidemia are 92 and 88% respectively [1], and similar after lung transplantation [2]. Overweight/obesity are known predictors for these conditions, and excessive weight gain occurs frequently post-transplantation [3, 4]. Several studies have shown dramatic upward weight trajectories in organ transplant recipients in the post-transplant period [5] with, for example, an average 10 kg weight gain in the first year in heart transplant recipients [3]. Factors contributing to this weight gain include altered energy metabolism [6] and side-effects of medications [7]. To prevent obesity and reduce the risk of associated chronic conditions in the general population, dietary modification is fundamental. Two dietary regimens have been shown to reduce CVD risk: the low-fat diet and the Mediterranean diet [8].

In contrast, in immunosuppressed populations, current CVD management focuses on tailoring immunosuppression and drug treatment [9]; only a limited number of studies have shown dietary approaches to be effective in organ transplant populations [10–12]. As a consequence, little is known about adherence to dietary interventions following transplantation [12], although it is recognized that in general, non-adherence to interventions is common and limits their overall effectiveness [13]. We therefore performed this study to assess adherence in thoracic transplant recipients randomly assigned to either of the two dietary interventions known to reduce CVD risk factors. We also assessed whether transplant recipients maintained these dietary changes after cessation of the intervention.

## Methods

The Assessment of the MEditerraneaN Diet In heart and lung Transplantation (AMEND-IT) study was a single-center parallel-randomized study designed to assess the feasibility and acceptability of two dietary interventions, namely the Mediterranean diet and low-fat diet among heart and lung transplant recipients. The 12-month study was conducted at the University Hospital of South Manchester. Eligible participants were clinically stable, aged ≥16 years, and a minimum 6 months post-transplant. Exclusion criteria included acute rejection, infection, prevalent cancer, diabetes, or chronic kidney disease (estimated glomerular filtration rate ≤ 30). Patients with any competing dietary issues (i.e. food allergies and following medically prescribed diets that conflicted with the interventions) were also excluded.

Study participants were identified through hospital records at the transplant outpatient clinic and recruitment commenced in February 2014 and ended in October 2014. A total of 116 heart or lung transplant recipients meeting the criteria were contacted. Each received an information package that included a participant information sheet, contact details and a return form. Among those contacted, 75 patients were not included (64 declined participation, 11 did not meet inclusion criteria) and the remaining 41 (20 heart, 21 lung) gave written consent to participate (Fig. 1). The study was approved by the NRES Committee North West (REC reference number 13/NW/0310) and was retrospectively registered on the IRAS trial registry (ISRCTN63500150).

Participants were stratified according to organ type and transplant date, and then randomly assigned to either a Mediterranean diet or a low-fat diet intervention using a computerized system with random block size and an equal 1:1 allocation ratio. To blind the investigator during recruitment, randomized codes

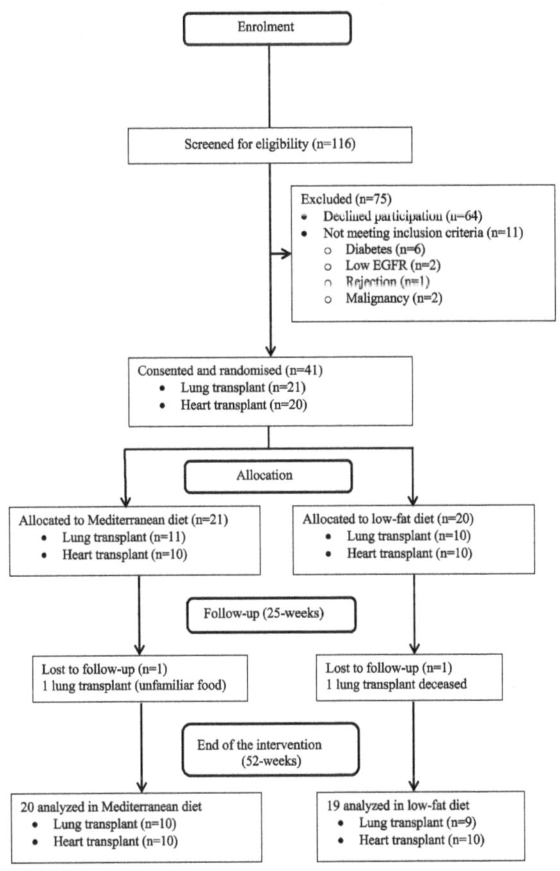


**Fig. 1** CONSORT flow diagram for AMEND-IT study. EGFR: estimated glomerular filtration rate

were sent to a third person who then allocated the randomized interventions to patients per protocol.

#### Dietary intervention

The study sought to change patients' overall dietary habits through behavioral modification. Several 5-h group education sessions were conducted for each diet group (with an accompanying family member if desired) on specified dates outside routine outpatient visits. A nutritionally-trained investigator administered the education sessions and explained the scientific rationale in a visual, interactive manner, and advice given about preparation and storage of fresh, whole foods as relevant. A trained chef demonstrated practical methods for Mediterranean or low-fat meal preparation. Attendance at each session was restricted to maximum of 10–12 participants (excluding family members). Energy intake restriction was not explicit, but portion sizes were discussed throughout the study. Each participant was encouraged to attend this baseline education session with an adult member of the same household [14]. All participants received a printed booklet containing advice about shopping, food preparation, hygiene, storage, dining out and recipes. Additional advice and support were provided at 6- and 12-month outpatient visits, and during six 15-min telephone consultations spaced evenly through the intervention period, when participants could raise any questions or concerns and when key dietary recommendations (e.g. plant-based diet, consume minimally processed food) were reinforced. SMS messaging was also used to remind patients of clinic study requirements.

Participants allocated to the Mediterranean diet received information and encouragement to follow an eating pattern representative of a traditional Mediterranean diet [15]. The key dietary recommendations were: daily mixed consumption of a range of vegetables, fruit, wholegrains, fish/seafood, raw nuts and legumes; abundant use of extra-virgin olive oil (a free 5-l container of extra-virgin olive oil was provided to each participant); moderate consumption of dairy products and red wine; low intake of red and processed meats, of sweets, sweet-baked pastries and sweetened beverages.

Participants assigned to the low-fat diet were advised to follow modified British Heart Foundation low-fat guidelines [8] with an emphasis on consuming mainly plant-based wholefoods similar to the Mediterranean diet,with advice to minimize high-fat foods such as processed meats, commercially baked pastries and desserts, and vegetable oils and spreads. Advice was given on how to identify and avoid different types of fat. Each participant received a low-fat recipe book. The main difference between the two diets was the intake of oil and fat which was encouraged to a moderate degree in the Mediterranean diet but discouraged in the low-fat diet.

#### Dietary assessment

Participants were asked to complete intervention-specific short dietary questionnaires at baseline, 6- and 12-months and again 6-weeks after the intervention to determine short-term post-study adherence. These questionnaires were completed at the hospital during routine visits, except for the post-intervention questionnaire that was sent by mail and completed at home.

Adherence to the Mediterranean diet was measured using a 14-point Mediterranean diet-screening questionnaire, adapted from the previously developed and validated version used in the Prevención con Dieta Mediterránea (PREDIMED) study conducted in a high CVD risk population [15]. The short Mediterranean diet questionnaire contains 14 questions characterizing key food groups commonly consumed in a traditional Mediterranean diet (Additional file 1) [15]. Favorable responses ('yes') were assigned a value of '1'; 'no' was assigned '0' and answers were summed to a total Mediterranean diet score ranging from 0 to 14, with higher scores indicating greater adherence. A validation study among a separate sample of 16 heart and lung transplant outpatients demonstrated good agreement with the Mediterranean diet score derived from the 183-item previously validated self-administered semi-quantitative food frequency questionnaire (FFQ) [16]. The mean agreement expressed as a ratio (short questionnaire: FFQ) was 0.99 (95% limits of agreement 0.60–1.38) (ratio of 1.00 indicating perfect agreement) and the two one-sided t-test showed the scores derived from the two methods were equivalent.

For participants assigned to the low-fat diet, the 9-point short questionnaire also adapted from the PREDIMED study [15] was used to measure adherence. The 9-point low-fat diet questionnaire assessed consumption frequencies or serving size of seven food items and two items assessed dietary habits (Additional file 2). For questions that assessed food intake, there were three possible answers scoring '0–2'; with favorable responses receiving higher scores. For the two questions that assessed dietary habits, favorable responses ('yes') were assigned '1'and 'no' was assigned '0'. Resultant low-fat diet scores ranged from 0 to 16 with a higher score indicating greater adherence. The same validation study that assessed validity of the Mediterranean diet questionnaire also showed good agreement between the low-fat short questionnaire with the FFQ: mean agreement 1.04, 95% limits of agreement 0.12–0.79; and the two one-sided t-test showed results from the two methods were equivalent [16].

### Adherence index

A diet adherence index was created for each diet using the scores from the short adherence questionnaire rescaled to range from 0 to 100, to reflect percentage of score achieved. For example, low-fat diet participants scoring 16 received an adherence index of 100 (16/16 × 100), whereas those who scored 9 in the Mediterranean diet achieved an adherence index of 64 (9/14 × 100). This enabled comparisons of the patterns of adherence between the two dietary regimens.

### Anthropometric and laboratory measurements

We measured body weight and serum triglycerides at baseline and at the end of the intervention to provide objective measures of adherence to the allocated diets. Weight was measured wearing light clothing with calibrated scales. Body mass index (BMI) was calculated (kg/m$^2$). Fasting blood samples were collected and processed immediately and stored at − 80 °C for later analysis. Triglycerides were quantified on an Architect c16000 immunoassay analyzer.

As a potential indicator of clinical effectiveness of the interventions, a biomarker of inflammatory state, namely high sensitive C-reactive protein (hs-CRP), was measured. However, hs-CRP values were highly skewed because inflammation status was heavily influenced by other factors, especially the background morbidity (generally high inflammation) and routine medication (Prednisolone, lowering inflammation) in these patients. Consequently, these data did not provide useful information by diet group.

### Statistical analysis

As this was a feasibility study, no formal sample size calculation was carried out. However, we aimed to enroll 40 to 50 participants, a number sufficient to indicate if the interventions were acceptable and the clinical evaluations feasible.

Statistical analyses were performed with SAS, version 9.4 (SAS Institute Inc. Cary, NC). Descriptive statistics were carried out and median (interquartile range (IQR)) was used for the continuous variables, and number (%) for ordinal or categorical variables. The Wilcoxon signed rank sum test was used to compare differences in the median baseline Mediterranean diet or low-fat diet scores, and the scores at each follow-up time. Taking into account the potential imbalanced baseline indices within the groups, ANCOVA was also used to assess adherence indices at each follow-up time compared with baseline indices [17]. Since this is a feasibility study, significance tests of differences between the two diet groups were not performed [18].

## Results

Among the 41 participants, one lung transplant recipient assigned to the Mediterranean diet was lost to follow-up due to dislike of unfamiliar food types and one lung transplant recipient in the low-fat diet group died from chronic rejection. As a result, $n = 20$ in the Mediterranean diet group (10 heart, 10 lung) and $n = 19$ in the low-fat diet group (10 heart, 9 lung) completed the study. In the Mediterranean diet group, 13 (65%) had a family member attend the education session and in the low-fat diet group 16 (84%) were accompanied by a family member. At baseline, the mean age of those randomized to the Mediterranean diet and low-fat diet groups was 56 and 54 years, respectively (Table 1). While body weight was slightly higher in the Mediterranean diet group, BMI was no different (29 kg/m$^2$ for both groups). Similarly, the two groups had comparable waist circumference, systolic and diastolic blood pressure, and heart rates. All participants were on immunosuppressive medication and most were prescribed antihypertensive and/or cholesterol-lowering medications.

At baseline, the median Mediterranean diet score was 4 (IQR 2) overall (Table 2). The score significantly increased to 10 at 6 months (IQR 3; $p < 0.001$) and

**Table 1** Baseline characteristics of Mediterranean and low-fat diet groups ($N = 41$)

| | Mediterranean ($n = 21$) | Low-fat ($n = 20$) |
|---|---|---|
| Age (year)[median (range)] | 58 (33–65) | 59 (27–65) |
| Male [n (%)] | 15 (71) | 14 (70) |
| Weight (kg ± SD) | 87 ± 15 | 82 ± 16 |
| BMI (kg/m$^2$ ± SD) | 29 ± 4 | 29 ± 5 |
| Waist circumference (cm ± SD) | 102 ± 12 | 100 ± 13 |
| Systolic BP (mm Hg ± SD) | 138 ± 13 | 141 ± 14 |
| Diastolic BP (mm Hg ± SD) | 86 ± 11 | 88 ± 8 |
| Heart rate (bpm ± SD) | 80 ± 13 | 79 ± 11 |
| Immunosuppressive medication [n (%)] | | |
| Cyclosporine | 14 (67) | 17 (85) |
| Tacrolimus | 7 (33) | 3 (15) |
| Everolimus | 1 (5) | 0 (0) |
| Mycophenolate | 13 (62) | 12 (60) |
| Azathioprine | 5 (24) | 5 (25) |
| Prednisolone | 21 (100) | 20 (100) |
| Other medication [n (%)] | | |
| Antihypertensive agents | 17 (81) | 15 (75) |
| Cholesterol lowering medication | 17 (81) | 16 (80) |
| Organ transplantation [n (%)] | | |
| Heart | 10 (48) | 10 (50) |
| Lung | 11 (52) | 10 (50) |

**Table 2** Median scores (interquartile range) from short dietary questionniare[1] at each time point and the score differences from the baseline to each time point[2]

| | Mediterranean diet ($n = 20$) | | Low fat diet ($n = 19$) | |
|---|---|---|---|---|
| | Scores at each point | Differences from baseline | Scores at each point | Differences from baseline |
| Baseline | | | | |
| All | 4 (2) | – | 11 (5) | – |
| Heart | 4 (1) | – | 11 (5) | – |
| Lung | 4 (4) | – | 10 (5) | – |
| 6 months | | | | |
| All | 10 (3) | 5 (3)*** | 12 (2) | 2 (3)*** |
| Heart | 10 (3) | 5 (3)** | 13 (2) | 3 (6)* |
| Lung | 10 (3) | 5 (2)** | 12 (2) | 2 (2)* |
| 12 months | | | | |
| All | 9 (4) | 4 (2)*** | 13 (3) | 2 (4)** |
| Heart | 11 (4) | 5 (3)** | 13 (3) | 3 (3)* |
| Lung | 9 (2) | 4 (4)** | 13 (3) | 2 (2)* |
| 6 weeks post-intervention | | | | |
| All | 10 (3) | 5 (3)*** | 12 (2) | 2 (4)* |
| Heart | 10 (3) | 5 (4)** | 13 (2) | 3 (5)* |
| Lung | 10 (3) | 5 (2)** | 11 (2) | 1 (3) |

* $p < 0.05$; ** $p < 0.01$; *** $p < 0.001$
[1]Mediterranean diet score ranged from 0 to 14; low-fat diet score ranged from 0 to 16; higher scores indicate greater adherence
[2]$p$-values from Wilcoxon signed rank sum test

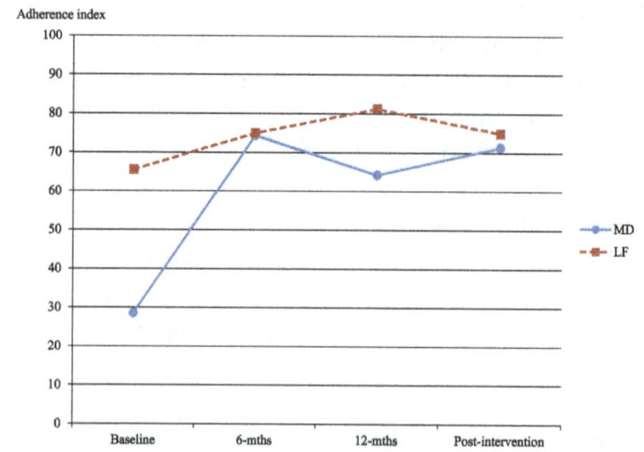


**Fig. 2** Median adherence indices by diet type over 58-weeks. MD: Mediterranean diet; LF: low-fat diet. Mediterranean diet $n = 20$ (10 heart, 10 lung); low-fat diet $n = 19$ (10 heart, 9 lung). Adherence index ranged from 0 to 100, reflecting % of score achieved. Mediterranean diet adherence index = (actual score observed/14) × 100; low-fat diet adherence index = (actual score observed/16) × 100. ANCOVA was used to assess adherence indices at each follow-up time point compared with baseline

remained elevated at 12 months and at 6 weeks post-intervention. For the low-fat diet group, the median baseline score was 11 (IQR 5); and increased to 12 (IQR 2; $p < 0.001$) at 6 months. The score remained high during and after the intervention.

The median adherence index at baseline was lower for the Mediterranean diet group (median 29) compared with the low-fat diet group (median 66) (Fig. 2). However, the Mediterranean diet adherence index increased to a level comparable to the low-fat diet group at each follow-up time point; and was maintained 6-weeks after the intervention ceased. A significant increase in indices at each time point from baseline were observed for both diet groups (all $p < 0.001$) and there were no statistically significant differences in transplant organ types in either intervention (all $p > 0.05$).

Adherence was objectively assessed by changes in body weight, BMI and serum triglycerides in the 12 months from baseline to the end of the intervention period. Compared with baseline body weight, there was a mean weight loss of 1.8 kg in the Mediterranean diet group (– 1.8 kg; 95% CI –4.6, 1.1) at 12 months, and negligible weight loss in the low-fat diet group (mean – 0.2 kg; 95% CI –2.4, 2.1). Similarly, BMI decreased in Mediterranean diet group from 29.0 to 28.5 kg/m$^2$ (mean change – 0.5 kg/m$^2$, 95% CI –1.4, 0.4) whereas no change was observed in the low-fat group over the 12 months (28.6 kg/m$^2$ at both time point, mean change 0.0 kg/m$^2$, 95% CI –0.8, 0.7). Over the same period, the serum triglycerides levels declined in both groups: Mediterranean diet – 0.17 mmol/L (mean – 9%, 95% CI –20, 4); low-fat diet – 0.44 mmol/L (mean – 21%, 95% CI –33 to – 7).

## Discussion

In this feasibility study comparing two dietary interventions in a thoracic transplant outpatient setting, both groups reported changes in their normal eating pattern and adhered to their allocated dietary regimen. In both Mediterranean diet and low-fat diet groups, the change from baseline eating habits was evident at 6 and 12 months; and this change was maintained 6 weeks after intervention.

The current evidence regarding dietary intervention and adherence among solid organ transplant recipients is limited [12]. Indeed this is the first known randomized study reporting adherence to different dietary interventions in heart or lung transplant recipients. One previous non-randomized study was conducted in 42 heart transplant recipients who were encouraged to follow the American Heart Foundation Step 1 Diet and adherence was assessed after 3 months, with only 50% adhering to the diet in that short-term study [10].

Non-adherence to dietary regimens in intervention studies is common and clearly hinders effectiveness [13]. Type of diet prescribed may influence adherence as a low-fat diet appears more difficult to follow and maintain compared with a moderate-fat diet [19]. However, in our study adherence did not differ between the groups and this may be partly due to the detailed advice given to the low-fat diet group. Overall fat and oil intake reduction was emphasized and practical advice was given about how to achieve this (e.g. shopping and cooking). Thus, the actual dietary advice, its delivery methods, and whether close patient support is on hand, appears very important. As highlighted by Zeltzer et al. [12], nutritional support following transplantation is currently sub-optimal and dietary advice is often too general and too-often provided without visual or practical information. To increase adherence, we used several methods: ensuring family support, practical and visual cooking advice, and educational sessions designed to emphasize the reasons why specific foods are beneficial whilst others contribute to disease progression. Our integrated and highly supportive approach may also explain the very low attrition observed during the 12-month intervention.

The PREDIMED study showed a 2-point increase in the Mediterranean diet score in a non-transplant population which was associated with a 14% reduction of all-cause mortality [20]. Similarly, a one-point increase in the Mediterranean diet adherence score was associated with an 18% reduction of myocardial infarction amongst a high risk CVD Mediterranean population [21]. Although there are differences in how diet adherence was assessed in these previous studies, our finding of a 5-point improvement is potentially clinically important among heart and lung transplant recipients.

The previous dietary intervention study of 42 heart transplant recipients encouraged consumption of a low-fat diet for 12 months [10]. This coincided with a reported beneficial effects on lipid and glucose regulation, weight loss and statin use in those who adhered, compared with non-adherent patients at 12 months and at 48-months follow-up [10]. These findings highlight the importance of adherence to diet regimens to help optimize health status. Further, in the present study we found baseline adherence index was much lower for the Mediterranean diet than the low-fat diet, likely reflecting the unfamiliarity of the Mediterranean diet in the UK as a non-Mediterranean European population [22] and the standard low-fat dietary advice previously given to study participants [23].

Adherence measured by body weight and serum triglycerides was further evidence of participants' dietary changes. While the weight reduction observed appears small, without any intervention, post-operative organ transplant recipients weight changes are typically relentlessly upward [5]. Similarly, a rising trajectory of blood lipids including triglycerides is well documented among organ transplant recipients [1, 2]. Nonetheless, the level of triglycerides decreased in both diet groups indicating participants had followed their allocated diets. In particular, the findings of lowered serum triglycerides suggest our participants reduced energy intakes that were excessive.

Limitations included the assessment of adherence using short diet questionnaires. Although short questionnaires have been widely used and reflect adherence of specific diets in non-transplant population [24]; method has not yet been validated with biomarkers of dietary intakes among transplant population. The repeatability has also not been assessed. However, the relative validity of the diet short questionnaires was assessed against a FFQ and showed good agreement [16]. In addition, adherence was assessed using body weight and serum triglycerides as objectively measured clinical and biomarker outcomes: these indicated adherence had been maintained. Finally, although the results from this feasibility study may not be widely generalizable because of small sample size and thus likely not representative, the methods and findings should assist in planning similar intervention studies using short index-based adherence questionnaires.

## Conclusion

Based on our findings, implementation of Mediterranean diet or low-fat diet interventions among clinically stable heart or lung transplant recipients can be achieved, adhered to, and maintained throughout a 12-month period, and even in the short-term, post-intervention. Dietary interventions based on education sessions targeting both patients and family members are crucial for the interventions' success. The educational approach with visual aids and practical information, along with the comprehensive support strategy, are likely to have assisted in patients' adoption and maintenance of their allocated diets during and after the intervention. Findings from this study provide new evidence to inform nutritional support strategies in thoracic transplant recipients.

**Abbreviations**

AMEND-IT study: Assessment of the MEditerraneaN Diet In heart and lung Transplantation study; BMI: Body mass index; CI: Confidence intervals; FFQ: Food frequency questionnaire; hs-CRP: High sensitive C-reactive protein; IQR: Interquartile range; PREDIMED study: Prevención con Dieta Mediterránea study

**Acknowledgements**

Not applicable.

**Funding**

TRE was supported by New Start Transplant Charity for PhD studentship. KM was supported by The National Health and Medical Research Council of Australia Program Grant Nos 552429 & 1073898.

**Authors' contributions**
The authors' responsibilities were as follows: TRE conceptualised and conducted the study, collected and managed the data, and wrote the manuscript. ACG assisted with study conception and design, data interpretation and supervised the study. JEF assisted in the study conception and design, helped obtain the funding, and supervised the study. KM analysed the data, assisted in the data interpretation, and wrote the manuscript. All authors critically reviewed the manuscript and approved the final version submitted for publication.

**Competing interests**
The authors declare that they have no competing interests.

**Author details**
[1]The Transplant Centre, University Hospital of South Manchester, Manchester M23 9LT, UK. [2]Cancer and Population Studies Group, QIMR Berghofer Medical Research Institute, 300 Herston Road, Herston, QLD 4006, Australia. [3]CRUK Manchester Institute, University of Manchester, Wilmslow Road, Manchester, UK. [4]Manchester Collaborative Centre for Inflammation Research, University of Manchester, Manchester, UK.

**References**

1. Lund LH, Edwards LB, Kucheryavaya AY, Benden C, Christie JD, Dipchand AI, Dobbels F, Goldfarb SB, Levvey BJ, Meiser B, et al. The registry of the International Society for Heart and Lung Transplantation: 31st official adult heart transplant report. J Heart Lung Transplant. 2014;33:996–1008. https://doi.org/10.1016/j.healun.2014.08.003.
2. Yusen RD, Edwards LB, Kucheryavaya AY, Benden C, Dipchand AI, Goldfarb SB, Levvey BJ, Lund LH, Meiser B, Rossano JW, Stehlik J. The registry of the International Society for Heart and Lung Transplantation: thirty-second official adult lung and heart-lung transplantation report. J Heart Lung Transplant. 2015;34:1264–77. https://doi.org/10.1016/j.healun.2015.08.014.
3. Williams JJ, Lund LH, LaManca J, Kunavarapu C, Cohen DJ, Heshka S, Heymsfield SB, Mancini DM. Excessive weight gain in cardiac transplant recipients. J Heart Lung Transplant. 2006;25:36–41. https://doi.org/10.1016/j.healun.2005.06.016.
4. Singer LG, Brazelton TR, Doyle RL, Morris RE, Theodore J. Weight gain after lung transplantation. J Heart Lung Transplant. 2003;22:894–902. https://doi.org/10.1016/S1053-2498(02)00807-0.
5. Kugler C, Einhorn I, Gottlieb J, Warnecke G, Schwarz A, Barg-Hock H, Bara C, Haller H, Haverich A. Postoperative weight gain during the first year after kidney, liver, heart, and lung transplant: a prospective study. Prog Transplant. 2015;25:49–55. https://doi.org/10.7182/pit2015668.
6. Forli L, Bollerslev J, Simonsen S, Isaksen GA, Godang K, Pripp AH, Bjortuft O. Disturbed energy metabolism after lung and heart transplantation. Clin Transpl. 2011;25:E136–43. https://doi.org/10.1111/j.1399-0012.2010.01379.x.
7. Mehra MR. Contemporary concepts in prevention and treatment of cardiac allograft vasculopathy. Am J Transplant. 2006;6:1248–56. https://doi.org/10.1111/j.1600-6143.2006.01314.x.
8. British Heart Foundation: Eating Well. In Healthy eating for you and your heart. pp. 98. London: British Heart Foundation 2012:98.
9. Laederach-Hofmann K, Bunzel B. Noncompliance in organ transplant recipients: a literature review. Gen Hosp Psychiatry. 2000;22:412–24.
10. Guida B, Perrino NR, Laccetti R, Trio R, Nastasi A, Pesola D, Maiello C, Marra C, De Santo LS, Cotrufo M. Role of dietary intervention and nutritional follow-up in heart transplant recipients. Clin Transpl. 2009;23:101–7. https://doi.org/10.1111/j.1399-0012.2008.00915.x.
11. Zaffari D, Losekann A, Santos AF, Manfroi WC, Bittar AE, Keitel E, Souza VB, Costa M, Prates VC, Kroth L, Braun ML. Effectiveness of diet in hyperlipidemia in renal transplant patients. Transplant Proc. 2004;36:889–90. https://doi.org/10.1016/j.transproceed.2004.03.115.
12. Zeltzer SM, Taylor DO, Tang WHW. Long-term dietary habits and interventions in solid-organ transplantation. J Heart Lung Transplant. 2015;34:1357–65. https://doi.org/10.1016/j.healun.2015.06.014.
13. Desroches S, Lapointe A, Ratte S, Gravel K, Legare F, Turcotte S. Interventions to enhance adherence to dietary advice for preventing and managing chronic diseases in adults. Cochrane Database Syst Rev. 2013;2: Cd008722. https://doi.org/10.1002/14651858.CD008722.pub2.
14. Miller TA, Dimatteo MR. Importance of family/social support and impact on adherence to diabetic therapy. Diabetes Metab Syndr Obes. 2013;6:421–6. https://doi.org/10.2147/dmso.s36368.
15. Estruch R, Ros E, Salas-Salvadó J, Covas M-I, Corella D, Arós F, Gómez-Gracia E, Ruiz-Gutiérrez V, Fiol M, Lapetra J, et al. Primary prevention of cardiovascular disease with a Mediterranean diet. N Engl J Med. 2013;368:1279–90. https://doi.org/10.1056/NEJMoa1200303.
16. Miura K, Entwistle TR, Fildes JE, Green AC. Relative validity of short questionnaires to assess Mediterranean diet or low-fat diet adherence. J Aging Res Clin Practice. 2017;6:23–7. https://doi.org/10.14283/jarcp.2017.4.
17. Van Breukelen GJ. ANCOVA versus change from baseline: more power in randomized studies, more bias in nonrandomized studies. J Clin Epidemiol. 2006;59:920–5. https://doi.org/10.1016/j.jclinepi.2006.02.007.
18. Lancaster GA, Dodd S, Williamson PR. Design and analysis of pilot studies: recommendations for good practice. J Eval Clin Pract. 2004;10:307–12. https://doi.org/10.1111/j.2002.384.doc.x.
19. McManus K, Antinoro L, Sacks F. A randomized controlled trial of a moderate-fat, low-energy diet compared with a low fat, low-energy diet for weight loss in overweight adults. Int J Obes Relat Metab Disord. 2001;25: 1503–11. https://doi.org/10.1038/sj.ijo.0801796.
20. Trichopoulou A, Bamia C, Trichopoulos D. Anatomy of health effects of Mediterranean diet: Greek EPIC prospective cohort study. BMJ. 2009;338 https://doi.org/10.1136/bmj.b2337.
21. Martinez-Gonzalez MA, Fernandez-Jarne E, Serrano-Martinez M, Wright M, Gomez-Gracia E. Development of a short dietary intake questionnaire for the quantitative estimation of adherence to a cardioprotective Mediterranean diet. Eur J Clin Nutr. 2004;58:1550–2.
22. Trichopoulos D, Lagiou P. Mediterranean diet and overall mortality differences in the European union. Public Health Nutr. 2004;7:949–51.
23. Moore C, Chowdhury Z, Young JB. Heart transplant nutrition programs: a national survey. J Heart Lung Transplant. 1991;10:50–5.
24. England CY, Andrews RC, Jago R, Thompson JL. A systematic review of brief dietary questionnaires suitable for clinical use in the prevention and management of obesity, cardiovascular disease and type 2 diabetes. Eur J Clin Nutr. 2015;69:977–1003. https://doi.org/10.1038/ejcn.2015.6.

# 16

# Dietary quality linkage to overall competence at school and emotional disturbance in representative Taiwanese young adolescents: dependence on gender, parental characteristics and personal behaviors

Lin-Yuan Huang[1], Mark L. Wahlqvist[1,2,3,4], Meei-Shyuan Lee[2] and Po-Huang Chiang[1,4*]

**Abstract**

**Background:** Child school performance during puberty may be at increased risk through emotional disturbance. It is hypothesized that this may be mitigated by dietary quality.

**Methods:** In a nationally representative sample (Nutrition and Health Survey in Taiwan, NAHSIT), 1371 Taiwanese aged 11–16 years, overall competence at school, (OCS) and emotional status have been assessed by teachers with the SAED (Scale for Assessing Emotional Disturbance). Parents provided family socio-demographics and students completed a behavioral and dietary questionnaire (Youth Healthy Eating Index - Taiwan, YHEI-TW). Associations between emotional disturbance (ED), OCS and dietary quality (YHEI-TW) were assessed in multiple linear regression models with adjustments for covariates including parental characteristics, personal behaviors, body fatness and puberty.

**Results:** Boys or girls with ED had a less favorable OCS ($p < 0.001$), minimally dependent on YHEI-TW. On multivariable analysis there was a more positive association between OCS and YHEI-TW among boys ($\beta = 0.05$, $p < 0.01$) and girls ($\beta = 0.07$, $p < 0.001$). Poor dietary quality was associated with ED, especially in girls ($\beta = -0.06$, $p < 0.001$). Additionally, parental characteristics, body fatness, and personal behaviors are associated with OCS. Puberty is associated with ED and may be indirectly linked to OCS.

**Conclusions:** Unsatisfactory food intake is associated with the link between emotional disturbance and impaired school performance, as assessed by OCS, especially among girls. For both genders, socio-economic and behavioral factors including parenteral income, reading, screen viewing and smoking are modulators of this association. Puberty was a modifying factor in girls. Dietary quality is a relevant factor for health (ED) as well as education (OCS) during early adolescence.

**Keywords:** Gender, Parental characteristics, Personal behaviors, Dietary quality, Puberty, Junior high school, School performance

* Correspondence: chiangp@nhri.org.tw
[1]Division of Preventive Medicine and Health Services Research, Institute of Population Health Sciences, National Health Research Institutes, 35 Keyan Road, Zhunan Town, Miaoli County 350, Taiwan, Republic of China
[4]College of Public Health, China Medical University, Taichung, Taiwan, Republic of China
Full list of author information is available at the end of the article

## Background

Adolescence, nowadays considered the transitional period between childhood and adulthood, is a critical time in human development when pubertal change is underway, personal identity is being formatted and when future livelihood prospects are being established [1], especially through the education system. Minimizing emotional disturbance (ED) [2, 3] and optimizing school performance [4] at this time is a desirable research and policy objective. However, associations between ED and school performance are poorly documented [5, 6]. There is a growing recognition that items in the SAED (scale for assessing emotional disturbance) methodology [7] may be linked to overall competence at school (OCS) as a surrogate for school performance [8, 9] or learning disability [10]. A number of factors could affect any association between ED and OCS. These include home environment, school environment [11, 12], personal behaviors such as recreation and physical activity, cigarette smoking & alcohol usage [11], dietary quality [8, 13] nutritional status insofar as body fatness is concerned [14], and pubertal development [11].

*Diet* may also be a key factor in the expression of emotional disturbance [13, 14] and in cognitive and school performance [8, 15–18]. It may operate through energy regulation in conjunction with physical activity and sedentariness given that cognitive function appears amenable to measures which alter cellular energy regulation [19, 20], particularly in relation to the increasing burden of the metabolic syndrome and diabetes [21, 22]. Dietary quality has also been shown to play a role in emotion, mood [23] and mental performance [13] where limited food biodiversity, notably of plant foods, and degree of processing, with more ready-to-eat low nutrient density food items are the riskier consumption patterns [18, 23, 24]. However, there are limited observations about the connectedness of dietary patterns and brain function in relation to the child-adult transition. Partly, this is because of the biological heterogeneity and its secular trends at this time of reproductive transition.

*Parents* have the potential to affect both ED and OCS in many ways which reflect their continuing, if declining, role as providers of care, support and resources during their offspring's adolescence [25]. This is likely to include pathways like diet [24, 26]. This is the case during elementary school where, particularly in girls vulnerable through low birth weight, nutritious diets have been associated with less likelihood of both emotional disturbance and poor school performance [13]. Further documentation and understanding of these phenomena may prompt guardians and mentors of young people to identify and act preventatively in regard to them, especially in regard to food choice and diet [2, 27].

*Our principal hypothesis* is that emotional disturbance (ED) during the child-to-adult transition is adversely associated with school performance as represented by overall competence (OC) and that dietary quality may mitigate such a linkage This association may, nevertheless, be modulated by various factors. The opportunity has been taken to study emotional disturbance and school performance among junior high school boys and girls in Taiwan in regard to diet and puberty, taking into account parental and various personal behavioral characteristics.

## Methods

### Study participants

Participants were adolescents aged 11–16 years (grade 7–9) who participated in the Nutrition and Health Survey in Taiwan (NAHSIT) 2010–2011. The original study is a national representative cross-sectional survey. All of Taiwan's 358 townships/districts were classified into 5 strata (northern 1, northern 2, central, southern and eastern area) by geographical location and population density. The survey used the PPS (probabilities proportional to sizes) sampling method to select 1620 students from 30 junior high schools (6 schools from each stratum) randomly. NAHSIT comprises questionnaires administered by face-to-face interview of parents and students (including a food frequency questionnaire, 24-h dietary recall, pubertal development, personal behaviors from students; and family socio-demographics from parents). Physical examination (including body composition, blood pressure) was conducted and plasma metabolic analytes obtained though venipuncture by a health care professional. Thus, the questionnaire covered both dietary and non-dietary health factors [28].

The present study excluded participants who did not complete the emotional disturbance questionnaire, leaving 1371 (656 boys and 715 girls) junior high school students eligible for analysis. The survey was approved by the Institutional Review Board of the National Health Research Institutes, Taiwan.

### Measures

#### *The scale for assessing emotional disturbance (SAED)*

The modified Scale for Assessing Emotional Disturbance (SAED) was used to assess the NAHSIT students' school and social performance, the original questionnaires being developed by Epstein and Cullinan [13, 29, 30]. The SAED scales for students were assessed by their teachers using the SAED questionnaire. The SAED is a rating scale designed to help identify students with emotional and/or behavioral difficulties at school. Its test-retest reliability coefficient is above > 0.80, and most of its subscales have inter-rater reliability coefficients over 0.79 [7]. The Chinese modification of SAED as used in this study has a high overall reliability of 0.92 and validity of

0.76 [29]. The SAED consist of a total of seven subscales including OC considered in this study as OCS and six other subscales. These are: Inability to Learn (IL, 8 items), Relationship Problems (RP, 6 items), Inappropriate Behavior (IB, 10 items), Unhappiness or Depression (UD, 7 items), Physical Symptoms or Fears (PF, 8 items)), Social Maladjustment (SM, 6 items), and Overall Competence at school (OCS, 7 items). OCS has been treated separately from SAED in this study (see below). Within the above subscales, items were scored by each student's Class Mentor teacher. As previously described, the first six subscales (52 items) were scored on a four-point scale (0 = not a problem, 1 = mild problem, 2 = considerable problem, 3 = severe problem), and five-point scale for OCS (0 = far below average, 1 = below average, 2 = average, 3 = above average, and 4 = far above average). The raw scores for the SAED subscales were summed and converted into standardized scores (mean = 10 and SD = 3). Compared with the Taiwanese Non-Emotional Disturbance Norms, a substantially deviant SAED score (except OCS) is indicated by a score that above the 91 percentile (>90th percentile), which corresponds to Z-scores ≥13 [29]. Therefore, a score of 13 was chosen as the cut point. Children with a Z-score ≥ 13 were considered to have emotional disturbance (ED). IL, RP, IB, UD, and PF scores could be combined to produce a total score of ED characteristics. These five subscale scores plus SM score can be combined to yield an "SAED total" score [30, 31].

#### *Overall competence at school (OCS)*

OCS was used to assess the students' overall performance and adaptation at school. The questions for OCS included (1) intellectual functioning, (2) family support for school, (3) overall level of academic functioning, (4) motivation for schoolwork, (5) level of peer support, (6) personal hygiene (e.g. grooming, dressing), and (7) interest in activities outside of school. Students with an OCS Z-score less than or equal to 6 (fell below the 9th percentile) were considered to have an unfavorable overall school performance [29, 30].

#### *Dietary quality (YHEI-TW)*

The Youth Healthy Eating Index-Taiwan (YHEI-TW) is a diet quality scoring system modified from the U.S. YHEI, which captures the adolescent's diet quality by assessing his or her adherence to dietary guidelines [32]. The YHEI–TW scores were obtained from daily consumption of 11 components derived from food frequency questionnaires and a 24–hour dietary recall employed during NAHSIT: (1) whole grains (0 to ≥ 2 servings, 0–10 points), (2) vegetables (0 to ≥ 3 servings, 0–10 points), (3) fruits (0 to ≥ 3 servings, 0–10 points), (4) dairy (0 to ≥ 3 servings, 0–10 points), (5) meat ratio (0 to ≥ 20, 10–0 points), (6) snack foods (i.e., salty snacks and snacks with added sugar, 0 to ≥ 3 servings, 10–0 points), (7) sweetened beverages (0 to ≥3 servings, 10–0 points), (8) multivitamins (never-daily, 5–0 points), (9) fried foods outside of home (never-daily, 0–5 points), (10) consumption of breakfast (never to > 5 times/week, 0–5 points) and (11) dinner with family (prepared by family member, 5 points). It does not take into account butter/margarine and visible animal fat, which were part of the original YHEI (US), since consumption of these items has been negligible in Taiwan. In all cases, except component 11 (dinner patterns), scores were derived in a proportionate manner. Thus, total scores range from 0 to 90, where higher scores indicate better dietary quality [13, 33, 34].

#### *Covariate measurements*

Covariates were derived from questionnaires, by anthropometry and from laboratory measurements of metabolic analytes in the NAHSIT survey. Those considered in the present study included mother's education (lower than university, university and above), household income (0–30,000, 30,000–50,000, 50,000–80,000, > 80,000 NTD/month where US$1 = NTD 30), ever smoking (no, yes), read during weekdays (0–1, 1–3, ≥3 h/day), watch TV during weekdays (0–1, 1–3, ≥3 h/day), play computer games during weekdays (0–1, 1–3, ≥3 h/day), moderate or heavy physical activity (0–30, ≥30 min/day; in accordance with Taiwanese recommendations) [35], BMI (underweight, normal, overweight, obesity; (the Childhood Obesity Expert Panel of the Taiwanese Department of Health defines 'obesity' and 'overweight' (≥95th and ≥85th percentile value of body mass index (BMI), respectively) using age- and gender-specificity percentiles for BMI (each gender and year of age from 2 to 18 had its own cut-off point for overweight and for obesity) [36], and puberty (boys: beard growth (not yet, at first, in progress, completed); girls: menarche (yes, no)).

#### Statistical analysis

Chi-square tests were used to assess the significant differences between categorical variables. We used t tests to assess differences in continuous variables. Categorical variables are presented as percentages (%), and continuous variables are presented as means (standard errors, SE). Multiple linear regression models (MLRs) were used to test associations between the key determinants (household, personal behaviors, puberty, dietary quality, body fatness) and outcome measures (ED and OCS); and in the adjustments for mother's education, household income, ever smoking, reading during weekdays, watching TV during weekdays, playing computer games during weekdays, moderate or heavy physical activity, pubertal development and BMI. Full models were considered which included all relevant variables. The regression coefficients reported are from these models. Statistical significance was set at $p < 0.05$. Data were analyzed using SAS 9.3 for Windows, weighted by SUDAAN [37]. SUDAAN was also used to adjust for the study design effect of cluster sampling to obtain unbiased estimates of the standard errors.

An overview of the study design and models is provided in Fig. 1.

## Results

### Overall competence at school

Table 1 shows the junior high school students' characteristics by overall competence as an index of school performance. The mean age of the 1371 participants (51.7% are boys) was 13.6 years. There were 5.9% adolescents with unfavorable overall competence at school (OCS) (OCS Z-score ≤ 6). The percentage in boys was higher than girls (61.3% vs. 38.7%, $p = 0.042$). Adolescents had a better OCS when parents had a higher education. Adolescents in households where income was less than 30,000 NTD/month (about 1000 US dollars) had the most unfavorable OCS (34.5%), whereas this was only 11.2% in the > 80,000 NTD/month group ($p < 0.001$).

#### *Personal Behaviors*

Compared with favorable OCS, more smokers were found among unfavorable OCS (24.5%, $p = 0.019$), those who read only 0–1 h/day during weekdays (67.2%, $p = 0.01$), those who watched TV ≥3 h/day during weekdays (12.9%, $p = 0.006$), and those who played computer games ≥3 h/day during weekdays (13.6%, $p = 0.064$).

#### *Dietary Quality*

Participants with unfavorable OCS had lower dietary scores than did those with favorable OCS (44.0 ± 1.1 vs. 48.4 ± 0.5, $p < 0.001$) and also a higher consumption frequency (times/week) of fast foods (0.7 ± 0.1 vs. 0.4 ± 0.1, $p = 0.029$), sugary beverages (6.5 ± 0.6 vs. 5.3 ± 0.2, $p = 0.053$), and flavored milk (1.4 ± 0.3 vs. 0.7 ± 0.1, $p = 0.015$), but a lower cheese consumption (0.6 ± 0.1 vs. 0.9 ± 0.1, $p = 0.035$) (Table 2).

#### *Puberty*

In regard to pubertal development, boys with 'completed' beard growth had the most unfavorable OCS (4.5%, $p = 0.036$) (Table 2). The means of YHEI-TW scores were not significant difference among onset of puberty in the present study (data not shown).

#### *Body fatness and Metabolic analytes*

Adolescents with an unfavorable OCS had a higher BMI and a lower HDL cholesterol than did those with a better OCS (BMI: 21.9 ± 0.5 vs. 20.8 ± 0.2, $p = 0.046$; HDL: 50.8 ± 1.9 vs. 55.6 ± 0.7, $p = 0.022$) (Table 2).

### Emotional disturbance

Figure 2 shows the SAED Z-scores of adolescents by dietary quality (< or ≥ YHEI-TW median). The median YHEI-TW for boys was 48.2, and 48.5 for girls.

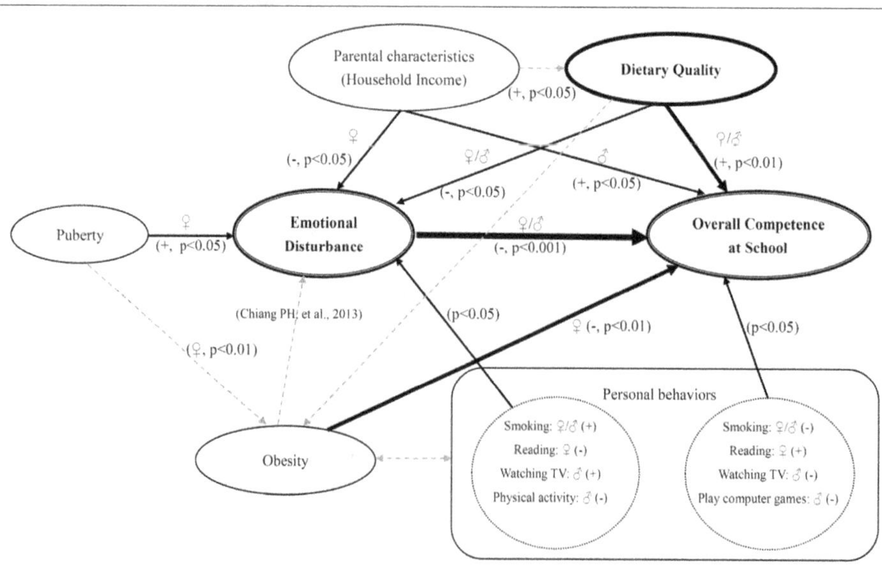


**Fig. 1** Pathways to emotional disturbance and overall competence at school in Taiwanese adolescents.
Where an association is significant, the level of significance is indicated with the relevant *p* value and in accordance with gender. The findings represented in this figure are those of the present report except for "obesity→emotional disturbance" which have been reported in Reference [14] for Taiwanese schoolchildren

**Table 1** Basic characteristics of junior high school students by Overall Competence (OCS) ($N = 1371$)

| Characteristics[a] | | OCS[b] | | *P* value |
|---|---|---|---|---|
| | Overall | Z-score ≤ 6 | Z-score > 6 | |
| Participants (%) | 1371 (100) | 98 (5.9) | 1273 (94.1) | |
| Mean age in years (SE) | 13.6 (0.1) | 13.3 (0.1) | 13.6 (0.1) | 0.130 |
| Gender (%) | | | | 0.042 |
| Boys | 51.7 | 61.3 | 51.1 | |
| Girls | 48.3 | 38.7 | 48.9 | |
| Father's ethnicity (%) | | | | 0.777 |
| Fukienese | 76.6 | 71.9 | 76.9 | |
| Hakka | 13.0 | 15.8 | 12.8 | |
| Mainlander | 8.3 | 9.2 | 8.2 | |
| Indigenes | 2.2 | 3.2 | 2.1 | |
| Father's educational level (%) | | | | 0.008 |
| Secondary education and below | 40.5 | 61.9 | 39.1 | |
| University and above | 59.5 | 38.1 | 60.9 | |
| Mother's educational level (%) | | | | 0.018 |
| Secondary education and below | 33.4 | 47.5 | 32.5 | |
| University and above | 66.6 | 52.5 | 67.5 | |
| Household income (%) | | | | <0.001 |
| 0–30,000 NTD/month[c] | 19.3 | 34.5 | 18.4 | |
| 30,000–50,000 NTD/month | 21.7 | 24.1 | 21.6 | |
| 50,000–80,000 NTD/month | 29.8 | 30.1 | 29.6 | |
| > 80,000 NTD/month | 29.2 | 11.2 | 30.3 | |
| Ever smoking (%) | | | | 0.019 |
| No | 89.9 | 75.5 | 90.8 | |
| Yes | 10.1 | 24.5 | 9.19 | |
| Drinking alcohol (%) | | | | 0.730 |
| No | 87.4 | 85.4 | 87.6 | |
| Yes | 12.6 | 14.6 | 12.4 | |
| Read during weekdays (%) | | | | 0.010 |
| 0–1 (h/day) | 45.6 | 67.2 | 44.3 | |
| 1–3 | 42.0 | 30.0 | 42.8 | |
| ≥ 3 | 12.4 | 2.9 | 13.0 | |
| Watch TV during weekdays (%) | | | | 0.006 |
| 0–1 (h/day) | 58.1 | 33.9 | 59.7 | |
| 1–3 | 33.7 | 53.2 | 32.5 | |
| ≥ 3 | 8.13 | 12.9 | 7.8 | |
| Play computer games during weekdays (%) | | | | 0.064 |
| 0–1 (h/day) | 62.3 | 48.8 | 63.2 | |
| 1–3 | 29.2 | 37.6 | 28.7 | |
| ≥ 3 | 8.45 | 13.6 | 8.1 | |
| Moderate or heavy physical activity (%) | | | | 0.734 |
| 0–30 (min/day) | 26.0 | 24.7 | 26.1 | |
| ≥ 30 | 74.0 | 75.3 | 73.9 | |

[a]Categorical variables are presented as percentage (%), and continuous variables are presented as mean (SE)
[b]Students with an OCS Z-score less than or equal to 6 were considered to have unfavorable overall school performance
[c]1 US dollars = 30 NTD

**Table 2** Student food intakes, physical examination and metabolic analytes by Overall Competence (OCS)

| | Overall | OCS[a] Z-score ≤ 6 | OCS[a] Z-score > 6 | p value |
|---|---|---|---|---|
| Mean (SE) Dietary score (YHEI-TW) | 48.1 (0.5) | 44.0 (1.1) | 48.4 (0.5) | <0.001 |
| Mean (SE) Food consumption (times/week) | | | | |
| Fast foods consumption | 1.7 (0.1) | 2.3 (0.3) | 1.7 (0.1) | 0.086 |
| Fast foods from fast food chain store | 0.5 (0.1) | 0.7 (0.1) | 0.4 (0.1) | 0.029 |
| Fast foods from non-fast food chain store | 1.3 (0.1) | 1.6 (0.3) | 1.2 (0.1) | 0.206 |
| Sugary beverages consumption | 5.4 (0.2) | 6.5 (0.6) | 5.3 (0.2) | 0.053 |
| Dairy products consumption | | | | |
| Milk | 3.5 (0.2) | 3.0 (0.7) | 3.6 (0.2) | 0.499 |
| Flavored milk | 0.7 (0.1) | 1.4 (0.3) | 0.7 (0.1) | 0.015 |
| Yoghurt | 0.5 (0.1) | 0.7 (0.2) | 0.5 (0.1) | 0.342 |
| Cheese | 0.9 (0.1) | 0.6 (0.1) | 0.9 (0.1) | 0.035 |
| Development of puberty | | | | |
| Menarche (girls only) (%) | | | | 0.929 |
| Yes | 94.0 | 93.5 | 94.0 | |
| No | 6.0 | 6.5 | 6.0 | |
| Beard growth (boys only) (%) | | | | 0.036 |
| Not yet | 33.4 | 45.3 | 32.4 | |
| At first | 31.4 | 36.9 | 30.9 | |
| In progress | 33.8 | 13.2 | 35.4 | |
| Completed | 1.5 | 4.5 | 1.2 | |
| Mean (SE) Body compositions | | | | |
| Height (cm) | 161 (0.3) | 160 (1.2) | 161 (0.3) | 0.716 |
| Weight (kg) | 54.2 (0.5) | 56.7 (1.7) | 54.0 (0.5) | 0.146 |
| Body mass index (BMI, kg/m$^2$) | 20.8 (0.2) | 21.9 (0.5) | 20.8 (0.2) | 0.046 |
| Triceps skin fold thickness (TSF, mm) | 16.6 (0.4) | 17.2 (0.9) | 16.6 (0.4) | 0.496 |
| Mid Arm Muscle Circumference (MAMC, cm) | 20.0 (0.2) | 21.5 (1.2) | 19.9 (0.2) | 0.221 |
| waist circumference (WC, cm) | 74.2 (0.5) | 76.2 (1.2) | 74.1 (0.5) | 0.114 |
| Mean (SE) Blood pressure (mmHg) | | | | |
| Systolic blood pressure (SBP) | 105 (0.5) | 106 (1.5) | 105 (0.5) | 0.520 |
| Diastolic blood pressure (DBP) | 60.5 (0.7) | 61.5 (1.2) | 60.4 (0.7) | 0.301 |
| Mean (SE) Plasma metabolic analytes | | | | |
| Fasting glucose (mg/dL) | 95.4 (0.4) | 95.2 (0.9) | 95.4 (0.4) | 0.835 |
| Total cholesterol (mg/dL) | 158 (1.4) | 155 (3.3) | 159 (1.4) | 0.191 |
| Triglycerides (mg/dL) | 71.4 (1.8) | 78.3 (5.5) | 71.0 (1.7) | 0.150 |
| HDL cholesterol (mg/dL) | 55.3 (0.7) | 50.8 (1.9) | 55.6 (0.7) | 0.022 |
| LDL cholesterol (mg/dL) | 88.8 (1.2) | 87.9 (3.2) | 88.8 (1.2) | 0.761 |
| Uric acid (mg/dL) | 5.8 (0.1) | 6.2 (0.2) | 5.74 (0.1) | 0.063 |

[a]Students with an OCS Z-score less than or equal to 6 were considered to have unfavorable overall school performance
YHEI-TW, Youth Healthy Eating Index-Taiwan

Whether boys or girls, those with better diet quality had higher overall competence at school ($p < 0.001$). Boys with poorer diet quality had higher IL, IB, UD, SM, ED and total SAED Z-scores compared to those with better diet quality ($p < 0.05$). Among girls, those with poorer diet quality demonstrated more emotional disturbance (except SM) compared to those with better diet quality ($p < 0.01$).

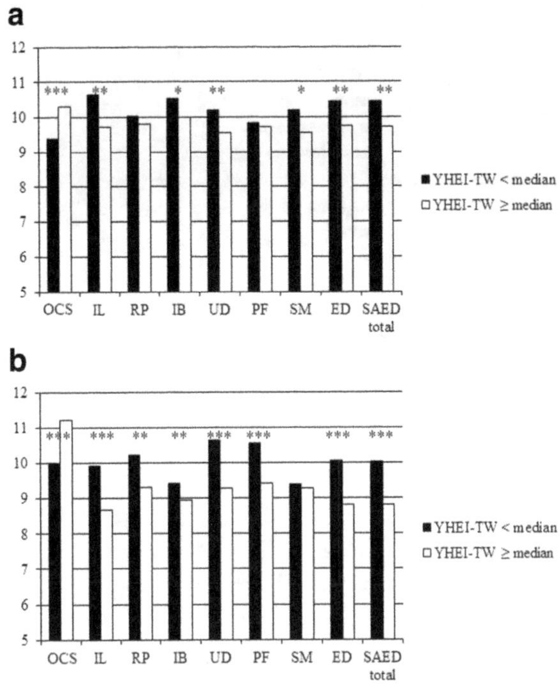


**Fig. 2** Gender-specific distribution of SAED Z-scores by YHEI-TW group. The median YHEI-TW for boys was 48.2, and 48.5 for girls. SAED, the Scale for Assessing Emotional Disturbance; OCS, Overall Competence at School; IL, Inability to Learn; RP, Relationship Problems; IB, Inappropriate Behavior; UD, Unhappiness or Depression; PF, Physical symptoms or Fears; SM, Socially Maladjusted; ED, Emotional Disturbance. * $p < 0.05$; ** $p < 0.01$; *** $p < 0.001$. **a** Boys SAED Z-score. **b** Girls SAED Z-score

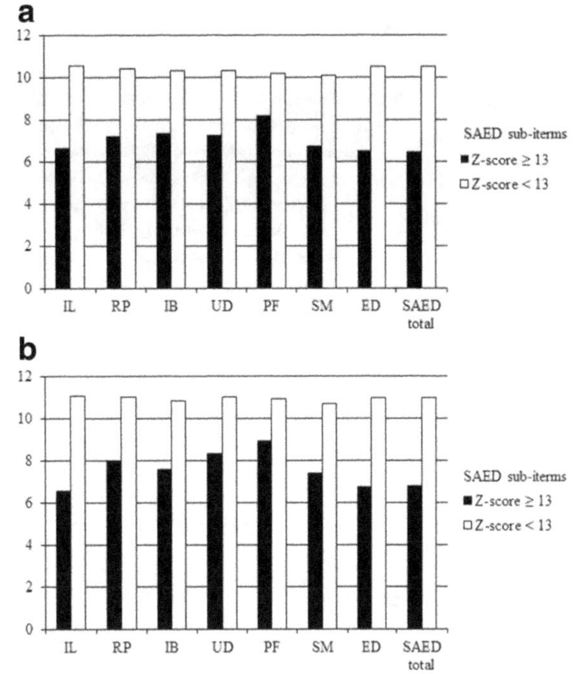


**Fig. 3** Z-scores of Overall Competence at school (OCS) by SAED sub-items and gender.
Students with Z-scores ≥13 in any subscale were classified as having emotional disturbance. The t-test was used to compared the difference between two SAED sub-items groups; all of the results were significant ($p < 0.001$). **a** Boys OCS Z-score. **b** Girls OCS Z-score

## Emotional disturbance and overall competence at school

Figure 3 shows the significant difference between total SAED and its sub-types with OCS as Z-scores < or ≥13. Whether boys or girls, students with emotional disturbance (Z-score ≥ 13) had significantly lower OCS Z-scores. Students without emotional disturbance had a better overall competence at school than those with emotional disturbance ($p < 0.001$). There were significant inverse associations between OCS and SAED and its sub-items among boys and girls (Additional file 1). When these relationships for SAED itself and its sub-items were adjusted for dietary quality, the β coefficients in the range of − 0.32 to − 0.85 were marginally reduced by the order of 0.01–0.05 in boys and girls, but remained significant; this indicated that a contribution from dietary quality to ED-linked OCS was small (Additional file 1).

## Predictive models for OCS

The multiple linear regression analysis for OCS Z-scores, with reference to YHEI-TW and relevant co-variates, is shown in Fig. 4. In conjunction with other co-variates, there was a significant positive association between OCS and YHEI-TW among boys (β = 0.05, $p < 0.01$) and girls (β = 0.07, $p < 0.001$). Boys with a household income of 50–80,000 NTD/month had an OCS Z-score which was 1.02 greater than for those with < 30,000 NTD/ month ($p < 0.05$). Compared with not smoking, not watching TV, and not playing computer games 0–1 h/day during weekdays, boys who did had lower OCS Z-scores (β = − 1.26 ($p < 0.05$), − 0.76 ($p < 0.05$), and − 0.93 ($p < 0.001$) respectively. For girls, ever smoking and obesity were associated with lower OCS Z-scores than their non-smoking and normal weight counterparts (β was − 0.97 (p < 0.05) and − 1.34 ($p < 0.01$) respectively). Girls who read ≥3 h/day during weekdays had higher OCS Z-scores than did those who read 0–1 h/day (β = 1.23, $p < 0.05$).

The $R^2$ for the complete model to predict OCS was 0.21 for boys and 0.22 for girls, explaining 21% and 22% of the variance respectively; without YHEI-TW in the model, $R^2$ was 0.18 and 0.16 (18% and 16% of the variance respectively) (Fig. 4).

## Predictive models for SAED

Tables 3 and 4 show the multiple linear regressions for SAED subscales with reference to YHEI-TW and relevant co-variates. There was a significant inverse association between IL and YHEI-TW (β = − 0.05, $p < 0.01$) among boys. In the multivariable models, boys who had ever smoked had higher IL (β = 1.87, $p < 0.05$), IB (β = 1.88, $p < 0.01$),

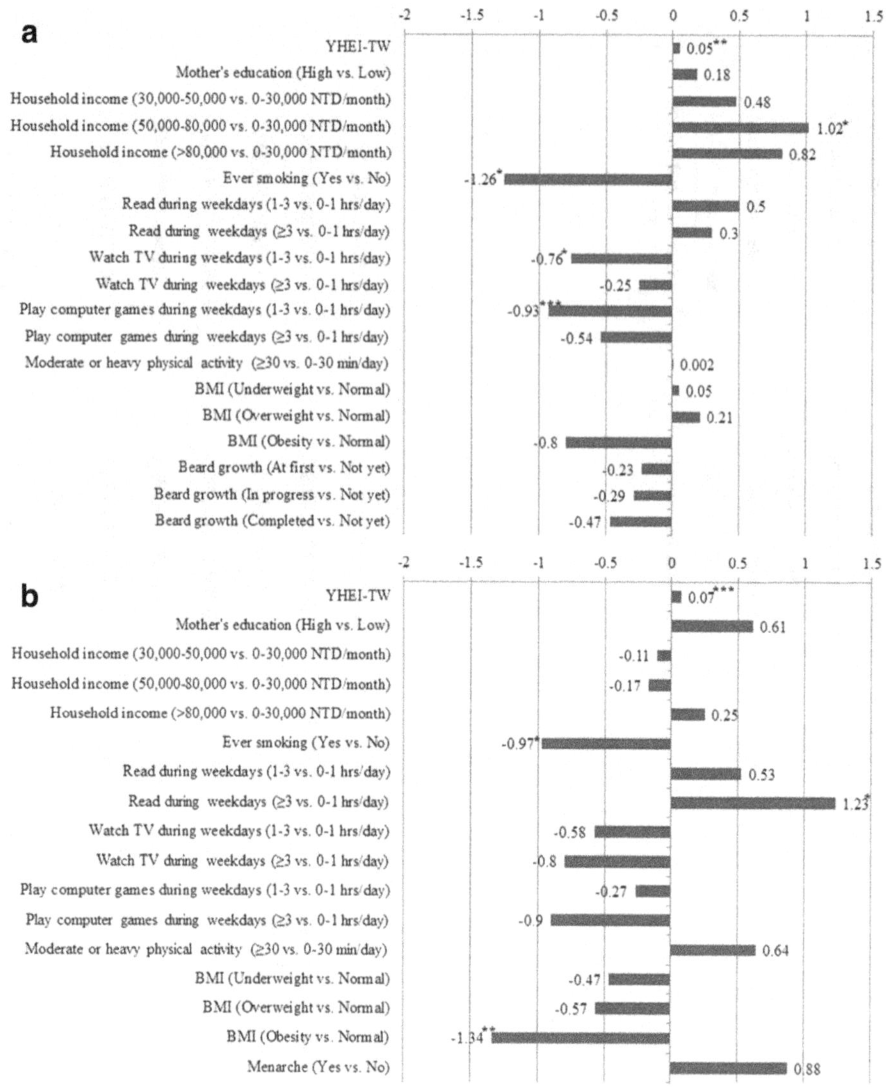


**Fig. 4** Socio-demographic, behavioral, nutritional and pubertal β-coefficients from MLRs[a] for the Overall Competence Z-score by gender. [a] MLRs, Multiple Linear Regressions. The $R^2$ for the complete model to predict OCS was 0.21 for boys and 0.22 for girls. * $p < 0.05$; ** $p < 0.01$; *** $p < 0.001$. **a** Boys. **b** Girls

SM (β = 2.15, $p < 0.05$), ED (β = 1.65, $p < 0.05$), and SAED total (β = 1.73, $p < 0.05$) Z-scores. Compared with 0–1 h/day, boys who watched TV ≥ 3 h/day during weekdays were positively associated with PF (β = 2.03, $p < 0.01$) and ED (β = 1.53, $p < 0.05$) Z-scores, but negatively associated with the SM (β = − 0.99, $p < 0.05$) Z-score. Boys who engaged in moderate or heavy physical activity (≥ 30 min/day) had lower PF Z-scores than did those who reported 0–30 min/day (β = − 0.75, $p < 0.05$). Among girls, there were significant inverse associations between SAED subscale (except IB and SM) and YHEI-TW Z-scores. Girls' households with 50,000–80,000 NTD/month income had lower IB, ED, and SAED total Z-scores (β values were − 0.69 ($p < 0.05$), − 0.97 ($p < 0.01$), and − 0.95 ($p < 0.01$), respectively) compared with those from the lowest household income group (0–30,000 NTD/month). Girls who had ever smoked had greater IL (β = 1.62, $p < 0.01$), IB (β = 1.96, $p < 0.01$), ED (β = 1.78, $p < 0.05$), and SAED total (β = 1.78, $p < 0.05$) Z-scores than those who never smoked. Unlike boys, there were significant negative associations between reading and IL, IB, SM, ED, and SAED total Z-scores among girls. In addition, girls who had entered menarche had higher PF (β = 1.2, $p < 0.01$) and SM (β = 0.34, $p < 0.05$) Z-scores than those who had not.

The $R^2$ for the complete model to predict SAED was 0.13 for boys and 0.21 for girls, explaining 13.4% and 20.6% of the variance respectively; without YHEI-TW in the model, $R^2$ was 0.13 and 0.15 (12.9% and 15.0% of the variance).

Dietary quality (YHEI-TW) is associated with overall competence at school (OCS) as shown in Figs. 1 and 4 (β =

**Table 3** Socio-demographic, behavioral, nutritional and pubertal β-coefficients from MLRs[a] with R-square for SAED sub-items[b] in boys

| Characteristics | SAED Z-score | | | | | | | |
|---|---|---|---|---|---|---|---|---|
| | IL | RP | IB | UD | PF | SM | ED | SAED total |
| YHEI-TW | −0.05** | − 0.02 | − 0.01 | − 0.01 | 0.0002 | − 0.02 | − 0.03 | − 0.03 |
| Mother's education (Ref: Low) | | | | | | | | |
| High (University and above) | − 0.36 | 0.45 | 0.25 | 0.01 | −0.08 | 0.25 | −0.002 | 0.01 |
| Household income (Ref: 0–30,000 NTD/month)[c] | | | | | | | | |
| 30,000–50,000 NTD/month | − 0.56 | − 0.40 | − 0.26 | 0.56 | 0.35 | 0.51 | − 0.21 | − 0.16 |
| 50,000–80,000 NTD/month | − 0.92 | − 0.78 | − 1.13 | − 0.30 | − 0.06 | − 0.28 | − 0.91 | − 0.89 |
| > 80,000 NTD/month | − 0.67 | − 0.37 | − 0.55 | − 0.15 | 0.36 | − 0.53 | − 0.47 | − 0.48 |
| Ever smoking (Ref: No) | | | | | | | | |
| Yes | 1.87* | 0.22 | 1.88** | 1.23 | 0.38 | 2.15* | 1.65* | 1.73* |
| Read during weekdays (Ref: 0–1 h/day) | | | | | | | | |
| 1–3 h/day | − 0.26 | −0.24 | − 0.59 | − 0.50 | − 0.12 | − 0.03 | −0.44 | − 0.42 |
| ≥ 3 h/day | − 0.22 | −0.45 | − 0.49 | −0.30 | 0.05 | 0.11 | −0.36 | −0.34 |
| Watch TV during weekdays (Ref: 0–1 h/day) | | | | | | | | |
| 1–3 h/day | 0.31 | 0.21 | −0.40 | 0.45 | 0.05 | −0.38 | 0.14 | 0.11 |
| ≥ 3 h/day | 1.19 | 0.50 | 1.02 | 1.61 | 2.03** | −0.99* | 1.53* | 1.40 |
| Play computer games during weekdays (Ref: 0–1 h/day) | | | | | | | | |
| 1–3 h/day | 0.46 | 0.26 | 0.72 | 0.66 | 0.49 | 0.55 | 0.65 | 0.66 |
| ≥ 3 h/day | 0.002 | 0.41 | 0.78 | 0.08 | −0.71 | −0.35 | 0.20 | 0.17 |
| Moderate or heavy physical activity (Ref: 0–30 min/day) | | | | | | | | |
| ≥ 30 min/day | 0.07 | 0.35 | −0.40 | 0.08 | −0.75* | −0.37 | − 0.14 | −0.16 |
| BMI (Ref: Normal weight) | | | | | | | | |
| Underweight | 0.08 | 0.10 | −0.19 | −0.22 | − 0.35 | 0.35 | − 0.11 | −0.08 |
| Overweight | −0.15 | 1.32 | 0.66 | 0.46 | 0.02 | 0.74 | 0.46 | 0.49 |
| Obesity | 0.88 | 0.50 | −0.22 | −0.06 | −0.15 | − 0.38 | 0.34 | 0.30 |
| Beard growth (Boys only) (Ref: Not yet) | | | | | | | | |
| At first | −0.39 | 0.004 | −0.09 | 0.07 | 0.04 | −0.03 | −0.16 | − 0.16 |
| In progress | −0.62 | − 0.74 | −0.63 | − 0.31 | −0.43 | − 0.34 | −0.70 | − 0.70 |
| Completed | −0.02 | − 0.50 | 0.55 | − 0.70 | −0.13 | − 0.16 | −0.09 | − 0.10 |
| $R^2$ with YHEI-TW | 0.175 | 0.049 | 0.124 | 0.097 | 0.083 | 0.123 | 0.133 | 0.134 |
| $R^2$ without YHEI-TW | 0.159 | 0.047 | 0.124 | 0.096 | 0.083 | 0.119 | 0.128 | 0.129 |

[a]MLRs, Multiple Linear Regressions
[b]The Scale for Assessing Emotional Disturbance (SAED) sub-items including Inability to learn (IL), Relationship problems (RP), Inappropriate behavior (IB), Unhappiness or depression (UD), Physical symptoms or fears (PF), Socially maladjusted (SM), and Emotional Disturbance (ED)
[c]1 US dollars = 30 NTD
* $p < 0.05$; ** $p < 0.01$; *** $p < 0.001$

0.05, $p < 0.01$ for boys; 0.07 with $p < 0.001$ for girls). It is also associated with ED in boys and girls. In particular, there is a significant inverse association between IL and YHEI-TW (β = − 0.05, $p < 0.01$) among boys (Table 3). Among girls, there are significant inverse associations between the SAED subscales (except IB and SM) and YHEI-TW Z-scores (β for IL = − 0.05 ($p < 0.001$), for RP β = − 0.05 ($p < 0.001$), for UD β = − 0.07 ($p < 0.001$), for PF β = − 0.06 (p < 0.01), for ED β = − 0.06 ($p < 0.001$), and for SAED β = − 0.06 ($p < 0.001$)) (Fig. 1 and Table 4).

Thus, dietary quality appears to be linked to OCS directly and also indirectly via ED. The possibility that it might have been linked indirectly through an association with obesity was not evident in the present study (regression Model for BMI on YHEI-TW, β = 0.004 for boys and − 0.002 for girls, $p > 0.05$ (data not shown)).

In turn, dietary quality may have many determinants of the food system and choice. In this study, we only report household income as a surrogate for socio-economic status. It was positively correlated

**Table 4** Socio-demographic, behavioral, nutritional and pubertal β-coefficients from MLRs[a] with R-square for SAED sub-items[b] in girls

| Characteristics | SAED Z-score | | | | | | | |
|---|---|---|---|---|---|---|---|---|
| | IL | RP | IB | UD | PF | SM | ED | SAED total |
| YHEI-TW | −0.05*** | −0.05*** | −0.03 | − 0.07*** | −0.06** | − 0.004 | −0.06*** | − 0.06*** |
| Mother's education (Ref: Low) | | | | | | | | |
| High (University and above) | −0.19 | 0.14 | 0.45 | 0.15 | 0.88 | 0.17 | 0.26 | 0.26 |
| Household income (Ref: 0–30,000 NTD/month)[c] | | | | | | | | |
| 30,000–50,000 NTD/month | 0.12 | −0.51 | −0.41 | −0.66 | − 0.91 | 0.06 | − 0.44 | −0.42 |
| 50,000–80,000 NTD/month | −0.59 | − 0.92 | −0.69* | − 0.91 | −1.09 | −0.33 | − 0.97** | −0.95** |
| > 80,000 NTD/month | 0.01 | 0.02 | −0.27 | −0.35 | − 0.59 | −0.17 | − 0.24 | −0.24 |
| Ever smoking (Ref: No) | | | | | | | | |
| Yes | 1.62** | 0.45 | 1.96** | 1.38 | 1.13 | 1.16 | 1.78* | 1.78* |
| Read during weekdays (Ref: 0–1 h/day) | | | | | | | | |
| 1–3 h/day | −0.32 | 0.36 | − 0.39 | 0.34 | − 0.12 | −0.07 | − 0.13 | −0.13 |
| ≥ 3 h/day | −1.35** | −0.44 | − 0.73* | −0.17 | − 0.20 | −0.38* | − 0.91* | −0.90* |
| Watch TV during weekdays (Ref: 0–1 h/day) | | | | | | | | |
| 1–3 h/day | 0.19 | −0.38 | 0.25 | −0.17 | − 0.40 | 0.16 | − 0.02 | −0.01 |
| ≥ 3 h/day | 0.33 | −0.08 | −0.20 | 0.01 | −0.56 | 0.04 | −0.03 | − 0.03 |
| Play computer games during weekdays (Ref: 0–1 h/day) | | | | | | | | |
| 1–3 h/day | 0.21 | 0.10 | 0.02 | 0.12 | 0.13 | −0.16 | 0.15 | 0.14 |
| ≥ 3 h/day | 0.96 | 1.19 | 1.66 | 0.92 | 0.81 | 0.10 | 1.40 | 1.35 |
| Moderate or heavy physical activity (Ref: 0–30 min/day) | | | | | | | | |
| ≥ 30 min/day | −0.49 | −0.54 | −0.84 | 0.18 | −0.49 | − 0.46 | −0.59 | − 0.60 |
| BMI (Ref: Normal weight) | | | | | | | | |
| Underweight | 0.61 | −0.31 | 0.24 | 0.61 | 0.32 | 0.33 | 0.43 | 0.44 |
| Overweight | 0.78 | 0.44 | 0.15 | 0.68 | −0.14 | 0.27 | 0.54 | 0.54 |
| Obesity | 0.38 | 1.21 | 0.43 | 0.62 | 0.34 | 0.01 | 0.67 | 0.65 |
| Menarche (Girls only) (Ref: No) | | | | | | | | |
| Yes | −0.23 | 0.50 | 0.63 | 0.85 | 1.20** | 0.34* | 0.55 | 0.55 |
| $R^2$ with YHEI-TW | 0.207 | 0.122 | 0.173 | 0.152 | 0.143 | 0.079 | 0.207 | 0.206 |
| $R^2$ without YHEI-TW | 0.167 | 0.094 | 0.160 | 0.092 | 0.091 | 0.078 | 0.150 | 0.150 |

[a]MLRs, Multiple Linear Regressions
[b]The Scale for Assessing Emotional Disturbance (SAED) sub-items including Inability to learn (IL), Relationship problems (RP), Inappropriate behavior (IB), Unhappiness or depression (UD), Physical symptoms or fears (PF), Socially maladjusted (SM), and Emotional Disturbance (ED)
[c]1 US dollars = 30 NTD
* $p < 0.05$; ** $p < 0.01$; *** $p < 0.001$

with YHEI-TW for boys and girls respectively (Fig. 1). Compared with those from lowest income group (0–30,000 NTD/month), students' household income over 80,000 NTD/month had higher YHEI-TW scores (β = 5.45 ($p < 0.001$) for boys, and 3.19 ($p < 0.05$) for girls) (data not shown).

## Discussion

Unsatisfactory food intake is associated with the link between emotional disturbance and impaired school performance, as assessed by OCS, especially among girls. For both genders, socio-economic and behavioral factors including parenteral income, reading, screen viewing, and smoking are modulators of this association. Puberty was a modifying factor in girls. Dietary quality is a relevant factor for health (ED) as well as educational (OCS) during early adolescence.

### Emotional disturbance and overall competence at school (OCS)

For the various measures of emotional disturbance reflected in SAED, there were consistently negative associations with OCS. These findings confirm several published studies [38–41]. Even so, a number of factors may be contributory to this relationship. The focus of the present investigation is how dietary quality might affect any such linkage. Linear regression for this association for boys and girls explains 44% and 42% of the variance, respectively (data not shown). There is a small contribution of dietary quality to OCS via ED evident in the β coefficients of the MLRs which are uniformly less when these models are adjusted for YHEI-TW However, dietary quality in boys and girls is directly associated with OCS in our analysis. This link remains independent of other covariates on MLRs. Thus OCS is dependent on ED, YHEI-TW and various independent covariates, namely, in boys, household income (favorably, screen viewing (unfavorably)) along with smoking (unfavorably) and, in girls, weekday reading (favorably) and body fatness (unfavorably along with smoking (unfavorably)).

#### Dietary quality and pattern

The present study has found that better dietary quality is associated with better overall competence at school and lower emotional disturbance. This supports reports, like that among Australian adolescents, that 'Western' dietary patterns characterized by energy-dense take-away 'fast' foods, plentiful red and processed meat, soft drinks, and other deep-fried and refined foods scores are associated with poorer academic performance (especially in mathematics and reading) [42]. For 14-year olds, this dietary pattern is associated with diminished cognitive performance 3 years later, at age 17 [43]. On the other hand, fruit and vegetable intake has a positive association with school performance among adolescents, as found in the Palestinian Gaza Strip [44]. Insofar as dairy foods are concerned, there may be differences within the category since OCS was less with flavored milk and greater with cheese; since all dairy products were treated together in the YHEI-TW, this may have accounted for non-significant associations on multiple linear regression for dairy. There is evidence that vitamin K-2 as found in cheese may play a role in brain function [45–47]. Of particular interest, regular breakfast, in its own right, is associated with better school performance, suggesting a role for diurnal dietary pattern in brain function [8, 17].

Previous studies in Taiwan show a dose-response for food diversity scores and health outcomes in adults, but comparable data are not available for children [48]. There is a gradient across the range, so that the upper quartile probably constitutes a desirable goal for food diversity at all ages. UN system data for dietary diversity and household food security support this position [49, 50].

The present study adds to a growing literature on the utility of YHEI-TW in children of dominantly Chinese ancestry and culture in the evaluation of diet in child development. These include studies of birth weight, food patterns and school performance [13] and of intergenerational dietary interplay in communities [34].

#### Parental characteristics

In this study, adolescents who had a better OC in school had parents with higher educational achievements. Children's school performance has previously been found to be strongly and positively associated with parental education [51].

Where household incomes were less, OCS was correspondingly less good. Similarly, in the US, youths with serious emotional disturbance have been observed to come from lower income families than for those youths without disturbance [52].

#### Personal behaviors

Smoking, reading, watching TV, playing computer games, and limited physical activity in the present study were associated with less OCS and with emotional disturbance. Likewise, smoking among adolescents has been associated with poor school performance and less study time [53]. Although causality is difficult to ascertain, clustering of riskier behaviors among adolescents is found with mood disturbance and includes smoking, substance use and self-harm or suicidal attempts [54].

#### Who are the students at risk-puberty and gender?

Although it is a difficult life stage to evaluate, because of its variable and changing time of onset, it is one of the most socio-biologically critical developmental periods. It is known that school environments in Taiwan, including their food systems and recreational settings, are associated with pubertal development, although differentially in girls and boys [11]. In the present study, the peri-pubertal period is evidently one of emotional and educational vulnerability, notably in girls, judged by both the indices of learning and mood examined. After the menarche, PF and SM were increased. However, dietary quality is a mitigating factor and food intake an addressable behavior.

#### What are the factors of greatest concern for adolescents in development and schooling?

Of the potential independent risk factors for emotional disturbance or school performance (OCS or sub-scales), diet (YHEI-TW), socio-economic advantage (household income) and reading were favorable, while screen viewing, smoking, puberty and greater BMI were unfavorable. These findings closely correspond to a Korean study of health behaviors and academic performance in adolescents, especially for diet and smoking, except that it found physical activity to be significant [26]. In the present study, for girls, we found BMI to be independently associated with OCS, which may have captured physical activity information.

In an Australian study of children and adolescents 4–17 years of age, internet usage and electronic gaming was found to be a mental health risk [55]. There are likely to be different internet usage patterns in a dominantly

Chinese as opposed to multicultural, but mainly European, Australian society with different cultural restraints and expectations of young adolescents. The gender difference in Taiwan of internet associations would also suggest this in the present study. It is an area in which more detailed analysis is required.

### Strengths and weaknesses

The adolescent population studied was representative of that in Taiwan, albeit dominantly Han Chinese with ancient and recent origins in mainland China. Indigenes were also studied and no differences in findings were apparent; this may represent a sampling limitation as previously observed, even though over-sampling of minorities, with SUDAAN adjustment for representativeness, has been undertaken in the present study [56]. Further cross-cultural extrapolation may be unwarranted, especially to other food cultures and educational systems. Other studies suggest limited generalizability to North-East Asian settings in general, but not dominantly European settings as in Australia, as discussed above. The cross-sectionality of the study begs the question of the medium to long-term health and performance outcomes of diet, along with other significant associated factors. As always with observational studies, residual confounding may be a problem in interpretation.

### Implications for health and nutrition policy and practice

Population-wide and representative evidence is provided in this study for children of dominantly Chinese ancestry and culture that dietary quality, along with parental input and personal behaviors is associated with emotional status and school performance. Intervention studies in support of these findings would add confidence to policy and practice which sought to enhance school performance by diet. In the meantime, household, school and community encouragement for healthier dietary patterns should be a low risk-high benefit option.

## Conclusions

The most supportable link of dietary quality to OCS is apparently direct rather than through ED to which it is also related in the present study. While ED is associated with OCS, and the intake of foods of limited nutritional value is seen with ED, the linkage of ED to OCS is minimally dependent on dietary quality. For both genders, socio-economic, parental education, reading or screen viewing, and smoking were associated with ED and OCS These factors may modulate the association between ED and OCS. Thus, the ways by which diet may affect OCS as a basis of school performance are likely to be complex.

#### Abbreviation

ED: Emotional disturbance; IB: Inappropriate behavior; IL: Inability to learn; NAHSIT: Nutrition and health survey in Taiwan; OC: Overall competence; OCS: Overall competence at school; PF: Physical symptoms or fears; RP: Relationship problems; SAED: Scale for assessing emotional disturbance; SM: Social maladjustment; UD: Unhappiness or depression; YHEI-TW: Youth healthy eating index – Taiwan

#### Acknowledgements

Prof Wen-Harn Pan is the coordinator of the Nutrition and Health Surveys in Taiwan (NAHSIT) on which the project was based.

#### Funding

The present study was funded internally by the National Health Research Institutes in Taiwan (PH-106-PP-18).

#### Authors' contributions

PHC and MLW designed the study. LYH performed the analyses. MSL provided assistance with interpretation. MLW and LYH wrote the paper. All authors critically read and approved the manuscript. The data were available to all authors.

#### Competing interests

The authors declare that they have no competing interests.

#### Author details

[1]Division of Preventive Medicine and Health Services Research, Institute of Population Health Sciences, National Health Research Institutes, 35 Keyan Road, Zhunan Town, Miaoli County 350, Taiwan, Republic of China. [2]School of Public Health, National Defense Medical Center, No.161, Sec. 6, Minchuan East Road, Taipei 114, Taiwan, Republic of China. [3]Monash Asia Institute, Monash University, 5th Floor, H Building, 900 Dandenong Road, Caulfield East, Melbourne, VIC 3145, Australia. [4]College of Public Health, China Medical University, Taichung, Taiwan, Republic of China.

#### References

1. WHO. HEALTH FOR THE WORLD'S ADOLESCENTS: A second chance in the second decade. 2014. http://apps.who.int/adolescent/second-decade/section4/page1/Mental-health-issues.html. Accessed 12 May 2017.
2. McGorry PD, Goldstone S. Is this normal? Assessing mental health in young people. Aust Fam Physician. 2011;40:94–7.
3. Rickwood DJ, Deane FP, Wilson CJ. When and how do young people seek professional help for mental health problems? Med J Aust. 2007;187(7 Suppl):S35–9.
4. Serbin LA, Stack DM, Kingdon D. Academic success across the transition from primary to secondary schooling among lower-income adolescents: understanding the effects of family resources and gender. J Youth Adolesc. 2013;42:1331–47.
5. Wiley AL, Siperstein GN, Forness SR, Brigham FJ. School context and the problem behavior and social skills of students with emotional disturbance. J Child Fam Stud. 2010;19:451–61.
6. Wagner MM. Outcomes for youths with serious emotional disturbance in secondary school and early adulthood. Futur Child. 1995;5:90–112.
7. Epstein MH, Cullinan D, Harniss M, Ryser G. The scale for assessing emotional disturbance: test-retest and Interrater reliability. Behav Disord. 1999;24:222–30.

8. Ho CY, Huang YC, Lo YT, Wahlqvist ML, Lee MS. Breakfast is associated with the metabolic syndrome and school performance among Taiwanese children. Res Dev Disabil. 2015;43-44:179–88.
9. Fu ML, Cheng L, Tu SH, Pan WH. Association between unhealthful eating patterns and unfavorable overall school performance in children. J Am Diet Assoc. 2007;107:1935–43.
10. Lane KL, Carter EW, Pierson MR, Glaeser BC. Academic, social, and behavioral characteristics of high school students with emotional disturbances or learning disabilities. J Emot Behav Disord. 2006;14:108–17.
11. Chiang PH, Huang LY, Lee MS, Tsou HC, Wahlqvist ML. Fitness and food environments around junior high schools in Taiwan and their association with body composition: gender differences for recreational, reading, food and beverage exposures. PLoS One. 2017;12:e0182517.
12. Chiang PH, Wahlqvist ML, Lee MS, Huang LY, Chen HH, Huang ST. Fast-food outlets and walkability in school neighbourhoods predict fatness in boys and height in girls: a Taiwanese population study. Public Health Nutr. 2011;14: 1601–9.
13. Lee MS, Huang LY, Chang YH, Huang ST, Yu HL, Wahlqvist ML. Lower birth weight and diet in Taiwanese girls more than boys predicts learning impediments. Res Dev Disabil. 2012;33:2203–12.
14. Chiang PH, Huang LY, Lo YT, Lee MS, Wahlqvist ML. Bidirectionality and gender differences in emotional disturbance associations with obesity among Taiwanese schoolchildren. Res Dev Disabil. 2013;34:3504–16.
15. Kim SY, Sim S, Park B, Kong IG, Kim JH, Choi HG. Dietary habits are associated with school performance in adolescents. Medicine. 2016;95:e3096.
16. Leventakou V, Roumeliotaki T, Sarri K, Koutra K, Kampouri M, Kyriklaki A, et al. Dietary patterns in early childhood and child cognitive and psychomotor development: the Rhea mother-child cohort study in Crete. Br J Nutr. 2016; 115:1431–7.
17. Adolphus K, Lawton CL, Dye L. The effects of breakfast on behavior and academic performance in children and adolescents. Front Hum Neurosci. 2013;7:425.
18. Burrows T, Goldman S, Pursey K, Lim R. Is there an association between dietary intake and academic achievement: a systematic review. J Hum Nutr Diet. 2017;30:117–40.
19. Hardman RJ, Kennedy G, Macpherson H, Scholey AB, Pipingas A. Adherence to a Mediterranean-style diet and effects on cognition in adults: a qualitative evaluation and systematic review of longitudinal and prospective trials. Front Nutr. 2016;3:22.
20. Santomauro F, Lorini C, Tanini T, Indiani L, Lastrucci V, Comodo N, Bonaccorsi G. Adherence to Mediterranean diet in a sample of Tuscan adolescents. Nutrition. 2014;30:1379–83.
21. Esposito K, Chiodini P, Maiorino MI, Bellastella G, Panagiotakos D, Giugliano D. Which diet for prevention of type 2 diabetes? A meta analysis of prospective studies. Endocrine. 2014;47:107–16.
22. Lee AM, Gurka MJ, DeBoer MD. Trends in metabolic syndrome severity and lifestyle factors among adolescents. Pediatrics. 2016;137:e20153177.
23. Isasi CR, Ostrovsky NW, Wills TA. The association of emotion regulation with lifestyle behaviors in inner-city adolescents. Eat Behav. 2013;14:518–21.
24. Burrows T, Goldman S, Olson RK, Byrne B, Coventry WL. Associations between selected dietary behaviours and academic achievement: a study of Australian school aged children. Appetite. 2017;116:372–80.
25. Farooq MS, Chaudhry AH, Shafiq M, Berhanu G. Factors affecting students' quality of academic performance: a case of secondary school level. JQTM. 2011;7:1–14.
26. So ES, Park BM. Health behaviors and academic performance among Korean adolescents. Asian Nurs Res (Korean Soc Nurs Sci). 2016;10:123–7.
27. Undheim AM, Lydersen S, Kayed NS. Do school teachers and primary contacts in residential youth care institutions recognize mental health problems in adolescents? Child Adolesc Psychiatry Ment Health. 2016;10:19.
28. Nutrition and Health Survey in Taiwan 2010. Health promotion administration. Taiwan: Ministry of Health and Welfare; 2016. https://obesity.hpa.gov.tw/TC/researchList.aspx?cid=164. Accessed 12 May 2017
29. Cheng LY. Scale for assessing emotional disturbance: Examiner's manual (Chinese edition). Taipei: Psychological Publishing Co.; 2001.
30. Epstein MH, Cullinan D. Scale for assessing emotional disturbance: Examiner's manual. Austin: Texas: PRO-ED, Inc; 1998.
31. Epstein MH, Cullinan D, Ryser G, Pearson N. Development of a scale to assess emotional disturbance. Behav Disord. 2002;28:5–22.
32. Feskanich D, Rockett HR, Colditz GA. Modifying the healthy eating index to assess diet quality in children and adolescents. J Am Diet Assoc. 2004;104:1375–83.
33. Yu XL. Overall dietary quality indices and nutritional knowledge, attitude, and status in the children of Taiwan. Taipei, Taiwan: National Defense Medical Center; 2007.
34. Wahlqvist ML, Huang LY, Lee MS, Chiang PH, Chang YH, Tsao AP. Dietary quality of elders and children is interdependent in Taiwanese communities: a NAHSIT mapping study. Ecol Food Nutr. 2014;53:81–97.
35. Ku PW, Fox KR, McKenna J, Peng TL. Prevalence of leisure-time physical activity in Taiwanese adults: results of four national surveys, 2000-2004. Prev Med. 2006;43:454–7.
36. Chu NF, Pan WH. Prevalence of obesity and its comorbidities among schoolchildren in Taiwan. Asia Pac J Clin Nutr. 2007;16(Suppl 2):601–7.
37. Shah BV, Barnwell BG, Bieler GS. SUDDAN. User's manual. In: Research Triangle Park, NC: Research Triangle Institute. 8th ed; 2001.
38. Mazzone L, Ducci F, Scoto MC, Passaniti E, D'Arrigo VG, Vitiello B. The role of anxiety symptoms in school performance in a community sample of children and adolescents. BMC Public Health. 2007;7:347.
39. Moksnes UK, Espnes GA, Haugan G. Stress, sense of coherence and emotional symptoms in adolescents. Psychol Health. 2013;29:32–49.
40. Vuontela V, Carlson S, Troberg AM, Fontell T, Simola P, Saarinen S, Aronen ET. Working memory, attention, inhibition, and their relation to adaptive functioning and behavioral/emotional symptoms in school-aged children. Child Psychiatry Hum Dev. 2013;44:105–22.
41. Wood JJ. Effect of anxiety reduction on children's school performance and social adjustment. Dev Psychol. 2006;42:345–9.
42. Nyaradi A, Li J, Hickling S, Foster JK, Jacques A, Ambrosini GL, Oddy WH. A western dietary pattern is associated with poor academic performance in Australian adolescents. Nutrients. 2015;7:2961–82.
43. Nyaradi A, Foster JK, Hickling S, Li J, Ambrosini GL, Jacques A, Oddy WH. Prospective associations between dietary patterns and cognitive performance during adolescence. J Child Psychol Psychiatry. 2014;55:1017–24.
44. Abudayya A, Shi Z, Abed Y, Holmboe-Ottesen G. Diet, nutritional status and school performance among adolescents in Gaza strip. East Mediterr Health J. 2011;17:218–25.
45. Ferland G. Vitamin K, an emerging nutrient in brain function. Biofactors. 2012;38:151–7.
46. Li J, Lin JC, Wang H, Peterson JW, Furie BC, Furie B, et al. Novel role of vitamin k in preventing oxidative injury to developing oligodendrocytes and neurons. J Neurosci. 2003;23:5816–26.
47. Walther B, Karl JP, Booth SL, Boyaval P. Menaquinones, bacteria, and the food supply: the relevance of dairy and fermented food products to vitamin K requirements. Adv Nutr. 2013;4:463–73.
48. Lee MS, Huang YC, Su HH, Lee MZ, Wahlqvist ML. A simple food quality index predicts mortality in elderly Taiwanese. J Nutr Health Aging. 2011;15:815–21.
49. Ruel MT. Operationalizing dietary diversity: a review of measurement issues and research priorities. J Nutr. 2003;133:3911S–26S.
50. Hoddinott J, Yohannes Y. Dietary diversity as a food security indicator. Food consumption and nutrition division discussion paper no. 136. Washington, D.C: IFPRI; 2002.
51. Ruijsbroek A, Wijga AH, Gehring U, Kerkhof M, Droomers M. School performance: a matter of health or socio-economic background? Findings from the PIAMA birth cohort study. PLoS One. 2015;10:e0134780.
52. Mark TL, Buck JA. Characteristics of U.S. youths with serious emotional disturbance: data from the National Health Interview Survey. Psychiatr Serv. 2006;57:1573–8.
53. Yorulmaz F, Akturk Z, Dagdeviren N, Dalkilic A. Smoking among adolescents: relation to school success, socioeconomic status nutrition and self-esteem. Swiss Med Wkly. 2002;132:449–54.
54. Pan PY, Yeh CB. Mood disturbance in adolescents screened by the mood disorder questionnaire predicts poorer social adjustment. J Adolesc Health. 2015;56:652–7.
55. Rikkers W, Lawrence D, Hafekost J, Zubrick SR. Internet use and electronic gaming by children and adolescents with emotional and behavioural problems in Australia - results from the second child and adolescent survey of mental health and wellbeing. BMC Public Health. 2016;16:399.
56. Chiang PH, Wahlqvist ML, Huang LY, Chang YC. Leisure time physical activities and dietary quality of the general and indigenous Taiwanese populations are associated with fat distribution and sarcopenia. Asia Pac J Clin Nutr. 2013;22:599–613.

# 17

# Vegetarian-style dietary pattern during adolescence has long-term positive impact on bone from adolescence to young adulthood

Elham Z. Movassagh[1], Adam D. G. Baxter-Jones[2], Saija Kontulainen[2], Susan Whiting[1], Michael Szafron[3] and Hassan Vatanparast[1,3*]

**Abstract**

**Background:** The amount of bone accrued during adolescence is an important determinant of later osteoporosis risk. Little is known about the influence of dietary patterns (DPs) on the bone during adolescence and their potential long-term implications into adulthood. We examined the role of adolescent DPs on adolescent and young adult bone and change in DPs from adolescence to young adulthood.

**Methods:** We recruited participants from the Saskatchewan Pediatric Bone Mineral Accrual Study (1991–2011). Data from 125 participants (53 females) for adolescent analysis (age 12.7 ± 2 years) and 115 participants (51 females) for adult analysis (age 28.2 ± 3 years) were included. Bone mineral content (BMC) and areal bone mineral density (aBMD) of total body (TB), femoral neck (FN) and lumbar spine (LS) were measured using dual-energy X-ray absorptiometry. Adolescent dietary intake data from multiple 24-h recalls were summarized into 25 food group intakes and were used in the principal component analysis to derive DPs during adolescence. Associations between adolescent DPs and adolescent or adult BMC/BMD were analyzed using multiple linear regression and multivariate analysis of covariance while adjusting for sex, age, the age of peak height velocity, height, weight, physical activity and total energy intake. Generalized estimating equations were used for tracking DPs.

**Results:** We derived five DPs including "Vegetarian-style", "Western-like", "High-fat, high-protein", "Mixed" and "Snack" DPs. The "Vegetarian-style" DP was a positive independent predictor of adolescent TBBMC, and adult TBBMC, TBaBMD ($P < 0.05$). Mean adolescent TBaBMD and young adult TBBMC, TBaBMD, FNBMC and FNaBMD were 5%, 8.5%, 6%, 10.6% and 9% higher, respectively, in third quartile of "Vegetarian-style" DP compared to first quartile ($P < 0.05$). We found a moderate tracking (0.47–0.63, $P < 0.001$) in DP scores at individual levels from adolescence to adulthood. There were an upward trend in adherence to "Vegetarian-style" DP and an downward trend in adherence to "High-fat, high-protein" DP from adolescence to young adulthood ($P < 0.01$).

**Conclusion:** A "Vegetarian-style" DP rich in dark green vegetables, eggs, non-refined grains, 100% fruit juice, legumes/nuts/seeds, added fats, fruits and low-fat milk during adolescence is positively associated with bone health.

**Keywords:** Dietary patterns, Vegetarian, Adolescence, Bone mineral content, Bone mineral density, Young adulthood

* Correspondence: vatan.h@usask.ca
[1]College of Pharmacy and Nutrition, University of Saskatchewan, 104 Clinic place, Saskatoon, SK S7N 2Z4, Canada
[3]School of Public Health, University of Saskatchewan, 104 Clinic place, Saskatoon, SK S7N 5E5, Canada
Full list of author information is available at the end of the article

## Background

Peak bone mass (PBM) attained by the end of adolescence is an early determinant of osteoporosis risk in older populations [1]. During adolescence, bone linear growth, and subsequent mineral deposition increase substantially [2]. The greatest rate of growth in height during this time is termed as peak height velocity (PHV). The PHV is considered as one of the main indicators of somatic maturation, the stage during which males and females are at a comparable sexual development milestone [3]. More than 39% of total body PBM is acquired during a 5-year period around PHV, and around 99% is attained by 6 years after attainment of PBM [4]. This suggests that modification of the factors that contribute to PBM attainment during adolescence might impact the risk of osteoporosis later in life [1].

Nutrition is an important modifiable factor, which could influence bone accrual, maintenance, and loss during one's lifetime [1, 5]. Diet is a complex combination of nutrients and dietary components that correlate or interact with each other. Even though the separate role of key nutrients, or foods, on bone health has been reported previously, these associations might be confounded by any change in the other dietary components. Dietary pattern (DP) approaches describe and quantify the whole diet and consider contributions from various dietary aspects [6]. Findings from DP studies could complement those from studies of single nutrients and foods on bone accrual and may be translated into public health recommendations, which better suit real world dietary habits.

In adults and elderly, several studies have investigated the association between DPs derived by an exploratory method, mainly factor analysis, and bone health [7–20]. However, little is known about the DPs influencing bone health during adolescence [21–24], and their potential long-term implications. Therefore, longitudinal studies that follow participants from adolescence to adulthood are of immense importance because they could bridge the current gap in knowledge.

The objectives of our study are: 1) to examine the association between adolescent DPs and adolescent and young adult bone measurements including total body (TB), femoral neck (FN) and lumbar spine (LS) bone mineral content (BMC) and areal bone mineral density (aBMD), and 2) to evaluate the stability of DPs from adolescence to young adulthood. We hypothesized that a "healthy" DP, with an emphasis on higher intake of fruits, vegetables would be beneficial for adolescence and young adulthood bone health; and DPs remain relatively stable over time from adolescence to young adulthood.

## Methods

### Participants

We recruited participants from the Saskatchewan Pediatric Bone Mineral Accrual Study (PBMAS) (1991–2011). The mixed longitudinal design of the study has been described in detail elsewhere [3, 4, 25]. In brief, the PBMAS cohort consists of 251 individuals (133 girls and 118 boys; aged 8 to 15 years) recruited from two elementary schools in the city of Saskatoon between 1991 and 1993 who were subsequently followed with annual follow-ups until 2011. There were two four-year breaks in annual measurements: one between 1997 and 2002 and one between 2005 and 2010. The ages of the participants at the final follow-up were between 24 to 32 years. At each measurement occasion, participants underwent dual-energy X-ray absorptiometry (DXA) scans for bone and body composition. Anthropometry, dietary intake, and physical activity were also assessed at each measurement point.

For the present study, the first measurement within the age of PHV ± 2 years was considered as the adolescent measurement. For most participants ($n = 105$), the data collected during 1992 or 1993 were included in the analysis as adolescent data. The data collected during 2010 or 2011 were included in the analysis as young adult data. We included data from 125 participants (age 12.7 ± 2 years, 53 females) for adolescent analysis (cross-sectional) and 115 participants (age 28.2 ± 3 years, 51 females) for adolescence to young adult analysis (longitudinal). All participants or their parents provided informed written consent. Ethics approval was obtained from the University of Saskatchewan and Royal Hospital advisory boards on ethics in human experimentation [25].

### Dietary intake

The dietary intakes of participants were assessed using 24-h recalls. To determine accurate estimates of portion sizes, participants had access to pictures of foods. Adolescent dietary intakes were assessed by two to four (mostly three) 24-h recalls collected over a year and were analyzed using the Canadian compatible nutrition assessment software: NUTS Nutritional Assessment System, version 3.7 (Quilchena Consulting Ltd., Victoria, BC, 1988) to estimate the daily total energy and nutrient intakes. The average dietary intakes per day during the study year were stratified with the other annual measurements during the same year. To include in DP analysis, first, we converted quantities of all consumed foods and beverages into grams per day; then, all items were assigned into 25 pre-defined non-overlapping food groups, manually, based on similar nutrient content or culinary usage of them (Table 1). Young adult dietary intakes were assessed using one 24-h recall and estimates of total energy and nutrient intakes were obtained using Food Processor version 8.0 and its revisions (ESHA Research Inc., Salem, Ore, 2003).

### Bone mineral content and areal density

Adolescent and young adult BMC and aBMD of TB, FN and LS (L1–L4) were measured using DXA (Hologic

**Table 1** Food groupings used for principal component analysis to identify dietary patterns during adolescence

| Food groups | Food items |
|---|---|
| Dark green vegetables | Asparagus, green beans, broccoli, lettuce, green pepper, seaweed, spinach, mixed greens, snow peas |
| Eggs | Eggs |
| Non-refined grains | Whole grains and partially whole grains (60%) mostly cereals, mixed granola/grain bar, cracker, oat flakes, wheat germ, whole wheat breads, puffed wheat, brown and wild rice, popcorn, barley |
| Fruit juice 100% | Apple cider, apple, lemon, lime, orange juice canned or bottled, unsweetened cranberry, etc. |
| Legumes, nuts and seeds | Beans (black, kidney, lima, navy, small white, soy), chickpeas, hummus, tofu, brazil nuts, coconut, almond, hazelnuts, walnuts, cashew, peanuts, mixed nuts, pecans, peanut butter, sunflower seeds |
| Added fats | Saturated fats such as butter, margarine, meatless bacon bits and coconut oil, and unsaturated fats such as vegetable oil, cooking oil, mayonnaise, olive oil, pesto |
| Fruits | All fresh and dried fruits, canned fruits (not sweetened), avocado, olives |
| Low-fat milk | 1%, skim, rice beverage, soy beverage |
| Fruit drinks | Fruit juice (sweetened), fruit drinks, iced tea |
| Refined grains | Refined cereals, white bread, white rice, refined pasta, noodles, pop corns, pie crust, pizza pop |
| Cream | Sour cream, cream (10%, whipped or low fat) |
| Poultry | Chicken and turkey |
| Processed meats | Burger patties (beef, ham, chicken, etc.), sausages, bacon, canned meat, dry ribs, fried chicken, nugget |
| High-fat milk | 2%, whole or almond milk |
| Tomato | Tomato and its products |
| Red meat | Beef, ham, pork, bison (ground, loin, rib, steak, stew, fried, pot roast, balls, loaf, chop) |
| Cheese | Cheddar, cream cheese, feta, gouda, mozzarella, parmesan, Swiss, cottage, ricotta, cheese sauce |
| Yogurt | Yogurt (plain, vanilla or fruit) |
| Desserts and sweets | Sweet baked products, milk desserts, jelly, chocolate, sugar, jam, syrups, honey and candies |
| Fish and seafood | Fish, shrimp, lobster, mussels, pickerel, prawns, scallops |
| Dressings, sauces, gravy | Gravy, dressings, Caesar, French, ranch, Italian, 1000 island, Alfredo, blue cheese, chip dip, Greek, honey garlic, white sauce, sandwich spread, tartar, teen, sundried tomato |
| Vegetables, others | Carrots, snap beans, cabbage, cauliflower, celery, cucumber, garlic, mushroom, pepper, squash, bean sprouts, beets, onion, eggplant, radish, zucchini, potato, green peas, corn, sweet potato and soups |
| Chips & fries | Potato chips, fries, corn chips, nacho, hash brown |
| Soft drinks | Soft drinks (sugar-sweetened or diet) |
| Others | Salt, spices, seasonings, additives, pickles (dill, beet), low fat sauces (mustard, hot, soy, teriyaki), vinegar |

QDR 2000, Hologic, Inc., Waltham, MA, USA) in the array mode; and analysis was conducted using enhanced global software version 7.1 [26]. To minimize operator-related variability in the scan analysis over the years, the same trained person analyzed all scans. The TB scans were analyzed using software version 5.67A and scans of the FN and LS were analyzed using software version 4.66A. The in vivo coefficients of variations, which represent short-term precision, were comparable to the values from other studies employing the QDR 2000 in the array mode (0.60, 0.91 and 0.61 for TB, FN, and LS BMC, respectively).

#### Physical activity

Physical activity was defined as sports, games, or dance that makes you breathe hard, makes your legs feel tired, or makes you sweat. The physical activity questionnaire (PAQ) was used to assess adolescent physical activity during spare time in the previous 7 days by rating nine items in elementary schools or eight items in high schools (excluding the item regarding activity at recess) scored on a five-point scale [27]. Six of these questions were related to scaling the level of different activities in physical education classes, recess, lunch, right after school, in the evenings and on the weekend. Other three questions were asking about the frequency of physical activity during each day, the number of hours spent for watching TV, and describing the whole week activity from low to very high activity levels [28]. The average score derived from each PAQ ranged from one to five, with higher scores indicating higher levels of physical activity. To assess young adult physical activity, PAQ was modified to a 7-item questionnaire including more age-relevant activities. The school-day structure of questions was replaced with a day section structure (i.e., morning, after lunch, before supper, evening) in the PAQ for adults [28]. The PAQ was administered three times a year during first 3 years of study and two times a year thereafter. The average PA scores derived from PAQs collected during each year were aligned with the other annual measurements [26].

### Anthropometry and age of PHV

Weight and stature were measured following standard protocols for each participant while wearing lightweight clothing and no shoes [25]. To control for somatic maturity, the age of PHV for each participant was estimated. The process for determining PHV has been described elsewhere [26]. In brief, whole-year height increase velocity was computed using serial measurements of height for each participant by age. Using a cubic spline procedure, a growth curve was fitted to each individual's annual height velocities (GraphPad Prism Version 3.00) and the age of PHV was determined from the estimated growth curve [26].

### Statistical analysis

The DPs were identified using factor analysis via principal component analysis (PCA). The PCA aggregates the food groups into a smaller number of the distinct factors based on inter-correlation between them [6, 29]. To achieve a simpler structure with higher interpretability, orthogonal rotation (Varimax option) was applied. Overall, 11 factors were extracted using PCA with an eigenvalue > 1 accounting for 66% of the total variance in all food group intakes. Based on the breakpoint in scree plot, we retained 5 major factors (accounting for almost 40% of the total variance) for further evaluation and reran the analysis with a five-factor solution. Factor loadings represent the correlation between food groups and the factors (Table 2). The absolute value represents the strength of the correlation. A positive loading shows a direct association and a negative loading shows an inverse association between the food group intake and DP score. Food groups with a factor loading ≥0.35 or ≤ −0.35 were considered informative for interpretation of DPs in our study. Regression scores for each DP were calculated using the regression scores option in SPSS. Calculating regression scores enhances the validity of DP scores and reduces the probability of biased estimates of the true scores [30].

Descriptive statistics for all bone variables (TBBMC, TBaBMD, FNBMC, FNaBMD, LSBMC, LSaBMD), and covariate variables (age, the age of PHV, height, weight, physical activity score and total energy intake) were presented as mean ± SD in adolescence and young adulthood. We used independent Student's t-test to compare variables of interest between females and males. Multiple linear regression using stepwise procedure were conducted to evaluate associations between adolescence DP and adolescence bone measurements. To assess the long-term impact of DPs on the bone, we also ran the same modeling with adolescent DP scores as predictor variables, and young adulthood bone measurements as outcome variables. All models were adjusted for sex, the age of PHV, age, height, weight, physical activity score and total energy intake. Covariates measured during adolescence and young

**Table 2** Factor loading of food groups in five dietary patterns identified by principal component analysis during adolescence, in participants of Pediatric Bone Mineral Accrual Study (PBMAS), $n$ = 125[1]

| | Factor Loadings for Dietary Patterns | | | | |
|---|---|---|---|---|---|
| | Vegetarian-Style | Western-Like | High-Fat, High-Protein | Mixed | Snack |
| Dark green vegetables | **0.64** | 0.02 | − 0.00 | 0.07 | − 0.22 |
| Eggs | **0.63** | − 0.18 | 0.23 | − 0.05 | − 0.15 |
| Non-refined grains | **0.54** | − 0.13 | − 0.11 | 0.10 | 0.20 |
| Added fats | **0.41** | **0.39** | − 0.03 | − 0.04 | − 0.00 |
| Fruits | **0.40** | 0.24 | − 0.16 | 0.13 | 0.23 |
| Others | − 0.28 | 0.03 | 0.08 | 0.08 | 0.04 |
| Fruit drinks | 0.00 | **0.73** | − 0.04 | − 0.03 | 0.04 |
| Refined grains | 0.06 | **0.66** | 0.21 | − 0.10 | − 0.03 |
| Cream | − 0.06 | **0.55** | − 0.01 | 0.13 | − 0.02 |
| Poultry | − 0.27 | **0.41** | − 0.04 | − 0.10 | **0.40** |
| Processed meats | − 0.05 | **0.35** | − 0.12 | 0.01 | − 0.09 |
| High-fat milk | − 0.12 | − 0.17 | **0.74** | − 0.04 | 0.18 |
| Tomato | 0.22 | 0.30 | **0.59** | − 0.14 | − 0.34 |
| Red meat | − 0.07 | − 0.05 | **0.52** | 0.14 | − 0.07 |
| Low fat milk | 0.35 | 0.03 | **− 0.48** | − 0.01 | − 0.16 |
| Legumes, nuts, and seeds | **0.45** | 0.11 | **0.47** | − 0.09 | 0.06 |
| Cheese | 0.03 | 0.12 | 0.06 | **0.72** | **− 0.36** |
| Yogurt | − 0.11 | 0.04 | − 0.12 | **0.61** | 0.19 |
| Desserts and sweets | − 0.18 | − 0.05 | 0.23 | **0.59** | 0.08 |
| Fish and seafood | 0.24 | − 0.10 | −0.08 | **0.52** | − 0.13 |
| Fruit juice 100% | **0.46** | 0.02 | − 0.04 | **0.49** | 0.18 |
| Dressings, sauces, gravy | 0.09 | − 0.30 | 0.24 | 0.08 | **0.64** |
| Vegetables, others | − 0.03 | 0.22 | 0.06 | − 0.03 | **0.58** |
| Chips & fries | − 0.03 | − 0.09 | − 0.02 | 0.00 | **0.40** |
| Soft drinks | 0.00 | − 0.02 | − 0.16 | − 0.20 | 0.20 |
| % Of variance explained | 9.2 | 8.5 | 7.8 | 7.7 | 6.7 |

[1]Factor loadings ≥0.35 or ≤ − 0.35 have been presented

The bold numbers represent the foods with significant positive or negative loading in each pattern

adulthood were used in the adolescence and young adulthood models, respectively.

Comparisons of the mean adolescence or young adult bone variables across the quartile categories of adolescent DP score were conducted via a multivariate analysis of covariance (MANCOVA) (with a Bonferroni adjustment for multiple comparisons) while adjusting for scores of the other four DPs (as continuous variables), sex, age of PHV, age, height, weight, physical activity score and total energy intake.

To evaluate the stability of DPs from adolescence to young adulthood, we calculated applied DP scores during adolescence and young adulthood, based on the factor loadings for 25 food groups in five DPs derived during adolescence. To control for the overall increase in consumption of food groups by age from adolescence to young adulthood, we computed the consumed amount (g) per 1000 kcal of total energy intake for each food group. Then, these energy-adjusted intakes were multiplied by their corresponding factor loading in each DP and were summed up as the DP score. We standardized adolescence and young adulthood DP scores for mean and standard deviation of adolescence DP scores in our sample. Then we calculated tracking coefficients using generalized estimating equations (GEE). Tracking coefficient represents how position of participants in a study population distribution is maintained from baseline to the last follow-up [31]. We regressed adolescence standardized DP scores (independent variable) against young adulthood standardized DP scores (dependent variable) while adjusting for chronological age as the time-dependent variable, and sex and age at adolescence as time-independent variables. The ß coefficient of adolescence standardized DP scores takes values between 0 to 1, representing no tracking and strong tracking, respectively. The ß coefficient for chronological age indicates the change in DP score as z-score or SD for each year increase in age.

The DP analysis and all other statistical analyses were performed using SPSS software, version 24.0 (SPSS, Chicago, lL, USA). $P < 0.05$ was considered significant.

**Table 3** Descriptive characteristics during adolescence and young adulthood by sex[1]

| | Females | Males | Total |
|---|---|---|---|
| Adolescence | *n* = 53 | *n* = 72 | n = 125 |
| Biologic age[2] (year) | 0.2 ± 1.7 | −0.1 ± 1.8 | 0.0 ± 1.7 |
| Age (year) | 12.0 ± 1.8 | 13.2 ± 1.8* | 12.7 ± 1.9 |
| Age of PHV (year) | 11.8 ± 0.8 | 13.2 ± 0.9 | 12.6 ± 1.2 |
| Physical activity (score) | 2.9 ± 0.7 | 3.0 ± 0.6 | 3.0 ± 0.7 |
| Total energy intake (kcal/d) | 1714 ± 461 | 1978 ± 615* | 1867 ± 569 |
| Height (cm) | 153 ± 11 | 162 ± 14** | 158 ± 13 |
| Weight (kg) | 46.0 ± 14 | 52.4 ± 14* | 49.8 ± 14 |
| TBBMC (g) | 1402 ± 452 | 1751 ± 612** | 1604 ± 575 |
| TBaBMD (g/cm²) | 0.87 ± 0.10 | 0.94 ± 0.12* | 0.91 ± 0.11 |
| FNBMC (g) | 3.3 ± 0.8 | 4.1 ± 1.0** | 3.8 ± 1.0 |
| FNaBMD (g/cm²) | 0.73 ± 0.13 | 0.81 ± 0.13* | 0.77 ± 0.13 |
| LSBMC (g) | 35.8 ± 13.4 | 40.8 ± 16.0 | 38.7 ± 15.1 |
| LAaBMD (g/cm²) | 0.76 ± 0.15 | 0.75 ± 0.14 | 0.76 ± 0.14 |
| Young adulthood | *n* = 51 | *n* = 64 | n = 115 |
| Biologic age[2] (year) | 16.1 ± 3.5 | 15.0 ± 3.3 | 15.5 ± 3.4 |
| Age (year) | 27.9 ± 3.4 | 28.3 ± 3.4 | 28.2 ± 3.4 |
| Physical activity (score) | 2.3 ± 0.6 | 2.3 ± 0.7 | 2.3 ± 0.6 |
| Total energy intake (kcal/d) | 1823 ± 698 | 2823 ± 1235** | 2401 ± 1151 |
| Height (cm) | 166 ± 7 | 179 ± 7** | 174 ± 9 |
| Weight (kg) | 70.7 ± 16 | 87.0 ± 14** | 80.3 ± 16 |
| TBBMC (g) | 2286 ± 321 | 3020 ± 413** | 2706 ± 523 |
| TBaBMD (g/cm²) | 1.12 ± 0.09 | 1.22 ± 0.10** | 1.18 ± 0.11 |
| FNBMC (g) | 4.3 ± 0.7 | 5.6 ± 0.8** | 5.0 ± 0.9 |
| FNaBMD (g/cm²) | 0.86 ± 0.10 | 0.95 ± 0.128** | 0.91 ± 0.12 |
| LSBMC (g) | 62.0 ± 12.6 | 76.2 ± 12.8** | 70.3 ± 14.5 |
| LSaBMD (g/cm²) | 1.04 ± 0.12 | 1.06 ± 0.12 | 1.05 ± 0.12 |

*Abbreviations*: *aBMD* areal bone mineral density, *BMC* bone mineral accrual, *FN* femoral neck, *LS* lumber spine, *PBMAS* the pediatric bone mineral accrual study, *PHV* the peak height velocity, *TB* total body

[1]Values are Mean ± SD. *P* values were obtained using independent samples Student's *t* test. *Different from females, $P < 0.01$. **Different from females, $P < 0.001$

[2]Biologic age is calculated as chronologic age minus the age of PHV

## Results

The characteristics of the study population during adolescence and young adulthood are shown in Table 3. Our estimated mean ± SD follow-up period from adolescence to young adulthood was 15.5 ± 3.4 years. The first factor, labeled as "Vegetarian-style" DP, was rich in dark green vegetables, eggs, non-refined grains, 100% fruit juice, legumes, nuts and seeds, added fats, fruits and low-fat milk (including non-dairy milk). The second factor, a "Western-like" DP was associated with higher intakes of fruit drinks, refined grains, cream, poultry and processed meats. The most significant characteristic of the third factor, "high fat, high protein" DP, was high positive loadings for High-fat milk, tomato, red meat and legumes, nuts and seeds and a negative loading for low-fat milk. The fourth factor, a "Mixed" DP, was characterized by a high intake of yogurt, cheese, desserts and sweets, fish and seafood and 100% fruit juice. Dressings and sauces, vegetables (excluding dark green vegetables), chips and fries and poultry had high positive loadings and cheese had a negative loading in the fifth factor, labeled a "Snack" DP (Table 2).

After controlling for covariates (sex, age of PHV and adolescent age, height, weight, physical activity score and total energy intake), multiple linear regression showed that the "Vegetarian-style" DP was a positive independent predictor of adolescent TBBMC (β =35.2, $P$ = 0.025; $R^2$ = 0.84) and young adult TBBMC (β = 55.8, $P$ = 0.021; $R^2$ = 0.78), TBaBMD (β = 0.016, $P$ = 0.041; $R^2$ = 0.67). No other adolescent DP was found to be an independent predictor for any of the adolescent or young adult bone variables.

Comparison of adolescent or young adult bone variables across adolescent DP score quartiles showed that, those in the third quartile of "Vegetarian-style" DP had 5.7%, 8.5%, 6%, 10.6% and 9% higher adolescent TBaBMD (Table 4), and young adult TBBMC, TBaBMD, FNBMC and FNaBMD (Table 5), respectively, compared to their peers in the lowest quartile, after adjusting for covariates and other four DP scores as continuous variables.

Tracking coefficients for standardized scores of five DPs and change in the score by age from adolescence to young adulthood are presented in Table 6. The greater tracking coefficients show the higher stability of DPs at the individual level. Since DP scores have been standardized for the baseline DP scores, ß coefficient for age variable represents the amount of change in z-score. Overall, energy-adjusted scores increased for "Vegetarian-style" and decreased for "High-fat, high-protein" DP, from adolescence to young adulthood (Table 6).

## Discussion

In our prospective study, we found that a "Vegetarian-style" DP rich in dark green vegetables, eggs, non-refined grains, 100% fruit juice, legumes, nuts and seeds, added fats, fruits and low-fat milk during adolescence was associated positively with adolescent TBBMC and TBaBMD. We also found that participants who had higher adherence to the "Vegetarian-style" DP during adolescence had higher TBBMC, TBaBMD, FNBMC and FNaBMD during young adulthood, average 15 years later. Tracking DP scores showed that participants moderately maintained their position in the study population distribution from adolescence to young adulthood, which means DPs were relatively stable over time. However, the overall adherence to "Vegetarian-style" DP increased from adolescence to young adulthood.

In the present study, the favorable effects of the "Vegetarian-style" DP were only observed in TB and FN bone measurements, but not in LS bone. This might be due to the different proportions of cortical and trabecular bone compartments in different skeletal sites. The trabecular bone is the predominant bone compartment in LS, while TB and FN mainly contain cortical bone [32, 33]. Trabecular bone is metabolically more active than cortical bone and might be influenced by everyday changes in hormone or environmental factors. Hence adaptations in bone might last longer in cortical compared to trabecular bone [34].

Our study is unique as it evaluated the long-term impact of adolescent DPs on young adult bone. To our knowledge, there are only four studies that evaluated the DPs during adolescence in association with bone health [21–24]. Even though three of these studies were similar to our study in their prospective design (follow-up period ranged from 22 months to 6 years) [21, 23, 24], identified DPs are not directly comparable, because of the differences in DP approaches, food groupings and dietary habits and other characteristics of the study population [3, 6]. However, our findings of a positive association between "Vegetarian-style" DP and bone measurements are in accordance with the results from two studies which used reduced-rank regression (RRR) to derive DPs. The RRR has the advantage of deriving DPs associated with bone variables such as BMD and BMC [21] or intermediate factors such as protein, calcium, and potassium [2], as response variables. In Korean girls (aged 9–11 years, $n$ = 198), the RRR-derived "fruits, nuts, milk beverages, eggs, and grains" DP was associated positively and "egg and rice" DP was associated negatively with BMC gain after 22 months [21]. Also, a higher intake of low-fat dairy, whole grains, and vegetables, as components of a DP rich in protein, calcium and potassium in Australian adolescents (aged 14 years, $n$ = 1024) was associated with higher BMD and BMC at age 20 years [24]. Overall, higher intakes of fruit and vegetables, milk and alternatives, nuts and grains were the common components in all DPs which determined to be beneficial for bone [2, 21]).

Our results are also in line with the findings from previous DP studies in adults and elderly populations suggesting that a high intake of fruit and vegetables, whole grains, poultry and fish, nuts and legumes and low-fat dairy products labeled as "healthy" DP is beneficial for bone health [7–10, 12–14, 16, 17]. Vegetables, fruits, and 100% fruit juices are rich in potassium, magnesium, vitamins C, K and folate and carotenoids [35]. Potassium and magnesium may contribute to acid-base balance [35] and calcium metabolism [36, 37] to prevent bone loss. Vitamin C, carotenoids, and other antioxidants may affect bone health through their antioxidant properties, which suppress osteoclast activity [38, 39]. Vitamin C also acts as a cofactor for osteoblast differentiation and collagen formation [38, 40]. Vitamin K also plays a role in bone matrix formation where mineralization happens [41]. Low-fat milk and its alternatives are the main contributors of calcium and magnesium in diet [42], which have a structural role in bone health [43]. Calcium from vegetable sources also has been shown to be positively effective in bone maintenance in older ages [44]. They are also a source of protein, vitamin D, vitamin B12, zinc and riboflavin [42]. An adequate protein intake is essential for bone matrix formation and maintenance. Eggs, legumes, nuts and seeds, as meat alternatives, are good

**Table 4** Adolescence bone variables across the quartile groups of each dietary patterns derived during adolescence[1]

| | Dietary pattern score quartiles[2] | | | | *P* value |
|---|---|---|---|---|---|
| | Quartile1 (n = 31) | Quartile2 (*n* = 31) | Quartile3 (n = 31) | Quartile4 (*n* = 32) | |
| Vegetarian-style | | | | | |
| TBBMC | 1555.34 ± 33.15 | 1579.43 ± 31.58 | 1649.63 ± 32.15 | 1634.61 ± 32.15 | 0.18 |
| TBaBMD | 0.88 ± 0.01[a] | 0.90 ± 0.01[a,b] | 0.93 ± 0.01[b] | 0.91 ± 0.01[a,b] | 0.025 |
| FNBMC | 3.64 ± 0.01 | 3.69 ± 0.01 | 3.86 ± 0.01 | 3.79 ± 0.01 | 0.31 |
| FNaBMD | 0.75 ± 0.01 | 0.78 ± 0.01 | 0.80 ± 0.01 | 0.76 ± 0.01 | 0.22 |
| LSBMC | 37.08 ± 1.18 | 39.68 ± 1.18 | 39.03 ± 1.19 | 38.9 ± 1.19 | 0.52 |
| LSaBMD | 0.73 ± 0.01 | 0.77 ± 0.01 | 0.77 ± 0.01 | 0.75 ± 0.01 | 0.20 |
| Western-like | | | | | |
| TBBMC | 1612.62 ± 33.61 | 1623.64 ± 31.58 | 1594.61 ± 32.25 | 1588 ± 33.32 | 0.86 |
| TBaBMD | 0.91 ± 0.01 | 0.91 ± 0.01 | 0.91 ± 0.01 | 0.90 ± 0.01 | 0.74 |
| FNBMC | 3.78 ± 0.11 | 3.68 ± 0.11 | 3.8 ± 0.12 | 3.8 ± 0.12 | 0.92 |
| FNaBMD | 0.79 ± 0.01 | 0.76 ± 0.01 | 0.77 ± 0.01 | 0.78 ± 0.01 | 0.82 |
| LSBMC | 39.21 ± 1.22 | 39.52 ± 1.14 | 38.18 ± 1.21 | 37.79 ± 1.21 | 0.73 |
| LSaBMD | 0.76 ± 0.01 | 0.76 ± 0.01 | 0.76 ± 0.01 | 0.75 ± 0.01 | 0.93 |
| High-fat, high-protein | | | | | |
| TBBMC | 1630.53 ± 32.15 | 1597.64 ± 32.14 | 1586.65 ± 32.15 | 1603.71 ± 34.28 | 0.82 |
| TBaBMD | 0.91 ± 0.01 | 0.90 ± 0.01 | 0.90 ± 0.01 | 0.91 ± 0.01 | 0.92 |
| FNBMC | 3.79 ± 0.01 | 3.88 ± 0.01 | 3.67 ± 0.01 | 3.68 ± 0.01 | 0.40 |
| FNaBMD | 0.77 ± 0.01 | 0.79 ± 0.01 | 0.77 ± 0.01 | 0.77 ± 0.01 | 0.74 |
| LSBMC | 38.91 ± 1.19 | 38.91 ± 1.19 | 39.08 ± 1.28 | 37.79 ± 1.28 | 0.91 |
| LSaBMD | 0.74 ± 0.01 | 0.76 ± 0.01 | 0.77 ± 0.01 | 0.76 ± 0.01 | 0.77 |
| Mixed | | | | | |
| TBBMC | 1580.01 ± 32.38 | 1608 ± 30.28 | 1657 ± 30.73 | 1572 ± 32.75 | 0.22 |
| TBaBMD | 0.89 ± 0.01 | 0.91 ± 0.01 | 0.92 ± 0.01 | 0.90 ± 0.01 | 0.24 |
| FNBMC | 3.79 ± 0.01 | 3.68 ± 0.01 | 3.88 ± 0.01 | 3.69 ± 0.01 | 0.41 |
| FNaBMD | 0.77 ± 0.01 | 0.77 ± 0.01 | 0.80 ± 0.01 | 0.76 ± 0.01 | 0.50 |
| LSBMC | 38.68 ± 1.21 | 37.77 ± 1.10 | 40.86 ± 1.10 | 37.31 ± 1.21 | 0.16 |
| LSaBMD | 0.75 ± 0.01 | 0.75 ± 0.01 | 0.78 ± 0.01 | 0.75 ± 0.01 | 0.37 |
| Snack | | | | | |
| TBBMC | 1587.11 ± 30.77 | 1639.27 ± 30.22 | 1590.44 ± 31.17 | 1601.11 ± 32.54 | 0.59 |
| TBaBMD | 0.90 ± 0.01 | 0.92 ± 0.01 | 0.90 ± 0.01 | 0.91 ± 0.01 | 0.37 |
| FNBMC | 3.81 ± 0.09 | 3.85 ± 0.09 | 3.68 ± 0.09 | 3.88 ± 0.09 | 0.43 |
| FNaBMD | 0.79 ± 0.01 | 0.78 ± 0.01 | 0.75 ± 0.01 | 0.78 ± 0.01 | 0.31 |
| LSBMC | 38.09 ± 1.12 | 41.05 ± 1.12 | 37.31 ± 1.12 | 38.44 ± 1.22 | 0.12 |
| LSaBMD | 0.76 ± 0.01 | 0.79 ± 0.01 | 0.73 ± 0.01 | 0.75 ± 0.01 | 0.055 |

*Abbreviations*: *aBMD* areal bone mineral density, *BMC* bone mineral accrual, *FN* femoral neck, *LS* lumber spine, *TB* total body

[1]Values are Mean ± SE. Mean adolescence bone variables were adjusted for sex and adolescent age of peak height velocity, age, height, weight, physical activity score, total energy intake and other four dietary pattern scores as continuous variables and were compared across quartiles of adolescence dietary pattern scores using MANCOVA with Bonferroni adjustment for multiple comparisons. Labeled means in a row without a common superscript letter differ, $P < 0.05$

[2]Participants in Quartile four have the highest adherence to the DPs in adolescence

sources of protein [45]. Dietary fiber from non-refined grains and other plant sources might also have a beneficial impact on bone through decreasing glycemic load and inhibiting hyperinsulinemia which in turn prevents urinary calcium loss induced by insulin [46]. Added fats including, mainly, butter, margarine, and mayonnaise as one of components of the "Vegetarian-style" DP might play a role in providing adequate dietary energy for adolescents during their growth spurt, when they are consumed along with other components of "Vegetarian-style" DP. Lower intake

**Table 5** Young adulthood bone variables across the quartile groups of each dietary patterns derived during adolescence[1]

| | Dietary pattern score quartiles[2] | | | | *P* value |
|---|---|---|---|---|---|
| | Quartile1 (n = 29) | Quartile2 (*n* = 29) | Quartile3 (n = 29) | Quartile4 (*n* = 28) | |
| Vegetarian-style | | | | | |
| TBBMC | 2592.38 ± 46.12[a] | 2693.36 ± 46.12[a,b] | 2813.68 ± 47.22[b] | 2709.64 ± 49.25[a,b] | 0.016 |
| TBaBMD | 1.14 ± 0.01[a] | 1.18 ± 0.01[a,b] | 1.21 ± 0.01[b] | 1.18 ± 0.01[a,b] | 0.017 |
| FNBMC | 4.69 ± 0.12[a] | 5.02 ± 0.12[a,b] | 5.19 ± 0.12[b] | 5.08 ± 0.12[a,b] | 0.042 |
| FNaBMD | 0.87 ± 0.02[a] | 0.92 ± 0.02[a,b] | 0.95 ± 0.02[b] | 0.89 ± 0.02[a,b] | 0.020 |
| LSBMC | 66.27 ± 1.91 | 71.75 ± 1.91 | 72.17 ± 2.04 | 68.91 ± 2.04 | 0.14 |
| LSaBMD | 1.00 ± 0.02 | 1.06 ± 0.02 | 1.08 ± 0.02 | 1.04 ± 0.02 | 0.09 |
| Western-like | | | | | |
| TBBMC | 2742.45 ± 47.45 | 2688.48 ± 47.62 | 2745.88 ± 48.22 | 2629.84 ± 48.24 | 0.28 |
| TBaBMD | 1.18 ± 0.01 | 1.17 ± 0.01 | 1.20 ± 0.01 | 1.15 ± 0.01 | 0.24 |
| FNBMC | 5.04 ± 0.11 | 4.91 ± 0.11 | 5.15 ± 0.12 | 4.90 ± 0.12 | 0.39 |
| FNaBMD | 0.91 ± 0.02 | 0.90 ± 0.02 | 0.93 ± 0.02 | 0.90 ± 0.02 | 0.71 |
| LSBMC | 70.10 ± 2.01 | 71.31 ± 1.90 | 71.34 ± 2.02 | 66.12 ± 2.02 | 0.25 |
| LSaBMD | 1.05 ± 0.02 | 1.05 ± 0.02 | 1.07 ± 0.02 | 1.01 ± 0.02 | 0.35 |
| High-fat, high-protein | | | | | |
| TBBMC | 2715.42 ± 48.68 | 2692.14 ± 50.25 | 2684.42 ± 48.58 | 2712.85 ± 47.85 | 0.96 |
| TBaBMD | 1.18 ± 0.01 | 1.18 ± 0.01 | 1.17 ± 0.01 | 1.18 ± 0.01 | 0.98 |
| FNBMC | 5.02 ± 0.11 | 5.20 ± 0.11 | 4.74 ± 0.11 | 5.08 ± 0.12 | 0.07 |
| FNaBMD | 0.90 ± 0.02 | 0.93 ± 0.02 | 0.88 ± 0.02 | 0.92 ± 0.02 | 0.27 |
| LSBMC | 67.90 ± 2.01 | 72.40 ± 2.11 | 66.60 ± 2.01 | 70.0 ± 2.04 | 0.45 |
| LSaBMD | 1.02 ± 0.02 | 1.07 ± 0.02 | 1.04 ± 0.02 | 1.06 ± 0.02 | 0.41 |
| Mixed | | | | | |
| TBBMC | 2713.25 ± 48.32 | 2700.38 ± 48.32 | 2721.25 ± 48.32 | 2668 ± 49.12 | 0.88 |
| TBaBMD | 1.17 ± 0.01 | 1.19 ± 0.01 | 1.18 ± 0.01 | 1.17 ± 0.01 | 0.78 |
| FNBMC | 5.11 ± 0.12 | 5.11 ± 0.12 | 4.90 ± 0.12 | 4.88 ± 0.12 | 0.28 |
| FNaBMD | 0.91 ± 0.02 | 0.93 ± 0.02 | 0.89 ± 0.02 | 0.89 ± 0.02 | 0.46 |
| LSBMC | 68.67 ± 2.02 | 70.18 ± 2.02 | 72.52 ± 2.02 | 67.52 ± 2.02 | 0.36 |
| LSaBMD | 1.04 ± 0.02 | 1.06 ± 0.02 | 1.07 ± 0.02 | 1.02 ± 0.02 | 0.50 |
| Snack | | | | | |
| TBBMC | 2673.32 ± 45.45 | 2780.77 ± 47.32 | 2652 ± 46.87 | 2699 ± 47.35 | 0.24 |
| TBaBMD | 1.17 ± 0.01 | 1.20 ± 0.01 | 1.17 ± 0.01 | 1.17 ± 0.01 | 0.58 |
| FNBMC | 5.01 ± 0.12 | 5.01 ± 0.12 | 4.80 ± 0.13 | 5.07 ± 0.13 | 0.64 |
| FNaBMD | 0.92 ± 0.02 | 0.90 ± 0.02 | 0.88 ± 0.02 | 0.92 ± 0.02 | 0.41 |
| LSBMC | 68.22 ± 1.9 | 72.04 ± 2.02 | 68.11 ± 2.02 | 70.51 ± 2.02 | 0.45 |
| LSaBMD | 1.05 ± 0.02 | 1.07 ± 0.02 | 1.03 ± 0.02 | 1.04 ± 0.02 | 0.58 |

*Abbreviations*: *aBMD* areal bone mineral density, *BMC* bone mineral accrual, *FN* femoral neck, *LS* lumber spine, *TB* total body

[1]Values are Mean ± SE. Mean young adulthood bone variables were adjusted for sex and age of peak height velocity and young adult age, height, weight, physical activity score, total energy intake and other four adolescence dietary pattern scores as continuous variables and were compared across quartiles of adolescence dietary pattern scores using MANCOVA with Bonferroni adjustment for multiple comparisons. Labeled means in a row without a common superscript letter differ, $P < 0.05$

[2]Participants in Quartile 4 have the highest adherence to the DPs in adolescence

of meat seems to be beneficial, as this seems to be one of the key differences between "Vegetarian-style" DP and other four DPs. Taken together, the "Vegetarian-style" DP represents a combination of beneficial nutrients and dietary components with potential synergic or interacting effects. Therefore no single nutrient or dietary components could be pointed out as the one responsible for the beneficial impact of the DP on bone.

**Table 6** Tracking coefficients and change in score by age for dietary patterns derived during adolescence[1]

| | Tracking dietary patterns | | | Change in dietary pattern score | | |
|---|---|---|---|---|---|---|
| | ß (adolescence score) | 95% CI | *P* value | ß (age) | 95% CI | *P* value |
| Vegetarian-style | 0.59 | 0.48, 0.71 | < 0.001 | 0.026 | 0.00, 0.04 | 0.008 |
| Western-like | 0.47 | 0.40, 0.53 | < 0.001 | – 0.008 | – 0.029, 0.012 | 0.42 |
| High-fat, high-protein | 0.51 | 0.41, 0.60 | < 0.001 | – 0.019 | –0.034, – 0.005 | 0.009 |
| Mixed | 0.54 | 0.39, 0.69 | < 0.001 | –0.003 | –0.033, 0.028 | 0.85 |
| Snack | 0.63 | 0.55, 0.70 | < 0.001 | –0.003 | –0.023, 0.018 | 0.80 |

*Abbreviations*: *CI* confidence intervals

[1]Generalized estimating equations was used for modeling association between adolescence and adulthood standardized and energy-adjusted dietary pattern scores while controlling for sex, age, and age at adolescence; $n = 115$. Tracking coefficient (ß coefficient for adolescent dietary pattern) shows how participants maintained their position in the study population distribution, between adolescence and young adulthood. Tracking coefficient for age represents z score change in dietary pattern score from adolescence to young adulthood

Our study has several strengths. This is the first study that evaluated DPs during adolescence in association with young adult bone health. In our sample, all participants during young adulthood had their PBM confirmed by a plateau in bone mineral accrual curve, representing a steady status of bone [4]. We also controlled for somatic maturity by including the age of PHV as a covariate in our models. Adolescent dietary intake data were collected using multiple, mostly three, 24-h recalls over a year for each participant, which is preferred to food frequency questionnaires [47], the method used by most previous studies. In addition, we analyzed the impact of the whole diet, instead of a single food or nutrient, on bone.

The main limitation of our study was the small sample size ($n = 125$ for adolescent analysis, and $n = 115$ for young adult analysis), which did not allow us to run the separate analysis for females and males or run other DP approaches such reduced-rank regression method. Small sample size also limited us from adding more covariates in the model such as young adult DPs, smoking status, oral contraceptive use or reproductive history (in females). Even though we did not control the models for young adult DPs, we assessed change in DPs from adolescence to young adulthood to overcome this limitation. Two further limitations of our study are reliance on only one 24-h recall in young adulthood and using two different nutrient assessment systems from adolescence to young adulthood. However, our focus was food group intake and these two systems were only used to measure total energy intake.

## Conclusions

Our results suggest that a diverse and well-balanced DP, rich in dark green vegetables, eggs, non-refined grains, 100% fruit juice, legumes, nuts and seeds, added fats, fruits and low-fat milk during adolescence has a beneficial impact on bone health during adolescence and this positive impact on bone accrual can be carried into young adulthood. Further population-based studies are needed to confirm our findings and generalize these results to other populations.

#### Abbreviations

aBMD: areal bone mineral density; BMC: Bone mineral content; DP: dietary pattern; DXA: dual-energy X-ray absorptiometry; FN: femoral neck; LS: lumbar spine; MANCOVA: multivariate analysis of covariance; PAQ: physical activity questionnaire; PBM: peak bone mass; PBMAS: Pediatric Bone Mineral Accrual Study; PCA: principal component analysis; PHV: peak height velocity; TB: total body

#### Acknowledgments

Not applicable.

#### Funding

This study was supported by the Canadian Institutes of Health Research (grant number MOP 98002; MOP57671). Dairy Farmers of Canada provided funding for PhD student support (E.Z.M., grant number DFC- 417283).

#### Authors' contributions

All authors contributed to the conception and design of the study. HV, SJW, ABJ and SK contributed to the research conduction and data collection. EZM analyzed the data, interpreted the results and wrote the first draft of the manuscript under HV's guidance. All authors contributed to interpretation of results and reviewing and revising the manuscript. All authors read and approved the final version of the paper. None of the authors revealed any conflict of interest regarding present study.

#### Competing interests

The authors declare that they have no competing interests.

#### Author details

[1]College of Pharmacy and Nutrition, University of Saskatchewan, 104 Clinic place, Saskatoon, SK S7N 2Z4, Canada. [2]College of Kinesiology, University of Saskatchewan, 87 Campus Drive, Saskatoon, SK S7N5B2, Canada. [3]School of Public Health, University of Saskatchewan, 104 Clinic place, Saskatoon, SK S7N 5E5, Canada.

## References


1. Weaver CM, Gordon CM, Janz KF, Kalkwarf HJ, Lappe JM, Lewis R, et al. The National Osteoporosis Foundation's position statement on peak bone mass development and lifestyle factors: a systematic review and implementation recommendations. Osteoporos Int. 2016;27:1281–386.
2. Weaver CM. Adolescence: the period of dramatic bone growth. Endocrine. 2002;17:43–8.
3. Baxter-Jones AD, Mirwald RL, McKay HA, Bailey DA. A longitudinal analysis of sex differences in bone mineral accrual in healthy 8-19-year-old boys and girls. Ann Hum Biol. 2003;30:160–75.
4. Baxter-Jones AD, Faulkner RA, Forwood MR, Mirwald RL, Bailey DA. Bone mineral accrual from 8 to 30 years of age: an estimation of peak bone mass. J Bone Miner Res. 2011;26:1729–39.
5. Tucker KL. Osteoporosis prevention and nutrition. Curr Osteoporos Rep. 2009;7:111–7.
6. Kant AK. Dietary patterns and health outcomes. J Am Diet Assoc. 2004;104:615–35.
7. Tucker KL, Chen H, Hannan MT, Cupples LA, Wilson PW, Felson D, et al. Bone mineral density and dietary patterns in older adults: the Framingham osteoporosis study. Am J Clin Nutr. 2002;76:245–52.
8. Okubo H, Sasaki S, Horiguchi H, Oguma E, Miyamoto K, Hosoi Y, et al. Dietary patterns associated with bone mineral density in premenopausal Japanese farm women. Am J Clin Nutr. 2006;83:1185–92.
9. Kontogianni MD, Melistas L, Yannakoulia M, Malagaris I, Panagiotakos DB, Yiannakouris N. Association between dietary patterns and indices of bone mass in a sample of Mediterranean women. Nutrition. 2009;25:165–71.
10. Langsetmo L, Poliquin S, Hanley DA, Prior JC, Barr S, Anastassiades T, et al. Dietary patterns in Canadian men and women ages 25 and older: relationship to demographics, body mass index, and bone mineral density. BMC Musculoskelet Disord. 2010;11:20.
11. Fairweather-Tait SJ, Skinner J, Guile GR, Cassidy A, Spector TD, MacGregor AJ. Diet and bone mineral density study in postmenopausal women from the TwinsUK registry shows a negative association with a traditional English dietary pattern and a positive association with wine. Am J Clin Nutr. 2011; 94:1371–5.
12. McNaughton SA, Wattanapenpaiboon N, Wark JD, Nowson CA. An energy-dense, nutrient-poor dietary pattern is inversely associated with bone health in women. J Nutr. 2011;141:1516–23.
13. Hardcastle AC, Aucott L, Fraser WD, Reid DM, Macdonald HM. Dietary patterns, bone resorption and bone mineral density in early post-menopausal Scottish women. Eur J Clin Nutr. 2011;65:378–85.
14. Whittle CR, Woodside JV, Cardwell CR, McCourt HJ, Young IS, Murray LJ, et al. Dietary patterns and bone mineral status in young adults: the Northern Ireland young hearts project. Br J Nutr. 2012;108:1494–504.
15. Karamati M, Jessri M, Shariati-Bafghi SE, Rashidkhani B. Dietary patterns in relation to bone mineral density among menopausal Iranian women. Calcif Tissue Int. 2012;91:40–9.
16. Chen Y, Xiang J, Wang Z, Xiao Y, Zhang D, Chen X, et al. Associations of bone mineral density with lean mass, fat mass, and dietary patterns in postmenopausal Chinese women: a 2-year prospective study. PLoS One. 2015;10:e0137097.
17. Shin S, Sung J, Joung H. A fruit, milk and whole grain dietary pattern is positively associated with bone mineral density in Korean healthy adults. Eur J Clin Nutr. 2015;69:442–8.
18. de França NA, Camargo MB, Lazaretti-Castro M, Peters BS, Martini LA. Dietary patterns and bone mineral density in Brazilian postmenopausal women with osteoporosis: a cross-sectional study. Eur J Clin Nutr. 2016;70:85–90.
19. Mangano KM, Sahni S, Kiel DP, Tucker KL, Dufour AB, Hannan MT. Bone mineral density and protein-derived food clusters from the Framingham offspring study. J Acad Nutr Diet. 2015;115:1605–13. e1
20. Ward KA, Prentice A, Kuh DL, Adams JE, Ambrosini GL. Life course dietary patterns and bone health in later life in a British birth cohort study. J Bone Miner Res. 2016;31:1167–76.
21. Noh HY, Song YJ, Lee JE, Joung H, Park MK, Li SJ, et al. Dietary patterns are associated with physical growth among school girls aged 9-11 years. Nutr Res Pract. 2011;5:569–77.
22. Shin S, Hong K, Kang SW, Joung H. A milk and cereal dietary pattern is associated with a reduced likelihood of having a low bone mineral density of the lumbar spine in Korean adolescents. Nutr Res. 2013;33:59–66.
23. Monjardino T, Lucas R, Ramos E, Lopes C, Gaio R, Barros H. Associations between a posteriori defined dietary patterns and bone mineral density in adolescents. Eur J Nutr. 2015;54:273–82.
24. van den Hooven EH, Ambrosini GL, Huang RC, Mountain J, Straker L, Walsh JP, et al. Identification of a dietary pattern prospectively associated with bone mass in Australian young adults. Am J Clin Nutr. 2015;102:1035–43.
25. Bailey DA. The Saskatchewan pediatric bone mineral accrual study: bone mineral acquisition during the growing years. Int J Sports Med. 1997;18(3):191–4.
26. Bailey DA, McKay HA, Mirwald RL, Crocker PR, Faulkner RA. A six-year longitudinal study of the relationship of physical activity to bone mineral accrual in growing children: the university of Saskatchewan bone mineral accrual study. J Bone Miner Res. 1999;14:1672–9.
27. Kowalski K, Crocker P, Faulkner R. Validation of the physical activity questionnaire for older children. Ped Exerc Sport. 1997;9:174–86.
28. Copeland J, Kowalski KC, Donen RM, Tremblay MS. Convergent validity of the physical activity questionnaire for adults: the new member of the PAQ family. J Phys Act Health. 2005;2:216–29.
29. Newby PK, Tucker KL. Empirically derived eating patterns using factor or cluster analysis: a review. Nutr Rev. 2004;62:177–203.
30. DiStefano C, Zhu M, Mindrila D. Understanding and using factor scores: considerations for applied researcher. Practical assessment, research and evaluation. 2009;14:1–11
31. Twisk JWR. Applied longitudinal data analysis for epidemiology. A practical guide. 1st ed. Cambridge: Cambridge University Press; 2003.
32. Eastell R, Mosekilde L, Hodgson SF, Riggs BL. Proportion of human vertebral body bone that is cancellous. J Bone Miner Res. 1990;5:1237–41.
33. Kuiper JW, Van Kuijk C, Grashuis JL. Distribution of trabecular and cortical bone related to geometry: a quantitative computed tomography study of the femoral neck. Investig Radiol. 1997;32:83–9.
34. Dodds RA, Emery RJ, Klenerman L, Chayen J, Bitensky L. Comparative metabolic enzymatic activity in trabecular as against cortical osteoblasts. Bone. 1989;10:251–4.
35. New SA. Intake of fruit and vegetables: implications for bone health. Proc Nutr Soc. 2003;62:889–99.
36. Rafferty K, Heaney RP. Nutrient effects on the calcium economy: emphasizing the potassium controversy. J Nutr. 2008;138:166S–71S.
37. Allgrove J. Physiology of calcium, phosphate and magnesium. Endocr Dev. 2009;16:8–31.
38. Gabbay KH, Bohren KM, Morello R, Bertin T, Liu J, Vogel P. Ascorbate synthesis pathway: dual role of ascorbate in bone homeostasis. J Biol Chem. 2010;285:19510–20.
39. Shewcita SA, Khoshhal KI. Calcium metabolism and oxidative stress in bone fractures: role of antioxidants. Curr Drug Metab. 2007;8(5):519–25.
40. Finck H, Hart AR, Jennings A, Welch AA. Is there a role for vitamin C in preventing osteoporosis and fractures? A review of the potential underlying mechanisms and current epidemiological evidence. Nutr Res Rev. 2014;27:268–83.
41. Gundberg CM, Lian JB, Booth SL. Vitamin K-dependent carboxylation of osteocalcin: friend or foe? Adv Nutr. 2012;3:149–57.
42. Heaney RP. Dairy and bone health. J Am Coll Nutr. 2009;28(1):82–90.
43. Peters BS, Martini LA. Nutritional aspects of the prevention and treatment of osteoporosis. Arq Bras Endocrinol Metabol. 2010;54:179–85.
44. Park HM, Heo J, Park Y. Calcium from plant sources is beneficial to lowering the risk of osteoporosis in postmenopausal Korean women. Nutr Res. 2011;31:27–32.
45. Bonjour JP. Protein intake and bone health. Int J Vitam Nutr Res. 2011;81:134–42.
46. Rosen CJ. Sugar and bone: a not-so-sweet story. J Bone Miner Res. 2008;23:1881–3.
47. Bingham SA, Gill C, Welch A, Day K, Cassidy A, Khaw KT, Sneyd MJ, Key TJ, Roe L, Day NE. Comparison of dietary assessment methods in nutritional epidemiology: weighted records vs. 24-h recalls, food-frequency questionnaires and estimated-diet records. Br J Nutr. 1994;72:619–43.

# 18

# Relationship between dietary patterns and risk factors for cardiovascular disease in patients with type 2 diabetes mellitus

Yusuke Osonoi[1], Tomoya Mita[1,2*], Takeshi Osonoi[5], Miyoko Saito[5], Atsuko Tamasawa[5], Shiho Nakayama[1], Yuki Someya[1], Hidenori Ishida[5], Akio Kanazawa[1,3], Masahiko Gosho[6], Yoshio Fujitani[1] and Hirotaka Watada[1,2,3,4]

**Abstract**

**Background:** While some dietary patterns are associated with the incidence of type 2 diabetes mellitus (T2DM) and cardiovascular disease (CVD), the relationship between dietary pattern and risk factors for CVD in patients with T2DM remains to be clarified. The aim of this study was to identify dietary patterns and investigate the relationship between dietary patterns and potential risk factors for CVD in patients with T2DM.

**Methods:** The study participants comprised 726 Japanese T2DM outpatients free of history of CVD. Life styles were analyzed using self-reported questionnaires. The relationship between dietary patterns, identified by factor analysis, and potential risk factors for CVD was investigated by linear and logistic regression analyses.

**Results:** Six dietary patterns were identified by factor analysis. Especially, three dietary patterns were associated with risk factors for CVD. The "Seaweeds, Vegetables, Soy products and Mushrooms" pattern, characterized by high consumption of seaweeds, soy products and mushrooms, was associated with lower use of diabetes medication and healthier lifestyles. The "Noodle and Soup" pattern, characterized by high consumption of noodle and soup was associated with higher body mass index, alanine aminotransferase, aspartate aminotransferase, γ-glutamyl transpeptidase and triglyceride levels. The "Fruit, Dairy products and Sweets" pattern was associated with lower γ-glutamyl transpeptidase levels, blood pressure, albuminuria and brachial-ankle pulse wave velocity.

**Conclusions:** The findings suggested that dietary patterns correlated with risk factors for CVD in T2DM patients.

**Keywords:** Dietary pattern, Type 2 diabetes mellitus, Risk factors for cardiovascular disease, Self-reported questionnaires

## Background

The onset of type 2 diabetes mellitus (T2DM) is associated with numerous lifestyle problems. Indeed, multiple lifestyle modifications, in addition to pharmacological intervention for classical risk factors, can reduce both the incidence of T2DM [1] in non-T2DM population and the development of cardiovascular disease (CVD) in patients with T2DM [2, 3]. However, a recent clinical trial showed that life style intervention, with a special focus on reduced calorie intake and increased physical activity, did not affect the rate of CVD in obese patients with T2DM [4]. In this regard, it is possible that not only caloric intake, but rather dietary composition, may need to be modified to achieve appropriate metabolism and prevent or delay CVD in patients with T2DM.

Recent studies showed that specific foods such as fruit and vegetables [5], nutritional supplements, such as magnesium and calcium [6–8], and quality of carbohydrate intake, such as high fibers, low glycemic index and whole grain intake [8–10], were associated with lower risk of T2DM. However, in real life, people do not consume certain foods or single nutrients, but rather mixed food that contains various nutrients. In this regard, the

* Correspondence: tom-m@juntendo.ac.jp
[1]Department of Metabolism & Endocrinology, Juntendo University Graduate School of Medicine, 2-1-1 Hongo, Bunkyoku, Tokyo 113-8421, Japan
[2]Center for Molecular Diabetology, Juntendo University Graduate School of Medicine, Bunkyoku, Tokyo 113-8421, Japan

dietary pattern should be taken into consideration, because it reflects the complexity of dietary intake, where the food contents usually have interactive and synergistic effects and occasionally even antagonistic effects [11]. In fact, it was suggested that dietary patterns may be more predictive of disease risks compared to specific food- and nutrient-based approaches [11].

Recent studies demonstrated that healthy Asian dietary patterns characterized by high consumption of vegetables, fruits, seaweeds, bonefishes, potatoes and/or soy foods were inversely associated with incidence of T2DM [12–14], metabolic syndrome [15], atherosclerosis [16] and related CVD [17] in non-T2DM general population, while western dietary pattern was associated with high incidence of T2DM [10, 18, 19] and metabolic syndrome [20]. Although it was demonstrated that the consumption of fruits, vegetable foods and meat was higher in patients with T2DM than non-T2DM subjects [21], only a few studies demonstrated that Korean Healthy diet pattern characterized by whole grains, legumes, vegetables and fruits was inversely associated with lipid metabolism [22], and vegetable and fish pattern was associated with better renal function in patients with T2DM [23]. Thus, there seems to be some gaps in our understanding of the relationship between dietary patterns and risk factors for CVD, especially arterial stiffness, in patients with T2DM. The aim of this cross-sectional study was to assess the above relationship in Japanese patients with T2DM free of history of CVD

## Research design and methods

### Subjects

The subjects of this cohort study were recruited from the Diabetes Outpatient Clinic of Juntendo University (Tokyo, Japan), Naka Memorial Clinic (Naka, Japan), and Secomedic Hospital (Funabashi, Japan) as reported previously [24]. Briefly, the inclusion criteria were as follows: *1)* T2DM patients, *2)* ≥25 years of age and <70 years of age (regardless of gender), and *3)* signing consent form for participation in the study. The following exclusion criteria were also applied: *1)* type 1 or secondary diabetes, *2)* presence of severe infectious disease, before or after surgery, or severe trauma, *3)* history of myocardial infarction, angina pectoris, cerebral stroke, or cerebral infarction, *4)* chronic renal failure requiring hemodialysis, *5)* liver cirrhosis, *6)* moderate or severe heart failure (NYHA/New York Heart Association stage III or higher), *7)* active malignancy, *8)* pregnant, lactating, or possibly pregnant women, or those planning to become pregnant during the study period, *9)* patients judged as ineligible by the clinical investigators.

A total of 1,032 consecutive subjects were screened between June 2013 and January 2014. Among them, 906 patients who met the above eligibility criteria were invited to participate in the present study. After providing information on the purpose and procedures of the study, 736 patients with T2DM accepted the invitation and were enrolled in this study. The study was approved by the Institutional Review Board of Juntendo University Hospital and conducted in accordance with the principles described in the Declaration of Helsinki. All patients provided written informed consent prior to participation. The study was registered on the University Hospital Medical Information Network Clinical Trials Registry (UMIN000010932).

### Questionnaire survey

Questionnaire survey was conducted using valid and reliable self-administered questionnaires described previously [24]. Briefly, dietary habits during the preceding month were assessed with the validated, Brief, self-administered Diet History Questionnaire (BDHQ). The BDHQ is a 4-page structured questionnaire that asks about consumption and frequency of selected foods to estimate the dietary intake of 56 food and beverage items with specified serving size described in terms of consumption in general Japanese populations [25].

We also used the Morning Evening Questionnaire (MEQ) [26], which is a self-assessment questionnaire developed primarily for screening candidates for sleep-related experiments to evaluate morningness and eveningness in individuals. A high MEQ score represents morning type.

The Pittsburg Sleep Quality Index (PSQI) [27] is a self-administered questionnaire designed to evaluate sleep quality and consists of 18 items that in turn are comprised of 7 components, which include subjective sleep quality, sleep duration, sleep onset, habitual sleep efficiency, sleep disturbances, use of sleeping medications, and daytime dysfunction, with each weighted equally on a 0–3 scale, to be summed to yield the global PSQI score ranging from 0 to 21, where the higher the scores, the worse the sleep quality. The PSQI has a high test-retest reliability and a good validity [28].

The participating patients also completed the BDI (Beck Depression inventory)-II, which is a 21-item questionnaire that assesses hopelessness, irritability, cognition, guilt, fatigue, weight loss, and sexual interest, representing depression-related symptoms in adults and adolescents [29]. A high BDI-II score represents depressive state.

Physical activity level was assessed with the International Physical Activity Questionnaire (IPAQ) that comprises four simple questions on physical activity [30]. The IPAQ results are expressed as metabolic equivalent scores (METs-hour-week$^{-1}$).

Workers were defined as full-time employees or shift workers by a question in the questionnaire, as described previously [24]. The subjects were also divided into non-smokers, former smokers or current smokers, as described previously [24].

### Blood and urine tests

Blood samples were obtained at visits to the Outpatients Clinic after overnight fast. Liver and renal function tests, lipids, HbA1c (National Glycohemoglobin Standardization Program), and glucose were measured with standard techniques. UAE was measured by the latex agglutination assay using a spot urine sample. The estimated glomerular filtration rate (eGFR) was calculated by the formula: eGFR (ml/min per 1.73 $m^2$) =194× $Age^{-0.287}$× serum $creatinine^{-0.1094}$ (×0.739 for females), as described previously [24] .

### Measurement of baPWV

baPWV was measured using an automatic waveform analyzer (BP-203RPE; Colin Medical Technology, Komaki, Japan), as described previously [24, 31]. Briefly, recording was performed with the patients in the supine position after resting for five minutes. Occlusion and monitoring cuffs were placed snugly around both areas in the upper and lower extremities. The pressure waveforms were then recorded simultaneously from the brachial arteries by the oscillometric method. All scans were automatically conducted by well-trained investigators who were blinded to the clinical information. The validity and reproducibility of baPWV measurements have been confirmed to be considerably high [32].

### Statistical analysis

Results are presented as mean ± SD or median (interquartile range: 25 % to 75 %) for continuous variables or number (proportion) of patients for categorical variables. Some parameters were logarithmically transformed to approximate normal distribution. We used factor analysis with varimax rotation to reduce the complexity of dietary patterns of patients with T2DM based on the results of BDHQ. Factors with an eigenvalue >1.25 were retained [33]. Individual food items with a factor loading of > |0.4| are highlighted as composing that factor for simplicity. The factor scores for each dietary pattern and for each subject were calculated by summing each dietary pattern score weighted by their factor loadings. The estimated factor scores were categorized into quintiles. Trend association across the quintile was evaluated by linear regression analysis for continuous variables or logistic regression analysis for categorical variables. We developed three models to evaluate the trend adjusted for age and gender or adjusted for age, gender, and body mass index (BMI), MEQ, PSQI, BDI-II, current smoking and physical activity. The model for eGFR was adjusted for BMI, MEQ, PSQI, BDI-II, current smoking and physical activity. Statistical tests were two-sided with 5 % significant level. All analyses were performed using the SAS software version 9.3 (SAS Institute, Cary, NC).

## Results

Among 736 patients, 10 patients did not complete the questionnaires, and were thus excluded from analysis. The study participants comprised 726 Japanese patients with T2DM who were being treated on an outpatient basis. Table 1 lists the characteristics of the study subjects. The mean age was 57.8 ± 8.6 years, 62.9 % male and HbA1c was 7.0 ± 1.0 %.

Factor analysis with varimax rotation identified six life style patterns (Table 2). Factor 1, with high loading for seaweeds, vegetables, soy products and mushroom, was labeled the "Seaweeds, Vegetables, Soy products and Mushrooms" pattern. Factor 2, which was characterized by fish, potatoes, meat and fats and oils, was labeled "Fish and Meat" pattern. Factor 3 seemed to load consumption of noodle and soup and thus it was named "Noodle and Soup" pattern. Factor 4 seemed to be characterized by meat, fats

**Table 1** Patients characteristics ($n = 726$)

| Demographic data | |
|---|---|
| Age (years) | 57.8 ± 8.6 |
| Gender (male) | 456 (62.9) |
| Estimated duration of diabetes (years) | 9.9 ± 7.2 |
| Body mass index (kg/$m^2$) | 24.6 ± 4.1 |
| HbA1c (%) | 7.0 ± 1.0 |
| Fasting blood glucose (mg/dl) | 134 ± 31 |
| Systolic blood pressure (mmHg) | 127 ± 14 |
| Diastolic blood pressure (mmHg) | 77 ± 11 |
| Total cholesterol (mg/dL) | 185 ± 28 |
| High-density lipoprotein-cholesterol (mg/dL) | 59 ± 14 |
| Triglyceride (mg/dL) | 100 [70, 152] |
| Aspartate aminotransferase (U/L) | 21 [18, 27] |
| Alanine aminotransferase (U/L) | 22 [16, 33] |
| γ-glutamyl transpeptidase (U/L) | 25 [17, 39] |
| Uric Acid (mg/dl) | 5.5 ± 1.2 |
| Estimated glomerular filtration rate (ml/min/ 1.73 $m^2$) | 78 ± 18 |
| Urinary albumin excretion (mg/g creatinine) | 10 [6, 23] |
| brachial-ankle pulse wave velocity (cm/s) | 1543 ± 279 |
| Morningness-Eveningness Questionnaire | 57.4 ± 7.3 |
| Pittsburg Sleep Quality Index | 5.1 ± 3.0 |
| Beck Depression inventory -II | 9.9 ± 7.6 |
| Energy intake (kcal/day) | 1713 ± 582 |
| Physical activity (Mets/h/week) | 42.8 ± 70.5 |
| Sleep duration (hours) | 6.4 ± 1.2 |
| Current smoker (yes) | 174 (24.0) |
| Alcohol (g/day) | 12.3 ± 21.5 |
| Treatment modality (n/%) | |
| Diabetes medication (yes) | 620 (85.5) |
| Hypertension medication (yes) | 346 (47.7) |
| Hyperlipidemia medication (yes) | 442 (61.0) |

Data are mean ± SD or number (percentage) of patients

**Table 2** Food items and factor analysis with varimax rotation

| Components and item labels | Factor 1 | Factor 2 | Factor 3 | Factor 4 | Factor 5 | Factor 6 |
|---|---|---|---|---|---|---|
| Rice | −0.07 | 0.07 | 0.00 | 0.06 | −0.15 | **0.80** |
| Noodle | 0.07 | 0.14 | **0.96** | 0.04 | 0.02 | 0.05 |
| Breads | 0.07 | −0.07 | 0.24 | 0.36 | **0.42** | −0.15 |
| Miso soup | 0.18 | 0.02 | 0.08 | −0.06 | 0.09 | **0.81** |
| Dairy products | 0.27 | −0.07 | −0.01 | 0.17 | **0.45** | 0.06 |
| Meats | 0.03 | **0.52** | 0.06 | **0.52** | −0.09 | 0.02 |
| Processed meats | 0.12 | 0.02 | 0.01 | **0.66** | 0.16 | −0.03 |
| Fish and shellfish | 0.32 | **0.63** | 0.17 | 0.16 | −0.03 | 0.05 |
| Processed fish | 0.23 | **0.60** | 0.10 | 0.16 | 0.07 | 0.14 |
| Eggs | 0.20 | 0.32 | 0.01 | **0.41** | 0.03 | −0.01 |
| Soy products | **0.63** | 0.10 | 0.13 | 0.13 | 0.13 | 0.08 |
| Green & dark yellow vegetables | **0.74** | 0.07 | −0.11 | 0.29 | 0.06 | −0.07 |
| White vegetables | **0.73** | 0.25 | 0.11 | 0.13 | 0.00 | −0.07 |
| Pickled vegetables | **0.51** | 0.18 | −0.03 | −0.07 | 0.04 | 0.10 |
| Fruit and vegetable Juices | 0.04 | 0.16 | −0.01 | −0.01 | 0.02 | −0.09 |
| Fruit | 0.21 | 0.35 | −0.01 | −0.03 | **0.56** | −0.05 |
| Sugary foods | 0.15 | **0.51** | 0.00 | −0.05 | 0.20 | 0.21 |
| Mushrooms | **0.55** | **0.41** | 0.01 | 0.01 | 0.13 | −0.14 |
| Seaweeds | **0.70** | 0.06 | 0.07 | 0.05 | −0.02 | 0.10 |
| Potatoes | 0.18 | **0.62** | 0.01 | 0.03 | 0.21 | −0.07 |
| Sweets | −0.03 | 0.21 | 0.13 | 0.17 | **0.62** | 0.06 |
| Fats and oils | −0.07 | **0.49** | 0.22 | **0.64** | −0.08 | 0.02 |
| Alcohol | 0.01 | 0.02 | 0.20 | 0.17 | **−0.53** | 0.15 |
| Tea | 0.04 | 0.06 | 0.03 | 0.13 | 0.34 | 0.11 |
| Coffee | 0.09 | 0.02 | 0.04 | 0.14 | 0.14 | 0.01 |
| Soft drinks | −0.05 | −0.09 | 0.21 | 0.19 | 0.07 | 0.03 |
| Seasonings | 0.32 | 0.05 | −0.09 | **0.60** | 0.03 | 0.06 |
| Soup | 0.08 | 0.11 | **0.96** | 0.02 | 0.01 | 0.04 |
| Contribution | 19 % | 8 % | 6 % | 6 % | 5 % | 4 % |

Individual food items with a factor loading of >|0.4| are shown in bold

and oils, seasonings and eggs, and was named "Meat, Fats and Oils, Seasonings and Eggs" pattern. Factor 5 seemed to be characterized by sweet, fruit and dairy products and was labeled "Fruit, Dairy products and Sweets" pattern. Factor 6 seemed to be characterized by rice and miso soups, and was named "Rice and Miso soups" pattern. Overall, these six diet patterns could account for 48 % of the variance in food intake.

The characteristics across quintile of dietary pattern are shown in Tables 3, 4, 5 and 6. Table 3 shows the characteristics of the study subjects according to the quintiles of "Seaweeds, Vegetables, Soy products and Mushrooms" pattern scores in age and gender adjusted model. Subjects with a higher score for this pattern were older, more morning type, higher consumption of food, higher physical activity and less depressive status. While HbA1c levels were comparable between the lowest quintile and the highest quintile, the lower prevalence of diabetes medication was found in the highest quintile in age- and gender-adjusted model. Subjects with a higher score for this pattern had lower aspartate aminotransferase (AST), γ-glutamyl transpeptidase (γ-GTP) and UAE values although these findings disappeared in multivariable adjusted model. Subjects with a higher score for "Fish and Meat" pattern were likely to be more female and higher consumption of food intake (Table 3). On the other hand, there were no significant trend in risk factors for CVD among quintiles in both age and gender, and multivariable adjusted model (Table 5). Table 3 also shows the characteristics of the study subjects according to the quintiles of "Noodle and Soup" pattern scores. Subjects with a higher score for this pattern were likely

**Table 3** Characteristics according to quintile categories based on dietary patterns

| Variable | Seaweeds, vegetables, soy products and mushrooms | | | Fish and meat | | | Noodle and soups | | |
|---|---|---|---|---|---|---|---|---|---|
| | Quintile 1 | Quintile 5 | Model 1 | Quintile 1 | Quintile 5 | Model 1 | Quintile 1 | Quintile 5 | Model 1 |
| Age (years) | 53.9 ± 8.9 | 59.5 ± 8.2 | - | 58.3 ± 8.6 | 57.9 ± 8.9 | - | 59.1 ± 7.9 | 57.6 ± 8.7 | - |
| Gender (male) | 92 (63.4) | 83 (57.2) | - | 108 (74.5) | 86 (59.3) | - | 83 (44.4) | 133 (85.3) | - |
| Body mass index (kg/m$^2$) | 25.8 ± 4.0 | 24.1 ± 4.2 | −1.64 | 24.7 ± 3.8 | 24.8 ± 4.3 | 0.40 | 23.9 ± 3.9 | 25.1 ± 4.1 | 3.04** |
| Estimated duration of diabetes (years) | 9.5 ± 6.8 | 9.4 ± 6.4 | −1.44 | 9.9 ± 6.8 | 10.4 ± 6.9 | 1.00 | 9.7 ± 7.3 | 9.5 ± 7.0 | 0.00 |
| MEQ | 55.3 ± 8.0 | 58.7 ± 6.8 | 2.55*** | 57.6 ± 7.5 | 57.6 ± 7.4 | −0.11 | 57.9 ± 7.4 | 57.5 ± 7.1 | −1.21 |
| PSQI | 5.8 ± 3.8 | 4.8 ± 2.6 | −1.53 | 5.0 ± 3.1 | 5.5 ± 3.4 | 1.35 | 5.1 ± 3.4 | 5.1 ± 2.8 | 1.03 |
| BDI-II | 11.4 ± 7.5 | 9.1 ± 7.4 | −2.18* | 10.0 ± 7.5 | 10.8 ± 8.0 | 0.71 | 9.8 ± 8.1 | 9.6 ± 7.9 | 0.47 |
| Energy intake (kcal/day) | 1614 ± 655 | 2000 ± 546 | 6.43*** | 1621 ± 506 | 2154 ± 658 | 10.90*** | 1542 ± 502 | 2055 ± 665 | 7.55 |
| Current smoker (%) | 34 (23.4) | 27 (18.6) | −0.28 | 41 (28.3) | 27 (18.6) | −0.64 | 42 (22.5) | 46(29.5) | 0.14 |
| Physical activity (kcal/day) | 37.2 ± 65.0 | 51.7 ± 84.1 | 2.17* | 44.5 ± 65.1 | 46.2 ± 85.6 | 1.14 | 40.3 ± 67.9 | 51.8 ± 95.2 | 1.73 |
| Worker (yes) | 114 (78.6) | 92 (63.4) | −1.22 | 105 (72.4) | 105 (72.4) | 1.31 | 132(70.6) | 118 (75.6) | −0.84 |
| Sleep duration (hours) | 6.4 ± 1.4 | 6.5 ± 1.2 | −1.15 | 6.5 ± 1.3 | 6.4 ± 1.3 | −0.14 | 6.4 ± 1.3 | 6.4 ± 1.1 | −0.27 |
| Diabetes medication (yes) | 130 (89.7) | 114 (78.6) | −2.50* | 122 (84.1) | 120 (82.8) | −033 | 155 (82.9) | 132 (84.6) | −0.21 |
| Hypertension medication (yes) | 74 (51.0) | 62 (42.8) | −1.84 | 71 (49.0) | 78 (53.8) | 1.60 | 85 (45.5) | 74 (47.4) | −0.03 |
| Hyperlipidemia medication (yes) | 90 (62.1) | 87 (60.0) | −0.93 | 89 (61.4) | 86 (59.3) | −1.10 | 106 (56.7) | 86 (55.1) | 1.37 |

Data are mean ± SD, median [range: 25 % to 75 %] or number of subjects (percentage) before adjustment. *$P < 0.05$, **$P < 0.01$, ***$P < 0.001$
Model 1: Trend estimation for linear trends across quintiles is based on linear regression analysis for continuous variables or logistic regression analysis for categorical variables adjusted for age and gender. Standardized regression coefficients are shown. *BDI* beck depression inventory, *MEQ* morningness-eveningness questionnaire, *PSQI*: Pittsburg sleep quality index

**Table 4** Characteristics according to quintile categories in each dietary pattern

| Variable | Meat, fats and oils, seasonings and eggs | | | Fruit, dairy products and sweets | | | Rice and miso soups | | |
|---|---|---|---|---|---|---|---|---|---|
| | Quintile 1 | Quintile 5 | Model 1 | Quintile 1 | Quintile 5 | Model 1 | Quintile 1 | Quintile 5 | Model 1 |
| Age (years) | 60.6 ± 6.7 | 54.9 ± 8.9 | - | 56.6 ± 9.1 | 58.7 ± 8.2 | - | 57.5 ± 8.8 | 58.3 ± 8.6 | - |
| Gender (male) | 104 (55.3) | 132 (72.9) | - | 134 (82.7) | 109(55.9) | - | 106 (55.5) | 137 (76.5) | - |
| Body mass index (kg/m$^2$) | 24.3 ± 3.9 | 25.3 ± 4.5 | −0.11 | 24.4 ± 3.8 | 24.6 ± 4.2 | 1.20 | 25.2 ± 4.3 | 24.4 ± 3.8 | −1.80 |
| Estimated duration of diabetes (years) | 10.0 ± 7.4 | 9.5 ± 6.5 | 0.47 | 9.4 ± 7.0 | 10.2 ± 7.8 | 0.76 | 9.5 ± 6.7 | 10.2 ± 7.0 | 0.83 |
| MEQ | 58.9 ± 7.4 | 56.5 ± 7.4 | −2.14* | 58.6 ± 7.8 | 56.3 ± 7.2 | −3.36*** | 57.1 ± 7.9 | 56.9 ± 7.5 | −0.91 |
| PSQI | 4.5 ± 2.6 | 5.3 ± 3.1 | 2.00* | 5.1 ± 3.0 | 5.2 ± 3.1 | 0.02 | 5.2 ± 2.9 | 5.0 ± 2.4 | −0.06 |
| BDI-II | 9.6 ± 8.1 | 10.0 ± 6.8 | 0.65 | 9.7 ± 7.1 | 10.6 ± 8.6 | 1.24 | 10.3 ± 7.9 | 10.4 ± 8.5 | 0.98 |
| Energy intake (kcal/day) | 1440 ± 479 | 2118 ± 651 | 12.94*** | 1781 ± 618 | 1909 ± 626 | 4.14*** | 1418 ± 456 | 2047 ± 568 | 11.01*** |
| Current smoker (%) | 39 (20.7) | 50 (27.6) | −0.03 | 55 (34.0) | 32 (16.4) | −2.54* | 46 (24.1) | 42 (23.5) | −1.00 |
| Physical activity (kcal/day) | 39.3 ± 65.3 | 39.1 ± 73.5 | 0.13 | 46.4 ± 78.9 | 45.5 ± 80.7 | −0.45 | 41.3 ± 62.8 | 47.8 ± 84.4 | 1.08 |
| Worker (yes) | 128 (68.1) | 150(82.9) | 0.11 | 134 (82.7) | 128 (65.6) | −2.51* | 131 (68.6) | 138 (77.1) | 1.91 |
| Sleep duration (hours) | 6.7 ± 1.2 | 6.3 ± 1.2 | −1.88 | 6.5 ± 1.3 | 6.5 ± 1.1 | −0.02 | 6.5 ± 1.1 | 6.4 ± 1.2 | −0.55 |
| Diabetes medication (yes) | 164(87.2) | 151 (83.4) | −0.58 | 140 (86.4) | 164 (84.1) | −1.12 | 167 (87.4) | 153 (85.5) | −0.80 |
| Hypertension medication (yes) | 92 (48.9) | 82 (45.3) | −0.75 | 95 (58.6) | 82 (42.1) | −2.86** | 94 (49.2) | 95 (53.1) | 0.01 |
| Hyperlipidemia medication (yes) | 122(64.9) | 99 (54.7) | −0.35 | 78 (48.1) | 131 (67.2) | 2.86** | 118 (61.8) | 95 (53.1) | −1.14 |

Data are mean ± SD, median [range: 25 % to 75 %] or number of subjects (percentages) before adjustment. *$P < 0.05$, **$P < 0.01$, ***$P < 0.001$
Model 1: Trend estimation for linear trends across quintiles is based on linear regression analysis for continuous variables or logistic regression analysis for categorical variables adjusted for age and gender. Standardized regression coefficients are shown. See Table 3 for abbreviations

**Table 5** Cardio-renal-metabolic parameters according to quintile categories in each dietary pattern

| Variable | Seaweeds, vegetables, soy products and mushrooms | | | | Fish and mea | | | | Noodle and soup | | | |
|---|---|---|---|---|---|---|---|---|---|---|---|---|
| | Quintile 1 | Quintile 5 | Model 1 | Model 2 | Quintile 1 | Quintile 5 | Model 1 | Model 2 | Quintile 1 | Quintile 5 | Model 1 | Model 2 |
| AST (U/L) | 22 [19, 29] | 22 [17, 26] | −2.07* | −1.71 | 21 [18, 27] | 23 [19, 28] | 1.14 | 0.98 | 21 [17, 25] | 23 [18, 29] | 3.25** | 2.60* |
| ALT (U/L) | 24 [17, 41] | 22 [16, 33] | −1.52 | −0.80 | 23 [16, 34] | 25 [17, 34] | 0.94 | 0.69 | 19 [15, 30] | 26 [18, 39] | 4.17*** | 3.29* |
| γ-GTP (U/L) | 28 [18,48] | 22 [15, 36] | −2.46* | −1.95 | 25 [18, 44] | 25 [18, 38] | 0.13 | −0.01 | 22 [16, 30] | 30 [21, 50] | 3.62*** | 2.75** |
| Uric Acid (mg/dl) | 5.5 ± 1.2 | 5.4 ± 1.2 | 0.12 | 0.51 | 5.6 ± 1.2 | 5.4 ± 1.2 | 0.75 | 0.63 | 5.2 ± 1.2 | 5.8 ± 1.2 | 0.85 | 0.27 |
| eGFR (ml/min/ 1.73 m$^2$) | 31 ± 18 | 77 ± 16 | - | 0.17 | 77 ± 18 | 78 ± 17 | - | 0.08 | 78 ± 19 | 79 ± 17 | - | −0.39 |
| Total cholesterol (mg/dl) | 190 ± 27 | 186 ± 29 | −1.64 | −1.70 | 184 ± 30 | 187 ± 27 | 0.16 | 0.09 | 188 ± 30 | 185 ± 27 | 0.39 | 0.22 |
| HDL-C (mg/dl) | 59 ± 14 | 62 ± 14 | 1.08 | 0.60 | 58 ± 13 | 59 ± 14 | −0.03 | −0.07 | 62 ± 15 | 57 ± 13 | −1.39 | −0.59 |
| Triglycerides (mg/dl) | 101 [71,163] | 96 [64, 144] | −1.74 | −1.06 | 94 [66, 144] | 112 [67, 152] | 0.88 | 0.78 | 89 [64, 135] | 116 [78, 164] | 2.82** | 1.73 |
| Fasting blood glucose (mg/dl) | 137 ± 34 | 131 ± 27 | 0.01 | 0.49 | 133 ± 32 | 138 ± 35 | 1.01 | 0.81 | 132 ± 31 | 137 ± 30 | 0.72 | 0.43 |
| HbA1c | 7.1 ± 1.1 | 6.9 ± 1.1 | −0.48 | −0.04 | 6.9 ± 0.9 | 7.1 ± 1.1 | 1.02 | 0.95 | 6.9 ± 1.0 | 7.0 ± 1.0 | 1.66 | 1.21 |
| Systolic BP(mmHg) | 128 ± 13 | 127 ± 15 | 0.12 | 0.83 | 127 ± 14 | 126 ± 15 | 0.09 | −0.10 | 126 ± 15 | 128 ± 13 | 1.83 | 0.92 |
| Diastolic BP (mmHg) | 79 ± 10 | 75 ± 10 | −1.00 | −0.53 | 78 ± 13 | 76 ± 11 | −0.19 | −0.33 | 75 ± 14 | 78 ± 10 | 0.99 | 0.27 |
| UAE (mg/g creatinine) | 10 [6, 21] | 10 [5, 17] | −2.12* | −1.74 | 10 [6, 24] | 10 [7, 23] | −0.80 | −0.88 | 11 [6, 30] | 9 [6, 19] | −0.39 | −1.18 |
| baPWV (cm/s) | 1528 ± 294 | 1556 ± 262 | −1.62 | −1.53 | 1536 ± 258 | 1535 ± 248 | 0.79 | 0.72 | 1549 ± 288 | 1536 ± 262 | −0.91 | −0.94 |

Data are mean ± SD, median [range: 25 % to 75 %] or number of subjects (percentage) before adjustment. $^*P < 0.05$, $^{**}P < 0.01$, $^{***}P < 0.001$

Model 1: Trend estimation for linear trends across quintiles is based on linear regression analysis for continuous variables or logistic regression analysis for categorical variables adjusted for age and gender. Model 2: Trend estimation for linear trends across quintiles is based on linear regression analysis for continuous variables or logistic regression analysis for categorical variables adjusted for age, gender, BMI, morningness-eveningness questionnaire, Pittsburg Sleep Quality Index, Beck Depression inventory, current smoking, and physical activity. Standardized regression coefficients are shown. *ALT* alanine aminotransferase, *AST* aspartate aminotransferase, *baPWV* brachial-ankle pulse wave velocity, *BP* blood pressure, *eGFR* estimated glomerular filtration rate, *HDL-C* high-density lipoprotein-cholesterol, *UAE* urinary albumin excretion, *γ-GTP* γ-glutamyl transpeptidase

**Table 6** Cardio-renal-metabolic parameters according to quintile categories in each dietary pattern

| Variable | Meat, fats and oils, seasonings and eggs | | | | Fruit, dairy products and sweets | | | | Rice and miso soups | | | |
|---|---|---|---|---|---|---|---|---|---|---|---|---|
| | Quintile 1 | Quintile 5 | Model 1 | Model 2 | Quintile 1 | Quintile 5 | Model 1 | Model 2 | Quintile 1 | Quintile 5 | Model 1 | Model 2 |
| AST (U/L) | 22 [19, 27] | 21 [17, 26] | −1.14 | −1.15 | 22 [18, 28] | 21 [18, 27] | 0.49 | 0.09 | 21 [17, 27] | 22[18, 27] | 1.05 | 1.45 |
| ALT (U/L) | 21 [16, 31] | 24 [17, 35] | −0.40 | −0.49 | 22 [16, 33] | 23 [17, 34] | 2.58* | 2.10* | 22 [15, 35] | 24 [17, 34] | 0.92 | 1.48 |
| γ-GTP (U/L) | 25 [16, 36] | 27 [17, 46] | −1.19 | −1.33 | 32 [20, 56] | 24 [17, 36] | −3.51*** | −4.20*** | 26 [17, 38] | 26 [19, 42] | 0.11 | 0.69 |
| Uric Acid (mg/dl) | 5.4 ± 1.2 | 5.5 ± 1.2 | −2.27* | −2.31* | 5.8 ± 1.3 | 5.3 ± 1.2 | −0.58 | −1.16 | 5.4 ± 1.3 | 5.6 ± 1.1 | 0.23 | 0.46 |
| eGFR (ml/min/ 1.73 $m^2$) | 75 ± 15 | 80 ± 19 | - | 1.24 | 78 ± 17 | 79 ± 19 | - | −0.56 | 79 ± 19 | 77 ± 17 | - | −0.87 |
| Total cholesterol (mg/dl) | 185 ± 26 | 188 ± 30 | 0.79 | 0.83 | 185 ± 27 | 185 ± 29 | −1.04 | −1.11 | 188 ± 29 | 183 ± 29 | −0.26 | −0.09 |
| HDL-C (mg/dl) | 59 ± 14 | 59 ± 16 | 1.25 | 1.35 | 61 ± 14 | 60 ± 14 | −2.87** | −2.65** | 59 ± 15 | 58 ± 13 | −0.50 | −1.05 |
| Triglycerides (mg/dl) | 98 [68,144] | 112 [72, 157] | −0.14 | −0.27 | 112 [70, 158] | 98 [71, 143] | −0.45 | −0.99 | 99 [71, 148] | 100 [70, 158] | −0.07 | 0.70 |
| Fasting blood glucose (mg/dl) | 130 ± 30 | 137 ± 33 | 0.93 | 0.64 | 136 ± 30 | 130 ± 31 | −1.22 | −1.74 | 135 ± 33 | 136 ± 31 | 0.28 | 0.21 |
| HbA1c | 6.8 ± 0.9 | 7.0 ± 1.0 | 1.55 | 1.25 | 6.8 ± 1.0 | 6.9 ± 0.9 | 0.56 | 0.12 | 7.0 ± 1.1 | 7.0 ± 0.9 | 0.65 | 0.79 |
| Systolic BP(mmHg) | 126 ± 15 | 127 ± 13 | 0.37 | 0.22 | 128 ± 13 | 125 ± 14 | −2.65** | −3.01** | 128 ± 15 | 127 ± 13 | −0.47 | 0.10 |
| Diastolic BP (mmHg) | 76 ± 10 | 79 ± 13 | −0.37 | −0.44 | 80 ± 11 | 76 ± 12 | −1.89 | −2.31* | 77 ± 11 | 78 ± 13 | 1.19 | 1.61 |
| UAE (mg/g creatinine) | 10 [6, 24] | 10 [5, 24] | −0.17 | −0.28 | 12[7, 36] | 9 [6, 18] | −3.20** | −3.44*** | 10 [6, 23] | 11 [6, 23] | −1.23 | −0.77 |
| baPWV (cm/s) | 1577 ± 282 | 1508 ± 265 | −0.07 | −0.33 | 1574 ± 314 | 1530 ± 259 | −3.04** | −3.14** | 1536 ± 256 | 1556 ± 277 | 0.18 | 0.15 |

Data are mean ± SD, median [range: 25 % to 75 %] or number of subjects (proportion) before adjustment. $^*P < 0.05$, $^{**}P < 0.01$, $^{***}P < 0.001$

Model 1: Trend estimation for linear trends across quintiles is based on linear regression analysis for continuous variables or logistic regression analysis for categorical variables adjusted for age and gender. Model 2: Trend estimation for linear trends across quintiles is based on linear regression analysis for continuous variables or logistic regression analysis for categorical variables adjusted for age, gender, BMI, morningness-eveningness questionnaire, Pittsburg Sleep Quality Index, Beck Depression inventory, current smoking, and physical activity. Standardized regression coefficients are shown. See Table 5 for abbreviations

to be males with higher BMI and consumption of food intake. Furthermore, patients with a higher score of this pattern had significantly higher AST, alanine aminotransferase (ALT) levels and γ-GTP compared to those with a lower score in both age- and gender-adjusted model, and multivariate adjusted model (Table 5). Furthermore, patients with a higher score of this pattern had significantly higher triglyceride levels compared to those with a lower score in the age- and gender-adjusted model.

Table 4 shows the characteristics of the study subjects according to the quintiles of "Meat, Fats and oils, Seasonings and Eggs" pattern scores in age- and gender-adjusted model. Subjects with a higher score for this pattern were younger males with lower score of MEQ, higher score of PSQI and higher consumption of food intake. On the other hand, there were no significant trend in risk factors for CVD except uric acid in both age- and gender-adjusted model and multivariable adjusted model (Table 6). Table 4 also displays the characteristics of the study subjects according to the quintiles of "Fruit, Dairy products and Sweets" pattern scores. This pattern was also characterized by lower consumption of alcohol. Subjects with a higher score for this pattern were more likely non-worker, non-smoker females with higher consumption of food intake, with lower score of MEQ. Lower use of hypertension medication and higher use of hyperlipidemia mediation were found in the highest quintile. Regarding risk factors for CVD, patients with higher a score of this pattern had lower γ-GTP level, HDL level, systolic BP, UAE and baPWV but slightly higher ALT level compared to those with a lower score in age- and gender-adjusted model, and multivariate adjusted model (Table 6). Table 4 shows the characteristics of the study subjects according to the quintiles of "Rice and Miso soups" pattern scores. Subjects with a higher score for this pattern were higher consumption of food while there was no significant trend in risk factors for CVD.

## Discussion

Among the six dietary patterns classified in this study, the "Seaweeds, Vegetables, Soy products and Mushrooms" pattern was associated with lower use of diabetes medications and healthier lifestyles. "Noodle and soup" pattern was associated with higher BMI, higher AST, ALT, γ-GTP and triglyceride levels. "Fruit, Dairy products and Sweets" pattern was associated with lower γ-GTP levels, BP, UAE and baPWV. On the other hand, the remaining three dietary patterns did not negatively affect risk factors for CVD.

Subjects with a higher score of "Seaweeds, Vegetables, Soy products and Mushrooms" pattern had healthier lifestyles, such as more morning type, less depressive symptoms and higher physical activity. Even after adjustment for those factors, the "Seaweeds, Vegetables, Soy products and Mushroom" pattern was associated with lower use of diabetes medication (data not shown), while there was no significant trend of HbA1c among their quintile categories. It is possible that the "Seaweeds, Vegetables, Soy products and Mushrooms" pattern positively affect glucose metabolism even in patients with T2DM, since a dietary pattern characterized by high consumption of vegetables, soy products and seaweed was reported to be inversely associated with lower incidence of T2DM [12–14] in the general population. Fiber [8], antioxidant vitamins [34], magnesium [6, 8] and phytoestrogens [35], which were abundant in those foods, have been reported to improve glucose metabolism and reduce insulin resistance. In addition, one previous study demonstrated that a healthy Japanese dietary pattern characterized by high consumption of vegetables, fruit, mushrooms and soy products was associated with fewer depressive symptoms in municipal employees [36]. Consistent with this finding, the almost similar type of "Seaweeds, Vegetables, Soy products and Mushrooms" pattern defined in this study was also associated with lower prevalence of depressive symptoms in patients with T2DM. Generally, vegetables and mushrooms contain vitamins and folate, which may reduce the prevalence of depression. In fact, it was demonstrated that antioxidant vitamins may protect neuropsychiatric disorders [37]. Similarly, folate intake was reported to be reduce depressive symptoms through metabolism of monoamines like serotonin and homocysteine in the brain [38]. Taken together, it seems that "Seaweeds, Vegetables, Soy products and Mushroom" dietary pattern is beneficial for patients with T2DM.

The "Fish and Meat" pattern was not associated with risk factors for CVD in this study. It was demonstrated that similar dietary pattern was also associated with the prevalence of the metabolic syndrome in Western populations [39] but not in Japanese workers [40]. These distinct results may be associated with relatively lower intake of meat and higher consumption of fish, vegetable and fruit in Japanese people compared to those in Western populations.

A higher score of "Noodle and Soup" pattern was associated with obesity characterized by high BMI, high AST, ALT, γ-GTP and triglyceride levels. Noodles including Japanese noodles, Chinese style noodles and pasta are one of the most favorite dishes in Japan. Higher intake of noodles, which contains high carbohydrate, may lead to obesity and fatty liver. Higher intake of oil included in the soup may be also associated with obesity and fatty liver.

We found that "Meat, Fats and Oils, Seasonings and Eggs" pattern represented by high intake of meat, fats and oils, seasonings and eggs was not related with risk factors for CVD, except high uric acid levels. On the other hand, a recent study reported that a similar dietary pattern, named high-fat pattern, was inversely associated with HbA1c levels in Japanese non-T2DM population [41]. The difference between our study and the above could be related to a number of differences among subjects, such as T2DM or non-T2DM, obesity, fat-derived energy intake and other dietary components. While frequent intake of meat, processed meat and eggs negatively affect lipid metabolism, "Meat, Fats and Oils, Seasonings and Eggs" pattern was not associated with lipid metabolism in this study. This may be related to the relatively higher intake of vegetables in addition to frequent intake of meat, processed meat and eggs. Indeed, it was reported that vegetable-rich diet seems to reduce cholesterol concentrations and other cardiovascular risk factors in patients with T2DM as effectively as in patients with non-T2DM [42].

The "Fruit, Dairy products and Sweets" pattern with less frequent consumption of alcohol and cigarette seemed to be preferred by females. Especially, this pattern was associated with lower BP, UAE and baPWV, even after adjustment for multivariate factors. These data may be reasonable because frequent dietary fruit intake was shown to be associated with lower BP and reduced atherosclerotic changes [43]. Also, previous studies demonstrated favorable preventive effects of dairy product on the incidence of hypertension, atherosclerosis and T2DM [44]. Antioxidant nutrients, such as vitamin C and E, carotene and dietary fiber are abundant in fruit. Similarly, dairy products contain calcium, magnesium, potassium, and vitamin D. These nutrients may have beneficial roles on risk factors for CVD in this pattern despite the co-presence of unhealthy diet pattern such as higher sweet consumption.

Recent studies showed that high consumption of rice contributed to the onset of T2DM in Chinese [9] and Japanese women, but not Japanese men [45]. While the mechanism by which frequent intake of rice increases the risk of T2DM remains largely unknown, the high glycemic index of white rice may affect glucose metabolism [46]. However, the "Rice and Soups" pattern was not associated with glycemic control in our patients with T2DM. Considering that subjects with high scores of this pattern showed higher consumption of fiber (data not shown), they may consume brown rice, which contains more dietary fiber, vitamin and minerals compared with white rice or fiber-rich foods with rice.

The present study has certain limitations. First, the cross-sectional design does not allow inference of a causal relationships between dietary patterns and risk factors for CVD. In addition, we could not confirm that the participating subjects adhered to the same dietary pattern throughout life. Especially, dietary patterns probably change depending on many factors such as status of glycemic control (good glycemic control vs. poor glycemic control) and estimated duration of T2DM (shorter duration vs. longer duration). This may cause reverse causality. Thus, it is not reasonable to conclude that our data could be generalized to a wider range of population, even in Japanese patients with T2DM. Second, we evaluated dietary pattern by self-reported questionnaires, though this method has been widely used in many studies. The results may be influenced by social desirability and recall bias. In addition, we evaluated only 56 food and beverage items. This could be associated with incomplete list of dietary patterns and an underestimation of energy intake. Finally, our results may be affected by several limiting features of factor analysis. It is not possible for investigators to avoid making judgmental decision at their discretion [47]. The results are dependent on the criterion to determine the number of factors to be retained and, the methods for rotation of factor axes and for labeling the dietary pattern. Therefore, our data should be interpreted with caution. For example, other remaining dietary patters or other remaining food items in each dietary pattern may be associated with risk factors for CVD.

## Conclusion

Our study showed the relationship between dietary patterns and risk factors for CVD in T2DM patients without history of CVD. Thus, dietary pattern could be a potentially important therapeutic target to achieve appropriate metabolic control and prevent the onset of future CVD in patients with T2DM.

#### Abbreviations

ALT: alanine aminotransferase; AST: aspartate aminotransferase; BaPWV: brachial-ankle pulse wave velocity; BDI: beck depression inventory; BDHQ: brief, self-administered diet history questionnaire; BMI: body mass index; BP: blood pressure; CVD: cardiovascular disease; eGFR: estimated glomerular filtration rate; γ-GTP: γ-glutamyl transpeptidase; HDL: high-density lipoprotein-cholesterol; IPAQ: International physical activity questionnaire; MEQ: morningness-eveningness questionnaire; PSQI: Pittsburg sleep quality index; T2DM: type 2 diabetes mellitus; UAE: urinary albumin excretion.

#### Competing interests

T.M. received research grand from Manpei Suzuki Diabetes Foundation. H.W. received lecture fees from Boehringer Ingelheim, Sanofi-Aventis, Ono Pharmaceutical Co., Novo Nordisk Pharma, Novartis Pharmaceuticals, Eli Lilly, Sanwakagaku Kenkyusho, Daiichi Sankyo Inc., Takeda Pharmaceutical Co., MSD, Dainippon Sumitomo Pharm., Kowa Co. and research funds from Boehringer Ingelheim, Pfizer, Mochida Pharmaceutical Co., Sanofi-Aventis, Novo Nordisk Pharma, Novartis Pharmaceuticals, Sanwakagaku Kenkyusho, Terumo Corp. Eli Lilly, Mitsubishi Tanabe Pharma, Daiichi Sankyo Inc., Takeda Pharmaceutical Co., MSD, Shionogi, Pharma, Dainippon Sumitomo Pharma, Kissei Pharma, and Astrazeneca.

#### Authors' contributions

All authors contribute to the study design and were involved at all stages of manuscript development. YO and TM mainly drafted the manuscript. MG, a statistician, contributed to analysis of research data. All authors were also involved in analysis and interpretation of data, reviewed/edited the manuscript and approved the final manuscript. HW is the principal guarantors of this work and has full access to all study data and takes responsibility for the integrity of the data and accuracy of data analysis. All authors have read and agreed to the publication of the manuscript.

The manuscript has not been submitted elsewhere. All authors read and approved the final manuscript.

**Acknowledgments**

This study was supported by research grand from Manpei Suzuki Diabetes Foundation (to T.M.). The authors thank the following staff who participated in this trial, including Mses Risa Yamamoto and Emi Ito (Department of Metabolism and Endocrinology, Juntendo University Graduate School of Medicine), Satako Douguchi, Chiyoko Sato, Yoko Ono, Norie Shiina, Nana Shiozawa, Mariko Kobori, Misato Ojima, Akiko Haginoya, and Kumiko Fujisaku, and Messrs Tadanori Koibuchi and Katuhiro Kawauchi (Naka Memorial Clinic) for the excellent technical support.

**Author details**

[1]Department of Metabolism & Endocrinology, Juntendo University Graduate School of Medicine, 2-1-1 Hongo, Bunkyoku, Tokyo 113-8421, Japan. [2]Center for Molecular Diabetology, Juntendo University Graduate School of Medicine, Bunkyoku, Tokyo 113-8421, Japan. [3]Center for Therapeutic Innovations in Diabetes, Juntendo University Graduate School of Medicine, Bunkyoku, Tokyo 113-8421, Japan. [4]Sportology Center, Juntendo University Graduate School of Medicine, Bunkyoku, Tokyo 113-8421, Japan. [5]Naka Memorial Clinic, 745-5, Nakadai, Naka, Ibaraki 311-0113, Japan. [6]Department of Clinical Trial and Clinical Epidemiology, Faculty of Medicine, University of Tsukuba, 1-1-1, Tennodai, Tsukuba, Ibaraki 305-8575, Japan.

**References**

1. Knowler WC, Barrett-Connor E, Fowler SE, Hamman RF, Lachin JM, Walker EA, et al. Reduction in the incidence of type 2 diabetes with lifestyle intervention or metformin. N Engl J Med. 2002;346(6):393–403. doi:10.1056/NEJMoa012512.
2. Sone H, Tanaka S, Iimuro S, Tanaka S, Oida K, Yamasaki Y, et al. Long-term lifestyle intervention lowers the incidence of stroke in Japanese patients with type 2 diabetes: a nationwide multicentre randomised controlled trial (the Japan Diabetes Complications Study). Diabetologia. 2010;53(3):419–28. doi:10.1007/s00125-009-1622-2.
3. Hu G, Jousilahti P, Barengo NC, Qiao Q, Lakka TA, Tuomilehto J. Physical activity, cardiovascular risk factors, and mortality among Finnish adults with diabetes. Diabetes Care. 2005;28(4):799–805.
4. Look ARG, Wing RR, Bolin P, Brancati FL, Bray GA, Clark JM, et al. Cardiovascular effects of intensive lifestyle intervention in type 2 diabetes. N Engl J Med. 2013;369(2):145–54. doi:10.1056/NEJMoa1212914.
5. Ford ES, Mokdad AH. Fruit and vegetable consumption and diabetes mellitus incidence among U.S. adults. Prev Med. 2001;32(1):33–9. doi:10.1006/pmed.2000.0772.
6. Song Y, Manson JE, Buring JE, Liu S. Dietary magnesium intake in relation to plasma insulin levels and risk of type 2 diabetes in women. Diabetes Care. 2004;27(1):59–65.
7. Fumeron F, Lamri A, Abi Khalil C, Jaziri R, Porchay-Balderelli I, Lantieri O, et al. Dairy consumption and the incidence of hyperglycemia and the metabolic syndrome: results from a french prospective study, data from the epidemiological study on the insulin resistance syndrome (DESIR). Diabetes Care. 2011;34(4):813–7. doi:10.2337/dc10-1772.
8. Schulze MB, Schulz M, Heidemann C, Schienkiewitz A, Hoffmann K, Boeing H. Fiber and magnesium intake and incidence of type 2 diabetes: a prospective study and meta-analysis. Arch Intern Med. 2007;167(9):956–65. doi:10.1001/archinte.167.9.956.
9. Villegas R, Liu S, Gao YT, Yang G, Li H, Zheng W, et al. Prospective study of dietary carbohydrates, glycemic index, glycemic load, and incidence of type 2 diabetes mellitus in middle-aged Chinese women. Arch Intern Med. 2007;167(21):2310–6. doi:10.1001/archinte.167.21.2310.
10. Liu S, Manson JE, Stampfer MJ, Hu FB, Giovannucci E, Colditz GA, et al. A prospective study of whole-grain intake and risk of type 2 diabetes mellitus in US women. Am J Public Health. 2000;90(9):1409–15.
11. Hu FB. Dietary pattern analysis: a new direction in nutritional epidemiology. Curr Opin Lipidol. 2002;13(1):3–9.
12. Montonen J, Knekt P, Harkanen T, Jarvinen R, Heliovaara M, Aromaa A, et al. Dietary patterns and the incidence of type 2 diabetes. Am J Epidemiol. 2005;161(3):219–27. doi:10.1093/aje/kwi039.
13. Odegaard AO, Koh WP, Butler LM, Duval S, Gross MD, Yu MC, et al. Dietary patterns and incident type 2 diabetes in chinese men and women: the singapore chinese health study. Diabetes Care. 2011;34(4):880–5. doi:10.2337/dc10-2350.
14. Morimoto A, Ohno Y, Tatsumi Y, Mizuno S, Watanabe S. Effects of healthy dietary pattern and other lifestyle factors on incidence of diabetes in a rural Japanese population. Asia Pac J Clin Nutr. 2012;21(4):601–8.
15. Cho YA, Kim J, Cho ER, Shin A. Dietary patterns and the prevalence of metabolic syndrome in Korean women. Nutrition, metabolism, and cardiovascular diseases: NMCD. 2011;21(11):893–900. doi:10.1016/j.numecd.2010.02.018.
16. Nettleton JA, Steffen LM, Schulze MB, Jenny NS, Barr RG, Bertoni AG, et al. Associations between markers of subclinical atherosclerosis and dietary patterns derived by principal components analysis and reduced rank regression in the Multi-Ethnic Study of Atherosclerosis (MESA). The American journal of clinical nutrition. 2007;85(6):1615–25.
17. Shimazu T, Kuriyama S, Hozawa A, Ohmori K, Sato Y, Nakaya N, et al. Dietary patterns and cardiovascular disease mortality in Japan: a prospective cohort study. Int J Epidemiol. 2007;36(3):600–9. doi:10.1093/ije/dym005.
18. van Dam RM, Rimm EB, Willett WC, Stampfer MJ, Hu FB. Dietary patterns and risk for type 2 diabetes mellitus in U.S. men. Ann Intern Med. 2002;136(3):201–9.
19. Fung TT, Schulze M, Manson JE, Willett WC, Hu FB. Dietary patterns, meat intake, and the risk of type 2 diabetes in women. Arch Intern Med. 2004;164(20):2235–40. doi:10.1001/archinte.164.20.2235.
20. Lutsey PL, Steffen LM, Stevens J. Dietary intake and the development of the metabolic syndrome: the atherosclerosis risk in communities study. Circulation. 2008;117(6):754–61. doi:10.1161/CIRCULATIONAHA.107.716159.
21. Murray AE, McMorrow AM, O'Connor E, Kiely C, Mac Ananey O, O'Shea D, et al. Dietary quality in a sample of adults with type 2 diabetes mellitus in Ireland; a cross-sectional case control study. Nutr J. 2013;12:110. doi:10.1186/1475-2891-12-110.
22. Lim JH, Lee YS, Chang HC, Moon MK, Song Y. Association between dietary patterns and blood lipid profiles in Korean adults with type 2 diabetes. J Korean Med Sci. 2011;26(9):1201–8. doi:10.3346/jkms.2011.26.9.1201.
23. Hsu CC, Jhang HR, Chang WT, Lin CH, Shin SJ, Hwang SJ, et al. Associations between dietary patterns and kidney function indicators in type 2 diabetes. Clin Nutr. 2014;33(1):98–105. doi:10.1016/j.clnu.2013.04.010.
24. Osonoi Y, Mita T, Osonoi T, Saito M, Tamasawa A, Nakayama S, et al. Morningness-eveningness questionnaire score and metabolic parameters in patients with type 2 diabetes mellitus. Chronobiol Int. 2014;31(9):1017–23. doi:10.3109/07420528.2014.943843.
25. Agency SaT. Standard Tables of Food Composition in Japan (in Japanese). 5th ed. Tokyo: Printing Bureau of the Ministry of Finance; 2005. doi:10.1007/s11136-007-9172-x.
26. Hone JA, Ostberg O. A self-assessment questionnaire to determine morningness-eveningness in human circadian rhythms. Int J Chronobiol. 1976;4:97–110. doi:10.1001/archinte.166.16.1768.
27. Buysse DJ, Reynolds 3rd CF, Monk TH, Berman SR, Kupfer DJ. The Pittsburgh sleep quality index: a new instrument for psychiatric practice and research. Psychiatry Res. 1989;28(2):193–213.
28. Backhaus J, Junghanns K, Broocks A, Riemann D, Hohagen F. Test-retest reliability and validity of the Pittsburgh sleep quality index in primary insomnia. J Psychosom Res. 2002;53(3):737–40.
29. Beck AT, Steer RA, Brown GK. Manual for the Beck Depression Inventory-II. San Antonio, TX: Psychological Corporation; 1996. doi:10.1207/s15327752jpa6703_13.
30. Craig CL, Marshall AL, Sjostrom M, Bauman AE, Booth ML, Ainsworth BE, et al. International physical activity questionnaire: 12-country reliability and validity. Med Sci Sports Exerc. 2003;35(8):1381–95. doi:10.1249/01.MSS.0000078924.61453.FB.
31. Takeno K, Mita T, Nakayama S, Goto H, Komiya K, Abe H, et al. Masked hypertension, endothelial dysfunction, and arterial stiffness in type 2 diabetes mellitus: a pilot study. Am J Hypertens. 2012;25(2):165–70. doi:10.1038/ajh.2011.158.
32. Yamashina A, Tomiyama H, Takeda K, Tsuda H, Arai T, Hirose K, et al. Validity, reproducibility, and clinical significance of noninvasive brachial-ankle pulse wave velocity measurement. Hypertension research : official journal of the Japanese Society of Hypertension. 2002;25(3):359–64.
33. Slattery ML, Boucher KM, Caan BJ, Potter JD, Ma KN. Eating patterns and risk of colon cancer. Am J Epidemiol. 1998;148(1):4–16.
34. Garcia-Bailo B, El-Sohemy A, Haddad PS, Arora P, Benzaied F, Karmali M, et al. Vitamins D, C, and E in the prevention of type 2 diabetes mellitus: modulation of inflammation and oxidative stress. Biologics: targets & therapy. 2011;5:7–19. doi:10.2147/BTT.S14417.

35. Bhathena SJ, Velasquez MT. Beneficial role of dietary phytoestrogens in obesity and diabetes. The American journal of clinical nutrition. 2002;76(6):1191–201.
36. Nanri A, Kimura Y, Matsushita Y, Ohta M, Sato M, Mishima N, et al. Dietary patterns and depressive symptoms among Japanese men and women. Eur J Clin Nutr. 2010;64(8):832–9. doi:10.1038/ejcn.2010.86.
37. Bilici M, Efe H, Koroglu MA, Uydu HA, Bekaroglu M, Deger O. Antioxidative enzyme activities and lipid peroxidation in major depression: alterations by antidepressant treatments. J Affect Disord. 2001;64(1):43–51.
38. Bottiglieri T. Homocysteine and folate metabolism in depression. Prog Neuro-Psychopharmacol Biol Psychiatry. 2005;29(7):1103–12. doi:10.1016/j.pnpbp.2005.06.021.
39. Denova-Gutierrez E, Castanon S, Talavera JO, Gallegos-Carrillo K, Flores M, Dosamantes-Carrasco D, et al. Dietary patterns are associated with metabolic syndrome in an urban Mexican population. The Journal of nutrition. 2010;140(10):1855–63. doi:10.3945/jn.110.122671.
40. Akter S, Nanri A, Pham NM, Kurotani K, Mizoue T. Dietary patterns and metabolic syndrome in a Japanese working population. Nutrition & metabolism. 2013;10(1):30. doi:10.1186/1743-7075-10-30.
41. Nanri A, Mizoue T, Yoshida D, Takahashi R, Takayanagi R. Dietary patterns and A1C in Japanese men and women. Diabetes Care. 2008;31(8):1568–73. doi:10.2337/dc08-0297.
42. Pischke CR, Weidner G, Elliott-Eller M, Scherwitz L, Merritt-Worden TA, Marlin R, et al. Comparison of coronary risk factors and quality of life in coronary artery disease patients with versus without diabetes mellitus. Am J Cardiol. 2006;97(9):1267–73. doi:10.1016/j.amjcard.2005.11.051.
43. Chan HT, Yiu KH, Wong CY, Li SW, Tam S, Tse HF. Increased dietary fruit intake was associated with lower burden of carotid atherosclerosis in Chinese patients with Type 2 diabetes mellitus. Diabetic medicine: a journal of the British Diabetic Association. 2013;30(1):100–8. doi:10.1111/j.1464-5491.2012.03764.x.
44. Chrysant SG, Chrysant GS. An update on the cardiovascular pleiotropic effects of milk and milk products. J Clin Hypertens. 2013;15(7):503–10. doi:10.1111/jch.12110.
45. Nanri A, Mizoue T, Noda M, Takahashi Y, Kato M, Inoue M, et al. Rice intake and type 2 diabetes in Japanese men and women: the Japan public health center-based prospective study. The American journal of clinical nutrition. 2010;92(6):1468–77. doi:10.3945/ajcn.2010.29512.
46. Foster-Powell K, Holt SH, Brand-Miller JC. International table of glycemic index and glycemic load values: 2002. The American journal of clinical nutrition. 2002;76(1):5–56.
47. Martinez ME, Marshall JR, Sechrest L. Invited commentary: factor analysis and the search for objectivity. Am J Epidemiol. 1998;148(1):17–9.

# 19

# Stability-based validation of dietary patterns obtained by cluster analysis

Nicolas Sauvageot[1*], Anna Schritz[1], Sonia Leite[2], Ala'a Alkerwi[1], Saverio Stranges[1], Faiez Zannad[3], Sylvie Streel[4], Axelle Hoge[4], Anne-Françoise Donneau[4], Adelin Albert[4] and Michèle Guillaume[4]

**Abstract**

**Background:** Cluster analysis is a data-driven method used to create clusters of individuals sharing similar dietary habits. However, this method requires specific choices from the user which have an influence on the results. Therefore, there is a need of an objective methodology helping researchers in their decisions during cluster analysis. The objective of this study was to use such a methodology based on stability of clustering solutions to select the most appropriate clustering method and number of clusters for describing dietary patterns in the NESCAV study (*Nutrition, Environment and Cardiovascular Health*), a large population-based cross-sectional study in the Greater Region ($N = 2298$).

**Methods:** Clustering solutions were obtained with K-means, K-medians and Ward's method and a number of clusters varying from 2 to 6. Their stability was assessed with three indices: adjusted Rand index, Cramer's V and misclassification rate.

**Results:** The most stable solution was obtained with K-means method and a number of clusters equal to 3. The "Convenient" cluster characterized by the consumption of convenient foods was the most prevalent with 46% of the population having this dietary behaviour. In addition, a "Prudent" and a "Non-Prudent" patterns associated respectively with healthy and non-healthy dietary habits were adopted by 25% and 29% of the population. The "Convenient" and "Non-Prudent" clusters were associated with higher cardiovascular risk whereas the "Prudent" pattern was associated with a decreased cardiovascular risk. Associations with others factors showed that the choice of a specific dietary pattern is part of a wider lifestyle profile.

**Conclusion:** This study is of interest for both researchers and public health professionals. From a methodological standpoint, we showed that using stability of clustering solutions could help researchers in their choices. From a public health perspective, this study showed the need of targeted health promotion campaigns describing the benefits of healthy dietary patterns.

**Keywords:** Dietary patterns, Cluster analysis, Stability

## Background

In recent years, the dietary patterns (DP) approach has been used extensively to describe overall eating patterns in populations. In the literature, the most famous methods for computing dietary patterns are cluster analysis (CA) and principal component analysis (PCA). However, both methods describe diet in quite different ways. In PCA, continuous factors are defined based on correlations between dietary intakes and each individual has a score for all derived factors [1]. However, an individual's DP is difficult to interpret as it is described by a score on several factors [2]. On the other hand, cluster analysis separates individuals into mutually exclusive groups (clusters) based on similarities between their diets. Compared to factors, individual DP are easier to interpret since individuals are assigned to one cluster only.

One major challenge in using cluster analysis is that the obtained solution strongly depends upon the choices made by the investigator. Among them, the choice of the clustering method and the optimal number of clusters are

* Correspondence: nicolas.sauvageot@lih.lu
[1]Luxembourg Institute of Health (LIH), CCMS (Competence center in methodology and statistics), 1A rue Thomas Edison, L-1445 Strassen, Luxembourg

particularly important [3]. Indeed, since different clustering methods make different assumptions about the structure of the data, the choice of the method should be done according to the group structure expected. However, researchers do not have any prior knowledge about the structure of the clusters and their number. As a result, it appears that researchers run different clustering methods with different number of clusters and tend to present the best interpretable solution [1, 2, 4]. Obviously, this solution may not be the best representative of dietary patterns in a population. As an alternative, some studies used indices measuring distances between clusters [3, 5–7]. However, since those indices assume a group structure, their use should be avoided when group structure is unknown [8].

Consequently, researchers need a method allowing objective selection of the most appropriate clustering method and number of clusters for describing their data. Lange et al. introduced an objective criterion to compare different clustering solutions and to choose the most appropriate [8]. This criterion measures the goodness of clustering solutions by assessing their stability. A stable clustering solution should be similar to solutions computed on other data sets drawn from the same source. The idea is that clustering solutions exhibiting higher stability are likely to be more appropriate for describing the data.

Therefore, the primary objective of this study was to test such objective procedure to select the optimal clustering method and the number of clusters describing dietary patterns, based on data from the interregional, cross-sectional population-based NESCaV study (Nutrition, Environment and Cardiovascular Health). For simplicity, we decided to limit its application to traditional clustering methods used in the field of dietary pattern analysis, namely K-means, K-medians and Ward's minimum variance. Secondly, description of the selected clustering solution and relationships with nutrients intakes, socio-demographic, lifestyle and cardiovascular risk factors (CVRF) were presented. Finally, a comparison was also made with PCA factors.

## Methods

Details concerning the NESCAV study have been presented previously [9–11]. Briefly, it is the first cross-border cardiovascular health population-based study, based on a stratified random sample of 3133 subjects, aged 18–69 years, recruited from three neighboring regions, namely Grand-Duchy of Luxembourg, Wallonia in Belgium, and Lorraine in France, constituting an important segment of the Greater Region population. Periods of recruitment were 2007 to 2008 for Grand-Duchy of Luxembourg and 2010 to 2011 for Wallonia and Lorraine. Pregnant women, people living in institutions, subjects outside the age range 18–69 years and those deceased before recruitment were excluded [10]. Sample sizes were computed in order to be able to estimate prevalence of cardiovascular risk factor with a level of confidence of 95% and a precision of 1%.

A 134-food frequency questionnaire (FFQ) was used to assess dietary intakes. Description and validation of this questionnaire have been detailed elsewhere [12, 13]. To facilitate the analysis, the 134 food items were merged into 45 broader food groups according to their similarities (unpublished observations). Daily food intakes were computed as the product of daily frequency of consumption and the amount consumed. Considered cardiovascular risk factors (CVRF) were body mass index (BMI, $kg/m^2$), waist to hip ratio (WHR), systolic blood pressure (SBP, mmHg), diastolic blood pressure (DBP, mmHg), fasting plasma glucose (FPG, mg/dl), glycated haemoglobin (HbA1c, %), low-density lipoprotein cholesterol (LDL, mg/dl), high-density lipoprotein cholesterol (HDL, mg/dl) and triglycerides (TG, mg/dl). Information on treatment for hypertension, diabetes and dyslipidaemia was also gathered. Collected lifestyle behaviours were smoking status and level of physical activity expressed as weekly energy expenditure in metabolic equivalent task minutes per week (METs min/week), based on self-reported data from the International Physical Activity Questionnaire (IPAQ) [14, 15]. Specific inclusion criteria for this particular study were also defined. Flowchart of participants who met inclusion criteria were described (see Additional file 1: Figure S1). First, 138 participants with non-reliable reporting in the FFQ and outlying values on nutrient intakes were excluded. Then, since relationships between dietary habits and CVRF may be biased by participants who had a serious cardiovascular event ($n = 327$) and/or who are under diet ($n = 312$), those individuals were excluded. In addition, participants who were not fasting at time of blood collection ($n = 58$) were also discarded. Thus, the final sample entailed 2298 individuals.

The protocol of the study was approved by the following institutional review boards: Comité National d'Ethique de Recherche (Grand-Duchy of Luxembourg), Comité de Protection des Personnes Est-III (Lorraine), Comité d'Ethique Hospitalo-Facultaire Universitaire de Liège (Wallonia) and Ethik-Kommission Ärztekammer des Saarlandes (Saarland). All participants provided written informed consent.

### Statistical analysis

#### *Transformation of the data*

Firstly, food groups and nutrient intake were adjusted for energy intake using the residuals methods of Willet and Stampfer [16]. Secondly, since extreme values may have a significant effect on clustering solutions, extreme intakes above six standard deviations were truncated

[17]. Of the 103,410 available intakes, only 294 (0.28%) were truncated. Thirdly, since food intakes with large scales tend to have a larger effect on clustering solutions, food intakes were standardized by subtracting the minimum intake and then dividing by the range [3, 18].

### *Formalization of cluster analysis*

Let $X = (X_1, \ldots, X_n)$ be the dataset of $n = 2298$ individuals to be clustered where $X_i$ is a 45-dimensional vector containing the 45 standardized food group intakes of the i-th individual. A clustering algorithm A with a predefined number of cluster k constructs a solution Y of the data set X into k clusters ($Y := A_k(X)$). This solution Y is represented by an n-dimensional vector of labels $Y = (Y_1, \ldots, Y_n)$ where $Y_i = v$ if the i-th individual is assigned to cluster v ($v \in \{1, \ldots, k\}$).

### The measure of stability

Cluster stability exploits the fact that when multiple datasets are sampled from the same distribution, the clustering algorithm is expected to behave in the same way and produce similar results. Based on this idea, Lange et al. introduced a stability measure computed on the comparison of solutions obtained on different datasets drawn from the same source [8]. This stability measure was then compared across clustering methods and numbers of clusters to select the model associated with the most stable solution. Since this concept and its use in practice were previously described in detail [8], the method is only summarized below.

Briefly, considering a solution $Y := A_k(X)$, the method consists in assessing its stability by randomly splitting the data X into two independent half sets $X_{tr}$ (training dataset) and $X_{te}$ (test dataset), and comparing the solutions obtained for these halves ($Y_{tr} := A_k(X_{tr})$ and $Y_{te} := A_k(X_{te})$). However, since dataset $X_{tr}$ and $X_{te}$ are disjoint, clustering solutions are not directly comparable. To make these solutions comparable, a solution transfer mechanism allows extension of the clustering solution $Y_{tr}$ of the dataset $X_{tr}$ to the dataset $X_{te}$. Technically, the training dataset ($X_{tr}, Y_{tr}$) is used to construct a classifier $\phi$ which is then used to predict label of individuals from the test sample $X_{te}$. Consequently, the two clustering solutions $A_k(X_{tr})$ and $A_k(X_{te})$ are made comparable by comparing $\phi\ (X_{te})$ and $A_k(X_{te})$. The stability measure between the two solutions is then computed as the empirical misclassification rate [8]. Lower misclassification rates indicate higher stability.

In order to reduce the effect of random splitting, the algorithm was repeated 20 times and the estimates of stability for a given solution were computed as the average of the 20 corresponding estimates. The highest estimate of stability indicates the optimal clustering method and number of clusters. Clustering methods considered were the Ward's minimum variance, K-means and K-medians and number of clusters k varying from 2 to 6. Since K-means and K-medians may return a local optimum, algorithms were always run 1000 times with different random starting seeds, and the solution that had the minimum total within-cluster sum of squares distances was selected. Concerning the choice of the classifier $\phi$ , since we want to measure the stability of clustering solutions, the influence of the classifier should be minimized. For this purpose, Lange suggested choosing a classifier using the same clustering method's grouping principle [8]. Therefore, K-nearest-means classifier was used when K-means and Ward's methods were assessed whereas the K-nearest-medians classifier was used for the K-medians algorithm. Moreover, as a sensitivity analysis for assessing the impact of the stability indices used, others measures, namely Cramer's V and Adjusted Rand index (ARI) were also computed. Contrary to the misclassification rate, higher values on Cramer's V and ARI indicate higher stability.

### Description of dietary patterns

According to the stability indices values, the optimal clustering method for describing dietary patterns in our dataset was K-means with a number of clusters equal to 3. Clusters were described with mean of daily food intakes relative to corresponding overall mean intake. Cluster names were assigned based on food groups with high consumption. Clusters were also presented according to nutrient intake, socio-demographic and lifestyle factors. Continuous variables were presented as mean ± standard deviation (SD). Since most of the variables describing food and nutrient intake were not normally distributed, differences across clusters were evaluated using Kruskal-Wallis test. Categorical variables were presented as percentages (%) and differences were tested by the Chi-square test. A multinomial logistic regression was run to assess the relationships between clusters (dependent variables) and all socio-demographics and lifestyle characteristics as independent variables. Finally, separate multivariable-adjusted regression models for each CVRF (dependent variables) were also used to assess relationships with clusters (independent variables). Models were adjusted for gender, age, educational level, smoking status and the level of physical activity and medication use for the corresponding CVRF. Interaction between DP and gender were tested and if significant, results were stratified by gender. In order to take into account the sampling design of the study, individuals were weighted by the reciprocal of the probability of selection. All analyses were conducted with SAS version 9.4 (SAS Institute Inc., Cary, NC, USA). Ward's method was performed with the procedure PROC CLUSTER and K-means and K-medians with the procedure PROC FASTCLUS. *P*-values < 0.05 were considered as significant.

### Comparison with PCA-DP

Continuous dietary patterns were also computed with PCA method. PCA-DP scores were calculated as a sum of the food intake variables weighted by the loadings generated by the method. Food groups with absolute loadings values superior to 0.2 were considered as contributing highly to the pattern [2]. According to the elbow method, three dietary patterns were selected. Both methods PCA and cluster analysis were compared by comparing means of PCA-DP across clusters with the Kruskal-Wallis test.

## Results

### Choice of clustering method and number of clusters

Figure 1 presents the distribution of the three stability indices across clustering methods and number of clusters. Distributions were described with box-plots and average values computed on 20 repetitions of the algorithm. Regardless of stability indices and number of clusters, more stable solutions were obtained with K-means. In addition, the most stable solution was obtained with 3 clusters. Therefore, dietary patterns were computed with K-means algorithm and a predefined number of clusters equal to three.

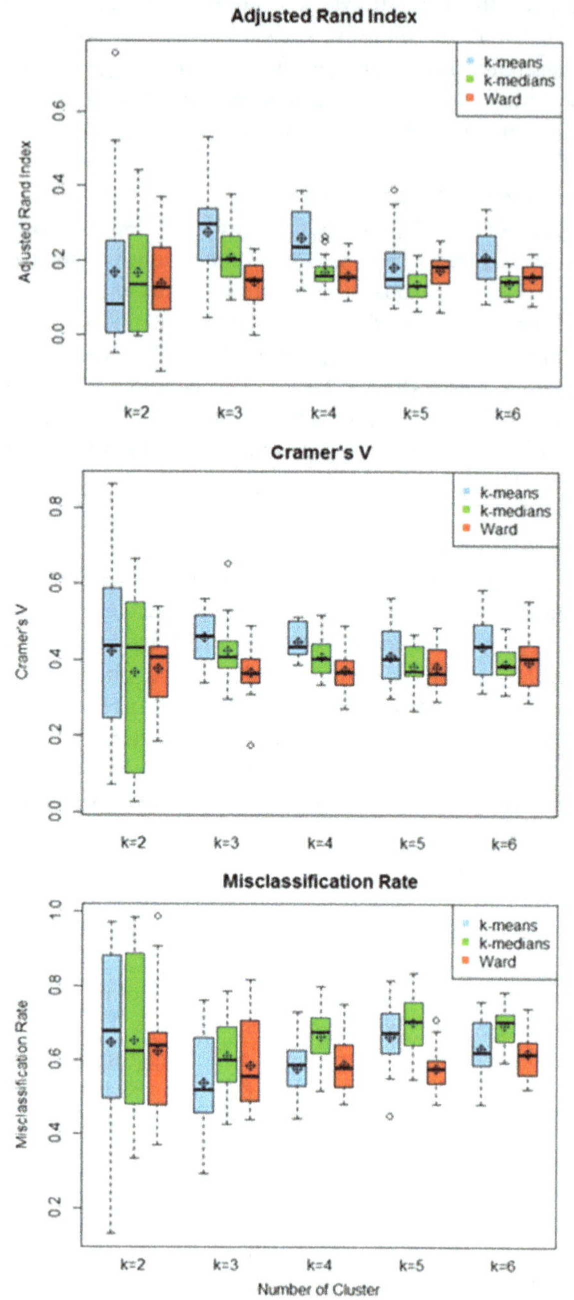


**Fig. 1** Distribution of stability indices across clustering methods and number of clusters

### Dietary patterns

The description of each cluster is given in Table 1. Clusters were described with mean of daily food intakes relative to corresponding overall mean intake. The cluster labelled "**Prudent**" was characterized by high intakes of brown bread, fruits, oleaginous fruits, dried fruits, soups, vegetables, pulses, preserved vegetables, offal, fish, smoked and canned fish, shellfish and mussels, dairy products, soya products, olive oil, oil-rich in omega 3 or 6, water and tea. In contrast, individuals in this cluster had low intakes of white bread, pastries, rice and pasta, fried foods, lean and fatty meat, processed smoked meat, processed meat, ready meals, minarine and margarine, fresh cream and dressing, sugar and sweets, salty biscuits, soft drinks, diet soft drinks, beer and aperitifs and spirits. Concerning the "**Non-Prudent**" cluster, individuals in this cluster consumed less cereals, rice/pasta, fruits, oleaginous fruits, dried fruits, vegetables, pulses, preserved vegetables, fish, smoked and canned fish, dairy products, soya products, olive oil and oil-rich in omega 3 or 6, light fresh cream and dressings, sugar and sweets, water, fruit or vegetable juice and tea. In contrast, the "Non-Prudent" cluster had high intakes of white bread, potatoes, fried foods, lean and fatty meat, offal, processed meat, shellfish and mussels, minarine and margarine, fresh cream and dressings, coffee, diet soft drinks, beer and wine. Finally, the "**Convenient**" cluster was characterized by consumption of convenient fast foods that require little preparation like cereals, pastries, rice and pasta, preserved vegetables, smoked and canned fish, ready meals, high-fat dairy products, soya products, fresh cream and dressings, sugar and sweets, salty biscuits, fruit or vegetable juice, soft drinks and aperitifs and spirits. In contrast, individuals in this cluster had low consumption of brown bread, potatoes, oleaginous

**Table 1** Description of clusters according to daily food intakes relative to corresponding overall mean intake (Mean (SD))

| Food groups | Clusters | | | *p*-value |
|---|---|---|---|---|
| | Convenient (*n* = 1005;46%) | Prudent (*n* = 718;29%) | Non-Prudent (*n* = 575;25%) | |
| White bread | **−2.9 (27.6)[ab]** | 1.4 (41.6)[a] | **3.4 (36.4)[b]** | 0.003 |
| Brown bread | **−9.6 (50.4)[a]** | 6.4 (69.4)[b] | **8.7 (76.1)[ab]** | 0.003 |
| Cereals | **19.5 (104.6)[a]** | −0.2 (95.9)[b] | **−33.9 (43)[c]** | <0.0001 |
| Pastries | **5.6 (29.8)[a]** | **−6.1 (27.2)[b]** | −2.2 (27.8)[c] | <0.0001 |
| Potatoes | **−12.2 (39.3)[a]** | 0.6 (54.2)[b] | **20.6 (55.8)[c]** | <0.0001 |
| Rice pasta | **7.6 (47.5)[a]** | **−5.1 (45.8)[b]** | **−6.9 (38.4)[b]** | <0.0001 |
| Fried foods | 2.2 (27.7)[a] | **−10.3 (21.2)[b]** | **9.1 (38.7)[c]** | <0.0001 |
| Fruits | −10.6 (30.2)[a] | **26.2 (63.4)[b]** | **−14.2 (29.5)[c]** | <0.0001 |
| Oleaginous fruits | **−6.2 (40.6)[a]** | **13.9 (71.3)[b]** | **−6.3 (45)[a]** | <0.0001 |
| Dried fruits | −27.7 (69.6)[a] | **63.4 (235.2)[b]** | **−30.7 (73.8)[c]** | <0.0001 |
| Soups | **−16.1 (40.2)[a]** | **23.2 (71.4)[b]** | −0.8 (53.9)[c] | <0.0001 |
| Vegetables | **−15.1 (30.3)[a]** | **30.9 (59.8)[b]** | **−12.1 (36.3)[a]** | <0.0001 |
| Pulses | **−7.6 (37.7)[a]** | **13.2 (56.3)[b]** | **−3.3 (56.5)[a]** | <0.0001 |
| Preserved vegetables | **−3.4 (67)[a]** | **12.1 (99.6)[a]** | **−9.2 (56.8)[b]** | 0.017 |
| Lean meat | −0.9 (28.7)[a] | **−6 (30.6)[b]** | **8.9 (31.6)[c]** | <0.0001 |
| Fatty meat | 4.4 (34.5)[a] | **−16.1 (30.9)[b]** | **12.3 (44.9)[c]** | <0.0001 |
| Offals | **−14.7 (50.4)[a]** | **16.3 (99.9)[b]** | **5.4 (96.6)[a]** | 0.006 |
| Processed smoked meat | −3.6 (37.7)[a] | **−7.1 (43.3)[b]** | **15.2 (57.6)[c]** | <0.0001 |
| Processed meat | 2.5 (37.1)[a] | **−12.7 (30.6)[b]** | **11.4 (49.3)[c]** | <0.0001 |
| Fish | **−11.1 (35.3)[a]** | **21.4 (56.1)[b]** | **−7.4 (40.7)[a]** | <0.0001 |
| Smoked and canned fish | **−2.9 (56.1)[a]** | **11.4 (83.4)[a]** | **−9.1 (51.9)[b]** | <0.0001 |
| Shellfish and mussels | **−8.4 (56)[a]** | **6.4 (71.4)[b]** | **6.8 (64.6)[b]** | <0.0001 |
| Eggs | −0.7 (42.5)[a] | −0.4 (45.6)[a] | 1.7 (45.2)[a] | 0.559 |
| Ready meal | **9.6 (31.9)[a]** | **−10.2 (24.2)[b]** | −4.1 (25.5)[c] | <0.0001 |
| High-fat dairy products | **2.3 (34.4)[a]** | **2.1 (38.4)[a]** | **−6.7 (32.7)[b]** | <0.0001 |
| Low-fat dairy products | −4.92 (62.8)[a] | **18.2 (84.9)[b]** | **−14.2 (57.3)[c]** | <0.0001 |
| Soya products | **−24.7 (233.9)[a]** | **83.1 (519)[a]** | **−60.6 (45)[b]** | <0.0001 |
| Butter and low fat butter | −8.1 (40.3)[a] | 2.2 (55.7)[a] | 11.5 (70.3)[a] | 0.080 |
| Minarine and margarine | −11.8 (53.1)[a] | **−21.1 (54.4)[b]** | **47.1 (117.8)[c]** | <0.0001 |
| Olive oil | −5.4 (49)[a] | **22.7 (76.4)[b]** | **−18.8 (40.7)[c]** | <0.0001 |
| Oil rich in omega6 | −12.2 (53.3)[a] | **27.7 (101)[b]** | **−13.3 (54.7)[c]** | <0.0001 |
| Oil rich in omega3 | **−6 (47.3)[a]** | **8.3 (69.6)[b]** | 0.1 (56.5)[ab] | 0.013 |
| fresh creamand dressing | **7.2 (43.5)[a]** | **−13 (32.9)[b]** | **3.6 (37.4)[a]** | <0.0001 |
| Light fresh cream and dressing | **4.2 (77.1)[a]** | **−4.4 (75.8)[b]** | **−1.9 (69)[b]** | <0.0001 |
| Sugar and sweets | **5.7 (27.1)[a]** | **−4.6 (24.5)[b]** | **−4.1 (25.1)[b]** | <0.0001 |
| Salty biscuits | **9.4 (65.5)[a]** | **−13.5 (38.3)[b]** | 0.4 (60.6)[c] | <0.0001 |
| Water | −2.1 (58.5)[a] | **14.8 (65.2)[b]** | **−14.8 (58.6)[c]** | <0.0001 |
| Coffee | **−23.1 (44.4)[a]** | −10.5 (52.8)[b] | **53.6 (85.8)[c]** | <0.0001 |
| Fruit or vegetable juice | **13.9 (67.8)[a]** | −4.7 (50.3)[b] | **−18.4 (38.5)[c]** | <0.0001 |
| Soft drinks | **15.6 (63.9)[a]** | **−18.9 (23)[b]** | −3.9 (48.5)[c] | <0.0001 |
| Diet soft drinks | **7.6 (192.1)[a]** | **−35.5 (108.2)[b]** | **31 (249.9)[a]** | <0.0001 |

**Table 1** Description of clusters according to daily food intakes relative to corresponding overall mean intake (Mean (SD)) *(Continued)*

| Beer | −4.6 (35.8)$^{a}$ | **−12.6 (28.5)$^{b}$** | **23.8 (82.7)$^{c}$** | <0.0001 |
|---|---|---|---|---|
| Wine | **−19.7 (54.6)$^{a}$** | −2.9 (80.6)$^{b}$ | **38.1 (134.9)$^{c}$** | <0.0001 |
| Aperitifs and spirits | **−2.6 (41.5)$^{a}$** | **−3.5 (52.5)$^{b}$** | **8.9 (63.2)$^{a}$** | <0.0001 |
| Tea | −53.6 (93.3)$^{a}$ | **135.2 (259.2)$^{b}$** | **−75.2 (68)$^{c}$** | <0.0001 |

Legend: $^{abc}$Means with same letters are not significantly different from each other; means that are in **bold** face are highest; means that are **underlined and bold** are lowest

fruits, soups, vegetables, pulses, offal, fish, shellfish and mussels, oil-rich in omega 3, coffee and wine.

The distribution of dietary patterns is also described in Table 1. The "Convenient" pattern was the most prevalent with 46% of the population assigned to this cluster. The remaining two clusters were smaller with 25% and 29% of the population belonging respectively to the "Non-Prudent" and "Prudent" cluster.

The description of dietary patterns according to nutrient intake is presented in Table 2. "Prudent" cluster was characterized by high intakes of all micronutrients, carbohydrates, total fiber and plant protein. In contrast, this cluster was associated with low intakes of alcohol, animal protein, added sugar and dietary cholesterol. Concerning fat profile, individuals in this cluster have higher MUFA: SFA (Ratio of monounsaturated fat to saturated fat) and PUFA: SFA (Ratio of polyunsaturated fat to saturated fat). On the opposite, "Non-Prudent" cluster had the highest intakes of alcohol, animal protein, and dietary cholesterol. It was also characterized by low intakes of carbohydrates, total fibre, added sugar, fat and all micronutrients and low MUFA: SFA and PUFA: SFA ratios. The "Convenient" pattern was associated with high intakes of carbohydrates, added sugar and fat and low intakes of alcohol, total fiber, plant and animal protein, β-carotene, vitamin E and iron.

### Association of DP with sociodemographic and lifestyle characteristics

The associations of DP with sociodemographic and lifestyle characteristics are shown in Table 3. "Non-Prudent" and "Convenient" clusters were compared to the "Prudent"

**Table 2** Description of clusters according to nutrient intakes relative to corresponding overall mean intake (Mean (SD))

| Nutrient | | Clusters | | | *p*-value |
|---|---|---|---|---|---|
| | | Convenient | Prudent | Non-Prudent | |
| Macro-nutrients | Alcohol | **−25.3 (89.0)$^{a}$** | **−19.6 (111.2)$^{a}$** | **69.4 (188.1)$^{b}$** | <0.0001 |
| | Carbohydrates | **2.2 (16.6)$^{a}$** | **1.1 (20.5)$^{a}$** | **−5.2 (18.3)$^{b}$** | <0.0001 |
| | Total fiber | **−9.3 (21.5)$^{a}$** | **19.3 (32.5)$^{b}$** | **−7.9 (26.4)$^{a}$** | <0.0001 |
| | Plant protein | **−5.5 (22.0)$^{a}$** | **8.3 (28.9)$^{b}$** | −0.6 (26.1)$^{c}$ | <0.0001 |
| | Animal protein | **−1.9 (29.7)$^{a}$** | **−1.4 (35.1)$^{a}$** | **5.1 (31.3)$^{b}$** | <0.0001 |
| | Added sugar | **27.6 (73.1)$^{a}$** | **−24.9 (52.1)$^{b}$** | **−17.0 (60.9)$^{b}$** | <0.0001 |
| | Fat | **0.9 (17.0)$^{a}$** | **−0.2 (21.7)$^{ab}$** | **−1.3 (19.7)$^{b}$** | 0.03 |
| | Cholesterol | 0.9 (26.2)$^{a}$ | **−4.8 (34.1)$^{b}$** | **4.4 (26.2)$^{c}$** | <0.0001 |
| | Monounsaturated fat | **−0.4 (21.5)$^{a}$** | **3.4 (27.4)$^{a}$** | **−3.6 (20.5)$^{b}$** | 0.0001 |
| | Polyunsaturated fat | **−6.1 (31.7)$^{a}$** | **13.2 (51.3)$^{b}$** | **−5.9 (29.4)$^{a}$** | <0.0001 |
| | Saturated fat | **0.9 (13.0)$^{a}$** | **−2.91 (15.9)$^{b}$** | **2.1 (12.8)$^{a}$** | <0.0001 |
| | Ratio of monounsaturated fat to saturated fat | −2.1 (36.0)$^{a}$ | **8.2 (49.5)$^{b}$** | **−6.5 (34.1)$^{c}$** | <0.0001 |
| | Ratio of polyunsaturated fat to saturated fat | **−8.3 (44.7)$^{a}$** | **19.4 (79.4)$^{b}$** | **−9.7 (39.9)$^{a}$** | <0.0001 |
| Micro-nutrients | β-caroten | **−17.5 (56.1)$^{a}$** | **39.9 (106.5)$^{b}$** | **−19.2 (58.5)$^{a}$** | <0.0001 |
| | Vitamin C | −8.3 (47.6)$^{a}$ | **31.4 (94.6)$^{b}$** | **−24.6 (43.8)$^{c}$** | <0.0001 |
| | Vitamin E | **−4.7 (34.3)$^{a}$** | **8.6 (43.2)$^{b}$** | **−2.4 (38.3)$^{a}$** | <0.0001 |
| | Iron | **−3.2 (16.5)$^{a}$** | **4.6 (19.3)$^{b}$** | −0.3 (18.2)$^{c}$ | <0.0001 |
| | Vitamin D | −8.7 (93.8)$^{a}$ | **25.0 (101.4)$^{b}$** | **−15.9 (64.8)$^{c}$** | <0.0001 |
| | Calcium | −2.5 (26.5)$^{a}$ | **13.3 (37.3)$^{b}$** | **−12.4 (28.0)$^{c}$** | <0.0001 |

$^{abc}$Means with same letters are not significantly different from each other; means that are in **bold** face are **highest**; means that are **underlined and bold** are **lowest**

**Table 3** Associations of clusters with sociodemographic and lifestyle characteristics (Mean(SD); Percentage) and odds-ratios)

| Sociodemographic and lifestyle characteristics | | Cluster | | | *p*-value | Odds ratio | |
|---|---|---|---|---|---|---|---|
| | | Convenient | Prudent | Non-Prudent | | Convenient vs Prudent | Non-Prudent vs Prudent |
| Age (years) | **(*n* = 2298)** | **36.9 (0.3)[a]** | **49.3 (0.5)[b]** | 48.9 (0.6)[c] | <0.0001 | 0.92 [0.91;0.93] | 1.00 [0.98;1.01] |
| Energy expenditure per week (MET/100) | **(*n* = 2298)** | **29.2 (1.21)[ac]** | **33.6 (1.8)[b]** | 32.4(1.6)[c] | 0.0075 | 0.993 [0.988;0.998] | 0.996 [0.99;1.002] |
| Gender (%) | **Men (*n* = 1158)** | 52.2% | **35.9%** | **66.0%** | <0.0001 | 2.2 [1.6;3.1] | 4.2 [2.9;5.9] |
| | **Women (*n* = 1140)** | 47.9% | **64.1%** | **34.0%** | | Reference | |
| Educational level (%) | **Primary (*n* = 331)** | **7.2%** | 10.1% | **10.5%** | <0.0001 | 1.3 [0.9;2.1] | 2.9 [1.4;3.8] |
| | **Secondary (*n* = 1127)** | 46.4% | **42.8%** | **57.6%** | | 1.9 [1.4;2.7] | 2.5 [1.7;3.7] |
| | **Tertiary (*n* = 818)** | **46.4%** | 41.1% | **32.0%** | | Reference | |
| Smokers (%) | **Smokers (*n* = 484)** | 21.6% | **15.3%** | **36.9%** | <0.0001 | 1 [0.6;1.6] | 3 [1.9;4.7] |
| | **Non smokers (n = 1814)** | 78.4% | **84.7%** | **63.1%** | | Reference | |
| Region (%) | **Luxembourg (*n* = 1071)** | **26.3%** | 23.0% | **19.1%** | <0.0001 | 1.7 [1.2;2.4] | 2.1 [1.3;3.4] |
| | **Wallonia (*n* = 750)** | 38.3% | **26.0%** | **60.0%** | | 2.7 [1.8;3.9] | 7.1 [4.5;11.4] |
| | **Lorraine (*n* = 477)** | 35.5% | **50.9%** | **20.9%** | | Reference | |

Legend: [abc] Means with same letters are not significantly different from each other; figures that are in **bold** face are **highest**; figures that are **underlined and bold** are **lowest**

cluster which was considered as the reference. Older subjects were less likely to adopt a "Convenient" pattern (OR = 0.92 [0.91; 0.93]). Indeed, individuals in the "Convenient" cluster were much younger (36.9 years) than those in the "Prudent" (49.3 years) and "Non-Prudent" (48.9 years) cluster. Men were also more likely to adopt a "Convenient" (OR = 2.2 [1.6; 3.1]) or "Non-Prudent" (OR = 4.2 [2.9; 5.9]) patterns rather than a "Prudent" one. Likewise, individuals with less education were also more likely to adopt a "Non-Prudent" pattern. Concerning the region, compared to Lorraine, individuals living in Luxembourg were more likely to adopt a "Convenient" (OR = 1.7 [1.2; 2.4]) or a "Non-Prudent" (OR = 2.1 [1.3; 3.4]) pattern. The difference was even larger when comparing with individuals living Wallonia with a net preference for the "Non-Prudent" (OR = 7.1 [4.5; 11.4]) and "Convenient" (OR = 2.7 [1.8; 3.9]) pattern. In details, 41% of individuals living in Lorraine adopted a "Prudent" pattern whereas they were only 28.7% in Luxembourg and 19.1% in Wallonia. On the opposite, only 14% of individuals in Lorraine adopted a "Non-Prudent" pattern whereas they were 19.9% in Luxembourg and 36.7% in Wallonia. Concerning lifestyle factors, smokers were more likely to adopt a "Non-Prudent" (OR = 3 [1.9; 4.7]) pattern. Regarding physical activity, individual in the "Convenient" cluster were engaged in significantly less physical activity (OR = 0.993 [0.988; 0.998]).

### Association of DP with CVRF

Multivariate-adjusted β-coefficients for CVRF according to DP are displayed in Table 4. Compared to the "Prudent" pattern, higher BMI was noticed in individuals who adopted the "Convenient" and the "Non-Prudent" pattern whereas higher WHR was only observed in men having adopted the "Non-Prudent" pattern. "Non-Prudent" and "Convenient" patterns also showed higher SBP and DBP values. Concerning diabetes, "Convenient" and especially "Non-Prudent" patterns were significantly associated with higher FPG but not HbA1c. Regarding cholesterol levels, "Non-Prudent" cluster was associated with higher LDL and HDL in men only. Further adjustment of treatment did not change the results.

### Comparison of dietary patterns obtained with PCA and K-means

Continuous dietary patterns were computed using the PCA method. According to the scree-plot, three dietary patterns were selected. The percentage of variance explained and loadings of food groups on DP are presented in Table 5. The three PCA-patterns accounted for 7.1%

**Table 4** Association of clusters with cardiovascular risk factors (β-coefficients (Standard error) of cluster on CVRF)

| | | Cluster | |
|---|---|---|---|
| | | Convenient | Non-Prudent |
| CVRF | Model | β (standard error) | |
| BMI | M1 | 0.49 (0.24)* | 1.20 (0.26)** |
| WHR | M1 men | 0.01 (0.01) | 0.02 (0.01)* |
| | M1 women | 0.01 (0.005) | −0.002 (0.01) |
| SBP | M1 | 2.58 (0.79)* | 4.41 (0.87)** |
| | M2 | 2.10 (0.77)* | 4.04 (0.85)** |
| DBP | M1 | 1.54 (0.55)* | 3.15 (0.61)** |
| | M2 | 1.29 (0.55)* | 2.95 (0.60)** |
| FPG | M1 | 1.77 (0.88)* | 3.10 (0.97)* |
| | M2 | 1.46 (0.78) | 2.30 (0.86)* |
| Hba1c | M1 | 0.01 (0.02) | 0.03 (0.03) |
| | M2 | 0.01 (0.02) | 0.01 (0.02) |
| HDL | M1 men | −0.78 (1.09) | 3.57 (1.10)* |
| | M1 women | 0.07 (1.17) | −1.59 (1.44) |
| | M2 men | −0.82 (1.09) | 3.62 (1.10)* |
| | M2 women | −0.11 (1.17) | −1.75 (1.44) |
| LDL | M1 men | 1.18 (2.70) | 6.63 (2.72)* |
| | M1 women | −2.77 (2.22) | −4.59 (2.73) |
| | M2 men | 1.02 (2.69) | 6.81 (2.71)* |
| | M2 women | −2.64 (2.22) | −4.47 (2.73) |
| TG | M1 | −1.77 (4.34) | 2.91 (4.78) |
| | M2 | −1.25 (4.34) | 2.94 (4.77) |

Prudent cluster is the reference category
M1 : adjusted on gender, age, educational level, smoking status, physical activity
M2 : M1 + treatment for the studied CVRF
*$p < 0.05$
**$p < 0.0001$

(3.1%, 2.1% and 1.9% respectively) of the total variance in food intakes. The first pattern was labelled "Prudent" as it was characterized by high intakes of fruits, oleaginous and dried fruits, soups, vegetables, pulses, fish, low-fat dairy products, soya products, olive oil, oil-rich in omega 6, water and tea and low intakes of fried foods, lean and fatty meat, processed meat, ready meals, minarine and margarine, fresh cream and dressing, salty biscuits, soft drinks, diet soft drinks and beer. The second PCA-pattern was named "Animal protein and alcohol" since it was positively associated with vegetables, pulses, all kinds of meat and fish and alcohol beverages and negatively associated with sugar and sweets, high-fat dairy products, pastries and cereals. The third pattern was labelled "Convenient" since this pattern was positively correlated with convenient foods that require little preparation like brown bread, cereals, rice, pasta, smoked and canned fish, shellfish and mussels, ready meals, low-fat dairy products, soya products, fresh cream and dressings, salty biscuits, fruit or vegetable juice. Moreover, it was also negatively correlated with white bread, potatoes and butter. Comparison of dietary patterns obtained through PCA and K-means are shown in Fig. 2. The three clusters were similar to the three continuous dietary patterns obtained through PCA. Indeed, the PCA-Prudent DP was highest in the "Prudent" cluster, the PCA-animal protein and alcohol DP was highest in the "Non-Prudent" cluster and the PCA-convenient DP was highest in the "Convenient" cluster.

## Discussion

The main objective of this study was to test a method allowing the objective selection of the most appropriate model among different clustering methods and numbers of clusters in the field of "dietary pattern analysis." The idea was to assess stability of different clustering solutions and choose the most stable solution as the most appropriate for describing the data. According to this method, three dietary patterns obtained with K-means algorithm were obtained. The "Non-Prudent" and "Convenient" patterns associated respectively with non-healthy food choices and convenient foods were both associated with a higher cardiovascular risk compared to the "Prudent" cluster characterized by healthier dietary habits and lower cardiovascular risk.

Among the clustering method considered in this article, K-means clearly showed more stable solutions regardless of the number of clusters. However, it is highly likely that other more sophisticated methods would have been more appropriate [3]. Indeed, clustering methods considered in this study were really simple and others methods with higher flexibility regarding cluster's characteristics are more likely to identify real complex structure. In addition, although K-means was found as the most appropriate method for describing dietary patterns in adults living in the Greater region, it may not be the case with other datasets. Indeed, group structures from other populations are likely to be different. Therefore, this should be explored in additional datasets across different populations.

In the field of dietary pattern analysis, we are aware of only two studies comparing different clustering methods. Like us, Lo Siou et al. assessed stability of solutions obtained with different clustering methods and number of clusters and also showed that K-means was the most appropriate method [3]. Contrary to our results, stability decreased with the number of clusters and therefore they were not able to identify an optimal number of clusters with this method. In addition, as proposed by Lange [8], the authors also used a classifier to transfer the solution obtained on one sample to another. However, the classifier should use the same clustering method's grouping principle. In accordance with Lange,

**Table 5** Factor loadings and explained variation of dietary patterns obtained with PCA

| Food groups | Dietary patterns | | |
|---|---|---|---|
| | Prudent | Animal protein and alcohol | Convenient |
| White bread | 0.02 | 0.01 | **−0.70** |
| Brown bread | 0.16 | 0.00 | **0.20** |
| Cereals | 0.13 | **−0.27** | **0.40** |
| Pastries | −0.16 | **−0.29** | 0.05 |
| Potatoes | 0.00 | 0.12 | **−0.28** |
| Rice pasta | −0.08 | 0.08 | **0.21** |
| Fried foods | **−0.39** | 0.13 | −0.09 |
| Fruits | **0.51** | −0.09 | 0.02 |
| Oleaginous fruits | **0.23** | 0.09 | 0.14 |
| Dried fruits | **0.35** | −0.02 | 0.06 |
| Soups | **0.25** | 0.09 | −0.11 |
| Vegetables | **0.56** | **0.25** | 0.19 |
| Pulses | **0.27** | **0.21** | −0.06 |
| Preserved vegetables | 0.05 | 0.14 | −0.12 |
| Lean meat | **−0.23** | **0.38** | −0.08 |
| Fatty meat | **−0.45** | **0.26** | 0.09 |
| Offal's | 0.15 | **0.29** | −0.11 |
| Processed smoked meat | −0.11 | **0.26** | 0.06 |
| Processed meat | **−0.36** | **0.27** | 0.08 |
| Fish | **0.43** | **0.39** | 0.16 |
| Smoked and canned fish | 0.17 | **0.37** | **0.24** |
| Shellfish and mussels | 0.06 | **0.47** | **0.22** |
| Eggs | −0.05 | 0.12 | −0.02 |
| Ready meal | **−0.38** | 0.08 | **0.41** |
| High-fat dairy products | 0.15 | **−0.23** | −0.11 |
| Low-fat dairy products | **0.26** | −0.04 | **0.20** |
| Soya products | **0.20** | −0.11 | **0.26** |
| Butter and low fat butter | 0.01 | −0.02 | **−0.30** |
| Minarine and margarine | **−0.26** | 0.04 | −0.07 |
| Olive oil | **0.35** | 0.05 | 0.16 |
| Oil rich in omega6 | **0.30** | 0.03 | −0.13 |
| Oil rich in omega3 | 0.15 | −0.01 | −0.15 |
| Fresh cream and dressing | **−0.38** | −0.03 | **0.24** |
| Light fresh cream and dressing | −0.03 | 0.05 | **0.31** |
| Sugar and sweets | −0.11 | **−0.49** | 0.08 |
| Salty biscuits | **−0.34** | 0.06 | **0.20** |
| Water | **0.24** | 0.08 | 0.15 |
| Coffee | −0.07 | 0.06 | −0.17 |
| Fruit or vegetable juice | −0.01 | −0.15 | **0.29** |
| Soft drinks | **−0.43** | −0.18 | 0.08 |
| Diet soft drinks | **−0.20** | 0.05 | 0.13 |
| Beer | **−0.26** | **0.34** | −0.03 |
| Wine | 0.03 | **0.38** | −0.07 |
| Aperitifs and spirits | −0.15 | **0.34** | −0.09 |
| Tea | **0.36** | −0.10 | −0.02 |
| Explained variation in food groups, % | 3.1% | 2.1% | 1.9% |

**Table 5** Factor loadings and explained variation of dietary patterns obtained with PCA *(Continued)*

Loading values superior to 0.2 or inferior to -0.2 were in bold

we used the nearest-means classifier for K-means and Ward's method and the nearest-medians classifier for K-medians. However, Lo Siou et al. used the nearest-neighbour classifier for K-means and Ward's method. In order to assess the effect of using a not optimal classifier, we compared stability indices computed on our data with optimal classifiers and the not optimal nearest-neighbour classifier. All stability indices were lower when the not optimal nearest-neighbour classifier was used (see Additional file 2: Figure S2). Therefore, stability values computed in the paper of Lo Siou et al. may have been underestimated.

In another study, Greve et al. use an inappropriate manner for choosing the optimal number of clusters [19]. Indeed, they selected as the optimal number of cluster the number maximizing the agreement between different clustering methods. However, agreement between methods is conditioned by the capability of methods to identify cluster's structure. Indeed, if a method is not able to distinguish clusters, it will never agree with another method even for the correct number of clusters. Therefore, although it is reassuring to have good agreement between solutions obtained with different algorithms, agreement should not be used for choosing the optimal number of clusters.

### Comparison with others studies

In accordance with the literature [2, 20], we also derived a "Prudent" dietary pattern characterized by plenty of plant foods and fish and a preference for vegetable oils and low-fat dairy products. In contrast, similar to Western DP described in others studies [2, 20], we also derived a "Non-Prudent" pattern characterized by intakes of red and processed meats, high fat content foods, refined grains, soft drinks and alcoholic beverages [21, 22]. However, contrary to most Western-DP described in the literature [2, 20], our "Non-Prudent" pattern was not associated with intakes of sweets and sugar.

Similar to some studies [4, 23, 24], we also found a cluster characterized by consumption of convenient fast foods. It showed high intakes of convenient unhealthy foods like pastries, ready meals, high-fat dairy products, fresh cream and dressings, sugar and sweets, salty biscuits, soft drinks and aperitifs and spirits. However, it was also characterized by high intakes of convenient

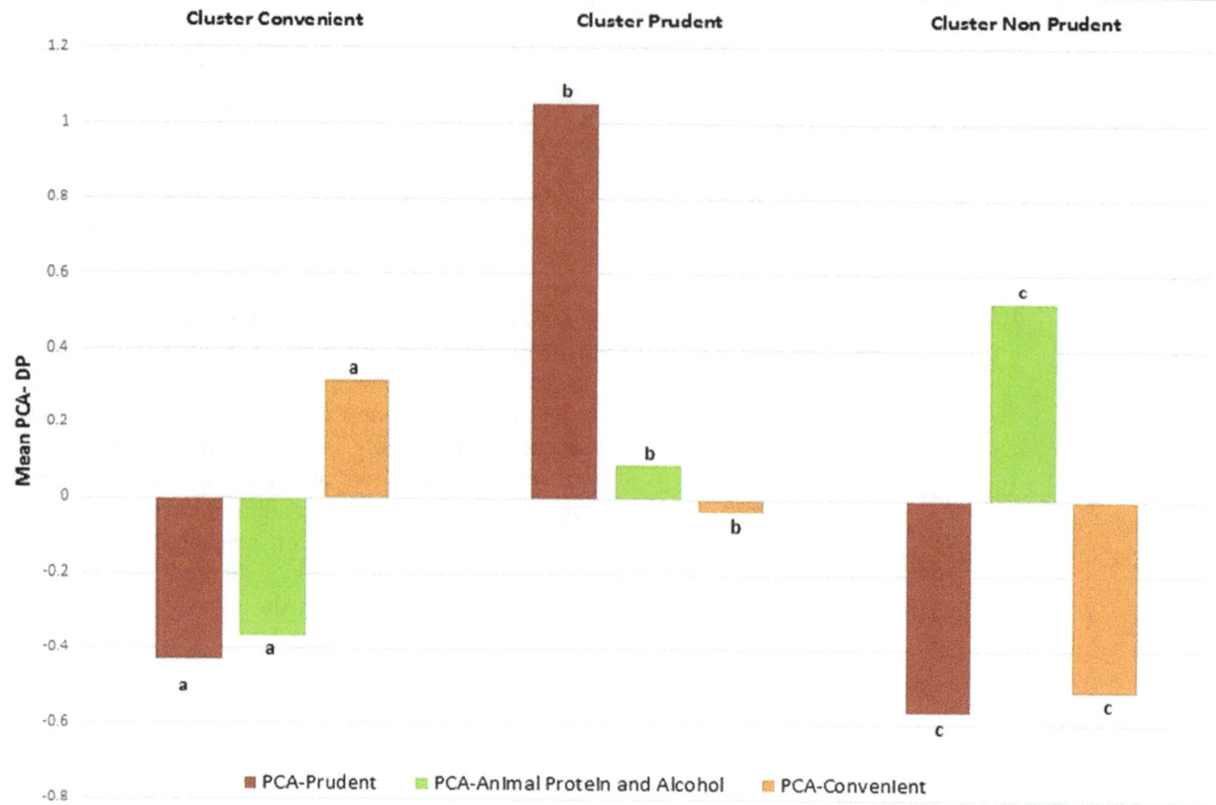


**Fig. 2** Mean PCA-DP across clusters. Legend: [abc]test if differences in mean for a PCA-DP were significantly different across clusters. Means with same letters are not significantly different from each other

healthy foods like cereals, preserved vegetables, smoked and canned fish, soya products, fruit or vegetable juice. Regarding nutrients, this pattern was associated with high intakes of carbohydrates, added sugar and fat.

The size of DP showed that the "Convenient" pattern was the most prevalent with 46% of the population assigned to this cluster. The "Prudent" and "Non-Prudent" patterns were adopted by 29% and 25% of the population respectively. However, striking differences were noticed across regions. Although, the "Convenient" pattern was the most adopted in all regions, the "Prudent" pattern was more frequent in Lorraine (41%) than in Luxembourg (28.7%) and Wallonia (19.1%). In sum, only a small part of the population has healthy dietary habits and this part is even smaller in Luxembourg and Wallonia. The adoption of a "Convenient" pattern may be due to the fact that people have less and less time for preparing and cooking foods and thus choose to consume prepared foods.

In line with others studies, we also found significant associations between dietary patterns and sociodemographic and lifestyle characteristics. We found that the "Convenient" pattern was more likely to be adopted by men and younger people [23]. Since the Luxembourg population is made up of more young active working people, this might explain the larger size of the "Convenient" cluster in Luxembourg compared to Wallonia and Lorraine [25]. In addition, as also shown by other studies [4], women and individuals with higher education were more likely to adopt a "Prudent" pattern. Moreover, in accordance with others studies [2, 4], we also found that people who choose unhealthy dietary habits are less likely to be engaged in healthy behaviours like doing physical activities and not smoking. It shows that the choice of a dietary pattern is in fact part of a larger pattern of lifestyle.

Concerning association with CVRF, we found that "Convenient" and "Non-Prudent" patterns were associated with higher BMI, WHR, SBP, DBP and FPG [4, 23, 26]. Moreover, the "Non-Prudent" pattern was also associated with higher HDL and LDL levels in men only. It is in accordance with others studies which also found that a cluster dominated by alcohol was directly associated with HDL [27–29]. The fact that the association was significant in men only might be explained by different level of alcohol consumption between men and women. Indeed, when clusters were described by gender, we observed that the "Non-Prudent" cluster was characterized by high intakes of alcohol in men but not in women (data not shown). Another explanation could be a different effect of diet on plasma lipids between men and women, possibly due to hormonal and sex differences in cholesterol metabolism [2, 30, 31]. Moreover, the genetic variation in lipoprotein metabolism may also have an effect [32].

### Comparison between PCA and cluster analysis

Despite clear differences in approaches and interpretation, PCA and cluster analysis gave similar results. A "Prudent" DP was identified with both methods. Indeed, a "Prudent" and "Non-Prudent" cluster with respectively high and low values on PCA-Prudent DP were found. Likewise, a convenient cluster was made of individuals with high values on PCA-convenient DP. Concerning PCA-Animal protein and alcohol pattern, we did not observe a cluster of individuals with only high intakes of meat, fish and alcohol. However, since this DP is characterized by high intakes of foods (meat and alcohol) usually consumed in a "Non-Prudent" pattern, it was significantly higher in the "Non-Prudent" cluster. Those results are in line with others studies, which also found differences in mean PCA-DP across clusters [33–35].

Although results between both methods were similar, they describe diet in different ways. Indeed, PCA aims to determine DP explaining variation in a set of food groups whereas cluster analysis aims to identify groups of people with different food intakes. Moreover, the format of DP is also different. An individual's dietary pattern is described through his/her membership to a group in cluster analysis whereas in PCA-DP the subject is described with his/her scores on all computed DP. Therefore, the choice of a method depends on both the desired format of the outcome but also hypothesis and aims of the study. Advantages of PCA are that it may be easier to perform as it requires less subjective researchers' decisions. However, findings from cluster analysis are easier to interpret because an individual is assigned to one cluster only whereas PCA-DP do not refer to identifiable groups within the population, and hence do not give an indication of the prevalence of a particular type of diet [35]. On the other hand, continuous factors determined by PCA may be advantageous when relationships between DP and others variables are assessed since a gradient is formed between individuals with low, medium or high values on factors. Moreover, they do not require the use of a reference category [26]. As other authors have suggested, unless the choice of one method is justified, it is advisable to use both factor and cluster analysis in order have complementary insights [36].

### Strength and limitations

The main strength of this study was the use of an objective procedure to select the most appropriate clustering method and number of clusters. Compared to other internal validity indices, the stability measure has the advantage to be model free and not being optimized by any clustering method. Moreover, comparison of cluster solution and PCA-derived factors were also made. Further, this study used a recent and homogeneous design of data collection including three large randomly selected samples from three neighbour regions. Shortcomings of this study were that considered clustering methods were all heuristic-based and make basic assumptions on group structure. The reason is that since the main objective of this study was to test the objective procedure, we decided to limit its application to traditional clustering methods used in the field of dietary pattern analysis [2]. Therefore, we will also consider more sophisticated methods in the future. In addition, although the method allows distinguishing between stable and spurious clustering solutions, stability is not the only aspect of a good solution. Indeed, a stable clustering solution may still be meaningless if it does not discriminate useful subset of the overall data [37]. However, unstable solutions should not be interpreted and thus stability is an indispensable requirement [37]. For this reason, the interpretation and criticism of the clustering solution by the researcher and comparison with results obtained with PCA are still important. In addition, many others subjective decisions have still been made that are likely to influence the final solution, namely the pooling of different food items into specific food groups, the quantification of the input variables, the adjustment for total energy intake and the method of standardization. However, the robustness of the chosen solution and the consistency of the results with PCA-DP gave confidence in our results. Other limitations are the cross-sectional design of the study and the probable measurement error linked with the FFQ. Finally, although we identified dietary pattern associated with disease risk, we still do not know if this effect comes from certain component only or is the product of the addition or interaction of several food groups.

## Conclusion

In summary, we used an objective methodology based on the stability of clustering solutions allowing selection of the most appropriate clustering method and number of cluster for describing dietary patterns in a population. Three main dietary patterns were identified in the Greater region. A "Convenient" and a "Non-Prudent" pattern associated with a higher cardiovascular risk and a "Prudent" pattern associated with a decreased cardiovascular risk. Those results flag the need for targeted public health initiatives promoting the benefit of a prudent dietary pattern and other healthy behaviours to relevant subgroups like men, young and less educated people, at interregional level.

### Abbreviations

ARI: Adjusted rand index; BMI: Body mass index; CA: Cluster analysis; CVRF: Cardiovascular risk factors; DBP: Diastolic blood pressure; DP: Dietary patterns; FFQ: Food frequency questionnaire; FPG: Fasting plasma glucose; HbA1c: Glycated hemoglobin; HDL: plasma high density cholesterol; LDL: Plasma low density cholesterol; MUFA: Monounsaturated fat; OR: Odds-ratio; PCA: Principal component analysis; PUFA: Polyunsaturated fat; RRR: Reduced rank regression; SBP: Systolic blood pressure; SD: Standard deviation; SFA: Saturated fat; TC: Plasma total cholesterol; TG: Triglycerides; WHR: Waist to hip ratio

### Acknowledgements

The cross-border NESCAV project is supported by INTERREG IV A program "Greater Region", 2007–2013, which aims to stimulate inter-regional cooperation. The four regions receive a co-funding from the European Regional Development Fund (ERDF), in addition to their own or public health authorities financial support.

### Funding

European Regional Development Fund : The funder had no role in study design, data collection and analysis, decision to publish, or preparation of the manuscript. National Fund of Research of Luxembourg : The funder had no role in study design, data collection and analysis, decision to publish, or preparation of the manuscript.

### Availability of data and materials

The data that support the findings of this study cannot be made publicly available for ethical and legal reasons. In fact, we are not authorized to share our NESCaV dataset with external researchers, as this condition had not been requested in the informed consent signed by the participants in 2007–2011. In addition, the NESCaV project is an interregional study that has been run in three different neighbor regions (Wallonia, Lorraine and Luxembourg). The current collaboration convention does not allow sharing the data with another party. However, any aggregated data in tables can be provided in case of request.

### Authors' contributions

NS, SL, AS, SS, AH, MG, AFD, AAlbert defined the methodology of this study. NS, SL, AS performed the statistical analysis. NS wrote the original draft. NS, SL, AAlkerwi, AS, FZ, SS, AFD, AAlbert, MG reviewed the draft. All authors read and approved the final manuscript.

### Competing interests

The authors declare no conflict of interest.

### Author details

[1]Luxembourg Institute of Health (LIH), CCMS (Competence center in methodology and statistics), 1A rue Thomas Edison, L-1445 Strassen, Luxembourg. [2]Ministry of Health, Luxembourg, Service épidémiologie & statistique, Allée Marconi, Villa Louvigny, L-2120 Luxembourg city, Luxembourg. [3]Département des maladies cardiovasculaires, Hypertension Unit, Centre Hospitalier Universitaire, 5, Rue du Morvan, 54500 Vandœuvre-lès-Nancy, France. [4]Ecole de Santé Publique, Université de Liège, 7, Place du 20 Août, 4000 Liège, Belgium.

### References

1. Kim J, et al. Dietary patterns derived by cluster analysis are associated with cognitive function among Korean older adults. Nutrients. 2015;7(6):4154–69.
2. Newby PK, Tucker KL. Empirically derived eating patterns using factor or cluster analysis: a review. Nutr Rev. 2004;62(5):177–203.
3. Lo Siou G, et al. Exploring statistical approaches to diminish subjectivity of cluster analysis to derive dietary patterns: the tomorrow project. Am J Epidemiol. 2011;173(8):956–67.
4. Berg CM, et al. Food patterns and cardiovascular disease risk factors: the Swedish INTERGENE research program. Am J Clin Nutr. 2008;88(2):289–97.
5. Anderson AL, et al. Relationships of dietary patterns with body composition in older adults differ by gender and PPAR-gamma Pro12Ala genotype. Eur J Nutr. 2010;49(7):385–94.
6. Michels KB, Schulze MB. Can dietary patterns help us detect diet-disease associations? Nutr Res Rev. 2005;18(2):241–8.
7. Thorpe MG, et al. A comparison of the dietary patterns derived by principal component analysis and cluster analysis in older Australians. Int J Behav Nutr Phys Act. 2016;13(1):30.
8. Lange T, et al. Stability-based validation of clustering solutions. Neural Comput. 2004;16(6):1299–323.
9. Alkerwi A, et al. Nutrition, environment and cardiovascular health (NESCAV): protocol of an inter-regional cross-sectional study. BMC Public Health. 2010;10:698.
10. Alkerwi A, et al. Comparison of participants and non-participants to the ORISCAV-LUX population-based study on cardiovascular risk factors in Luxembourg. BMC Med Res Methodol. 2010;10:80.
11. Alkerwi A, et al. First nationwide survey on cardiovascular risk factors in Grand-Duchy of Luxembourg (ORISCAV-LUX). BMC Public Health. 2010;10:468.
12. Sauvageot N, et al. Use of food frequency questionnaire to assess relationships between dietary habits and cardiovascular risk factors in NESCAV study: validation with biomarkers. Nutr J. 2013;12(1):143.
13. Sauvageot N, et al. Validation of the food frequency questionnaire used to assess the association between dietary habits and cardiovascular risk factors in the NESCAV study. J Nutr Food Sci. 2013;3(208):2.
14. Sjöström M, B A, Bauman A, et al. Guidelines for data processing and analysis of the International Physical Activity Questionnaire (IPAQ). Stockholm: Karolinka Institute; 2005.
15. Alkerwi A, et al. Adherence to physical activity recommendations and its associated factors: an interregional population-based study. J Public Health Res. 2015;4(1):406.
16. Willett W, Stampfer MJ. Total energy intake: implications for epidemiologic analyses. Am J Epidemiol. 1986;124(1):17–27.
17. Fransen HP, et al. A posteriori dietary patterns: how many patterns to retain? J Nutr. 2014;144(8):1274–82.
18. Gnanadesikan R, Kettenring JR, Tsao SL. Journal of Classification. 1995;12(1): 113–36.
19. Greve B, et al. A comparison of heuristic and model-based clustering methods for dietary pattern analysis. Public Health Nutr. 2016;19(2):255–64.
20. Wirfält E, Drake I, Wallström P. What do review papers conclude about food and dietary patterns? Food & Nutrition Research. 2013;57. doi:10.3402/fnr.v57i0.20523.
21. Slattery ML, et al. Eating patterns and risk of colon cancer. Am J Epidemiol. 1998;148(1):4–16.
22. Hu FB, et al. Prospective study of major dietary patterns and risk of coronary heart disease in men. Am J Clin Nutr. 2000;72(4):912–21.
23. Barker ME, et al. Dietary behaviours and sociocultural demographics in Northern Ireland. Br J Nutr. 1990;64(2):319–29.
24. Kerver JM, et al. Dietary patterns associated with risk factors for cardiovascular disease in healthy US adults. Am J Clin Nutr. 2003;78(6):1103–10.
25. Region, o.s.d.l.g.r.G., Statistiques en bref 2014. http://www.grande-region.lu/portal/.
26. Thorpe MG, Milte CM, Crawford D, McNaughton SA. A Revised Australian Dietary Guideline Index and Its Association with Key Sociodemographic Factors, Health Behaviors and Body Mass Index in Peri-Retirement Aged Adults. Nutrients. 2016;8(3):160.

27. Millen BE, et al. Dietary patterns and the odds of carotid atherosclerosis in women: the Framingham Nutrition Studies. Prev Med. 2002;35(6):540–7.
28. Huijbregts PP, Feskens EJ, Kromhout D. Dietary patterns and cardiovascular risk factors in elderly men: the Zutphen elderly study. Int J Epidemiol. 1995; 24(2):313–20.
29. Tucker KL, Dallal GE, Rush D. Dietary patterns of elderly Boston-area residents defined by cluster analysis. J Am Diet Assoc. 1992;92(12):1487–91.
30. van Dam RM, et al. Patterns of food consumption and risk factors for cardiovascular disease in the general Dutch population. Am J Clin Nutr. 2003;77(5):1156–63.
31. Vega-Lopez S, et al. Sex and hormonal status influence the effects of psyllium on lipoprotein remodeling and composition. Metabolism. 2002; 51(4):500–7.
32. Masson LF, McNeill G, Avenell A. Genetic variation and the lipid response to dietary intervention: a systematic review. Am J Clin Nutr. 2003;77(5): 1098–111.
33. Newby PK, Muller D, Tucker KL. Associations of empirically derived eating patterns with plasma lipid biomarkers: a comparison of factor and cluster analysis methods. Am J Clin Nutr. 2004;80(3):759–67.
34. Smith AD, et al. A comparison of dietary patterns derived by cluster and principal components analysis in a UK cohort of children. Eur J Clin Nutr. 2011;65(10):1102–9.
35. Hearty AP, Gibney MJ. Dietary patterns in Irish adolescents: a comparison of cluster and principal component analyses. Public Health Nutr. 2013;16(5):848–57.
36. Hoffman K, et al. Dietary patterns: report of an international workshop. Public Health Nutr. 2002;5(1):89–90.
37. Hennig C. Cluster-wise assessment of cluster stability. Computational Statistics & Data Analysis. 52(1):258–71

# 20

# Several grain dietary patterns are associated with better diet quality and improved shortfall nutrient intakes in US children and adolescents: a study focusing on the 2015–2020 Dietary Guidelines for Americans

Yanni Papanikolaou[1*], Julie Miller Jones[2] and Victor L. Fulgoni III[3]

## Abstract

**Background:** The present study identified the most commonly consumed grain food patterns in US children and adolescents (2–18 years-old; $N = 8,367$) relative to those not consuming grains and compared diet quality and nutrient intakes, with focus on 2015–2020 Dietary Guidelines for Americans (2015–2020 DGA) shortfall nutrients.

**Methods:** Cluster analysis using data from the National Health and Nutrition Examination Survey 2005–2010, identified 8 unique grain food patterns: a) no consumption of main grain groups, b) cakes, cookies and pies, c) yeast bread and rolls, d) cereals, e) pasta, cooked cereals and rice, f) crackers and salty snacks, g) pancakes, waffles and French toast and other grains, and h) quick breads.

**Results:** Energy intake was higher for all grain cluster patterns examined, except 'cereals', compared to no grains. Children and adolescents in the 'yeast bread and rolls', 'cereals', 'pasta, cooked cereals and rice', and 'crackers and salty snacks' patterns had a higher diet quality relative to no grains (all $p < 0.01$). Energy adjusted (EA) dietary fiber intake was greater in five of the seven grain patterns, ranging from 1.8 – 2.8 g more per day (all $p < 0.01$), as compared to those consuming no grains. All grain patterns, except cakes, cookies and pies had higher EA daily folate relative to children in the no grains pattern (all $p < 0.0001$). EA total fat was lower in 'cereals', 'pasta, cooked cereals and rice', and 'pancakes, waffles, French toast and other grains' in comparison to the no grains food pattern (all $p < 0.01$). EA magnesium intakes were greater in children and adolescents consuming 'yeast bread and rolls', 'pasta, cooked cereals and rice', and 'quick breads', while EA iron was higher in all grain patterns relative to no grains (all $p < 0.01$). EA vitamin D intake was higher only in children consuming 'cereals' vs. no grain group ($p < 0.0001$). There were no significant differences in total or added sugar intake across all grain clusters as compared to no grains.

**Conclusions:** Consumption of several, but not all, grain food patterns in children and adolescents were associated with improved 2015–2020 DGA shortfall nutrient intakes and diet quality as compared to those consuming no grains.

**Keywords:** NHANES, Grains, Children, Adolescents, Nutrient intakes, Diet quality

* Correspondence: papanikolaou.yanni@gmail.com
[1]Nutritional Strategies Inc., 59 Marriott Place, Paris, ON N3L 0A3, Canada
Full list of author information is available at the end of the article

## Background

The 2015–2020 Dietary Guidelines for Americans (2015–2020 DGA) policy report states that several nutrients are under-consumed relative to requirement levels set by the Institute of Medicine (IOM). These have been characterized as shortfall nutrients and include vitamin A, vitamin D, vitamin E, vitamin C, folate, calcium, magnesium, fiber, and potassium. For adolescent, premenopausal females and women who are pregnant, iron is also deemed an under-consumed nutrient of public health concern largely due to increased risk of iron-deficiency in these populations. Of the shortfall nutrients, calcium, vitamin D, fiber, and potassium also are classified as nutrients of public health concern because their under-consumption has been linked in the scientific literature to adverse health outcomes [1]. The report further identified that a healthy dietary pattern is higher in fruits, vegetables, whole grains, low- and non-fat dairy, seafood, legumes, and nuts; and lower in red and processed meat, sugar-sweetened foods and beverages and refined grains. However, a variety of grain-based food products, of which include refined/enriched grains, are sources for several shortfall nutrients identified by the DGA, including dietary fiber, folate, iron, and magnesium [1]. With mandatory folic acid fortification commencing in 1998 by the Food and Drug Administration [2], specific grain foods became leading sources for folate; breads, rolls, and crackers are the largest contributor of total folate to the US diet, contributing nearly 16% of total intake, which exceeds contribution of folate from vegetables [3]. Similarly, using data from the National Health and Nutrition Examination Survey (NHANES) 2003–2006, researchers have reported that fortification of grain foods substantially contributes nutrient adequacy for U.S. children and adolescents aged 2–18 years-old, without excessive intakes for most vitamins and minerals [4].

While certain grain food products are contributors of nutrients to limit in the diet, including added sugar, total and saturated fat [5, 6], grain foods also contribute positive nutrients to the diet, including dietary fiber, iron, magnesium, and B vitamins (thiamin, riboflavin, niacin and folate). Food sources of energy and nutrients data in children showed that while three of the top ten ranking foods for calorie contribution to the diet were grain-based foods, the top ten ranking food sources of dietary fiber included six grain-based products, collectively contributing 40% of total daily dietary fiber intake [4]. Others have argued that while three of the top ten sources of energy provided no nutritional value, the remaining sources of energy, including milk, beef, poultry, cheese and baked goods are significant contributors of nutrients of concern and other essential nutrients, postulating the premise that elimination of these foods from food patterns could potential have inadvertent effects on diet quality in the US population [6].

Recent NHANES data in adults showed that some, but not all, grain food patterns were associated with better nutrient intakes, improved diet quality and beneficial obesity-related parameters [7]. While 2015–2020 DGA identify several healthy dietary food patterns, and encourage increased whole grain consumption and reduced refined grain intake, at present, there are no data that evaluate the association of different grain food patterns on nutrient intakes and diet quality outcomes in children and adolescents. Further, some popular diet plans encourage diet patterns that omit gluten- containing or grain-based foods (e.g. Paleolithic diet) as healthier patterns [8, 9]. As such, the objective of the current analyses was to isolate the most commonly consumed grain food patterns in U.S. children and adolescents and compare nutrient intakes and diet quality of those consuming various grain food patterns to those not consuming grain foods using data from the National Health and Nutrition Examination Survey (NHANES) 2005–2010. The hypothesis for the present analysis was that certain grain food patterns are associated with improved diet quality and can significantly contribute nutrients, including shortfall nutrients, while concurrently lowering nutrients to limit in the diet.

## Methods

Data were obtained from What We Eat in America, the dietary intake component of NHANES. NHANES is a government-directed program led by the Center for Disease Control and Prevention in collaboration with US Department of Agriculture. Written informed consent was obtained for all participants or proxies, and the survey protocol was approved by the Research Ethics Review Board at the National Center for Health Statistics. **The distribution of the civilian non-institutionalized US population, as well as response rate percentages and population totals in NHANES 2005–2010 data by age and gender, can be viewed at www.cdc.gov/nchs/nhanes/response_rates_cps.htm.** Data from the current NHANES are released every two years and for the current analyses, we used three data releases, namely 2005–2006, 2007–2008, and 2009–2010 [10, 11].

**The dietary intake data were obtained from an in-person 24-hour dietary recall (Day 1) by trained specialists using the Automated Multiple-Pass Method [12] as a means to reduce bias in reporting energy and nutrient intakes in the Mobile Examination Center. The Multiple-Pass Method consisted of five steps: (1) the quick list, which included an uninterrupted list of foods and beverages consumed by the subject; (2) the forgotten foods list, which queried the subject on categories of foods that have been documented as frequently forgotten; (3) a time and occasion where foods were consumed; (4) the detail cycle, which elicited descriptions of foods and amounts consumed with the**

**aid of an interactive Food Model Booklet and measuring guides; and (5) final probe review.** USDA's Food and Nutrient Database for Dietary Studies, 3.0, 4.1, and 5.0 was used to code dietary intake data and calculate nutrient intakes [13–15].

Cluster analysis was used to develop patterns of grain consumption—a statistical procedure that analyses large data sets to identify various patterns while trying to maximize differences among the patterns. **Cluster analysis allows for the focus on a specifically defined aspect (i.e., grain food consumption) and then forces maximal differences in clusters for assessments. Cluster analysis also allows for group comparisons rather than factor analysis which are generally associations.** The USDA food coding system was used to define categories of grain foods [15]. Grain foods intake patterns were identified using SAS 9.2 (SAS Institute, Cary, NC, 2013) PROC CLUSTER using a single 24-hour dietary recall in NHANES 2005–2010. **SUDAAN v.11.0 (Research Triangle Institute; Raleigh, NC) was used to adjust analyses for sampling weights and the sampling units and strata information as provided by NHANES.** Clusters were developed based on the percentage of calories consumed from the grain products as the centroid for each cluster. Grains from flour and dry mixes, mixed dishes, and meat substitutes were not included in development of grain clusters. Cluster analyses provides the ability to focus on a particular defined aspect (e.g. calories from grains) and then forces maximal differences in clusters for assessment. For these analyses, the USDA grains products main categories were used to identify the grain cluster patterns of intake (see Table 1).

All main grain food codes fit into one and only one of the grain foods groupings. The patterns identified by the cluster analysis were then identified by percent calories within each grain food grouping (only groups that contributed 5% or more of calories were used to define the clusters) at the centroid of each cluster. Using this method resulted in seven readily identifiable grain food patterns and a no consumption of main grain groups (i.e., no grains group); creating eight unique patterns of **grain food** consumption. With grain food cluster patterns identified, and using the output from the cluster procedure, each subject was then placed in the cluster that matched most closely to the pattern of calories across the food categories.

Adjusted **least-square means ± SE** values for subjects were determined in each cluster using PROC REGRESS and LOGREGRESS in SUDAAN 11.0 **for dietary intakes and diet quality [Healthy Eating Index (HEI)-2010]** with various sets of covariates. Covariates for analyses of energy intake, HEI-2010 and HEI sub-components [16] were age, gender, and ethnicity. **The poverty income ratio (PIR) grouped into three categories (<1.25, 1.25-3.49, and >3.49) and physical activity (sedentary, moderate or vigorous based on questionnaire responses), current smoking status, alcohol intake (g/d), and energy intake for nutrient-related variables (with the exception of energy intake itself or HEI-2010) also served as covariates. The PIR values reflected the federally established poverty criteria, thus a PIR of <1.25 equated to below 125% of poverty, while higher values represented the subject was from a higher income status.** The HEI-2010 provides a measure of diet quality and measures conformance to federal dietary guidance and has been predominantly used to monitor dietary practices of the US population and the low-income subpopulation. Nutrient intakes were also adjusted for energy intakes. The main comparison of interest was to compare results between the no consumption of main grain groups (cluster 0) and all other clusters. A conservative *P*-value of $p < 0.01$ was set for significance.

**Table 1** Grain cluster pattern based on percentage of calories from grains in children and adolescents 2–18 years-old of age using data from NHANES 2005–2010

| Cluster Number | Grain Foods Pattern | Description |
|---|---|---|
| 0 | No Grains | 4.0% of the population |
| 1 | Cakes, Cookies and Pies | (5.1% of the population) with approximately 92% of grains coming from this grain group) |
| 2 | Yeast Breads and Rolls | (33.8% of the population) with over 68% of grains coming from this grain group; |
| 3 | Cereals | (4.0% of the population) with over 95% of grains coming from this grain group; |
| 4 | Pasta, Cooked Cereals and Rice | (4.9% of the population) with over 67% of grains coming from this grain group; |
| 5 | Crackers and Salty Snacks | (26.1% of the population) with over 53% of grains coming from this grain group; |
| 6 | Pancakes, Waffles, French Toast and Other Grains | (9.4% of the population) with over 51% of grains coming from this grain group and approximately 23% of grains coming from yeast bread and rolls. |
| 7 | Quick Breads | (12.8% of the population) with approximately 57% of grains coming from this group. |

## Results

Eight grain clusters were identified, one of which included isolating a group of children and adolescents that did not consume any of the identified grains (4.0% of the population). The eight clusters are defined as outlined in Table 1, namely: 1) no consumption of main grain groups, 2) cakes, cookies and pies 3) yeast breads and rolls, 4) cereals, 5) pasta, cooked cereal and rice, 6) crackers and salty snacks, 7) pancakes, waffles, French toast, and 8) quick breads.

### Energy and nutrient intakes

Energy intake was significantly higher for children and adolescents in all grain pattern clusters, with the exception of 'cereals' ($p = 0.089$), when compared to the no grains group. The higher energy intake ranged from 416 – 524 kcal/d with 'pancakes, waffles, French toast and other grains' and 'quick breads' clusters representing the greatest increase in kcal/day (Table 2).

Energy adjusted nutrient intakes in the eight grain food patterns are presented in Table 2. When examining nutrients of concern, as outlined by the 2015–2010 DGA [1], no differences in calcium intake was observed in children all of the grain clusters compared to those not consuming grain foods, while dietary fiber was higher in children consuming 'yeast breads and rolls', 'cereals', 'pasta, cooked cereals and rice', 'crackers and salty snacks', and 'quick breads', ranging from 1.8 – 2.8 g/day greater daily fiber than children and adolescents in the no grains group.

In terms of nutrients (i.e., vitamins and minerals) present naturally or added to grain foods, via either enrichment or fortification practices, nutrient intakes were higher for those in certain grain clusters. Iron intake was greater across all seven grain clusters examined, thus demonstrating the relevance of both the naturally occurring and added iron in contributing to this 2015–2020 DGA shortfall nutrient. Daily vitamin D (D2 + D3) was significantly greater only in children and adolescents consuming a 'cereals' grain pattern, while no significant differences were observed with potassium intakes in any of the grain clusters as compared to those not consuming grain food products. Intakes of thiamin were significantly higher for children and adolescents consuming all grain clusters, except for 'cakes, cookies and pies', while daily intakes of riboflavin were significantly greater all grain patterns, with the exception of 'cakes, cookies and pies', 'pasta, cooked cereals and rice' and 'crackers and salty snacks' when compared to those not consuming grain foods. Similarly, folate was higher (76 – 411 µg/d; all $p < 0.0001$) in those in all grain food clusters, except 'cakes, cookies and pies', relative to the no grains cluster. Zinc intake was higher only in children and adolescents consuming 'yeast breads and rolls', 'cereals' and 'pasta, cooked cereals and rice' and significantly lower in those consuming 'cakes, cookies and pies' compared to those in the no grains cluster. Magnesium intakes were greater in children and adolescents consuming 'yeast bread and rolls', 'pasta, cooked cereals and rice', and 'quick breads' relative to the no grains group (Table 2).

Regarding nutrients to limit, daily saturated fat intake was significantly lower in all grain patterns examined, with the exception of 'yeast breads and rolls' and 'quick breads', compared to those not consuming grain foods, with a range of difference in saturated fat ranging from 1.5 – 4.8 g less per day. Daily sodium intake was only lower (approximately 350 mg/day) in children and adolescents consuming 'cakes, cookies and pies' compared to the no grains cluster pattern. There were no significant differences in total and added sugar intake across all grain clusters as compared to the no grain cluster (Table 2).

### Diet quality assessment

Diet quality, as measured by USDA's HEI-2010 is depicted in Table 3. Four of the grain clusters had significantly greater scores when compared to the no grains cluster. Specifically, those in the 'pasta, cooked cereals and rice' had the greatest score at 50.6 ± 1.0, while children and adolescents consuming 'yeast breads and rolls', 'cereals' and 'crackers and salty snacks' had scores of 46.1 ± 0.5, 48.5 ± 1.2, and 46.0 ± 0.4, respectively (all $p < 0.001$) compared to the no grains cluster (42.7 ± 0.9).

When examining the subcomponents of HEI-2010 (Table 3), children and adolescents in the 'crackers, salty snacks', 'pancakes, waffles, French toast and other grains' and 'quick breads' had significantly lower total vegetable scores than subjects in the no grains pattern. Children and adolescents in all grain clusters examined had significantly greater scores for whole grains as compared to those not consuming grain foods, which indicated higher consumption of whole grains (see Table 3). Children and adolescents in the 'cakes, cookies and pies' grain cluster were the only cluster to show significantly higher scores for sodium intake relative to individuals not consuming grains. The lower HEI-2010 sub-component scores were more than offset with increased scores for those in the 'yeast breads and rolls', 'cereal', 'pasta, cooked cereals and rice' and 'crackers and salty snacks' clusters for total fruit, whole fruit and whole grains as compared to those not consuming grain foods. Additionally, children and adolescents consuming 'yeast breads and rolls', 'pasta, cooked cereals, and rice', 'crackers and salty snacks' and 'quick breads' had significantly higher scores for greens and beans, while the 'cereals' cluster showed higher dairy scores in comparison to children and adolescents in the no grains pattern. The significantly greater score for empty calories in the 'pasta, cooked cereals, and rice' cluster translates as fewer calories from solid fats, alcohol and added sugars), while those consuming 'cakes, cookies and pies' ingested more calories from solid fats, alcohol and added sugars relative to the no grains dietary pattern.

## Discussion

This is the first study that has identified various grain food patterns in US children and adolescents with

**Table 2** Adjusted mean (SE) nutrient and energy intake for all grain clusters using NHANES 2005–2010, 2–18 years of age

| | No Grains | | Cakes, Cookies & Pies | | | Yeast Breads and Rolls | | | Cereals | | | Pasta, Cooked Cereals & Rice | | | Crackers & Salty Snacks | | | Pancakes, Waffles, French Toast and Other Grains | | | Quick Breads | | |
|---|---|---|---|---|---|---|---|---|---|---|---|---|---|---|---|---|---|---|---|---|---|---|---|
| Energy or Nutrient | Cluster 0 | | Cluster 1 | | | Cluster 2 | | | Cluster 3 | | | Cluster 4 | | | Cluster 5 | | | Cluster 6 | | | Cluster 7 | | |
| | LSM | SE | LSM | SE | P | LSM | SE | P | LSM | SE | P | LSM | SE | P | LSM | SE | P | LSM | SE | P | LSM | SE | P |
| Energy (kcal) | 1497 | 90 | 1931 | 65 | 0.0009 | 1961 | 22 | <0.0001 | 1694 | 65 | 0.0887 | 1913 | 62 | 0.0005 | 1946 | 29 | <0.0001 | 2021 | 39 | <0.0001 | 2021 | 36 | <0.0001 |
| Carbohydrate (g) | 245 | 6.0 | 268 | 3.4 | 0.0016 | 256 | 1.2 | 0.0679 | 269 | 4.2 | 0.0012 | 272 | 3.4 | 0.0004 | 262 | 1.4 | 0.0046 | 265 | 2.2 | 0.0014 | 255 | 2.1 | 0.1542 |
| Total sugars (g) | 134 | 6.7 | 149 | 3.6 | 0.0594 | 130 | 1.4 | 0.6016 | 139 | 4.9 | 0.5190 | 130 | 4.4 | 0.6484 | 128 | 1.7 | 0.3738 | 130 | 2.3 | 0.6479 | 124 | 1.9 | 0.1674 |
| Added sugars (tsp eq) | 22 | 2.0 | 25 | 0.5 | 0.1791 | 20 | 0.3 | 0.2535 | 21 | 1.0 | 0.7195 | 19 | 1.1 | 0.1331 | 20 | 0.4 | 0.2152 | 20 | 0.6 | 0.3609 | 18 | 0.4 | 0.0874 |
| Protein (g) | 72 | 2.2 | 59 | 1.1 | <0.0001 | 72 | 0.5 | 0.7474 | 70 | 1.5 | 0.2823 | 72 | 1.7 | 0.9931 | 65 | 0.6 | 0.0004 | 67 | 1.3 | 0.0301 | 68 | 0.9 | 0.0685 |
| Total fat (g) | 76 | 1.9 | 72 | 1.2 | 0.0958 | 71 | 0.4 | 0.0296 | 67 | 1.5 | 0.0004 | 64 | 1.3 | <0.0001 | 72 | 0.5 | 0.0727 | 70 | 0.8 | 0.0022 | 74 | 0.8 | 0.4128 |
| Total monounsaturated fatty acids (g) | 27 | 0.8 | 28 | 0.6 | 0.7623 | 26 | 0.2 | 0.0648 | 24 | 0.7 | 0.0003 | 23 | 0.5 | <0.0001 | 26 | 0.3 | 0.1789 | 26 | 0.4 | 0.0958 | 27 | 0.4 | 0.7836 |
| Total saturated fatty acids (g) | 27 | 0.7 | 25 | 0.5 | 0.0080 | 26 | 0.2 | 0.0313 | 25 | 0.6 | 0.0049 | 22 | 0.7 | <0.0001 | 25 | 0.2 | 0.0001 | 24 | 0.5 | 0.0001 | 26 | 0.4 | 0.0311 |
| Cholesterol (mg) | 261 | 23.5 | 184 | 8.0 | 0.0018 | 229 | 4.5 | 0.1745 | 198 | 9.4 | 0.0163 | 211 | 8.1 | 0.0771 | 189 | 4.2 | 0.0074 | 240 | 9.7 | 0.4133 | 233 | 9.9 | 0.2342 |
| Dietary fiber (g) | 11 | 0.5 | 12 | 0.4 | 0.4815 | 13 | 0.2 | 0.0007 | 13 | 0.6 | 0.0052 | 13 | 0.5 | <0.0001 | 13 | 0.2 | 0.0006 | 12 | 0.3 | 0.1014 | 14 | 0.3 | <0.0001 |
| Calcium (mg) | 962 | 53.5 | 863 | 28.2 | 0.1005 | 1054 | 12.6 | 0.0898 | 1092 | 31.5 | 0.0388 | 964 | 31.0 | 0.9737 | 968 | 13.6 | 0.8987 | 1056 | 32.4 | 0.1635 | 1043 | 19.1 | 0.1526 |
| Magnesium (mg) | 208 | 8.7 | 204 | 5.0 | 0.6863 | 232 | 2.1 | 0.0089 | 231 | 4.9 | 0.0158 | 257 | 6.7 | <0.0001 | 230 | 2.3 | 0.0141 | 209 | 2.9 | 0.8743 | 237 | 4.5 | 0.0009 |
| Iron (mg) | 10.6 | 0.3 | 11.8 | 0.3 | 0.0097 | 14.17 | 0.15 | <0.0001 | 19.03 | 0.67 | <0.0001 | 15.45 | 0.39 | <0.0001 | 14.16 | 0.21 | <0.0001 | 13.34 | 0.23 | <0.0001 | 13.44 | 0.25 | <0.0001 |
| Zinc (mg) | 9.4 | 0.3 | 8.2 | 0.2 | 0.0016 | 10.97 | 0.16 | 0.0001 | 12.74 | 0.41 | <0.0001 | 11.00 | 0.37 | 0.0050 | 10.12 | 0.12 | 0.0322 | 9.23 | 0.22 | 0.7165 | 9.93 | 0.19 | 0.2085 |
| Sodium (mg) | 2996 | 87.24 | 2645 | 44.20 | 0.0018 | 3137 | 23.94 | 0.1432 | 3004 | 71.10 | 0.9403 | 3429 | 150.37 | 0.0107 | 3066 | 38.87 | 0.4346 | 3129 | 45.06 | 0.2079 | 3118 | 55.97 | 0.2002 |
| Potassium (mg) | 2148 | 91.60 | 2021 | 69.94 | 0.2406 | 2243 | 21.46 | 0.3103 | 2333 | 46.88 | 0.0663 | 2365 | 51.12 | 0.0385 | 2070 | 23.24 | 0.3637 | 2044 | 33.81 | 0.3037 | 2209 | 39.34 | 0.5443 |
| Folate, DFE (µg) | 361 | 12.60 | 393 | 13.48 | 0.0694 | 526 | 10.60 | <0.0001 | 772 | 36.39 | <0.0001 | 636 | 29.86 | <0.0001 | 523 | 11.21 | <0.0001 | 438 | 9.85 | <0.0001 | 498 | 12.04 | <0.0001 |
| Riboflavin (Vitamin B2) (mg) | 1.8 | 0.1 | 1.8 | 0.0 | 0.9836 | 2.1 | 0.03 | 0.0001 | 2.6 | 0.04 | <0.0001 | 2.0 | 0.05 | 0.0171 | 2.0 | 0.03 | 0.0154 | 2.1 | 0.04 | 0.0014 | 2.1 | 0.05 | 0.0031 |
| Thiamin (Vitamin B1) (mg) | 1.3 | 0.0 | 1.3 | 0.1 | 0.7019 | 1.6 | 0.02 | <0.0001 | 1.9 | 0.04 | <0.0001 | 1.7 | 0.04 | <0.0001 | 1.5 | 0.03 | 0.0003 | 1.5 | 0.03 | 0.0024 | 1.5 | 0.03 | <0.0001 |
| Total choline (mg) | 266 | 14.4 | 215 | 5.5 | 0.0007 | 260 | 3.4 | 0.6977 | 245 | 7.7 | 0.2363 | 264 | 6.9 | 0.9240 | 225 | 2.7 | 0.0053 | 260 | 7.4 | 0.6825 | 256 | 5.8 | 0.5145 |
| Vitamin A, RAE (µg) | 481 | 34.5 | 536 | 29.2 | 0.1948 | 599 | 9.8 | 0.0016 | 736 | 21.5 | <0.0001 | 666 | 39.2 | 0.0008 | 551 | 12.2 | 0.0592 | 650 | 21.7 | 0.0001 | 578 | 18.6 | 0.0192 |
| Vitamin B12 (µg) | 4.2 | 0.2 | 3.8 | 0.1 | 0.1470 | 5.3 | 0.1 | 0.0001 | 6.8 | 0.3 | <0.0001 | 4.7 | 0.2 | 0.1237 | 4.7 | 0.1 | 0.0246 | 4.9 | 0.1 | 0.0255 | 4.8 | 0.2 | 0.0529 |
| Vitamin B6 (mg) | 1.4 | 0.1 | 1.4 | 0.0 | 0.7590 | 1.7 | 0.03 | 0.0004 | 2.2 | 0.1 | <0.0001 | 1.9 | 0.1 | <0.0001 | 1.6 | 0.03 | 0.0059 | 1.7 | 0.04 | 0.0031 | 1.7 | 0.1 | 0.0045 |

**Table 2** Adjusted mean (SE) nutrient and energy intake for all grain clusters using NHANES 2005–2010, 2–18 years of age *(Continued)*

| | | | | | | | | | | | | | | | | | | | | | | | |
|---|---|---|---|---|---|---|---|---|---|---|---|---|---|---|---|---|---|---|---|---|---|---|---|
| Vitamin C (mg) | 70.0 | 5.0 | 78.0 | 6.0 | 0.2829 | 80.0 | 2.0 | 0.0690 | 83.9 | 6.1 | 0.0575 | 103.6 | 9.0 | 0.0025 | 80.0 | 2.6 | 0.0846 | 72.3 | 3.1 | 0.7126 | 78.7 | 3.0 | 0.1833 |
| Vitamin D (D2 + D3) (μg) | 5.0 | 0.5 | 4.7 | 0.3 | 0.5028 | 6.0 | 0.2 | 0.0753 | 7.6 | 0.4 | <0.0001 | 6.0 | 0.2 | 0.1363 | 5.3 | 0.1 | 0.5640 | 5.3 | 0.3 | 0.6946 | 5.8 | 0.2 | 0.1939 |
| Vitamin E as alpha-tocopherol (mg) | 5.8 | 0.3 | 5.6 | 0.2 | 0.6583 | 5.9 | 0.2 | 0.6465 | 5.1 | 0.1 | 0.0198 | 5.9 | 0.4 | 0.7239 | 6.2 | 0.1 | 0.1437 | 5.4 | 0.1 | 0.1511 | 6.1 | 0.2 | 0.3859 |
| Vitamin K (μg) | 52.7 | 4.0 | 57.4 | 5.4 | 0.4934 | 58.2 | 2.6 | 0.3003 | 52.2 | 5.5 | 0.9396 | 76.7 | 9.8 | 0.0277 | 52.4 | 1.9 | 0.9567 | 55.9 | 3.3 | 0.5779 | 55.4 | 1.7 | 0.5403 |

NHANES 2005–2010, $N = 8{,}367$

*LSM*: least square mean; *SE*: standard error; $P = p$ value of difference as compared to cluster 0 (No grains)

Covariates include age, gender, ethnicity, poverty income ratio, physical activity, current smoking status, alcohol and for all variables except Energy, the covariate of energy (kcal)

**Table 3** Adjusted mean (SE) Total healthy eating index-2010 (HEI) and component scores for all grain clusters using NHANES 2005–2010, 2–18 years of age

| | No Grains | | Cakes, Cookies & Pies | | | Yeast Breads and Rolls | | | Cereals | | | Pasta, Cooked Cereals & Rice | | | Crackers & Salty Snacks | | | Pancakes, Waffles, French Toast and Other Grains | | | Quick Breads | | |
|---|---|---|---|---|---|---|---|---|---|---|---|---|---|---|---|---|---|---|---|---|---|---|---|
| HEI-2010 Component | Cluster 0 | | Cluster 1 | | | Cluster 2 | | | Cluster 3 | | | Cluster 4 | | | Cluster 5 | | | Cluster 6 | | | Cluster 7 | | |
| | LSM | SE | LSM | SE | P | LSM | SE | P | LSM | SE | P | LSM | SE | P | LSM | SE | P | LSM | SE | P | LSM | SE | P |
| Total Vegetables | 2.52 | 0.13 | 2.13 | 0.10 | 0.0327 | 2.16 | 0.05 | 0.0121 | 2.44 | 0.16 | 0.7002 | 2.56 | 0.17 | 0.8395 | 1.93 | 0.06 | 0.0001 | 1.74 | 0.10 | <0.0001 | 2.06 | 0.07 | 0.0024 |
| Greens and Beans | 0.30 | 0.07 | 0.50 | 0.10 | 0.0784 | 0.62 | 0.05 | 0.0002 | 0.61 | 0.16 | 0.0617 | 1.32 | 0.20 | <0.0001 | 0.54 | 0.04 | 0.0064 | 0.52 | 0.09 | 0.0808 | 0.77 | 0.08 | 0.0004 |
| Total Fruit | 1.97 | 0.11 | 2.28 | 0.14 | 0.0468 | 2.58 | 0.07 | <0.0001 | 2.51 | 0.17 | 0.0039 | 2.72 | 0.16 | 0.0007 | 2.55 | 0.06 | <0.0001 | 2.60 | 0.12 | 0.0002 | 2.57 | 0.10 | 0.0003 |
| Whole Fruit | 1.72 | 0.17 | 1.96 | 0.19 | 0.3720 | 2.31 | 0.08 | 0.0004 | 2.38 | 0.23 | 0.0073 | 2.51 | 0.18 | 0.0081 | 2.21 | 0.07 | 0.0038 | 2.33 | 0.14 | 0.0079 | 2.25 | 0.09 | 0.0087 |
| Whole Grains | 0.26 | 0.06 | 0.57 | 0.10 | 0.0033 | 2.11 | 0.08 | <0.0001 | 2.24 | 0.17 | <0.0001 | 2.58 | 0.28 | <0.0001 | 2.36 | 0.12 | <0.0001 | 1.44 | 0.15 | <0.0001 | 1.66 | 0.12 | <0.0001 |
| Dairy | 6.84 | 0.26 | 6.53 | 0.25 | 0.3773 | 7.20 | 0.09 | 0.2028 | 8.09 | 0.29 | 0.0029 | 6.78 | 0.22 | 0.8751 | 6.76 | 0.11 | 0.7361 | 6.89 | 0.21 | 0.8796 | 7.12 | 0.16 | 0.3282 |
| Total Protein Foods | 3.65 | 0.14 | 3.03 | 0.14 | 0.0002 | 3.74 | 0.05 | 0.4854 | 3.38 | 0.16 | 0.1844 | 3.66 | 0.15 | 0.9260 | 3.36 | 0.05 | 0.0363 | 3.59 | 0.09 | 0.7878 | 3.47 | 0.08 | 0.3256 |
| Seafood and Plant Protein | 0.98 | 0.13 | 1.10 | 0.16 | 0.4806 | 1.46 | 0.08 | <0.0001 | 0.98 | 0.18 | 0.9839 | 1.45 | 0.21 | 0.1112 | 1.37 | 0.06 | 0.0161 | 1.14 | 0.09 | 0.2582 | 1.47 | 0.09 | 0.0018 |
| Fatty Acid Ratio | 3.31 | 0.23 | 3.84 | 0.23 | 0.1020 | 3.30 | 0.08 | 0.9556 | 3.06 | 0.34 | 0.5560 | 4.15 | 0.31 | 0.0378 | 4.34 | 0.11 | 0.0001 | 3.74 | 0.18 | 0.1540 | 3.81 | 0.16 | 0.1028 |
| Sodium | 4.98 | 0.34 | 6.78 | 0.23 | 0.0002 | 4.69 | 0.09 | 0.4418 | 4.98 | 0.35 | 1.0000 | 3.97 | 0.34 | 0.0330 | 5.00 | 0.14 | 0.9503 | 4.69 | 0.20 | 0.4555 | 4.93 | 0.18 | 0.8815 |
| Refined Grains | 6.78 | 0.30 | 5.72 | 0.23 | 0.0054 | 5.40 | 0.12 | 0.0001 | 7.02 | 0.33 | 0.5979 | 6.55 | 0.26 | 0.5711 | 4.95 | 0.08 | <0.0001 | 4.63 | 0.21 | <0.0001 | 4.20 | 0.16 | <0.0001 |
| SoFAAS Calories | 9.42 | 0.58 | 6.46 | 0.41 | 0.0003 | 10.50 | 0.21 | 0.0992 | 10.80 | 0.63 | 0.1216 | 12.33 | 0.54 | 0.0004 | 10.65 | 0.16 | 0.0250 | 10.19 | 0.36 | 0.2374 | 10.00 | 0.34 | 0.3755 |
| HEI-2010 Total Score | 42.72 | 0.85 | 40.90 | 0.92 | 0.1926 | 46.06 | 0.48 | 0.0003 | 48.48 | 1.19 | 0.0005 | 50.58 | 1.02 | <0.0001 | 46.02 | 0.44 | 0.0009 | 43.49 | 0.60 | 0.4102 | 44.33 | 0.65 | 0.1534 |

NHANES 2005–2010, $N = 8{,}367$

*LSM*: least square mean; *SE*: standard error; $P = p$: value of difference as compared to cluster 0 (no grains)

*SoFAAS*: solid fat, alcohol, added sugars

Covariates include age, gender, ethnicity, poverty income ratio, physical activity, current smoking status, and alcohol

reported associations between grain pattern consumption, energy and nutrient intakes and diet quality. The current data support that a variety of grain food patterns, including those recommended by dietary guidance and those that focus on enriched and fortified grain staples, are associated with greater nutrient intakes, including higher consumption of shortfall nutrients and nutrients of public health concern as identified by the 2015–2020 DGA [1], in comparison to an alternative dietary pattern that does not emphasize grain-based foods in children and adolescents. The findings from the present study are aligned with recently published data in American adults, where consumption of specific grain foods were associated with greater nutrient intakes, including greater consumption of shortfall nutrients and nutrients of public health concern. Several, but not all grain food patterns, were associated with improved diet quality compared to adults not consuming main grain groups. Adults consuming pasta, cooked cereals and rice also had lower body weights and smaller waist circumferences when compared to individuals not consuming grain foods [7].

**Several nutrients contributed by grain foods naturally or via fortification/enrichment, including folate, calcium, magnesium, fiber and iron are under consumed relative to IOM nutrition standards [17]. Dietary patterns that encourage nutrient-dense grain foods, with the concept of limiting sodium, total fat and sugar, may help shift population consumption in children and adolescents toward recommended intake levels for several shortfall nutrients identified by 2015 DGAC [17]. Additionally, creating positive habits including nutrient-dense dietary patterns that include whole and enriched grain consumption in earlier years may benefit health outcomes into adulthood [18, 19].** Indeed, the current research in children and adolescents provides a sound rationale to support more specific dietary guidance for American children and adolescents about grain consumption rather than simply having two broad categories of recommended intakes that revolve around refined/enriched and whole grains. The current data illustrates how various enriched grain products contribute to daily nutrient intakes and overall diet quality. For example, we observed that children and adolescents consuming 'yeast breads and rolls,' 'cereals,' 'pasta, cooked cereals and rice,' and 'crackers and salty snacks' grain patterns had a significantly higher diet quality, as measured by USDA's HEI-2010 and dietary fiber intake was significantly greater in five of the eight patterns, ranging from 1.8 – 2.8 g more daily fiber, as compared to those consuming no grain foods. It is rationale to suggest that these daily increases in dietary fiber can have a meaningful impact on public health initiatives by helping to minimize gaps in fiber consumption in children and adolescents. In fact, a recent study evaluating ten-year trends in fiber intakes using NHANES data from 2001–2010 in children and adolescents reported mean fiber intake to be $13.2 \pm 0.1$ g/day [20]. Thus, dietary fiber intake levels in children and adolescents continue to fall short of meeting dietary guidance based on recommendations set forth by the Institute of Medicine where fiber Adequate Intake in children 1 – 8 years and children and adolescents 9–18 years is set at 19 – 25 g/day and 26 – 38 g/day, respectively [21].

Collaborative efforts from the American Heart Association, American College of Cardiology and The Obesity Society state that nearly one-third of children and youth are overweight or obese, further exacerbating poor health profiles and increasing risks for chronic diseases and their co-morbidities [22, 23]. In the current analyses, total fat intake was lower in, 'cereals' and 'pasta, cooked cereals and rice,' and daily saturated fat intake was lower in many of the grain patterns examined, in comparison to the no grains food pattern. The range of saturated fat lowering per day translates to meaningful reductions when considering the U.S. Food and Drug Administration's Daily Value (DV) for saturated fat; the mean lowering of saturated fat ranged from 1.5 – 4.8 g per day which represents 7.5 – 24% of the DV for adults and children ≥4 years of age consuming 2000 kcal/day. Taken collectively, some grain food patterns, comprised of both whole and enriched grains, can be beneficial in children and adolescents when considering dietary guidance and health outcomes.

Our results are aligned with previous observational findings that considered sources of nutrients in the US diet. When identifying the top food sources of nutrients, including both intrinsic and added to foods via fortification, results showed that grain foods represented the top five ranking food sources for folate, such that ready-to-eat cereals, yeast breads and rolls, pizza, pasta and crackers, popcorn, pretzels, and chips contributed 56.7 and 54.4% of folate to the diet of children and adolescents, respectively. Results were similar another shortfall nutrient, such that grain foods represented the top five food sources for iron in the diet of US children and adolescents, with ready-to eat cereals, yeast breads, pizza, cakes, cookies, and pies, and crackers, popcorn, pretzels, and chips cumulatively contributing 52.1 and 48.7% of iron [24].

The 2015–2020 DGA and 2015 Dietary Guidelines Advisory Committee (2015 DGAC) report further states 'of the shortfall nutrients, calcium, vitamin D, fiber, and potassium also are classified as nutrients of public health concern because their under consumption has been linked in the scientific literature to adverse health outcomes" [21], a principle carried forward from the DGA 2010 policy document [25]. The 2015 DGAC [17] also reports that "if whole grains were consumed in the amounts recommended in the recommended food patterns, whole grains would provide substantial percentages of several key nutrients, such as about 32% of dietary fiber, 42% of iron, 35% of folate, 29% of magnesium and 16% of vitamin A". While these nutrients levels represent significant contributions from whole grains, whole grain consumption alone can still leave a gap between consumption and recommendation levels. The 2005 DGAC reported that refined grains contribute substantial levels of key nutrients to food patterns, naming folate, iron, calcium, dietary fiber, thiamin, riboflavin and niacin [26], thus demonstrating the importance of consuming both enriched and whole grains. The committee further acknowledged that including only three ounce equivalents of whole grains daily with no refined grains in recommended food patterns would lower intake of many of key nutrients and potentially place specific populations at risk for nutrient inadequacy [26]; an argument which led the 2015 DGAC to conclude that consumption of whole grains with no substitutions would result in nutrient shortfalls [17]. The current analysis provides data linking different grain food patterns with nutrient intakes and concurrently we observe the adverse nutrient- and health-related outcomes when grain foods as a whole are eliminated from the diet. In many of the grain patterns examined, we see a better overall nutrient intake profile, which demonstrates the important dietary contributions made by different grain foods and emphasizes the importance of consuming a balance of whole grains, enriched and fortified grain products. Indeed, while some of the grain food clusters contributed nutrients to limit in the diet as identified by the 2015–2020 DGA [1], including saturated fat, added sugars, and sodium, several of the grain food patterns were associated with lower intakes of these nutrients and improved shortfall nutrients and diet quality. Such findings provide a rationale for more specific, evidence-based dietary guidance around grain consumption.

There are several limitations to the present analysis that deserve recognition. Data for energy and nutrient intakes, including values reported for diet quality, were obtained using 24-hour dietary recalls, which rely on study participant memory. While validated procedures are used to collect the data, recalled information may be inaccurate and biased from misreporting or memory challenges [27]. In addition, the current evidence, being observational, cannot establish a causal link between the different grain foods patterns examined and improvements in nutrient intakes and diet quality. However, a large strength of the current work stems from the use of NHANES, which is a large continuous survey that examines a nationally representative sample of about 5,000 individuals yearly by highly-trained medical personnel. Additionally, numerous covariates were used to adjust the data in an attempt to remove potential confounding scenarios. However, residual confounding may still exist and may explain some of the results reported. Lastly, we identified a small percentage of the population with no consumption of the main grain groups investigated, which served as the comparison group. While the comparison group was relevant for research purposes, it only represented 4% of the population, suggesting that further research is required.

## Conclusions

Several grain food dietary patterns in U.S. children and adolescents are associated with greater nutrient intakes, including greater consumption of shortfall nutrients and nutrients of public health concern as identified by the 2015–2020 DGA. Improved diet quality, as measured by USDA's HEI-2010 was also linked to consumption of specific grain food patterns, including 'pasta, cooked cereals and rice, 'cereals,' 'yeast breads and rolls' and 'crackers and salty snacks,' when compared to those children and adolescents not consuming grain food dietary pattern. Improved diet quality was due not only to the contribution of nutrients inherent in the grain, but also to those added through enrichment and fortification practices and those provided by natural food pairings such as cereal and dairy foods (i.e., milk). Overall, while some grain food patterns were associated with elevated sodium and added sugar, the present data also support that several grain food patterns can serve as part of a healthy dietary food pattern in children and adolescents, that accounts for 2015–2020 DGA dietary recommendations to reduce total fat, saturated fat and added sugar consumption, while concurrently increasing intake of shortfall nutrients and/or nutrients of concern, including iron, magnesium, dietary fiber, vitamin D, potassium and folate.

#### Acknowledgments
Not Applicable.

#### Funding
This project has been funded by the Grain Foods Foundation. The funding group had no role in the design of the study and collection, analysis and interpretation of the data, nor in the writing of the manuscript.

#### Authors' contributions
YP and JMJ collaborated on the intellectual conception and interpretation of the research. VLF directed the intellectual conception and design of the research, conducted the analyses and provided interpretation. YP drafted the manuscript and all authors approved the final manuscript version of the present research.

#### Competing interests
YP as Vice President of Nutritional Strategics Inc. provides food, nutrition and regulatory affairs consulting services for numerous food and beverage companies and food-related associations and collaborates with VLF on NHANES analyses; JMJ as Professor Emerita of Food and Nutrition at St. Catherine University provides nutrition science research consulting to food companies and not-for-profit organizations. VLF as Senior Vice President of Nutrition Impact, LLC provides food and nutrition consulting services for numerous food and beverage companies. VLF also conducts analyses of NHANES data for members of the food industry.

**Author details**
[1]Nutritional Strategies Inc., 59 Marriott Place, Paris, ON N3L 0A3, Canada. [2]Distinguished Scholar and Professor Emerita of Food and Nutrition, Department of Foods and Nutrition, St. Catherine University, 4030 Valentine Ct. Arden Hills, Minnesota, MN 55112, USA. [3]Nutrition Impact, LLC, 9725 D Drive North, Battle Creek, MI, USA.

## References

1. United States Department of Health and Human Services and United States Department of Agriculture, "2015 – 2020 Dietary Guidelines for Americans, 8th Edition," U.S. Government Printing Office, December 2015. https://health.gov/dietaryguidelines/2015/resources/2015-2020_Dietary_Guidelines.pdf. Accessed 28 June 2016.
2. U.S. Food and Drug Administration. Food standards: amendment of standards of identity for enriched grain products to require addition of folic acid. Fed Reg. 1996;61(44). http://www.gpo.gov/fdsys/pkg/FR-1996-03-05/pdf/96-5014.pdf. Accessed 22 May 2016.
3. Dietrich M, Brown CJ, Block G. The effect of folate fortification of cereal-grain products on blood folate status, dietary folate intake, and dietary folate sources among adult non-supplement users in the United States. J Am Coll Nutr. 2005;24:266–74.
4. Keast DR, Fulgoni VL, Nicklas TA, O'Neil CE. Food sources of energy and nutrients among children in the United States: NHANES 2003–2006. Nutrients. 2013;5:283–301.
5. Reedy J, Krebs-Smith SM. Dietary sources of energy, solid fats, and added sugars among children and adolescents in the United States. J Am Diet Assoc. 2010;110:1477–84.
6. Huth PJ, Fulgoni VL, Keast DR, Park K, Auestad N. Major food sources of calories, added sugars, and saturated fat and their contribution to essential nutrient intakes in the U.S. Diet: data from the national health and nutrition examination survey (2003–2006). Nutr J. 2013;12:116. doi:10.1186/1475-2891-12-116.
7. Papanikolaou Y, Fulgoni VLF. Certain grain food patterns are associated with improved 2015 dietary guidelines shortfall nutrient intakes, diet quality, and lower body weight in US adults: results from the national health and nutrition examination survey, 2005–2010. Food Nutr Sci. 2016;7:772–81.
8. Jönsson T1, Granfeldt Y, Lindeberg S, Hallberg AC. Subjective satiety and other experiences of a Paleolithic diet compared to a diabetes diet in patients with type 2 diabetes. Nutr J. 2013;12. doi:10.1186/1475-2891-12-105.
9. Manheimer EW, van Zuuren EJ, Fedorowicz Z, Pijl H. Paleolithic nutrition for metabolic syndrome: systematic review and meta-analysis. Am J Clin Nutr. 2015;102:922–32.
10. National Health and Nutrition Examination Survey. Analytic and Reporting Guidelines. Available at http://www.cdc.gov/nchs/data/nhanes/nhanes_03_04/nhanes_analytic_guidelines_dec_2005.pdf. Accessed 17 June 2016.
11. National Health and Nutrition Examination Survey. Analytic Note Regarding 2007–2010 Survey Design Changes and Combining Data Across other Survey Cycles. Available at http://www.cdc.gov/nchs/data/nhanes/analyticnote_2007-2010.pdf. Accessed 17 June 2016.
12. Moshfegh AJ, Rhodes DG, Baer DJ, Murayi T, Clemens JC, Rumpler WV, Paul DR, Sebastian RS, Kuczynski KJ, Ingwersen LA, Staples RC, Cleveland LE. The US department of agriculture automated multiple-pass method reduces bias in the collection of energy intakes. Am J Clin Nutr. 2008;88:324–32.
13. USDA Food and Nutrient Database for Dietary Studies, 3.0. 2008. Beltsville: U.S. Department of Agriculture, Agricultural Research Service, Food Surveys Research Group. https://www.ars.usda.gov/ARSUserFiles/80400530/pdf/fndds/fndds3_doc.pdf. Accessed 17 June 2016.
14. USDA Food and Nutrient Database for Dietary Studies, 4.1. 2010. Beltsville: U.S. Department of Agriculture, Agricultural Research Service, Food Surveys Research Group. https://www.ars.usda.gov/ARSUserFiles/80400530/pdf/fndds/fndds4_doc.pdf. Accessed 17 June 2016.
15. Ahuja JKA, Montville JB, Omolewa-Tomobi G, Heendeniya KY, Martin CL, Steinfeldt LC, et al. USDA food and nutrient database for dietary studies, 5.0. Beltsville: U.S. Department of Agriculture, Agricultural Research Service, Food Surveys Research Group; 2012.
16. Guenther PM, Casavale KO, Reedy J, Kirkpatrick SI, Hiza HA, Kahle LL, Krebs-Smith SM. Update of the healthy eating index: HEI-2010. J Acad Nutr Diet. 2013;113:569–80.
17. U.S. Department of Agriculture and U.S. Department of Health and Human Services (USDA/HHS). Scientific Report of the 2015 Dietary Guidelines Advisory Committee: Advisory Report to the Secretary of Health and Human Services and Secretary of Agriculture. 2015. Washington: USDA, Agricultural Research Service; 2015. http://health.gov/dietaryguidelines/2015-scientific-report/PDFs/Scientific-Report-of-the-2015-Dietary-Guidelines-Advisory-Committee.pdf. Accessed 17 June 2016.
18. Jaaskelainen P, Magnussen CG, Pahkala K, Mikkila V, Kahonen M, Sabin MA, Fogelholm M, Hutri-Kahonen N, Taittonen L, Telama R, Laitinen T, Jokinen E, Lehtimaki T, Viikari JS, Raitakari OT, Juonala M. Childhood nutrition in predicting metabolic syndrome in adults: the cardiovascular risk in young Finns study. Diabetes Care. 2012;35:1937–43.
19. Qi Y, Niu J. Does childhood nutrition predict health outcomes during adulthood? evidence from a population-based study in china. J Biosoc Sci. 2015;47:650–66.
20. McGill CR, Fulgoni 3rd VL, Devareddy L. Ten-year trends in fiber and whole grain intakes and food sources for the united states population: national health and nutrition examination survey 2001–2010. Nutrients. 2015;7:1119–30.
21. Institute of Medicine of the National Academies, Food and Nutrition Board. Dietary reference intakes for energy, carbohydrate, fiber, Fat, fatty acids, cholesterol, protein, and amino acids. Washington: The National Academies Press; 2005.
22. Eckel RH, Jakicic JM, Ard JD, de Jesus JM, Houston Miller N, Hubbard VS, et al. AHA/ACC guideline on lifestyle management to reduce cardiovascular risk: a report of the american college of cardiology/american heart association task force on practice guidelines. J Am Coll Cardiol. 2014;63(25 Pt B):2960–84.
23. Jensen MD, Ryan DH, Apovian CM, Ard JD, Comuzzie AG, Donato KA, et al. American college of cardiology/american heart association task force on practice guidelines; obesity society. 2013 AHA/ACC/TOS guideline for the management of overweight and obesity in adults: a report of the american college of cardiology/american heart association task force on practice guidelines and the obesity society. J Am Coll Cardiol. 2014;63(25 Pt B):2985–3023.
24. Berner LA, Keast DR, Bailey RL, Dwyer JT. Fortified foods are major contributors to nutrient intakes in diets of US children and adolescents. J Acad Nutr Diet. 2014;114:1009–22.
25. U.S. Department of Agriculture and U.S. Department of Health and Human Services (USDA/HHS). Scientific report of the 2010 dietary guidelines advisory committee: advisory report to the secretary of health and human services and secretary of agriculture. Washington: USDA, Agricultural Research Service; 2010.
26. U.S. Department of Agriculture and U.S. Department of Health and Human Services (USDA/HHS). Scientific report of the 2005 dietary guidelines advisory committee: advisory report to the secretary of health and human services and secretary of agriculture. Washington: USDA, Agricultural Research Service; 2005.
27. Dwyer J, Picciano MF, Raiten DJ. Members of the steering committee; national health and nutrition examination survey. Collection of food and dietary supplement intake data: what We Eat in america-NHANES. J Nutr. 2003;133:590S–600S.

# Food choice motives including sustainability during purchasing are associated with a healthy dietary pattern in French adults

B. Allès[1,4*], S. Péneau[1], E. Kesse-Guyot[1], J. Baudry[1], S. Hercberg[1,2] and C. Méjean[1,3]

**Abstract**

**Background:** Sustainability has become a greater concern among consumers that may influence their dietary intake. Only a few studies investigated the relationship between sustainable food choice motives and diet and they focused on specific food groups.

**Objective:** This cross-sectional study aimed to assess the associations between food choice motives during purchasing, with a focus on sustainability, and dietary patterns in a large sample of French adults.

**Design:** Food choice motives were collected in 31,842 adults from the NutriNet-Santé study, using a validated 63 items questionnaire gathered into 9 dimension scores: ethics and environment, traditional and local production, taste, price, environmental limitation (i.e. not buying a food for environmental concerns), health, convenience, innovation and absence of contaminants. Dietary intake was assessed using at least three web-based 24-h food records. Three dietary patterns were obtained through factor analysis using principal component analysis. The associations between food choice motive dimension scores and dietary patterns were assessed using linear regression models, stratifying by sex.

**Results:** Individuals were more likely to have a "healthy diet" when they were more concerned by not buying a food for environmental concerns (only for 3rd tertile versus 1st tertile $\beta_{women}$=0.18, 95% CI=0.15–0.20, $\beta_{men}$=0.20 95% CI=(0.15–0.25)), ethics and environment (women only, β=0.05, 95% CI=0.02–0.08), absence of contaminants (women only, β=0.05, 95% CI=0.01–0.07), local production (women only, β=0.08, 95% CI=0.04–0.11), health (women only) and innovation (men only), and when they were less concerned by price. Individuals were also less likely to have traditional or western diets when they gave importance to food choice motive dimensions related to sustainability.

**Conclusion:** Individuals, especially women, having higher concerns about food sustainability dimensions such as ethics and environment and local production, appear to have a healthier diet. Further longitudinal studies are required to better understand how sustainable concerns may influence long-term nutritional quality of the diet.

**Keywords:** Sustainability, Food choice motives, Diet, Dietary patterns

* Correspondence: b.alles@eren.smbh.univ-paris13.fr
[1]Université Paris 13, Equipe de Recherche en Epidémiologie Nutritionnelle, Centre de Recherche en Epidémiologie et Statistiques, Inserm (U1153), Inra (U1125), Cnam, COMUE Sorbonne Paris Cité, F-93017 Bobigny, France
[4]EREN (Nutritional Epidemiology Research Unit), SMBH Paris 13, 74 rue Marcel Cachin, F-93017 Bobigny Cedex, France
Full list of author information is available at the end of the article

## Background

Food sustainability has become a critical political issue in societies as well as a matter of public health. Sustainable diets were defined by the Food and Agriculture Organization (FAO) as "diets protective and respectful of biodiversity and ecosystems, culturally acceptable, accessible, economically fair and affordable; nutritionally adequate, safe and healthy; while optimizing natural and human resources" [1]. Considering that sustainable diets could be health promoting, scientific communities in USA [2], Brazil [3], UK [4] and some Northern countries from Europe [5], have recently proposed dietary guidelines taking sustainability into account. In fact, it has been previously reported that some current diets, such as a western diet rich in high fat, high sugar processed foods and poor in fruit and vegetables, has negative effects on both health and environment [6]. Consumers can be considered as the main stakeholders in nutritional public health policies [7]. Public health strategies aiming at encouraging healthy and environmentally friendly food choices need to better understand consumer motives when purchasing. However, little is known about the relationship between their food choice motives including those related to sustainability and dietary intake. Previous studies suggest that the motivation to behave sustainably is frequently found among consumers, while its translation into actual sustainable food choices and consumptions seems more difficult [8–13]. Previous researches about dietary behaviors have indicated that food choice motives may play a mediating role between personal norms and values and dietary behaviors [14, 15]. Indeed some types of concerns (e.g.: health, environment, etc.) may be explained by a combination of values that could influence dietary behaviors such as purchases and food choices and thus diet quality [15].

Previous studies about food choice motives conducted in industrialized countries identified price [16–19], health [17, 19, 20], sensory appeal [19, 21], mood during purchasing [19], attitude toward foods [22] convenience [16, 17, 19, 23–25] and ethical concerns [16, 17, 19, 23–25] as main motives influencing consumers choice. Although sustainability is a rising concern in consumers, to date, only a few studies [23, 25–29] have investigated food choice motives covering all the dimensions of sustainability as defined by the FAO [1]. Those studies investigated motives such as environmental, animal welfare, local production and they mainly focused on organic products [26–29] or specific food groups [23, 25]. For example, a study conducted in Finland reported that health and ethical concerns were associated with a higher consumption of fruit and vegetables and a lower consumption of energy dense foods [23]. Another study, conducted among young adults in the USA, reported that a positive attitude toward organically grown and local food was associated with a higher consumption of fruit and vegetables, and a lower consumption of sugar-sweetened beverages [29]. Finally, another study conducted in six European countries did not report any association between food choice motives related to sustainability and consumption of traditional foods, except for France [25].

To the best of our knowledge, the relationship between sustainable food choice motives and the overall diet such as dietary patterns has not been reported yet. Dietary patterns have the two advantages of reflecting the complexity of the dietary habits and overall food intake [30] and to enhance the promotion of healthy food habits [31]. In addition, specific dimensions of sustainable food choice motives such as health in the context of sustainability were rarely reported in previous studies [19, 25].

This cross-sectional study aimed to investigate the relationships between food choice motives including sustainability during purchasing, and dietary patterns in a large sample of French adults from the NutriNet-Santé Study.

## Material and methods

Subjects were participants in the NutriNet-Santé Study, a large web-based prospective observational cohort launched in France in May 2009 with a scheduled follow-up of 10 years. Participants were Internet-using adult volunteers from the general population aged 18 years or more. The study was designed to investigate determinants of dietary behaviours and nutritional status, as well as the relationships between nutrition and health. The design, methods and rationale of this study have been previously described [32]. Briefly, participants had to fill in an initial set of questionnaires assessing dietary intake, physical activity, anthropometry, lifestyle and socio-economic conditions along with health status to be included in the cohort. Each month, they are invited to fill out other questionnaires related to determinants of food behaviour and various nutritional and health status issues.

This study was conducted according to guidelines laid down in the Declaration of Helsinki, and all procedures were approved by the Institutional Review Board of the French Institute for Health and Medical Research (IRB Inserm n° 0000388FWA00005831) and the Commission Nationale Informatique et Libertés (CNIL n° 908,450 and n° 909,216). Written electronic informed consent to participate in the study was obtained from all subjects.

### Data collection

#### *Assessment of food choice motives including sustainability*

As no study has simultaneously and thoroughly explored all dimensions of sustainability as defined by FAO [1], in consumer food-buying motives, in particular social dimension, a new questionnaire including all aspects of sustainability has been developed [33].

In September 2013, 122,091 subjects living in the French metropolitan area were invited to complete this optional validated questionnaire on food choice motives on the "Nutrinet-Santé" website (https://www.etude-nutrinet-sante.fr/). The development and validation of the questionnaire have been previously described [33]. Briefly, the final questionnaire included the 63 most relevant items, and was divided into 9 dimensions scores obtained by first-order analysis: ethics and environment (17 items, e.g.: production waste, impact on earth's resources, respect for working conditions), traditional and local production (12 items, e.g.: proximity of production, support for small-scale producers), taste (4 items), price (6 items), environmental limitations (4 items, e.g.: not buying meat for environmental reasons), health (6 items, e.g.: health impact, nutritional composition), convenience (4 items, e.g.: cooking convenience), innovation (4 items, e.g.: original of innovative product, innovative fabrication/conservation process) and absence of contaminants (5 items, e.g.: additives, exposure to chemicals). Four intercorrelated dimensions (ethics and environment, local and traditional production, health and absence of contaminants) formed a second-order factor interpreted as healthy and environmentally friendly consumption, corresponding to a sustainability dimension in food choices for consumers [33]. The other five uncorrelated dimensions do not directly relate to sustainable food choice motives.

Participants were first asked whether they were in charge of food supply in their household or not. Then, the questionnaire was divided into two main sections: one for general aspects of food purchasing and another one for purchasing of specific food groups (meat, fish, fruit and vegetable and dairy products). Participants were asked whether they were buying these products or not. If they were buying them, they answered all questions concerning their motives during purchasing. For each item, subjects were asked to rate on a 4-point Likert scale from "I strongly disagree" to "I strongly agree" (e.g.: "When I purchase [meat/fish/fruits and vegetables/dairy products], I take into account its impact on the environment: Strongly disagree / Disagree / Agree / Strongly agree / Undecided"). If they were not buying products from a food group, they had to answer specific questions on reasons for not buying them (e.g., "I avoid purchasing [meat/fish/fruits and vegetables/dairy products] for environmental issues: Strongly disagree / Disagree / Agree / Strongly agree / Undecided").

To control the quality of the data collected through such a questionnaire, feasibility, internal validity and reliability were assessed in 637 randomly selected subjects participating in the Nutrinet-Santé cohort study [33]. Feasibility was measured by assessing specific questions on the perceived complexity and difficulty of filling in the questionnaire, and whether the questionnaire was too long and redundant, using the same 4-point Likert scale from « I strongly disagree » to « I strongly agree » [33]. The feasibility assessment revealed that only one third of the sample found the questionnaire redundant before it was shortened. The shorter version used for this study may be even more feasible.

The underlying structure of the questionnaire was determined by exploratory factor analysis and then internally validated by confirmatory factor analysis. Reliability was also assessed by internal consistency of selected dimensions and test–retest repeatability. The model demonstrated excellent internal validity (adjusted goodness of fit index = 0.97; standardized root mean square residuals = 0.07) and satisfactory reliability (internal consistency = 0.96, test–retest repeatability coefficient ranged between 0.31 and 0.68 over a mean 4-week period).

Also, to improve quality of data collected, controls were implemented in the web-based questionnaire to avoid missing values implying that individuals had to fill in every question. In addition, at the end of the questionnaire, participants had access to all questions and given answers to check if their answers were right and had the possibility to modify them eventually.

#### *Dietary intake assessment*

Dietary data were collected using web-based 24 h dietary records. At enrolment and yearly thereafter, participants were invited to provide three 24 h records (1 weekend day and 2 weekdays) [32]. These records were randomly assigned over a two-week period. The dietary record is completed via an interactive interface and designed for self-administration on the Internet [34]. The web-based dietary assessment method relies on a meal-based approach, recording all foods and beverages (type and quantity) consumed at breakfast, lunch, dinner and all other eating occasions. First, participants fills in the names of all food items eaten. Then, they estimate portion sizes for each reported food and beverage item according to standard measurements (e.g. home containers, grams displayed on the package) or using photographs available via the interactive interface. These photographs, taken from a validated picture booklet [35], represent more than 250 foods (corresponding to 1000 generic foods) served in seven different portion sizes. The values for energy were estimated using a published nutrient database [36] and completed for recent market foods and recipes. The accuracy of web-based 24 h dietary records has been assessed by comparing to interviews by trained dietitians [34] and against 24 h urinary biomarkers [37, 38].

Participants in our sample were included if they had completed at least three 24 h dietary records during the two years before the questionnaire on food choice motives (September 2011–September 2013). For each participant, daily mean quantities of the food group (in grams for solid food or cL for beverages) were calculated from 24 h records, weighted according to the day (week or weekend). Diet-underreporting participants were identified by the method proposed by Black [39]. Briefly, basal metabolic rate (BMR) was estimated by Schofield eqs. [40] according to sex, age, weight and height collected at enrolment in the study. BMR was compared to energy intake taking into account the physical activity level [39]. Foods were classified according to the information provided in the French Nutrition and Health Program (Programme National Nutrition Santé) guides [41]. Twenty-five food groups were created: fruit, vegetables, legumes, potatoes and other tubers, refined starchy foods, whole starchy foods, cereals (non fatty), fish and seafood, meat, eggs, processed meat, cheese, dairy products low in sugar, cream based deserts, butter and other added animal fats, vegetable oils, margarine, salad dressing and other dressings, salty snacks, cereals (sweet and fatty) sweet and fatty foods (pastries, biscuits, cookies, chocolate), sweet products (honey, jam, candy), sugary drinks, non-alcoholic beverages and alcoholic beverages.

#### Statistical analysis

The present analyses focused on participants included in the NutriNet-Santé cohort study, included between May 2009 and October 2013, who completed the food choice motive questionnaires, who completed at least three 24 h dietary records, who are not diet-underreporting participants and with no missing socioeconomic data.

#### Dietary patterns analysis

To create dietary patterns, factor analysis using principal component analysis was performed on the correlation matrix of the 25 food groups. Three principal components representing three independent dietary patterns were identified according to their eigenvalues, interpretability and percentage of variance explained. Varimax rotation was performed to improve the interpretability of the factor loadings [42]. Component scores of dietary patterns were then adjusted for energy using the residual method described by Willett and Stampfer [43]. Mean intakes of 25 food groups and products were described according to the quartiles of dietary pattern factor scores to allow better interpretation of the food intake associated with each one the dietary pattern obtained.

#### Statistical analyses

Sociodemographic characteristics of the included and excluded samples were compared using $chi^2$ tests and t-tests. Since each factor consisted of different number of items (from 17 to 4 items), all factors were linearly transformed into values ranging from 0 (no concern) to 10 (strong concern) to standardize ratings. Those quantitative score variables were later converted into qualitative variable to ease interpretation of the results. Cut-offs, were either tertiles or median, depending on the distribution of the score. The association between the nine food choice motives dimension scores and the three dietary pattern factor scores were assesssed using ANCOVA models. Each factor of dietary pattern identified was used as a dependent variable. Because of a statistcally significant interaction between sex and the food choices motives, the analyses were stratified by sex. First, an univariable analysis was performed for each dietary pattern, to select food choice motive dimensions that were significantly associated with dietary pattern ($p < 0.05$, data not shown). Then, a multivariable analysis assessed the associaton between dimensions of food motives and each dietary pattern. This analysis included the retained food choice motives dimensions in univariable models, adjusted for energy intake, age and education. Mean scores of the nine dimension scores of food choice motives were also computed by sex to describe their ranking in stratified analyses. Mean dimension scores were compared between men and women using t-tests.

All tests of significance were two-sided, and a $P$ value <0.05 was considered significant. All statistical analyses were performed using SAS software (version 9.3, SAS Institute Inc.).

### Results

#### Characteristics of the sample

From the initial 122,091 subjects who received the questionnaire measuring food choice motives regarding sustainable foods, a total of 46,958 answered the questionnaire. Then, 15,113 subjects were excluded because of missing data on food intake (including 6650 underreporting) and 3 had missing data for age and education. The final sample was composed by 31,842 subjects (25,217 women and 6625 men).

As shown in Table 1, in both sexes, the sample of included subjects had a higher proportion of individuals with higher education, compared with excluded subjects. The proportion of women living with a partner was higher in the included sample as well as those living in an urban area of 20,000 to 200,000 inhabitants. The mean age was also lower in included subjects than in excluded subjects.

#### Description of food choice motive dimensions

Food choice motive dimensions ranked the same in men and women (Table 2). The highest mean scores were found for taste dimension, motives regarding health and absence of contaminants, followed by local and traditional production, price, ethics and environment and

**Table 1** Characteristics of the included and excluded subjects (*n* = 45,155, Nutrinet-Santé study, 2013)

| | Men (*n* = 9499) | | | | | Women (*n* = 35,656) | | | | |
|---|---|---|---|---|---|---|---|---|---|---|
| | Excluded (*n* = 2874) | | Included (*n* = 6625) | | p[a] | Excluded (*n* = 10,439) | | Included (*n* = 25,217) | | p[a] |
| Age (mean SD) | 54.4 | 13.3 | 51.4 | 13.9 | <0.001 | 47.1 | 14.1 | 44.8 | 14.1 | <0.001 |
| Educational level (n %) | | | | | <0.001 | | | | | <0.001 |
| Primary | 110 | 3.8 | 183 | 2.8 | | 361 | 3.5 | 529 | 2.1 | |
| Secondary | 1070 | 37.2 | 2065 | 31.2 | | 3756 | 36.0 | 7266 | 28.8 | |
| Higher education | 1685 | 58.6 | 4361 | 65.8 | | 6263 | 60.0 | 17,302 | 68.6 | |
| Missing data | 9 | 0.3 | 16 | 0.2 | | 59 | 0.6 | 120 | 0.5 | |
| Marital status (*n* %) | | | | | 0.78 | | | | | 0.001 |
| Single, divorced, separated or widowed | 578 | 20.1 | 1311 | 19.8 | | 3002 | 28.8 | 6717 | 26.6 | |
| Living with a partner | 2289 | 79.6 | 5300 | 80.0 | | 7420 | 71.1 | 18,456 | 73.2 | |
| Missing data | 7 | 0.2 | 14 | 0.2 | | 17 | 0.2 | 44 | 0.2 | |
| Size of the residential city (n %) | | | | | 0.63 | | | | | 0.015 |
| Rural | 584 | 20.3 | 1395 | 21.1 | | 2299 | 22.0 | 5519 | 21.9 | |
| Paris area | 542 | 18.9 | 1227 | 18.5 | | 1952 | 18.7 | 4396 | 17.4 | |
| Urban, 20,000–200,000 inhabitants | 518 | 18.0 | 1253 | 18.9 | | 1902 | 18.2 | 4660 | 18.5 | |
| Urban, < 20,000 inhabitants | 461 | 16.0 | 988 | 14.9 | | 1551 | 14.9 | 3737 | 14.8 | |
| Urban, > 200,000 inhabitants | 762 | 26.5 | 1748 | 26.4 | | 2694 | 25.8 | 6833 | 27.1 | |
| Missing data | 7 | 0.2 | 14 | 0.2 | | 41 | 0.4 | 72 | 0.3 | |

[a]: *p*-value for t-test for age and for chi$^2$ for every other categorical variables
*SD* Standard-deviation

convenience. The lowest scores observed were for innovation and environmental limitations. Women had higher scores for every dimension except for innovation and environmental limitations.

### Description of dietary patterns

Three dietary patterns explaining 24.9% of the total variance were derived (Table 3). The first dietary pattern was labelled healthy, it had the highest factor loadings for fruit, vegetables, legumes, whole starchy foods, fish and seafood, eggs, vegetable oils, non-alcoholic beverages and lowest factor loadings for cream based desserts, sweet and fatty food (pastries, biscuits, cookies and chocolate) and sugary drinks. The second dietary pattern was labelled traditional, it had the highest factor loadings for potatoes and other tubers, non-fatty cereals, meat, cheese, butter and other added animal fats, margarine and sweet products (honey, jam, candy) and the lowest factor loadings for fatty and sweet cereals. The third dietary pattern was labelled Western, it had the highest factor loadings for processed meat, cheese, salad dressings, salty snacks, sweet and fatty food, sugary drinks and alcoholic beverages and the lowest factor loadings for dairy products low in sugar and margarine. Mean daily intakes for food groups, according to quartiles of component scores obtained by FA-PCA, are presented in Additional file 1: Table S1.

**Table 2** Mean food choice dimension scores in the sample, sorted from high to low (n = 31,842, Nutrinet-Santé study, 2013)

| | Women | | Men | | p[1] |
|---|---|---|---|---|---|
| | Mean | SD | Mean | SD | |
| Taste | 9.0 | 0.9 | 8.8 | 0.9 | <0.001 |
| Health | 7.6 | 1.2 | 7.4 | 1.1 | <0.001 |
| Absence of contaminants | 7.5 | 1.5 | 7.4 | 1.3 | <0.001 |
| Local and traditional production | 7.4 | 1,0 | 7.2 | 0.8 | <0.001 |
| Price | 7.4 | 1.1 | 7.1 | 1.1 | <0.001 |
| Ethics and environment | 5.7 | 1,0 | 5.5 | 0.8 | <0.001 |
| Convenience | 5.5 | 1.6 | 5.2 | 1.5 | <0.001 |
| Innovation | 3.5 | 1.4 | 3.6 | 1.3 | <0.001 |
| Environmental limitations | 2.8 | 2.2 | 2.7 | 2.2 | 0.22 |

1:*p*-value for t-test
s-d: standard-deviation

### Associations between food choice motive dimension and dietary patterns

After univariable analyses, convenience dimension for the three dietary patterns and price dimension for the Western dietary pattern were excluded for multivariable analyses.

In both sexes, individuals with higher concern for environmental limitations (not buying specific food for environmental reasons), and those with lower concerns for price, were more likely to have a healthy dietary pattern

**Table 3** Dietary patterns obtained by factor analysis using principal component analysis of daily food intakes in the Nutrinet-Santé sample (*n* = 31,842, Nutrinet-Santé study, 2013)

| | Healthy dietary pattern | Traditional dietary pattern | Western dietary pattern |
|---|---|---|---|
| Fruit | 0.44 | 0.07 | −0.21 |
| Vegetables | 0.58 | 0.20 | −0.28 |
| Legumes | 0.27 | −0.09 | 0.05 |
| Potatoes and other tubers | 0.04 | 0.42 | 0.00 |
| Refined starchy food | −0.08 | −0.06 | 0.18 |
| Whole starchy food | 0.60 | −0.27 | −0.01 |
| Cereals, non fatty | −0.22 | 0.71 | 0.01 |
| Fish and seafood | 0.31 | −0.07 | 0.02 |
| Meat | −0.20 | 0.29 | 0.02 |
| Eggs | 0.14 | 0.05 | −0.06 |
| Processed meat | −0.11 | 0.24 | 0.40 |
| Cheese | 0.09 | 0.36 | 0.34 |
| Dairy products, low in sugar | −0.13 | 0.05 | −0.49 |
| Cream based deserts | −0.20 | −0.04 | 0.03 |
| Butter and other added animal fats | 0.08 | 0.43 | −0.05 |
| Vegetable oils | 0.38 | 0.11 | 0.11 |
| Margarine | 0.04 | 0.24 | −0.20 |
| Salad dressings and other dressings | −0.02 | 0.10 | 0.28 |
| Salty snacks | 0.00 | −0.04 | 0.48 |
| Cereals, sweet and fatty | −0.01 | −0.28 | −0.07 |
| Sweet and fatty foods (pastries, biscuits, cookies, chocolate) | −0.23 | −0.07 | 0.37 |
| Sweet products (honey, jam, candy) | 0.13 | 0.38 | 0.02 |
| Sugary drinks | −0.29 | −0.10 | 0.30 |
| Non-alcoholic beverages | 0.44 | 0.01 | 0.04 |
| Alcoholic beverages | 0.12 | 0.22 | 0.53 |
| variance explained (%) | 8.8 | 8.2 | 7.9 |

(tertile 3 vs 1 only) (Tables 4 and 5). Women with higher concern for ethics and environment, those with higher interest in traditional and local production, health, and those with higher concern for absence of contaminants were more likely to have a healthy dietary pattern as well (Tables 4 and 5). Men with higher concern for innovation were also more likely to have a healthy dietary pattern. In both sexes, individuals with lower concerns for environmental limitations were more likely to have a traditional dietary pattern. In addition, women with moderate concern for health (tertile 2 vs 1 only), men with moderate concern for the absence of contaminants (tertile 2 vs 1 only), and men with lower concern for innovation, were more likely to have a traditional dietary pattern. Finally, in both sexes, individuals with lower concerns for health (in men, tertile 2 vs 1 only) were more likely to have a western dietary pattern. In addition, women with higher concern for taste (tertile 3 vs 1 only) and those with lower concern for health, and men with lower concern for environmental limitations, were more likely to have a western dietary pattern.

## Discussion

To the best of our knowledge, this is the first study to investigate associations between sustainable food choice motives and dietary patterns. Individuals, and in particular women, having higher concerns about food sustainability motives such as ethics and environment, local and traditional production and health appear to have a healthier diet. Higher concern for taste was also associated with the traditional dietary pattern (in women) reflecting less healthy dietary habits.

Findings from previous studies support our results even if they focused on specific food groups instead of dietary patterns. They showed an association between sustainable food choice motives and fruit and vegetables [23, 29], lower consumption of high-fat high sugar food [29] and higher consumption of traditional food [25].

**Table 4** Associations between dietary patterns and food choice motives dimension scores ($n$ = 31,842, Nutrinet-Santé study, 2013)

| | Healthy[a] | | | | Traditional[a] | | | |
|---|---|---|---|---|---|---|---|---|
| | Women | | Men | | Women | | Men | |
| | β | 95% CI | β | 95% CI | β | 95% CI | β | 95% CI |
| ethics and environment | | | | | | | | |
| 2nd tertile of score vs. 1st tertile | **0.047** | **[0.018; 0.076]** | −0.002 | [−0.061; 0.058] | 0.009 | [−0.015: 0.034] | −0.007 | [−0.065;0.050] |
| 3rd tertile of score vs. 1st tertile | **0.033** | **[0.001; 0.065]** | −0.007 | [−0.077; 0.064] | 0.025 | [−0.002: 0.052] | −0.037 | [−0.106;0.030] |
| traditional and local production | | | | | | | | |
| 2nd tertile of score vs. 1st tertile | **0.080** | **[0.051; 0.109]** | 0.013 | [−0.046; 0.073] | 0.008 | [−0.016; 0.033] | 0.007 | [−0.050; 0.066] |
| 3rd tertile of score vs. 1st tertile | **0.081** | **[0.049; 0.112]** | −0.019 | [−0.089; 0.052] | −0.008 | [−0.035; 0.018] | −0.009 | [−0.078; 0.059] |
| taste | | | | | | | | |
| 2nd tertile of score vs. 1st tertile | 0.016 | [−0.010; 0.043] | 0.041 | [−0.018; 0.100] | −0.001 | [−0.024; 0.020] | 0.038 | [−0.018; 0.096] |
| 3rd tertile of score vs. 1st tertile | 0.022 | [−0.006; 0.050] | 0.011 | [−0.060; 0.083] | −0.011 | [−0.035; 0.012] | −0.002 | [−0.072; 0.067] |
| price | | | | | | | | |
| 2nd tertile of score vs. 1st tertile | −0.015 | [−0.043; 0.013] | −0.025 | [−0.086; 0.036] | −0.001 | [−0.025; 0.020] | 0.010 | [−0.048; 0.069] |
| 3rd tertile of score vs. 1st tertile | **−0.040** | **[−0.067; −0.013]** | **−0.074** | **[−0.141; −0.007]** | 0.004 | [−0.019; 0.027] | −0.014 | [−0.079; 0.051] |
| health | | | | | | | | |
| 2nd tertile of score vs. 1st tertile | **0.042** | **[0.014; 0.071]** | 0.003 | [−0.059; 0.065] | **0.027** | **[0.002; 0.052]** | 0.011 | [−0.049; 0.072] |
| 3rd tertile of score vs. 1st tertile | **0.069** | **[0.040; 0.099]** | **0.067** | **[0.001; 0.135]** | 0.003 | [−0.022; 0.029] | −0.059 | [−0.125; 0.006] |
| absence of contaminants | | | | | | | | |
| 2nd tertile of score vs. 1st tertile | **0.046** | **[0.017; 0.074]** | 0.017 | [−0.044; 0.079] | −0.001 | [−0.026; 0.023] | 0.084 | [0.024; 0.144] |
| 3rd tertile of score vs. 1st tertile | **0.038** | **[0.008; 0.069]** | 0.028 | [−0.040; 0.095] | −0.019 | [−0.045; 0.007] | −0.013 | [−0.079; 0.052] |
| environmental limitations (above median vs. under median) | **0.175** | **[0.153; 0.198]** | **0.202** | **[0.149; 0.255]** | **−0.087** | **[−0.107; −0.068]** | **−0.130** | **[−0.181; −0.078]** |
| innovation (above median vs. under median) | −0.010 | [−0.033;0.013] | **0.063** | **[0.010; 0.116]** | −0.011 | [−0.031; 0.008] | **−0.061** | **[−0.113; −0.009]** |

[a]: parameters estimated with multivariable linear regression models, 8 food choice dimension scores adjusted for age, education and total energy intake; in bold: statiscally significant
β: linear regression coefficient estimate; 95% CI = Confidence interval

The positive association between sustainable food choice motives and a healthy diet may be explained by a combination of both egoistic and altruistic values that could influence food behaviour and diet [26, 44]. Indeed, egoistic motives, such as health, have been reported as better predictors of the purchase of foods [26] compared with altruistic motives.

In general, self-perception regarding health or ethics concerns can influence food motives that in turn will have an effect on dietary intake. A review on determinants of healthy eating reported that individuals defining themselves as health and environmental conscious, or animal friendly, for example, may have healthier dietary habits [45]. Another study showed that food choice motives play a mediating role in the relationship between health concerns of developing diseases, and healthy eating attitudes [14]. In particular, the latter study highlighted that food choice motives regarding natural content and ethical concerns may have a mediating role between health concern and healthy eating attitude.

In our study, food choice motives regarding ethics and environment and environmental limitations specifically, were positively associated with a healthy dietary pattern and negatively associated with a western dietary pattern. In addition, the environmental limitation dimension was negatively associated with the traditional dietary pattern. Our results are suggesting that individuals that have a healthy diet may be more concerned by the environmental impact of their diet, independently from health concerns. Individuals having concerns for environment may not have conflicting concerns with health. Indeed, in another sample from the Nutrinet-Santé study, we reported that having environmental concerns is not contradictory with adherence to nutritional guidelines (data not shown).

Personal norms, especially those regarding ethics in food production and protection of the environment may induce healthy eating [45], explaining the association with healthy dietary habits. Previous work from de Boer et al. [15] showed that ethical and environmental concerns may relate to personal values and value-related

**Table 5** Associations between dietary patterns and food choice motives dimension scores (*n* = 31,842, Nutrinet-Santé study, 2013)

| | Western[b] | | | |
|---|---|---|---|---|
| | Women | | Men | |
| | β | 95% CI | β | 95% CI |
| ethics and environment | | | | |
| 2nd tertile of score vs. 1st tertile | 0.014 | [−0.013;0.041] | 0.052 | [−0.009; 0.114] |
| 3rd tertile of score vs. 1st tertile | −0.014 | [−0.043; 0.017] | 0.001 | [−0.071; 0.073] |
| traditional and local production | | | | |
| 2nd tertile of score vs. 1st tertile | −0.009 | [−0.036; 0.017] | 0.040 | [−0.021; 0.103] |
| 3rd tertile of score vs. 1st tertile | 0.012 | [−0.017; 0.042] | 0.064 | [−0.009; 0.014] |
| taste | | | | |
| 2nd tertile of score vs. 1st tertile | 0.007 | [−0.017; 0.033] | 0.002 | [−0.059; 0.063] |
| 3rd tertile of score vs. 1st tertile | **0.037** | **[0.011; 0.064]** | 0.046 | [−0.028; 0.119] |
| health | | | | |
| 2nd tertile of score | **−0.051** | **[−0.078; −0.023]** | **−0.114** | **[−0.178; −0.049]** |
| 3rd tertile of score | **−0.142** | **[−0.170; −0.114]** | −0.145 | [−0.214; 0.075] |
| absence of contaminants | | | | |
| 2nd tertile of score | 0.005 | [−0.021; 0.033] | 0.019 | [−0.045; 0.083] |
| 3rd tertile of score | −0.006 | [−0.034; 0.023] | −0.001 | [−0.070; 0.069] |
| environmental limitations (above median vs under median) | 0.011 | [−0.010; 0.032] | **−0.081** | **[−0.136; −0.026]** |
| innovation (above median vs under median) | −0.001 | [−0.021; 0.033] | 0.045 | [−0.010; 0.099] |

[b]; parameters estimated with multivariables linear regression models, 7 food choice dimensions scores + age, education and total energy intake; in bold: statiscally significant
β: linear regression coefficient estimate; 95% CI = Confidence interval; 95% CI = Confidence interval

attitudes in a prevention motivational system, influencing food choice motives, and then, food intakes. According to the Higgin's regulatory focus theory [46, 47], this motivational system is implying a higher level of concerns with safety and fulfilment of responsibilities, as well as concerns for security and avoidance of negative outcome. Following those theories, personal values such as ethics and environment protection may act as preventive psychological determinants of a healthier food behavior.

The traditional and local production dimension was also associated with a healthy dietary pattern. This dimension of food choice motives contains various concerns including proximity of production especially (for fruit and vegetables), artisanal or traditional production, support for small-scale producers (and cooperatives) or seasonality. Previous studies about food choice motives never assessed a dimension gathering those concerns.

Previous studies focusing on consumers' motives for buying local food highlighted that both organic and freshly locally grown characteristics of the products were important concerns [48, 49]. Indeed, individuals buying local food may have a particular interest in the seasonality and the origin of the products they buy, two personal values that may be on the motivational pathway to healthy eating attitudes [15]. This food choice motives dimension was not associated with the traditional dietary pattern. A possible explanation is that in our questionnaire, the traditional and local dimension was also representing altruistic values (e.g.: promoting local producers). These altruistic values may be associated with healthier diet [15] instead of traditional and less healthy dietary patterns.

Health dimension was positively associated with both healthy and traditional dietary patterns whereas it was inversely associated with a western dietary pattern. It has been shown that health as a food choice motive was positively correlated with better adherence to healthy nutritional guidelines [20]. The health concern, mediated by attitudes and personal values regarding the prevention of diseases or other health conditions, may be associated with healthier food choices as previously described [14].

The association between the absence of contaminants motive and a healthy dietary pattern observed in our study has not been previously assessed in the literature. This motive was also associated with a traditional dietary pattern in our study. A comparative study conducted across six European countries including France, investigated the relationship between food choice motives and consumption of traditional food [25]. In this study, natural content was a concern for consumers of traditional products [25]. Higher concerns for natural content [50] and natural products [14] were also previously related to higher consumptions of healthy food such as fruit and vegetables.

An association between the taste dimension and the western pattern in women was observed. Previous work that investigated food choice motives also reported that taste highly ranked among other dimensions of motives [19, 25, 27, 51]. Taste and food preferences (e.g.: fat, salt, sweet) have been reported as strong predictors of food intake [52–55]. The small variation of the taste dimension score within this sample may partially explain the absence of any other statistically significant association. This may be also be explained by the conceptual model proposed by De Boer et al. [15] implying that food choice motives influence taste-related attitudes and not directly food choices.

Lower concern for price, independently from other dimensions, is associated with healthy food intake. Previous study reported that food price is an obvious determinant of food choices [19] and a food choice motive positively associated with healthy eating [14]. However, to the best of our knowledge, lower concerns for price were never reported associated with healthy dietary patterns in previous studies. Individuals with healthier diet have higher incomes in the Nutrinet-Santé study (data not shown) and, they may therefore feel less concerned by price. This may explain the inverse relationships between price motive and healthy dietary pattern.

The innovation dimension was poorly associated with any of the dietary patterns, except with a healthy dietary pattern in men. The fact that individuals having those concerns have higher incomes, higher educational level and thus, healthier diets (data not shown), may explain this significant association with a healthy dietary pattern in men, similarly to price concerns.

Our results may not be generalizable to the general population. First, our study sample includes a greater proportion of women and participants with higher education. Those characteristics that have been previously reported as demographic predictors of greater concerns for health and sustainability [29, 56, 57]. Indeed, a previous study among older adults reported that individuals with higher income and higher level of educations were more likely to report health related motives [56]. Another studies highlighted that women were more likely to exhibit higher concerns for the environment, whereas individuals with lower levels of educations are less environmentally sensitive [57]. Women seemed to also report higher importance for local production and sustainable foods in a previous study among young adults [29]. Thus, individuals with greater concerns for health and sustainability may be over-represented in this sample. However, it may be difficult to estimate how it could have biased our study sample, as no data from studies using random samples in the general population are available. To prevent this bias, statistical models were stratified by sex and adjusted for education.

Secondly, a previous study assessed the representativity of the Nutrinet-Santé cohort study comparing the distribution of sociodemographic and economic characteristics to statistics from the French census data (58). Notable differences were reported concerning gender and educational level. Thus, women and individuals with higher level of education are over-represented in our sample from the Nutrinet-Santé study, as they are more likely to participate in voluntary-based health and epidemiological studies in many epidemiological fields [58]. A high interest in nutrition could also lead to this over-representation [58, 59].

Finally, a comparison study about dietary intake was conducted comparing the Nutrinet-Santé study cohort to a representative sample of the French population [60]. The authors reported a low magnitude of differences in food intakes between those studies, except for fruit and vegetables.

Food consumptions were self-reported using a self-administrated web-based tool, implying methodological constraints. However, a validation study [61] concluded that compared to interview with dietitian, web-based self-reported food intake seem to be valid and feasible method. A strength of this study is to provide an accurate estimation of overall dietary intakes. Indeed, dietary data used to derive dietary patterns were collected through a validated [37] interactive web-based self-reported dietary record tool. Moreover, the three non-consecutive-day dietary records are recommended methods in large epidemiological studies [62], especially because it allows a good estimation of usual diet [63]. Additionally, we used a data-driven method that enables the description of global dietary patterns instead of focusing on specific food items. This method enhanced a broader description of food habits within the sample that were later associated with food choice motives. Within our study sample, we were able to cover a good variety of food habits, and related dietary patterns, similar to previous studies using these methods (for example: opposite nutritional qualities of healthy and western diets [64, 65]).

Food choice motives were assessed using a validated questionnaire specifically designed for the French population [33]. As food choice motives were self-reported some difficulties may have appeared when participants completed it by themselves [33]. As the answers from the questionnaire were based on self-reporting, the reliability and validity of the questionnaire could be questioned. However, reliability tests were performed [33] and showed that both internal consistency for each factor and repeatability for most of the items were satisfying. In addition, the model demonstrated excellent internal validity. However, external validity may be limited because this questionnaire was developed in a French cultural setting and cross-cultural adaptations may be required before submitting it to other cultures [24]. To our knowledge, this is the first study using such a validated food choice motives questionnaire with a specific focus on sustainability. Indeed, additionally to an increasing number of items investigated compared to previous studies, this questionnaire also covered new themes such as local production and environmental limitations for example.

## Conclusion

In some countries, public health experts are already promoting sustainable diets that could allow reaching a better nutritional quality of the diet, but little is known about determinants of consumers' choices concerning sustainability. Our results support the idea that sustainable food motives during puchases are related to healthier dietary patterns. We also highlighted that sustainable concerns may influence dietary intake of individuals, and thus should not be neglected in the promotion of healthy dietary habits. Further longitudinal observational studies are also required to better understand how sustainable concerns may influence long term nutritional quality of diets.

### Abbreviations

BMR: Basal metabolic rate; FAO: Food and Agriculture Organization; FA-PCA: Factor analysis using principal component analysis

### Acknowledgements

We thank the scientists, dieticians, technicians, statisticians and assistants who helped carry out the NutriNet-Santé study, and all dedicated and conscientious volunteers.

### Funding

The OCAD project was supported by the French National Research Agency (Agence Nationale de la Recherche) in the context of the 2011 Systèmes Alimentaires Durables (OCAD project, ANR-11-ALID-002-06). The NutriNet-Santé cohort study is funded by the following public institutions: Ministère de la Santé, Institut de Veille Sanitaire (InVS), Institut National de la Prévention et de l'Education pour la Santé (INPES), Fondation pour la Recherche Médicale (FRM), Institut National de la Santé et de la Recherche Médicale, Institut National de la Recherche Agronomique (INRA), Conservatoire National des Arts et Métiers (CNAM) and Paris 13 University. The funders had no role in study design, data collection and analysis, decision to publish, or preparation of the manuscript.

### Authors' contributions

AB, MC, PS designed research. MC, PS and SH conducted research. AB analyzed data or performed statistical analysis. AB, MC and PS wrote paper. AB had primary responsibility for final content. AB, MC and BJ conducted the review of the litterature. All the authors were involved in the interpretation of the results and the critical review of the manuscript. All authors read and approved the final manuscript.

### Competing interests

The authors declare that they have no competing interests.

### Author details

[1]Université Paris 13, Equipe de Recherche en Epidémiologie Nutritionnelle, Centre de Recherche en Epidémiologie et Statistiques, Inserm (U1153), Inra (U1125), Cnam, COMUE Sorbonne Paris Cité, F-93017 Bobigny, France. [2]Department of Public Health, Hôpital Avicenne, F-93300 Bobigny, France. [3]INRA, UMR 1110 MOISA, F-34000 Montpellier, France. [4]EREN (Nutritional Epidemiology Research Unit), SMBH Paris 13, 74 rue Marcel Cachin, F-93017 Bobigny Cedex, France.

### References

1. FAO. Definition of sustainable diets. International scientific symposium. Biodiversity and sustainable diets united against hunger. Rome, Italy: FAO Headquarters.; 2010.
2. Dietary guidelines advisory committee. 2015 Advisory Report [Internet]. 2016. Accessed on may 19. Available online: http://health.gov/dietaryguidelines/2015-scientific-report/
3. Ministry of Health of Brazil. Dietary guidelines for the Brazilian popuation - 2nde Edition [Internet]. 2014. Accessed on 29 June 2015. Available online: http://www.fao.org/nutrition/education/food-dietary-guidelines/regions/brazil/en/
4. Global food security. The principle of healthy and sustainable eating patterns, Program Follow on the work of the Green food project focusing on sustainable consumptions [Internet]. 2015. Accessed on September 22 2016. Available online: https://www.foodsecurity.ac.uk/publications/principles-healthy-sustainable-eating-patterns.pdf
5. Niva M, Mäkelä J, Kahma N, Kjærnes U. Eating sustainably? Practices and background factors of ecological food consumption in four Nordic countries. J Consum Policy. 2014;37:465–84.
6. Johnston JL, Fanzo JC, Cogill B. Understanding sustainable diets: a descriptive analysis of the determinants and processes that influence diets and their impact on health, food security, and environmental sustainability. Adv Nutr Int Rev J. 2014;5:418–29.
7. FAO. Influencing food environments for healthy diets [Internet]. FAO; 2016. Accessed on June 6 2017. Available online: http://www.fao.org/documents
8. Bray J, Johns N, Kilburn D. An exploratory study into the factors impeding ethical consumption. J Bus Ethics. 2011;98:597–608.
9. de Boer J, Boersema JJ, Aiking H. Consumers' motivational associations favoring free-range meat or less meat. Ecol Econ. 2009;68:850–60.
10. Grunert KG, Hieke S, Wills J. Sustainability labels on food products: consumer motivation, understanding and use. Food Policy. 2014;44:177–89.
11. Krystallis A, de Barcellos MD, Kügler JO, Verbeke W, Grunert KG. Attitudes of European citizens towards pig production systems. Livest Sci. 2009;126:46–56.
12. van Dam YK, van Trijp HCM. Relevant or determinant: importance in certified sustainable food consumption. Food Qual Prefer. 2013;30:93–101.
13. Vermeir I, Verbeke W. Sustainable food consumption: exploring the consumer "attitude – behavioral intention" gap. J Agric Environ Ethics. 2006;19:169–94.
14. Sun Y-HC. Health concern, food choice motives, and attitudes toward healthy eating: the mediating role of food choice motives. Appetite. 2008;51:42–9.
15. de Boer J, Hoogland CT, Boersema JJ. Towards more sustainable food choices: value priorities and motivational orientations. Food Qual Prefer. 2007;18:985–96.

16. Blaylock J, Smallwood D, Kassel K, Variyam J, Aldrich L. Economics, food choices, and nutrition. Food Policy. 1999;24:269–86.
17. Eertmans A, Victoir A, Vansant G, Van Den Bergh O. Food-related personality traits, food choice motives and food intake : mediator and moderator relationships. Food Qual Prefer. 2005;16:714–26.
18. Lindeman M, Väänänen M. Measurement of ethical food choice motives. Appetite. 2000;34:55–9.
19. Steptoe A, Pollard TM, Wardle J. Development of a measure of the motives underlying the selection of food: the food choice questionnaire. Appetite. 1995;25:267–84.
20. Lê J, Dallongeville J, Wagner A, Arveiler D, Haas B, Cottel D, Simon C, Dauchet L. Attitudes toward healthy eating: a mediator of the educational level–diet relationship. Eur J Clin Nutr. 2013;67:808–14.
21. Januszewska R, Pieniak Z, Verbeke W. Food choice questionnaire revisited in four countries. Does it still measure the same? Appetite. 2011;57:94–8.
22. Rozin P. The socio-cultural context of eating and food choice. In: Meiselman HL, editor. MacFie HJH, editors. Food Choice: Acceptance and Consumption. Springer US; 1996. p. 83–104.
23. Konttinen H, Sarlio-Lähteenkorva S, Silventoinen K, Männistö S, Haukkala A. Socio-economic disparities in the consumption of vegetables, fruit and energy-dense foods: the role of motive priorities. Public Health Nutr. 2013;16:873–82.
24. Pula K, Parks CD, Ross CF. Regulatory focus and food choice motives. Prevention orientation associated with mood, convenience, and familiarity. Appetite. 2014;78:15–22.
25. Pieniak Z, Verbeke W, Vanhonacker F, Guerrero L, Hersleth M. Association between traditional food consumption and motives for food choice in six European countries. Appetite. 2009;53:101–8.
26. Magnusson MK, Arvola A, Hursti UKK, Aberg L, Sjödén P-O. Choice of organic foods is related to perceived consequences for human health and to environmentally friendly behaviour. Appetite. 2003;40:109–17.
27. Brown E, Dury S, Holdsworth M. Motivations of consumers that use local, organic fruit and vegetable box schemes in Central England and southern France. Appetite. 2009;53:183–8.
28. Kesse-Guyot E, Peneau S, Mejean C. Szabo de Edelenyi F, Galan P, Hercberg S. Lairon D Profiles of organic food consumers in a large sample of French adults: results from the Nutrinet-Sante cohort study PloS One. 2013;8:e76998.
29. Pelletier JE, Laska MN, Neumark-Sztainer D, Story M. Positive attitudes toward organic, local, and sustainable foods are associated with higher dietary quality among young adults. J Acad Nutr Diet. 2013;113:127–32.
30. Imamura F, Jacques PF. Invited commentary: dietary pattern analysis. Am J Epidemiol. 2011;173:1105–8.
31. Freeland-Graves JH. Nitzke S, academy of nutrition and dietetics. Position of the academy of nutrition and dietetics: total diet approach to healthy eating. J Acad Nutr Diet. 2013;113:307–17.
32. Hercberg S, Castetbon K, Czernichow S, Malon A, Mejean C, Kesse E, Touvier M, Galan P. The Nutrinet-Santé study: a web-based prospective study on the relationship between nutrition and health and determinants of dietary patterns and nutritional status. BMC Public Health. 2010;10:242.
33. Sautron V, Péneau S, Camilleri GM, Muller L, Ruffieux B, Hercberg S, Méjean C. Validity of a questionnaire measuring motives for choosing foods including sustainable concerns. Appetite. 2015;87:90–7.
34. Touvier M, Méjean C, Kesse-Guyot E, Pollet C, Malon A, Castetbon K, Hercberg S. Comparison between web-based and paper versions of a self-administered anthropometric questionnaire. Eur J Epidemiol. 2010;25:287–96.
35. Le Moullec N, Deheeger M, Preziosi P, Monteiro P, Valeix P, Rolland-Cachera M-F. Potier De Courcy G, Christides J-P, Cherouvrier F, Galan P, et al. Validation du manuel-photos utilisé pour l'enquête alimentaire de l'étude SU.VI.MAX. Cah Nutr Diététique. 1996;31:158–64.
36. Arnault N, Caillot L, Castetbon K, Coronel S, Deschamps V, Fezeu L. Table de Composition des aliments NutriNet-Santé. Paris: Editions Économica; 2013.
37. Lassale C, Castetbon K, Laporte F, Camilleri GM, Deschamps V, Vernay M, Faure P, Hercberg S, Galan P, Kesse-Guyot E. Validation of a web-based, self-administered, non-consecutive-day dietary record tool against urinary biomarkers. Br J Nutr. 2015;113:953–62.
38. Lassale C, Castetbon K, Laporte F, Deschamps V, Vernay M, Camilleri GM, Faure P, Hercberg S, Galan P, Kesse-Guyot E. Correlations between Fruit, Vegetables, Fish, Vitamins, and Fatty Acids Estimated by Web-Based Nonconsecutive Dietary Records and Respective Biomarkers of Nutritional Status. J Acad Nutr Diet. 2016;116:427–438.e5.
39. Black AE. Critical evaluation of energy intake using the Goldberg cut-off for energy intake:basal metabolic rate. A practical guide to its calculation, use and limitations. Int J Obes Relat Metab Disord J Int Assoc Study Obes. 2000; 24:1119–30.
40. Schofield WN. Predicting basal metabolic rate, new standards and review of previous work. Hum Nutr Clin Nutr. 1985;39(Suppl 1):5–41.
41. Hercberg S, Chat-Yung S, Chaulia M. The French National Nutrition and health program: 2001-2006-2010. Int J Public Health. 2008;53:68–77.
42. Kleinbaum DG, Kupper LL, Muller KE. Applied regression analysis and other multivariable methods. 3rd Revised edition. USA: Wadsworth Publishing Co Inc; 1997. 736 p.
43. Willett W, Stampfer MJ. Total energy intake: implications for epidemiologic analyses. Am J Epidemiol. 1986;124:17–27.
44. Sirieix L, Kledal PR, Sulitang T. Organic food consumers' trade-offs between local or imported, conventional or organic products: a qualitative study in shanghai. Int J Consum Stud. 2011;35:670–8.
45. Brug J. Determinants of healthy eating: motivation, abilities and environmental opportunities. Fam Pract. 2008;25:i50–5.
46. Higgins ET. Beyond pleasure and pain. Am Psychol. 1997;52:1280–300.
47. Higgins ET, Friedman RS, Harlow RE, Idson LC, Ayduk ON, Taylor A. Achievement orientations from subjective histories of success: promotion pride versus prevention pride. Eur J Soc Psychol. 2001;31:3–23.
48. O'Kane G. A moveable feast: contemporary relational food cultures emerging from local food networks. Appetite. 2016;105:218–31.
49. Conner D, Colasanti K, Ross RB, Smalley SB. Locally grown foods and farmers markets: consumer attitudes and behaviors. Sustainability. 2010;2:742–56.
50. Pollard TM, Steptoe A, Wardle J. Motives underlying healthy eating: using the food choice questionnaire to explain variation in dietary intake. J Biosoc Sci. 1998;30:165–79.
51. Glanz K, Basil M, Maibach E, Goldberg J, Snyder D. Why Americans eat what they do: taste, nutrition, cost, convenience, and weight control concerns as influences on food consumption. J Am Diet Assoc. 1998;98:1118–26.
52. Drewnowski A, Hann C, Henderson SA, Gorenflo D. Both food preferences and food frequency scores predict fat intakes of women with breast cancer. J Am Diet Assoc. 2000;100:1325–33.
53. Nagata C, Sugiyama C, Shimizu H. Nutrient intakes in relation to style of breakfast and taste preferences. J Epidemiol. 1999;9:91–8.
54. Mejean C, Deglaire A, Kesse-Guyot E, Hercberg S, Schlich P, Castetbon K. Association between intake of nutrients and food groups and liking for fat (the Nutrinet-Sante study). Appetite. 2014;78:147–55.
55. Drewnowski A, Hann C. Food preferences and reported frequencies of food consumption as predictors of current diet in young women. Am J Clin Nutr. 1999;70:28–36.
56. Dijkstra SC, Neter JE, Brouwer IA, Huisman M, Visser M. Motivations to eat healthily in older Dutch adults–a cross sectional study. Int J Behav Nutr Phys Act. 2014;11:141.
57. Ghvanidze S, Velikova N, Dodd TH, Oldewage-Theron W. Consumers' environmental and ethical consciousness and the use of the related food products information: the role of perceived consumer effectiveness. Appetite. 2016;107:311–22.
58. Andreeva VA, Salanave B, Castetbon K, Deschamps V, Vernay M, Kesse-Guyot E, Hercberg S. Comparison of the sociodemographic characteristics of the large NutriNet-Sante e-cohort with French census data: the issue of volunteer bias revisited. J Epidemiol Community Health. 2015;69:893–8.
59. Mejean C, Szabo de Edelenyi F, Touvier M, Kesse-Guyot E, Julia C, Andreeva VA, Hercberg S. Motives for participating in a web-based nutrition cohort according to sociodemographic, lifestyle, and health characteristics: the NutriNet-Sante cohort study. J Med Internet Res. 2014;16:e189.

60. Andreeva VA, Deschamps V, Salanave B, Castetbon K, Verdot C, Kesse-Guyot E, Hercberg S. Comparison of dietary intakes between a large online cohort study (etude NutriNet-Santé) and a nationally representative cross-sectional study (etude Nationale nutrition Santé) in France: addressing the issue of generalizability in E-epidemiology. Am J Epidemiol. 2016;184:660–9.
61. Touvier M, Kesse-Guyot E, Méjean C, Pollet C, Malon A, Castetbon K, Hercberg S. Comparison between an interactive web-based self-administered 24 h dietary record and an interview by a dietitian for large-scale epidemiological studies. Br J Nutr. 2011;105:1055–64.
62. Willett W. Nutritional epidemiology: Oxford University Press US; 1998. 538 p.
63. Brussaard JH, Löwik MRH, Steingrímsdóttir L, Møller A, Kearney J, De Henauw S, Becker W, EFCOSUM Group. A European food consumption survey method–conclusions and recommendations. Eur J Clin Nutr. 2002;56 Suppl 2:S89–94.
64. Gu Y, Scarmeas N. Dietary patterns in Alzheimer's disease and cognitive aging. Curr Alzheimer Res. 2011;8:510–9.
65. Popkin BM. Contemporary nutritional transition: determinants of diet and its impact on body composition. Proc Nutr Soc. 2011;70:82–91.

# PERMISSIONS

All chapters in this book were first published in NUTRITION, by BioMed Central; hereby published with permission under the Creative Commons Attribution License or equivalent. Every chapter published in this book has been scrutinized by our experts. Their significance has been extensively debated. The topics covered herein carry significant findings which will fuel the growth of the discipline. They may even be implemented as practical applications or may be referred to as a beginning point for another development.

The contributors of this book come from diverse backgrounds, making this book a truly international effort. This book will bring forth new frontiers with its revolutionizing research information and detailed analysis of the nascent developments around the world.

We would like to thank all the contributing authors for lending their expertise to make the book truly unique. They have played a crucial role in the development of this book. Without their invaluable contributions this book wouldn't have been possible. They have made vital efforts to compile up to date information on the varied aspects of this subject to make this book a valuable addition to the collection of many professionals and students.

This book was conceptualized with the vision of imparting up-to-date information and advanced data in this field. To ensure the same, a matchless editorial board was set up. Every individual on the board went through rigorous rounds of assessment to prove their worth. After which they invested a large part of their time researching and compiling the most relevant data for our readers.

The editorial board has been involved in producing this book since its inception. They have spent rigorous hours researching and exploring the diverse topics which have resulted in the successful publishing of this book. They have passed on their knowledge of decades through this book. To expedite this challenging task, the publisher supported the team at every step. A small team of assistant editors was also appointed to further simplify the editing procedure and attain best results for the readers.

Apart from the editorial board, the designing team has also invested a significant amount of their time in understanding the subject and creating the most relevant covers. They scrutinized every image to scout for the most suitable representation of the subject and create an appropriate cover for the book.

The publishing team has been an ardent support to the editorial, designing and production team. Their endless efforts to recruit the best for this project, has resulted in the accomplishment of this book. They are a veteran in the field of academics and their pool of knowledge is as vast as their experience in printing. Their expertise and guidance has proved useful at every step. Their uncompromising quality standards have made this book an exceptional effort. Their encouragement from time to time has been an inspiration for everyone.

The publisher and the editorial board hope that this book will prove to be a valuable piece of knowledge for researchers, students, practitioners and scholars across the globe.

# LIST OF CONTRIBUTORS

**Amare Worku**
Department of Public Health Sciences, Addis Continental Institute of Public Health, Addis Ababa, Ethiopia

**Yohannes Adama Melaku**
Department of Public Health Sciences, Addis Continental Institute of Public Health, Addis Ababa, Ethiopia
Adelaide Medical School, The University of Adelaide, Adelaide, Australia

**Tiffany K. Gill, Anne W. Taylor and Zumin Shi**
Adelaide Medical School, The University of Adelaide, Adelaide, Australia

**Robert Adams**
Health Observatory, Discipline of Medicine, The Queen Elizabeth Hospital Campus, The University of Adelaide, Adelaide, Australia

**Yonghua Li and Binggan Wei**
Key Laboratory of Land Surface Pattern and Simulation, Institute of Geographical Sciences and Natural Resources Research, Chinese Academy of Sciences, 11 A Datun Road, Beijing 100101, People's Republic of China

**Jing Wang, Linsheng Yang and Hairong Li**
Key Laboratory of Land Surface Pattern and Simulation, Institute of Geographical Sciences and Natural Resources Research, Chinese Academy of Sciences, 11 A Datun Road, Beijing 100101, People's Republic of China
College of Resources and Environment, University of Chinese Academy of Sciences, Beijing 100049, People's Republic of China

**Jacqueline Tereza da Silva, Ângela Cristine Bersch-Ferreira and Camila Ragne Torreglosa**
Department of Nutrition, School of Public Health, University of São Paulo, Avenida Doutor Arnaldo, 715, São Paulo, SP 01246904, Brazil
Research Institute, Hospital do Coração (HCor), Rua Abílio Sorares, 250, 12° andar, São Paulo, SP 04005-000, Brazil

**Renata Bertazzi Levy**
Department of Nutrition, School of Public Health, University of São Paulo,
Avenida Doutor Arnaldo, 715, São Paulo, SP 01246904, Brazil
Department of Preventive Medicine, School of Medicine, University of São Paulo, Avenida Doutor Arnaldo, 455, São Paulo, SP 01246903, Brazil

**Bernardete Weber**
Research Institute, Hospital do Coração (HCor), Rua Abílio Sorares, 250, 12° andar, São Paulo, SP 04005-000, Brazil

**Vijay Ganji**
Human Nutrition Department, College of Health Sciences, Qatar University, Doha, Qatar

**Bernadette Martineau**
Children Healthcare of Atlanta, Emory University, Atlanta, GA, USA

**William Edmund Van Fleit**
Georgia State University, Atlanta, GA, USA

**Mohamed Khalis, Meimouna Mint Sidi Deoula, Abdelilah Benslimane, Amran Ibrahim and Karima El Rhazi**
Department of Epidemiology and Public Health, Faculty of Medicine and pharmacy of Fez, Sidi Mohamed Ben Abdellah University, Fez, Morocco

**Khaoula El Kinany**
Department of Epidemiology and Public Health, Faculty of Medicine and pharmacy of Fez, Sidi Mohamed Ben Abdellah University, Fez, Morocco
Laboratory of Microbiology and Molecular Biology, Faculty of Science DharMehraz, Fez, Morocco

**Vanessa Garcia-Larsen**
Department of International Health, The Johns Hopkins Bloomberg School of Public Health, Baltimore, USA
Population Health and Occupational Disease, NHLI, Imperial College London, London, UK

**Mohamed Chakib Benjelloun**
Respiratory Department, Hassan II University Hospital Center of Fez, Fez, Morocco

**Qianling Zhou**
Division of Birth Cohort Study, Guangzhou Women and Children's Medical Center, Guangzhou Medical University, 9 Junsui Road, Zhujiang Newtown, Tianhe District, Guangzhou 510623, China

**Jian-Rong He, Jinhua Lu, Xueling Wei, Fanfan Chan, Lifang Zhang, Niannian Chen, Lan Qiu and Mingyang Yuan**
Division of Birth Cohort Study, Guangzhou Women and Children's Medical Center, Guangzhou Medical University, 9 Junsui Road, Zhujiang Newtown, Tianhe District, Guangzhou 510623, China
Department of Woman and Child Health Care, Guangzhou Women and Children's Medical Center, Guangzhou Medical University, Guangzhou, China

**Min-Shan Lu and Xiu Qiu**
Division of Birth Cohort Study, Guangzhou Women and Children's Medical Center, Guangzhou Medical University, 9 Junsui Road, Zhujiang Newtown, Tianhe District, Guangzhou 510623, China
Department of Woman and Child Health Care, Guangzhou Women and Children's Medical Center, Guangzhou Medical University, Guangzhou, China
Department of Obstetrics and Gynecology, Guangzhou Women and Children's Medical Center, Guangzhou Medical University, Guangzhou, China

**Huimin Xia**
Division of Birth Cohort Study, Guangzhou Women and Children's Medical Center, Guangzhou Medical University, 9 Junsui Road, Zhujiang Newtown, Tianhe District, Guangzhou 510623, China
Department of Neonatal Surgery, Division of Birth Cohort Study, Guangzhou Women and Children's Medical Center, Guangzhou Medical University, 9 Junsui Road, Zhujiang Newtown, Tianhe District, Guangzhou 510623, China

**Qiaozhu Chen**
Department of Obstetrics and Gynecology, Guangzhou Women and Children's Medical Center, Guangzhou Medical University, Guangzhou, China

**Kar Keung Cheng**
Institute of Applied Health Research, University of Birmingham, Birmingham, UK

**Farah Naja, Lamis Jomaa, Sibelle El Labban and Nahla Hwalla**
Nutrition and Food Sciences Department, Faculty of Agriculture and Food Sciences, American University of Beirut, Riad El Solh, Beirut 11072020, Lebanon

**Leila Itani**
Department of Nutrition & Dietetics, Faculty of Health Sciences, Beirut Arab University, Riad El Solh, Beirut 11072809, Lebanon

**Abla Mehio Sibai**
Department of Epidemiology and Population Health, Faculty of Health Sciences, American University of Beirut, Riad El Solh, Beirut 11072020, Lebanon

**Jeremy Zidek**
Futura Food LLC, 113 Creekside Drive, State College, PA 16801, USA

**Joachim Gæde, Trine Nielsen, Mia L. Madsen, Torben Hansen and Oluf Pedersen**
The Novo Nordisk Foundation Center for Basic Metabolic Research, Section of Metabolic Genetics, Faculty of Health and Medical Sciences, University of Copenhagen, Blegdamsvej 3B, DK-2200 Copenhagen, Denmark

**Kristine H. Allin**
The Novo Nordisk Foundation Center for Basic Metabolic Research, Section of Metabolic Genetics, Faculty of Health and Medical Sciences, University of Copenhagen, Blegdamsvej 3B, DK-2200 Copenhagen, Denmark
Department of Clinical Epidemiology, Bispebjerg and Frederiksberg Hospital, Copenhagen, the Capital Region of Denmark, Denmark

**Ulla Toft**
Research Centre for Prevention and Health, Copenhagen, the Capital Region of Denmark, Denmark

**Torben Jørgensen**
Research Centre for Prevention and Health, Copenhagen, the Capital Region of Denmark, Denmark
Department of Public Health, Faculty of Health and Medical Sciences, University of Copenhagen, Copenhagen, Denmark
Faculty of Medicine, Aalborg University, Aalborg, Denmark

**Kim Overvad and Anne Tjønneland**
Danish Cancer Society Research Center, Copenhagen, Denmark

**Amanda J Lee and Meron Lewis**
The Australian Prevention Partnership Centre, The Sax Institute, 10 Jones Street, Ultimo, NSW 2007, Australia

**Sarah Kane**
School of Public Health and Social Work, Queensland University of Technology, Brisbane, QLD, Australia

**Elizabeth Good and Mathew Dick**
Preventive Health Branch, Department of Health, Queensland Government, Brisbane, QLD, Australia

**Timothy J Landrigan**
School of Public Health, Curtin University, Kent Street, Perth 6845, Western Australia

**Christina M Pollard**
School of Public Health, Curtin University, Kent Street, Perth 6845, Western Australia
Public Health Division, Department of Health, Government of Western Australia, 189 Royal Street, East Perth 6004, Western Australia

**E. F. Sprake and P. Grabowski**
Human Nutrition Unit, Department of Oncology & Metabolism, The Medical School, University of Sheffield, Sheffield S10 2RX, UK

**J. M. Russell**
Corporate Information & Computing Service, University of Sheffield, Sheffield S10 2GU, UK

**J. E. Cecil**
Medical & Biological Sciences Building, University of St Andrews, St Andrews KY16 9TF, UK

**R. J. Cooper**
School of Health and Related Research, University of Sheffield, Sheffield S1 4DA, UK

**L. K. Pourshahidi**
Nutrition Innovation Centre for Food & Health (NICHE), Ulster University, Coleraine BT52 1SA, UK

**M. E. Barker**
Food & Nutrition Group, Business School, Sheffield Hallam University, Sheffield S1 1WB, UK

**Mikko Pänkäläinen and Erja Lappalainen**
Department of Psychiatry, Päijät-Häme Central Hospital, Keskussairaalankatu 7, FI-15850 Lahti, Finland

**Jukka Hintikka**
Department of Psychiatry, Päijät-Häme Central Hospital, Keskussairaalankatu 7, FI-15850 Lahti, Finland
School of Medicine, University of Tampere, Tampere, Finland

**Mikael Fogelholm and Raisa Valve**
Department of Food and Environmental Sciences, University of Helsinki, Helsinki, Finland

**Olli Kampman**
Department of Psychiatry, Seinäjoki Hospital District, Seinäjoki, Finland
School of Medicine, University of Tampere, Tampere, Finland

**Markku Kauppi**
School of Medicine, University of Tampere, Tampere, Finland
Department of Internal Medicine, Päijät-Häme Central Hospital, Lahti, Finland

**Ahmad Syauqy**
School of Nutrition and Health Sciences, College of Nutrition, Taipei Medical University, 250 Wu-Hsing Street, Taipei 110, Taiwan
Department of Nutrition Science, Faculty of Medicine, Diponegoro University, Semarang, Indonesia

**Jane C.-J. Chao**
School of Nutrition and Health Sciences, College of Nutrition, Taipei Medical University, 250 Wu-Hsing Street, Taipei 110, Taiwan
Master Program in Global Health and Development, College of Public Health, Taipei Medical University, Taipei, Taiwan
Nutrition Research Center, Taipei Medical University Hospital, Taipei, Taiwan

**Chien-Yeh Hsu**
Department of Information Management, National Taipei University of Nursing and Health Sciences, Taipei, Taiwan
Master Program in Global Health and Development, College of Public Health, Taipei Medical University, Taipei, Taiwan

**Hsiao-Hsien Rau**
Joint Commission of Taiwan, New Taipei City, Taiwan

**Wonjeong Chae and Yeong Jun Ju**
Department of Public Health, College of Medicine, Yonsei University, Seoul, Republic of Korea
Institute of Health Services Research, Yonsei University, 50 Yonsei-ro, Seodaemun-gu, Seoul 120-752, Republic of Korea

**Jaeyong Shin, Sung-In Jang and Eun-Cheol Park**
Institute of Health Services Research, Yonsei University, 50 Yonsei-ro, Seodaemun-gu, Seoul 120-752, Republic of Korea
Department of Preventive Medicine, College of Medicine, Yonsei University, 50 Yonsei-ro, Seodaemun-gu, Seoul 120-752, Republic of Korea

**Kentaro Murakami**
Interfaculty Initiative in Information Studies, University of Tokyo, Tokyo 113 0033, Japan

**M. Barbara E. Livingstone**
Northern Ireland Centre for Food and Health, Ulster University, Coleraine BT52 1SA, UK

**Timothy R. Entwistle**
The Transplant Centre, University Hospital of South Manchester, Manchester M23 9LT, UK

**James E. Fildes**
1The Transplant Centre, University Hospital of South Manchester, Manchester M23 9LT, UK
Manchester Collaborative Centre for Inflammation Research, University of Manchester, Manchester, UK

**Kyoko Miura**
Cancer and Population Studies Group, QIMR Berghofer Medical Research Institute, 300 Herston Road, Herston, QLD 4006, Australia

**Adèle C. Green**
Cancer and Population Studies Group, QIMR Berghofer Medical Research Institute, 300 Herston Road, Herston, QLD 4006, Australia
CRUK Manchester Institute, University of Manchester, Wilmslow Road, Manchester, UK

**Meei-Shyuan Lee**
School of Public Health, National Defense Medical Center, No.161, Sec. 6, Minchuan East Road, Taipei 114, Taiwan, Republic of China

**Lin-Yuan Huang**
Division of Preventive Medicine and Health Services Research, Institute of Population Health Sciences, National Health Research Institutes, 35 Keyan Road, Zhunan Town, Miaoli County 350, Taiwan, Republic of China

**Mark L. Wahlqvist**
Division of Preventive Medicine and Health Services Research, Institute of
Population Health Sciences, National Health Research Institutes, 35 Keyan Road, Zhunan Town, Miaoli County 350, Taiwan, Republic of China
School of Public Health, National Defense Medical Center, No.161, Sec. 6, Minchuan
East Road, Taipei 114, Taiwan, Republic of China
Monash Asia Institute, Monash University, 5th Floor, H Building, 900 Dandenong Road, Caulfield East, Melbourne, VIC 3145, Australia
College of Public Health, China Medical University, Taichung, Taiwan, Republic of China

**Po-Huang Chiang**
Division of Preventive Medicine and Health Services Research, Institute of Population Health Sciences, National Health Research Institutes, 35 Keyan Road, Zhunan Town, Miaoli County 350, Taiwan, Republic of China College of Public Health, China Medical University, Taichung, Taiwan, Republic of China

**Elham Z. Movassagh and Susan Whiting**
College of Pharmacy and Nutrition, University of Saskatchewan, 104 Clinic place, Saskatoon, SK S7N 2Z4, Canada

**Hassan Vatanparast**
College of Pharmacy and Nutrition, University of Saskatchewan, 104 Clinic place, Saskatoon, SK S7N 2Z4, Canada
School of Public Health, University of Saskatchewan, 104 Clinic place, Saskatoon, SK S7N 5E5, Canada

**Adam D. G. Baxter-Jones and Saija Kontulainen**
College of Kinesiology, University of Saskatchewan, 87 Campus Drive, Saskatoon, SK S7N5B2, Canada

**Michael Szafron**
School of Public Health, University of Saskatchewan, 104 Clinic place, Saskatoon, SK S7N 5E5, Canada

**Yusuke Osonoi, Yuki Someya, Shiho Nakayama and Yoshio Fujitani**
Department of Metabolism & Endocrinology, Juntendo University Graduate School of Medicine, 2-1-1 Hongo, Bunkyoku, Tokyo 113-8421, Japan

**Tomoya Mita**
Department of Metabolism & Endocrinology, Juntendo University Graduate School of Medicine, 2-1-1 Hongo, Bunkyoku, Tokyo 113-8421, Japan
Center for Molecular Diabetology, Juntendo University Graduate School of Medicine, Bunkyoku, Tokyo 113-8421, Japan

**Akio Kanazawa**
Department of Metabolism & Endocrinology, Juntendo University Graduate School of Medicine, 2-1-1 Hongo, Bunkyoku, Tokyo 113-8421, Japan
Center for Therapeutic Innovations in Diabetes, Juntendo University Graduate School of Medicine, Bunkyoku, Tokyo 113-8421, Japan

**Hirotaka Watada**
Department of Metabolism & Endocrinology, Juntendo University Graduate School of Medicine, 2-1-1 Hongo, Bunkyoku, Tokyo 113-8421, Japan
Center for Molecular Diabetology, Juntendo University Graduate School of Medicine, Bunkyoku, Tokyo 113-8421, Japan
Center for Molecular Diabetology, Juntendo University Graduate School of Medicine, Bunkyoku, Tokyo 113-8421, Japan
Sportology Center, Juntendo University Graduate School of Medicine, Bunkyoku, Tokyo 113-8421, Japan

**Nicolas Sauvageot, Anna Schritz, Ala'a Alkerwi and Saverio Stranges**
Luxembourg Institute of Health (LIH), CCMS (Competence center in methodology and statistics), 1A rue Thomas Edison, L-1445 Strassen, Luxembourg

**Sonia Leite**
Ministry of Health, Luxembourg, Service épidémiologie & statistique, Allée Marconi, Villa Louvigny, L-2120 Luxembourg city, Luxembourg

**Yanni Papanikolaou**
Nutritional Strategies Inc., 59 Marriott Place, Paris, ON N3L 0A3, Canada

**Julie Miller Jones**
Distinguished Scholar and Professor Emerita of Food and Nutrition, Department of Foods and Nutrition, St. Catherine University, 4030 Valentine Ct. Arden Hills, Minnesota, MN 55112, USA

**S. Péneau, E. Kesse-Guyot and J. Baudry**
Université Paris 13, Equipe de Recherche en Epidémiologie Nutritionnelle, Centre de Recherche en Epidémiologie et Statistiques, Inserm (U1153), Inra (U1125), Cnam, COMUE Sorbonne Paris Cité, F-93017 Bobigny, France

**S. Hercberg**
Université Paris 13, Equipe de Recherche en Epidémiologie Nutritionnelle, Centre de Recherche en Epidémiologie et Statistiques, Inserm (U1153), Inra (U1125), Cnam, COMUE Sorbonne Paris Cité, F-93017 Bobigny, France
Department of Public Health, Hôpital Avicenne, F-93300 Bobigny, France

**C. Méjean**
Université Paris 13, Equipe de Recherche en Epidémiologie Nutritionnelle, Centre de Recherche en Epidémiologie et Statistiques, Inserm (U1153), Inra (U1125), Cnam, COMUE Sorbonne Paris Cité, F-93017 Bobigny, France
INRA, UMR 1110 MOISA, F-34000 Montpellier, France

**B. Allès**
Université Paris 13, Equipe de Recherche en Epidémiologie Nutritionnelle, Centre de Recherche en Epidémiologie et Statistiques, Inserm (U1153), Inra (U1125), Cnam, COMUE Sorbonne Paris Cité, F-93017 Bobigny, France
EREN (Nutritional Epidemiology Research Unit), SMBH Paris 13, 74 rue Marcel Cachin, F-93017 Bobigny Cedex, France

**Franziska Jannasch and Matthias B. Schulze**
Department of Molecular Epidemiology, German Institute of Human Nutrition Potsdam-Rehbruecke (DIfE), Arthur-Scheunert-Allee 114-116, 14558 Nuthetal, Germany

**George Bedu-Addo**
Komfo Anokye Teaching Hospital, School of Medical Science, Kwame Nkrumah University of Science and Technology, Kumasi, Ghana

**Ina Danquah**
Department of Molecular Epidemiology, German Institute of Human Nutrition Potsdam-Rehbruecke (DIfE), Arthur-Scheunert-Allee 114-116, 14558 Nuthetal, Germany
Institute for Social Medicine, Epidemiology and Health Economics, Charité - Universitaetsmedizin Berlin, corporate member of Freie Universitaet Berlin, Humboldt-Universitaet zu Berlin, and Berlin Institute of Health, Campus Charité Mitte, 10098 Berlin, Germany

# Index

www.ingramcontent.com/pod-product-compliance
Lightning Source LLC
LaVergne TN
LVHW080921210926
848485LV00004B/697